/60101/

Nurse's Handbook of
I.V. Drugs

Third Edition

D0111388

JONES AND BARTLETT PUBLISHERS
Sudbury, Massachusetts
BOSTON   TORONTO   LONDON   SINGAPORE

World Headquarters

Jones and Bartlett Publishers
40 Tall Pine Drive
Sudbury, MA 01776
978-443-5000
info@jbpub.com
www.jbpub.com

Jones and Bartlett Publishers
Canada
6339 Ormindale Way
Mississauga, Ontario L5V 1J2
Canada

Jones and Bartlett Publishers
International
Barb House, Barb Mews
London W6 7PA
United Kingdom

Jones and Bartlett's books and products are available through most bookstores and online book-sellers. To contact Jones and Bartlett Publishers directly, call 800-832-0034, fax 978-443-8000, or visit our website www.jbpub.com.

Substantial discounts on bulk quantities of Jones and Bartlett's publications are available to corporations, professional associations, and other qualified organizations. For details and specific discount information, contact the special sales department at Jones and Bartlett via the above contact information or send an email to special-sales@jbpub.com.

Production Credits

Publisher: Kevin Sullivan
Acquisitions Editor: Emily Ekle
Acquisitions Editor: Amy Sibley
Associate Editor: Patricia Donnelly
Editorial Assistant: Rachel Shuster
Supervising Production Editor: Carolyn F. Rogers
Associate Marketing Manager: Ilana Goddess
Manufacturing Buyer: Therese Connell

Clinical Reviewer: Marlene Ciranowicz-Steenburg, RN, MSN, CDE
Composition: Catherine E. Harold
Interior Illustrations: Rolin Graphics, Inc.
Cover Design: Kristin E. Ohlin
Cover Image: © Rob Byron/ShutterStock, Inc.
Printing and Binding: Malloy, Inc.
Cover Printing: Malloy, Inc.

6048

Printed in the United States of America
12 11 10 09 08   10 9 8 7 6 5 4 3 2 1

CONTENTS

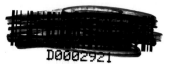

D0002921

Reviewers and Clinical Consultants iv
How to Use This Book v
Foreword xii
Overview of Pharmacology xv
Principles of I.V. Drug Administration xxiii
I.V. Drug Therapy and the Nursing Process xxxii

INDIVIDUAL DRUGS (organized alphabetically)

A 1
B 87
C 115
D 209
E • F 285
G • H 365
I • J 393
K • L 435
M 473
N • O 543
P 591
Q • R • S 673
T • U • V 703
W • X • Y • Z 763

APPENDICES

Equianalgesic Doses for Opioid Agonists 777
Calculating the Strength of a Solution 778
Calculating Parenteral Drug Dosages 780
Calculating I.V. Flow Rates 782
I.V. Antineoplastic Drugs 784
Body Mass Index Calculation 794
Abbreviations 796

Index 799

Reviewers and Clinical Consultants

Karen T. Bruchak, RN, MSN, MBA
Director, Medical-Surgical Nursing
The Chester County Hospital
Chester, PA

Terri Corbo, PharmD, BCPS
Clinical Specialist, Cardiology
Christiana Care Health System
Newark, DE

Kimberly Anne Boykin Couch, PharmD
Clinical Specialist
Christiana Care Health System
Adjunct Faculty
University of Delaware School of Nursing
Newark, DE

Reviewers and Clinical Consultants

Karen T. Bruchak, RN, MSN, MBA
Director, Medical-Surgical Nursing
The Chester County Hospital
Chester, PA

Terri Corbo, PharmD, BCPS
Clinical Specialist, Cardiology
Christiana Care Health System
Newark, DE

Kimberly Anne Boykin Couch, PharmD
Clinical Specialist
Christiana Care Health System
Adjunct Faculty
University of Delaware School of Nursing
Newark, DE

HOW TO USE THIS BOOK

Jones and Bartlett's Nurse's Handbook of I.V. Drugs, Third Edition, gives you what today's nurses and nursing students need: accurate, concise, and reliable facts about I.V. drug administration. This book emphasizes the vital information you need to know before, during, and after drug administration. The information is presented in easy-to-understand language and organized alphabetically, so you can find what you need quickly.

What's Special
In addition to the drug information you expect to find in each entry (see "Drug Entries" below for details), *Nurse's Handbook of I.V. Drugs,* Third Editon, boasts these special features:
- **Practical trim size and good-size type** give you a book that's easy to carry, easy to read, and easy to handle. You can hold the book in one hand, see complete pages at a glance, and use your other hand to document or perform other activities.
- **Introductory material** reviews essential general information you need to know to administer I.V. drugs safely and effectively, including an overview of pharmacology and the principles of I.V. drug administration. In addition, the five steps of the nursing process are reviewed and related specifically to drug therapy.
- **Useful illustrations** throughout the text help you visualize selected mechanisms of action by showing how drugs work at the cellular, tissue, and organ levels. In addition, the inside front cover features a table listing all the drugs whose mechanisms of action are illustrated—along with other drugs that have similar mechanisms of action.
- **No-nonsense writing style** uses the terms and abbreviations you're mostly likely to encounter in your practice and your studies. (See the *Abbreviations* appendix.) And to avoid sexist language, we alternate male and female pronouns as we move from letter to letter throughout the book.
- **Up-to-date drug information** includes the latest FDA-approved drugs, new and changed indications, new warnings, and newly reported adverse reactions.
- **Dosage adjustment,** highlighted in color, alerts you to expected dosage changes for patients with a specific condition or disorder, such as advanced age or renal impairment.
- **Warning,** highlighted in color, calls attention to important facts

that you need to know before, during, and after drug administration. For example, in the alatrofloxacin entry, a Warning reports that the drug usually is reserved for hospitalized patients and is given for no longer than 2 weeks because of the high risk of severe liver damage.

- **Easy-to-use tables** for route, onset, peak, and duration provide a timesaving way to track and check this important data. (See page viii for details on route, onset, peak, and duration tables.)
- **Useful appendices** provide you with even more handy information you can use every day in your practice and studies, such as the *I.V. Antineoplastic Drugs* appendix, where you can review generic and trade antineoplastic drug names and their indications, and dosages. You'll also find help calculating solution strengths, parenteral dosages, and flow rates. On the inside back cover is a handy table showing which drugs are compatible in a syringe.

Drug Entries
Nurse's Handbook of I.V. Drugs, Third Editon, clearly and concisely presents all the vital facts on the drugs that you'll typically administer. To help you find the information you need quickly, drug entries are organized alphabetically by generic drug name—from abatacept to zoledronic acid. For ease of use, every drug entry follows a consistent format.

Generic and Trade Names
First, each entry identifies the drug's main generic name and, if needed, alternate generic names. (For drugs prescribed by trade name, you can quickly check the comprehensive index, which refers you to the appropriate generic name and page.) Next, the entry lists the most commonly used U.S. trade names for each drug. It also includes common trade names available only in Canada, marked (CAN).

Class, Category, and Schedule
Each entry lists the drug's chemical and therapeutic classes. With this information, you can compare drugs in the same chemical class but in different therapeutic classes and vice versa.

The entry also lists the FDA's pregnancy risk category, which categorizes drugs based on their potential to cause birth defects. (For details, see *FDA pregnancy risk categories*.) Where appropriate, the entry also includes the drug's controlled substance schedule. (For details, see *Controlled substance schedules*, page viii.)

FDA PREGNANCY RISK CATEGORIES

Each drug may be placed in a pregnancy risk category based on the FDA's estimate of risk to the fetus. If the FDA hasn't provided a category, the *Nurse's Handbook of I.V. Drugs* notes that the drug is "Not rated." The categories range from A to X, signifying least to greatest fetal risk.

A Controlled studies show no risk

Adequate, well-controlled studies with pregnant women have failed to demonstrate a risk to the fetus in any trimester of pregnancy.

B No evidence of risk in humans

Adequate, well-controlled studies with pregnant women haven't shown increased risk of fetal abnormalities despite adverse findings in animals, or—in the absence of adequate human studies—animal studies show no fetal risk. The chance of fetal harm exists but is remote.

C Risk can't be ruled out

Adequate, well-controlled human studies are lacking, and animal studies are lacking as well or have demonstrated a risk to the fetus. A chance of fetal harm exists if the drug is administered during pregnancy, but the potential benefits may outweigh the potential risk.

D Positive evidence of risk

Studies in humans, or investigational or post-marketing data, have demonstrated fetal risk. Nevertheless, potential benefits from the drug's use may outweigh potential risks. For example, the drug may be acceptable if needed in a life-threatening situation or serious disease for which safer drugs can't be used or are ineffective.

X Contraindicated in pregnancy

Studies in animals or humans, or investigational or post-marketing reports, have demonstrated positive evidence of fetal abnormalities or risks; these risks clearly outweigh any possible benefit to the patient.

Indications and Dosages

This section lists FDA-approved therapeutic indications. For each indication, you'll find the applicable drug form or route, age-group (adults, adolescents, or children), and dosage (which includes amount per dose, timing, and duration).

CONTROLLED SUBSTANCE SCHEDULES

The Controlled Substances Act of 1970 mandated that certain prescription drugs be categorized in schedules based on their potential for abuse. The greater their abuse potential, the greater the restrictions on their prescription. The controlled substance schedules range from I to V, signifying highest to lowest abuse potential.

I High potential for abuse

No accepted medical use exists for Schedule I drugs, which include heroin and lysergic acid diethylamide (LSD).

II High potential for abuse

Use may lead to severe physical or psychological dependence. Prescriptions must be written in ink or typewritten and must be signed by the prescriber. Oral prescriptions must be confirmed in writing within 72 hours and may be given only in a genuine emergency. No renewals are permitted.

III Some potential for abuse

Use may lead to low-to-moderate physical dependence or high psychological dependence. Prescriptions may be oral or written. Up to five renewals are permitted within 6 months.

IV Low potential for abuse

Use may lead to limited physical or psychological dependence. Prescriptions may be oral or written. Up to five renewals are permitted within 6 months.

V Subject to state and local regulation

Abuse potential is low; a prescription may not be required.

Route, Onset, Peak, and Duration

Quick-reference tables show the drug's onset, peak, and duration (when known) for the applicable administration route. The *onset of action* is the time a drug takes to be absorbed, reach a therapeutic blood level, and cause an initial therapeutic response. The *peak therapeutic effect* occurs when a drug reaches its highest blood concentration and the greatest amount of drug reaches the site of action to produce the maximum therapeutic response. The *duration of action* is the amount of time a drug remains at a blood concentration that produces a therapeutic response.

Mechanism of Action

Set off by a box, this section concisely describes how a drug achieves its therapeutic effects at the cellular, tissue, or organ level, as appropriate. Illustrations of selected mechanisms of action lend exceptional detail and clarity to sometimes complex processes.

Incompatibilities

This section alerts you to drugs or solutions that are incompatible with the topic drug when mixed in a syringe or solution or infused through the same I.V. line.

Contraindications

An alphabetical list details conditions and disorders that preclude administration of the topic drug.

Interactions

This section presents the drugs, foods, and activities (such as alcohol use and smoking) that can cause important, problematic, or life-threatening interactions with the topic drug. For each interacting drug, food, or activity, you'll learn the effects of the interaction.

Adverse Reactions

Organized by body system, this section highlights common, serious, and life-threatening adverse reactions in alphabetical order.

Nursing Considerations

Warnings, general precautions, and key information that you must know before, during, and after drug administration are detailed in this section. Examples include whether you need to take special precautions when preparing a drug for administration and how to properly reconstitute, dilute, store, handle, or dispose of a drug.

Patient teaching information is also included here. You'll find important guidelines for patients, such as how to spot and manage adverse reactions, when to report them, which cautions to observe, and more. To save you time, however, this section doesn't repeat basic patient-teaching points. (For a summary of those, see *Teaching your patient about I.V. drug therapy,* pages x and xi.)

In short, *Nurse's Handbook of I.V. Drugs,* Third Edition, is designed expressly to give you more of what you need in a versatile and highly useful format. It puts vital drug information at your fingertips and helps you remain ALWAYS CURRENT in this critical part of your practice or studies.

TEACHING YOUR PATIENT ABOUT I.V. DRUG THERAPY

Your teaching about I.V. drug therapy will vary with your patient's needs and your practice setting. To help guide your teaching, each drug entry provides key information that you must teach your patient about that drug. For all patients, however, you should also:

☑ Teach the generic and trade names for each prescribed drug that he'll take after discharge—even if he took the drug before admission.

☑ Clearly explain why each drug was prescribed, how it works, and what it's supposed to do. To help your patient understand the drug's therapeutic effects, relate its action to her disorder or condition.

☑ Review the I.V. administration process, and inform the patient how often the drug will be administered. If the patient will be switched from an I.V. drug to another drug form (for example, from I.V. methyldopate hydrochloride to oral methyldopa for continuing treatment of hypertension), teach him how to administer the new form correctly. Also instruct him how often to take the drug and for what length of time. Emphasize that he should take the drug exactly as prescribed.

☑ If the patient is being switched to an oral drug, describe the drug's appearance. Explain that she may break scored tablets in half for safe, accurate dosing but *should not* break unscored tablets because doing so may alter the drug dosage. If the patient has difficulty swallowing capsules, explain that she can open ones that contain sprinkles and take them with food or a drink but that she shouldn't do this with capsules that contain powder. Also, warn her not to crush or chew enteric-coated, extended-release, sustained-release, or similar drug forms.

☑ Teach the patient common adverse reactions associated with his drug therapy, and advise him to immediately report any dangerous ones, such as syncope. Also instruct the patient to report changes at the I.V. site, such as pain, redness, or leaking fluid.

☑ If the patient experiences unpleasant adverse reactions, such as a rash or mild itching, inform her that her prescriber may adjust the dosage or substitute a drug that causes fewer adverse reactions. Tell her which adverse reactions resolve with time.

☑ Caution the patient that some adverse reactions, such as dizziness and drowsiness, can impair his ability to perform activities requiring alertness, such as driving a car or operating machinery. If the drug is known to have CNS effects, advise the patient to avoid such activities until the drug's full CNS effects are known or as directed by the prescriber.

☑ If your patient will be self-administering a drug, teach her how to store the drug properly. Let her know if the drug is sensitive to light or temperature and how to protect it from these elements. Instruct the patient to store the drug in its original container, if possible, with the drug's name and dosage clearly printed on the label.

☑ Inform the patient which devices are available for drug administration and which ones to avoid. For example, advise him to ask the prescriber about using an infusion control device for administering I.V. morphine sulfate infusions.

☑ Teach your patient who will be self-administering a drug what to do if she misses a dose. Generally, she should administer a once-daily drug as soon as she remembers—provided that she remembers within the first 24 hours. If 24 hours has elapsed, she should administer the next scheduled dose, but not double the dose. If she has questions or concerns about missed doses, advise her to contact the prescriber.

☑ Provide information that is specific to the prescribed drug. For example, if your patient takes a diuretic to manage heart failure, instruct him to weigh himself daily at the same time of day, using the same scale and wearing the same amount of clothing; or if the patient takes digoxin or an antihypertensive, teach him how to measure his pulse and blood pressure and how to record the measurements. Then instruct him to bring the diary to his regular appointments so that the prescriber can monitor his response to the drug.

☑ Advise the patient to refill prescriptions promptly, unless she no longer needs the drug. Also instruct her to discard expired drugs because they may become ineffective or even dangerous over time.

☑ Warn the patient to keep all drugs out of the reach of children at all times.

FOREWORD

As you know, administering I.V. drug therapy safely and effectively is a top priority for nurses in today's health care environment. In the past, I.V. drug therapy was administered primarily in acute care settings. However, as health care has expanded to include multiple specialties, the practice settings for I.V. drug therapy have also broadened. Today, nurses care for a diverse population of patients in hospitals, outpatient clinics, extended care facilities, surgical centers, and the patient's own home.

The types of drugs that can be administered by I.V. injection or infusion are wide ranging and include antibiotics, antivirals, antineoplastics, and opioids. New drugs are continually becoming available to manage various health problems, such as HIV infection and cancer, and to manage or prevent drug-induced complications. In addition, many patients have more than one health problem and are taking multiple medications.

Your Responsibilities in I.V. Drug Therapy

Your basic responsibilities in drug therapy—whether enteral or parenteral—include:

• administering the right drug in the right dose by the right route at the right time to the right patient
• knowing the therapeutic use, dosage, interactions, adverse effects, and warnings of each administered drug
• being aware of newly approved drugs that may be prescribed
• knowing about changes to existing drugs, such as new indications and dosages and recently reported adverse reactions and interactions
• concentrating fully when preparing and administering drugs
• responding promptly and appropriately to serious or life-threatening adverse reactions, interactions, and other complications.

Beyond these basic responsibilities, however, you also need additional nursing knowledge and skills to meet the demands of today's I.V. drug therapy—for example, knowing when and how to observe the I.V. insertion site and surrounding area for signs and symptoms of complications. *Jones and Bartlett's Nurse's Handbook of I.V. Drugs,* Third Edition, provides all this information in an accurate and easy-to-use reference that has been developed specifically for you.

Meeting Your Needs

This book offers a wealth of reliable and easy-to-understand information on virtually all of the I.V. drugs you're likely to administer. For example, you'll find:

- instructions on how to prepare a drug dose, including directions for reconstitution and further dilution when appropriate
- appropriate storage information, including specific temperatures required for storing drugs before preparation and, if indicated, after reconstitution and dilution, as well as recommended lighting conditions, if applicable
- important facts on drug stability, such as how long the drug remains stable after reconstitution and dilution, and drug compatibility
- instructions on which drugs require special equipment, such as specific filters or a diluent supplied directly by the manufacturer
- recommended administration rate, when applicable, and whether the drug is administered as a continuous infusion, an intermittent infusion, or an injection.
- appropriate guidelines for patient monitoring after drug administration—for example, for adverse reactions, such as tissue sloughing and necrosis.

You can depend on the accuracy and reliability of the information contained in *Nurse's Handbook of I.V. Drugs*, Third Edition, because each entry has been reviewed by experts in nursing and pharmacology. What's more, every drug fact has been checked against the most respected drug references today, including the *American Hospital Formulary Service Drug Information, Drug Facts and Comparisons, The Physician's Desk Reference,* and the USP DI's *Drug Information for the Health Care Professional.*

Nurse's Handbook of I.V. Drugs, Third Edition, is also more practical and convenient than many other drug references on the market. For example, it's organized alphabetically by generic drug name, each entry follows a consistent format, and the writing throughout is concise and clear. And its Nursing Considerations are rich in advice and guidance specific to your responsibilities.

Whether you work in a hospital, a clinic, or another setting, you face greater challenges than ever before: more patients who are acutely ill, tighter budgets and staffing, and more complex drug therapy. But your ultimate goal must remain to provide your patients with the best and safest care possible. That's why we highly recommend the new third edition of *Jones and Bartlett's Nurse's Hand-*

book of I.V. Drugs to help you provide that optimal care. We have found the information in this book so valuable and practical that we use it every day—in our practice and in the classroom. Just slip it in your pocket and take it with you. We're confident that you'll refer to this book again and again and that it will become one of your most essential tools.

Joseph P. Zbilut, RN,C, DNSc, PhD, ANP
Professor, Adult Health Nursing
Rush University College of Nursing
Professor, Molecular Biophysics and Physiology
Rush Medical College
Chicago, IL

Kimberly Anne Boykin Couch, PharmD
Clinical Specialist
Christiana Care Health System
Adjunct Faculty
University of Delaware School of Nursing
Newark, DE

OVERVIEW OF PHARMACOLOGY

Understanding the basics of pharmacology is an essential nursing responsibility. Pharmacology is the science that deals with the physical and chemical properties, and the biochemical and physiologic effects, of drugs. It includes the areas of pharmacokinetics, pharmacodynamics, pharmacotherapeutics, pharmacognosy, and toxicodynamics.

Jones and Bartlett's Nurse's Handbook of I.V. Drugs, Third Edition, deals primarily with pharmacokinetics, pharmacodynamics, and pharmacotherapeutics—the information you need to administer drug therapy safely and effectively (discussed below). *Pharmacognosy* is the branch of pharmacology that deals with the biological, biochemical, and economic features of naturally occurring drugs. *Toxicodynamics* is the study of the harmful effects that excessive amounts of a drug produce in the body; in a drug overdose or drug poisoning, large drug doses may saturate or overwhelm normal mechanisms that control absorption, distribution, metabolism, and excretion.

Drug Nomenclature
Most drugs are known by several names—chemical, generic, trade, and official—each of which serves a specific function. (See *How drugs are named,* page xvi.) However, multiple drug names can also contribute to medication errors. You may find a familiar drug packaged with an unfamiliar name if your institution changes suppliers or if a familiar drug is newly approved in a different dose or for a new indication.

Drug Classification
Drugs can be classified in various ways. Most pharmacology textbooks group drugs by their functional classification, such as psychotherapeutics, which is based on common characteristics. Drugs can also be classified according to their therapeutic use, such as antibiotics and sedative-hypnotics. Drugs within a certain therapeutic class may be further divided into subgroups based on their mechanisms of action. For example, the therapeutic class antineoplastics can be further classified as alkylating agents, antibiotic antineoplastics, antimetabolites, antimitotics, biological response modifiers, and hormonal antineoplastics.

HOW DRUGS ARE NAMED

A drug's chemical, generic, trade, and official names are developed at different phases of the drug development process and serve different functions. For example, the various names of the commonly prescribed diuretic chlorothiazide sodium are:

- Chemical name: 6-chloro-2H–1,2,4-benzothiadiazine-7-sulfonamide 1,1-dioxide monosodium salt, or $C_7H_5ClN_3NaO_4S_2$
- Generic name: chlorothiazide sodium
- Trade name: Diuril
- Official name: Chlorothiazide Sodium for Injection, USP

A drug's *chemical name* describes its atomic and molecular structures. The chemical name of chlorothiazide sodium indicates that the drug is a substituted ring structure with a sulfonamide group as well as a sodium salt.

Once a drug successfully completes several clinical trials, it receives a *generic name,* also known as the nonproprietary name. The generic name is usually derived from, but shorter than, the chemical name. The United States Adopted Names Council is responsible for selecting generic names, which are intended for unrestricted public use.

Before submitting the drug for FDA approval, the manufacturer creates and registers a *trade name* (or brand name) when the drug appears ready to be marketed. Trade names are copyrighted and followed by the symbol ® to indicate that they're registered and that their use is restricted to the drug manufacturer. Once the original patent on a drug has expired, any manufacturer may produce the drug and market it with its own trade name.

A drug's *official name* is the name under which it's listed in the United States Pharmacopoeia (USP) and the National Formulary (NF).

Pharmacokinetics

Pharmacokinetics is the study of a drug's actions—or fate—as it passes through the body during absorption, distribution, metabolism, and excretion.

Absorption

Before a drug can begin working, it must be transformed from its pharmaceutical dosage form to a biologically available (bioavailable) substance that can pass through various biological cell membranes to reach its site of action. This process is known as absorption. A drug's absorption rate depends on its route of administration, its circulation through the tissue into which it's administered, and its solubility—that is, whether it's more water-soluble (hydrophilic) or fat-soluble (lipophilic).

Although drugs may penetrate cellular membranes either actively or passively, most drugs do so by *passive diffusion,* moving inertly from an area of higher concentration to an area of lower concentration. Passive diffusion may occur through water or fat. Passive diffusion through water—*aqueous diffusion*—occurs in large water-filled compartments, such as interstitial spaces, and across epithelial membrane tight junctions and pores in the epithelial lining of blood vessels. Aqueous diffusion is driven by concentration gradients. Drug molecules that are bound to large plasma proteins, such as albumin, are too large to pass through aqueous pores in this way. Passive diffusion through fat—*lipid diffusion*—plays an important role in drug metabolism because of the large number of lipid barriers that separate the aqueous compartments of the body. The ability of a drug to move through lipid layers between aqueous compartments often depends on the pH of the medium—that is, the ability of the water-soluble or fat-soluble drug to form weak acid or weak base.

Drugs whose molecules are too large to readily diffuse may rely on *active diffusion,* in which special carriers on molecules, including peptides, amino acids, and glucose, transport the drug through the membranes. However, some molecules with selective membrane carriers can expel foreign drug molecules; this is why many drugs can't cross the blood-brain barrier.

Drug absorption begins at the administration route. The three main administration route categories are parenteral (I.M., I.V., subcutaneous, and intradermal routes), enteral (oral, nasogastric, and rectal routes), and transcutaneous. Depending on its nature or chemical makeup, a drug may be better absorbed from one site than another.

I.V. drug administration allows for rapid distribution throughout the body because a drug is injected or infused directly into the blood circulation. This route usually provides the greatest bioavailability and may be used whenever other routes are contraindicated or inadequate. Drug absorption is much faster and more predictable after parenteral administration than after enteral administration.

Distribution
Distribution is the process by which a drug is transported by the

circulating fluids to various sites, including its sites of action. To ensure maximum therapeutic effectiveness, the drug must permeate all membranes that separate it from its intended site of action. Drug distribution is influenced by blood flow, tissue availability, and protein binding.

Metabolism

Drug metabolism is the enzymatic conversion of a drug's structure into substrate molecules or polar compounds that are either less active or inactive and are readily excreted. Drugs can also be synthesized to larger molecules. Metabolism may also convert a drug to a more toxic compound. Because the primary site of drug metabolism is the liver, children, the elderly, and patients with impaired hepatic function are at risk for altered therapeutic effects.

Biotransformation is the process by which a drug changes into its active metabolite. Compounds that require metabolic biotransformation for activation are known as *prodrugs*. During phase I of biotransformation, the parent drug is converted into an inactive or partially active metabolite. Much of the original drug may be eliminated during this phase. During phase II, the inactive or partially active metabolite binds with available substrates, such as acetic acid, glucuronic acid, sulfuric acid, or water, to form its active metabolite. When biotransformation leads to synthesis, larger molecules are produced to create a pharmacologic effect.

Excretion

The body eliminates drugs by both metabolism and excretion. Drug metabolites—and, in some cases, the active drug itself—are eventually excreted from the body, usually through bile, feces, and urine. The primary organ for drug elimination is the kidney. Impaired renal function may cause excessive drug accumulation in the body, thus increasing the patient's risk of adverse drug reactions and toxicity. Other excretion routes include evaporation through the skin, exhalation from the lungs, and secretion into saliva and breast milk.

A drug's elimination *half-life* is the amount of time required for half of the drug to be eliminated from the body. The half-life roughly correlates with the drug's duration of action and is based on normal renal and hepatic function. Typically, the longer the half-life, the less often the drug has to be given and the longer it remains in the body after it's discontinued.

Pharmacodynamics

Pharmacodynamics is the study of the biochemical and physiologic effects of drugs and their mechanisms of action. A drug's actions may be structurally specific or nonspecific. Structurally specific drugs combine with cell receptors, such as proteins or glycoproteins, to enhance or inhibit cellular enzyme actions. Drug receptors are the cellular components affected at the site of action. Many drugs form chemical bonds with drug receptors, but a drug can bond with a receptor only if it has a similar shape—much the same way that a key fits into a lock. When a drug combines with a receptor, channels are either opened or closed and cellular biochemical messengers, such as cyclic adenosine monophosphate or calcium ions, are activated. Once activated, cellular functions can be turned either on or off by these messengers. Structurally nonspecific drugs, such as biological response modifiers, don't combine with cell receptors; rather, they produce changes within the cell membrane or interior.

The mechanisms by which drugs interact with the body are not always known. Drugs may work by physical action (such as the protective effects of a topical ointment) or chemical reaction (such as an antacid's effect on the gastric mucosa), or by modifying the metabolic activity of invading pathogens (such as an antibiotic) or replacing a missing biochemical substance (such as insulin).

Agonists

Agonists are drugs that interact with a receptor to stimulate a response. They alter cell physiology by binding to plasma membranes or intracellular structures. *Partial agonists* can't achieve maximal effects even though they may occupy all available receptor sites on a cell. *Strong agonists* can cause maximal effects while occupying only a small number of receptor sites on a cell. *Weak agonists* must occupy many more receptor sites than strong agonists to produce the same effect.

Antagonists

Antagonists are drugs that attach to a receptor but don't stimulate a response; instead, they inhibit or block responses that would normally be caused by agonists. *Competitive antagonists* bind to receptor sites that are also compatible with an agonist, thus preventing the agonist from binding to the site. *Noncompetitive antagonists* bind to receptor sites that aren't occupied by an agonist; this changes the receptor site so that it's no longer recognized by the agonist. *Irreversible antagonists* work in much the same way that noncompetitive ones do, except that they permanently bind with the receptor.

Antagonism plays an important role in drug interactions. When two agonists that cause opposite therapeutic effects, such as a vasodilator and a vasoconstrictor, are combined, the effects cancel each other out. When two antagonists, such as morphine and naloxone, are combined, both drugs may become inactive.

Pharmacotherapeutics

Pharmacotherapeutics is the study of how drugs are used to prevent or treat disease. Understanding why a drug is prescribed for a certain disease can assist you in prioritizing drug administration with other patient care activities. Knowing a drug's desired and unwanted effects may help you uncover problems not readily apparent from the admitting diagnosis. This information may also help you prevent such problems as adverse reactions and drug interactions.

A drug's *desired effect* is the intended or expected clinical response to the drug. This is the response you start to evaluate as soon as a drug is given. Dosage adjustments and the continuation of therapy often depend on your accurate evaluation and documentation of the patient's response.

An *adverse reaction* is any noxious and unintended response to a drug that occurs at therapeutic doses used for prophylaxis, diagnosis, or therapy. Adverse reactions associated with excessive amounts of a drug are considered drug overdoses. Be prepared to follow your institution's policy for reporting adverse drug reactions.

An *idiosyncratic response* is a genetically determined abnormal or excessive response to a drug that occurs in a particular patient. The unusual response may indicate that the drug has saturated or overwhelmed mechanisms that normally control absorption, distribution, metabolism, or excretion, thus altering the expected response. You may be unsure whether a reaction is adverse or idiosyncratic. Once you report the reaction, the pharmacist usually determines the appropriate course of action.

An *allergic reaction* is an adverse response that results from previous exposure to the same drug or to one that is chemically similar to it. The patient's immune system reacts to the drug as if it were a foreign invader and may produce a mild hypersensitivity reaction, characterized by localized dermatitis, urticaria, angioedema, or photosensitivity. Allergic reactions should be reported to the prescriber immediately and the drug should be discontinued. Follow-up care may include giving drugs, including antihistamines and corticosteroids, to counteract the allergic response.

An *anaphylactic reaction* is an immediate hypersensitivity response characterized by urticaria, pruritus, and angioedema. Left untreated, an anaphylactic reaction can lead to systemic involvement, resulting in shock. It's often associated with life-threatening hypotension and respiratory distress. Be prepared to assist with emergency life support measures, especially if the reaction occurs in response to I.V. drugs, which have the fastest rate of absorption.

A *drug interaction* occurs when one drug alters the pharmacokinetics of another drug—for example, when two or more drugs are given concurrently. Such concurrent administration can increase or decrease the therapeutic or adverse effects of either drug. Some drug interactions are beneficial. For example, when taken with penicillin G, probenecid decreases the excretion rate of penicillin G, resulting in higher blood levels of penicillin G. Drug interactions may also occur when a drug's metabolism is altered, often owing to the induction of or competition for metabolizing enzymes. For example, H_2-receptor agonists, which reduce secretion of the enzyme gastrin, may alter the breakdown of enteric coatings on other drugs. Drug interactions due to carrier protein competition typically occur when a drug inhibits the kidneys' ability to reduce excretion of other drugs. For example, probenecid is completely reabsorbed by the renal tubules and is metabolized very slowly. It competes with the same carrier protein as sulfonamides for active tubular secretion and so decreases the renal excretion of sulfonamides. This particular competition can lead to an increased risk of sulfonamide toxicity.

Special Considerations
Although every drug has a usual dosage range, certain factors—such as a patient's age, weight, culture and ethnicity, gender, pregnancy status, and renal and hepatic function—may contribute to the need for dosage adjustments. When you encounter special considerations such as these, be prepared to reassess the prescribed dosage to make sure that it's safe and effective for your patient.

Culture and Ethnicity
Certain drugs are more effective or more likely to produce adverse effects in particular ethnic groups or races. For example, blacks with hypertension respond better to thiazide diuretics than do patients of other races; on the other hand, blacks also have an increased risk of developing angioedema associated with angiotensin-converting enzyme (ACE) inhibitors. A patient's religious or cultural background may also call for special consideration. For example, a drug made from porcine products may be unacceptable to a Jewish or Muslim patient.

Elderly Patients

Because aging produces certain changes in body composition and organ function, elderly patients present unique therapeutic and dosing problems that require special attention. For example, the weight of the liver, the number of functioning hepatic cells, and hepatic blood flow all decrease as a person ages, resulting in slower drug metabolism. Renal function may also decrease with aging. These processes can lead to the accumulation of active drugs and metabolites as well as increased sensitivity to the effects of some drugs in elderly patients. Because they're also more likely to have multiple chronic illnesses, many elderly patients take multiple prescription drugs each day, thus increasing the risk of drug interactions.

Children

Because their bodily functions are not fully developed, children—particularly those under age 12—may metabolize drugs differently than adults. In infants, immature renal and hepatic function delay metabolism and excretion of drugs. As a result, pediatric drug dosages are very different from adult dosages.

The FDA has provided drug manufacturers with guidelines that define pediatric age categories. Use these categories as a guide when administering drugs, unless the manufacturer provides a specific age range:
- neonates—birth up to age 1 month
- infants—ages 1 month to 2 years
- children—ages 2 to 12
- adolescents—ages 12 to 16.

Pregnancy

The many physiologic changes that take place in the body during pregnancy may affect a drug's pharmacokinetics and alter its effectiveness. Additionally, exposure to drugs may pose risks for the developing fetus. Before administering a drug to a pregnant patient, be sure to check its assigned FDA pregnancy risk category and intervene appropriately.

Principles of I.V. Drug Administration

Administering I.V. drugs requires a combination of skills—not only knowing how to give drugs safely but also knowledge of anatomy (such as the location of veins in the body) and of assessment (for example, when and how to observe the insertion site, surrounding area, and the patient for complications).

In I.V. drug administration, a drug enters the circulatory system through a single, small-volume injection or a slow, large-volume infusion rather than through GI absorption. Because drugs injected I.V. don't encounter absorption barriers, this route produces the most rapid drug action, making it vital in emergency situations. The I.V. route is also used when the patient is uncooperative, unconscious, or unable to accept medication by the oral or I.M. route or when a drug is ineffective by other routes. Although it's the preferred route for certain situations, I.V. administration has several disadvantages: I.V. drugs are generally more expensive to administer than other dosage forms because they require strict sterility, and once the drug has been injected, it can't be removed and the dosage can't be reduced.

One way that you can enhance your understanding of the principles of I.V. drug administration is to *associate, ask,* and *predict* during the critical thinking process. For example, *associate* each drug with general information you may already know about the drug or drug class. *Ask* yourself why a drug may be given by the I.V. route or why it's given multiple times throughout the day rather than only once. Learn to *predict* a drug's actions, uses, adverse effects, and possible drug interactions based on your knowledge of the drug's mechanism of action. As you apply these principles to I.V. drug administration, you'll begin to intuitively know which facts you need to make rational clinical decisions.

Each facility or agency has its own protocols for I.V. drug administration, including care of the I.V. site. Many of them use the Intravenous Nurses Society's Standards of Practice to formulate their policies. Individual state nursing practice guidelines are another component that may be used to develop I.V. administration protocols.

"Rights" of Drug Administration

Always keep in mind the following "rights" of drug administration, which apply to all forms of drug administration, including I.V.: the right drug, right time, right dose, right patient, right route, and right preparation and administration.

Right Drug
Many drugs have similar spellings, a variety of concentrations, and several generic forms. Before administering any drug, compare the exact spelling and concentration of the prescribed drug that appears on the label with the information contained in the medication administration record or drug profile. Regardless of which drug distribution system your facility uses, you should read the drug label and compare it to the medication administration record at least three times:
- before removing the drug from the dispensing unit or unit-dose cart
- before reconstituting, diluting, or measuring the prescribed dose
- before opening a unit-dose package (just prior to administering the drug to the patient).

Right Time
Various factors can affect the time a drug is given, such as the timing of meals, other drugs, or scheduled diagnostic tests; standardized times used by the institution; and factors that may alter the consistency of blood levels and drug absorption. Before giving any p.r.n. drug, check the patient's chart to ensure that no one else has already administered it and that the specified time interval has passed. Also, document administration of a p.r.n. drug immediately.

Right Dose
Whenever you're dispensing an unfamiliar drug or in doubt about a dosage, check the prescribed dose against the range specified in a reliable reference. In addition, because many I.V. drugs come in different concentrations—such as urokinase, which is available in concentrations ranging from 5,000 to 250,000 international units—you must examine the label closely to make sure you're giving the proper strength. Also make sure you're using the appropriate concentration for the method of delivery. For example, the 5,000– and 9,000–international unit concentrations of urokinase are used only for clearing I.V. catheter occlusions, not for I.V. or intracoronary administration. Conversely, the 250,000–international unit concentration is used only for I.V. and intracoronary drug administration.

Be sure to consider any reasons for which your patient might need a dosage adjustment, such as age, preexisting medical conditions, or response to the drug. Also, be familiar with the standard abbreviations your institution uses for writing prescriptions.

Right Patient
Always compare the name on the medication record with the name on the patient's identification bracelet. When using a unit-dose system, compare the name on the drug profile with that on the identification bracelet.

Right Route
Each prescribed drug should specify the administration route. If the route is missing, consult the prescribing physician. Never substitute one route for another without a prescription for the change. Severe adverse reactions can result from administering a parenteral drug by the wrong route. For example, the antineoplastic drug vinblastine can cause potentially fatal paralysis when administered intrathecally and requires special labeling when it's being prepared.

Right Preparation and Administration
Be sure to maintain aseptic technique when handling drugs that need to be reconstituted, diluted, and measured. Follow any specific directions included in the manufacturer's insert regarding diluent type and amount and the use of filters, if needed. Clearly label any drug you've reconstituted with the patient's name, the strength or dose, the date and time you prepared the drug, the amount and type of diluent you used, the expiration date, and your initials. Be aware that certain drugs and diluents contain additives that have been known to cause adverse reactions. One example is benzyl alcohol, a preservative found in some drugs and diluents that may cause a fatal toxic syndrome in neonates and premature infants. It's characterized by CNS, respiratory, circulatory, and renal impairment and metabolic acidosis. Also, determine whether your patient has an allergy to a prescribed drug or its components, to similar drugs, or to a recommended diluent; if so, report it to the prescriber. If the patient is allergic to a diluent, discuss possible alternative diluents with the pharmacist.

Become familiar with the I.V. administration method being used. For example, if you're using an I.V. administration set, find out the accurate flow rate—usually between 10 and 60 drops/ml. If you're using an infusion device, know how to use it correctly. Also, check the infusion rate periodically to ensure that the appropriate amount of drug is being administered.

Types of Venous Access
I.V. drugs can be given through a peripheral or central venous access. The type of access depends on such factors as the patient's

overall medical condition, the type of drug to be given, and the amount of time the patient needs I.V. drug therapy.

Once I.V. access has been established, it is used for either continuous or intermittent injection or infusion. Intermittent infusion typically involves use of a saline, or heparin, lock. This device allows for immediate venous access and doesn't require continuous administration of fluids to maintain its patency.

Peripheral I.V. Drug Administration

In peripheral I.V. administration, a drug is injected or infused through a peripheral vein, usually one in the forearm. Peripheral access is used to administer various fluids and solutions, including antibiotics, chemotherapeutic drugs, blood products, and hydrating fluids. It is typically used for short-term drug administration in the hospital and in outpatient settings. For longer periods of drug administration, a midline catheter may be used. This is a longer catheter that remains in the peripheral venous system, typically in the larger veins of the arm below the axilla. A peripheral insertion site may also be used for a peripherally inserted central catheter (PICC), which delivers drugs directly into the central venous system.

Veins in the distal part of the arm are typically selected first, but the choice of vein depends on the type of drug being administered, possible adverse effects, the patient's age and medical condition, which hand is dominant, and the length of time the I.V. line will be in place. These factors also influence the choice of a venipuncture device, which may range from a winged infusion set to an over-the-needle catheter made of polyethylene, silicone, or other materials. Use the shortest needle and the smallest gauge that meet the needs of the drug or solution to be infused.

Central Venous Administration

Central venous therapy is commonly used to give long-term drug therapy to patients whose condition contraindicates placement of a peripheral I.V. line. Central venous access may be achieved via centrally or peripherally inserted catheters or implantable ports.

If venous access is placed in the upper part of the body, the central venous catheter tip lies in the superior vena cava; if femoral venous access is used, the catheter tip lies in the inferior superior vena cava. Common sites for centrally inserted catheters are the subclavian vein and the internal or external jugular veins. Common sites for PICCs are the basilic, cephalic, and median cubital veins in the arm. Surgically implanted central venous ports have a self-sealing septum with a catheter attached that leads to the superior vena cava.

Ports may be accessed using noncoring needles from above or at the side of the port, depending on the type used.

The type of central catheter used varies, depending on such factors as the type and number of drugs to be administered and the amount of time the central access will be in place. Single-lumen or multi-lumen catheters may be used, depending on the patient's needs. Tunneled catheters, such as the Hickman catheter, are used when long-term use is anticipated. These catheters are radiopaque and have a cuff at the end, near the body entrance site. Part of the tunneled catheter lies within subcutaneous tissue, which over time turns into a collagenous matrix that gradually adheres to the cuff, thus helping to secure the catheter and protect against infection.

Alternative Infusion Methods

Although the focus of this book is I.V. drug therapy, you should be aware of other methods used to infuse drugs, such as subcutaneous (sometimes called SubQ) and intraosseous infusion. One of the most common subcutaneous drugs is insulin. A programmed insulin pump administers small amounts of regular insulin throughout the day through a needle or catheter inserted into the patient's abdomen. Intraosseous infusions are administered by a needle inserted into the bone marrow. They're used in such conditions as shock, anaphylaxis, or trauma when venous access is not available.

Infusion Devices

I.V. drug therapy commonly requires the use of an infusion device to ensure that the appropriate dose is being administered—for example, when administering I.V. antiarrhythmics (such as lidocaine hydrochloride or procainamide hydrochloride) or when administering drugs to children. The type of infusion device can vary, depending on the drug used, the amount of fluid to be given, and the setting at which the drug is being administered.

Electronic infusion devices (also known as electronic infusion pumps and controllers) are powered by electricity or battery packs. These devices come in various sizes, from compact ambulatory versions designed for portable use to multidrug infusion pumps commonly used in acute care settings. Controller devices don't assist in drug delivery; rather they monitor the drop flow based on a programmed rate. Electronic infusion pumps provide a positive pressure flow to assist with drug delivery.

Electronic infusion devices may have alarms to signal increased pressure or air in the I.V. line or the completion of an infusion. Some devices prevent the solution from flowing if the line becomes disconnected from the device. Others contain a free-flow alarm, which can signal an uncontrolled rate of fluid administration stemming from accidental disconnection.

Patient-Controlled Analgesia

Patient-controlled analgesia (PCA) allows the patient to be actively involved in his own drug delivery. First, you administer the loading dose and program the pump to deliver additional bolus doses of the drug within predetermined limits for amount and frequency. The patient then presses a button when he wants to activate a bolus dose. You must clearly explain the drug delivery system to the patient, making sure he understands that there is a "lock-out" period during which he won't be able to administer additional doses.

Complications of I.V. Therapy

Because I.V. drug administration requires a break in the skin, it poses an increased risk of infection, ranging from local infection of surrounding tissues to sepsis. To prevent infection or detect it early, monitor the I.V. site, change dressings and tubing, and rotate the I.V. site in accordance with your facility's policy. Administration sets are typically changed every 24 to 48 hours (every 24 hours for intermittent infusion), and I.V. sites are rotated every 48 to 72 hours.

Two other potential complications of I.V. therapy are infiltration—the leakage of nonvesicant solution into surrounding tissues—and extravasation—the leakage of a vesicant solution, such as certain chemotherapeutic drugs, into surrounding tissues. To detect these complications, frequently assess the I.V. site and surrounding area. If you observe either of these conditions, restart the I.V. line at another site. Extravasation can cause tissue necrosis, gangrene, and other reactions around the injection site. If extravasation occurs, expect to use a drug such as phentolamine to antagonize vasoconstriction and minimize sloughing and tissue necrosis.

Other risks of I.V. drug therapy include catheter occlusion, circulatory overload, phlebitis, thrombosis, hematoma, pulmonary or air embolism, and venous spasm. Some complications are specific to the route. For example, central venous catheters increase the risk of arterial puncture, pneumothorax, and hemothorax.

The rapid distribution and greater bioavailability in I.V. therapy mean that you must watch for adverse reactions diligently. Too-rapid delivery of a drug can result in a reaction called speed shock. Anaphylactic reactions can occur within a few minutes of drug administration or several days afterward. Become familiar with the potential adverse effects of each drug you administer.

Safe Handling of Toxic Agents

I.V. drug administration may expose you to toxic agents, such as many antineoplastic drugs. To protect yourself from potential carcinogenic, mutagenic, and teratogenic effects of these drugs, learn how to handle them safely. Because no standard procedure exists, follow your facility's protocols for preparing and handling antineoplastic drugs and for appropriate disposal of used equipment. In addition, before you prepare a toxic drug, consult the manufacturer's package insert for specific recommendations, such as the use of a biological containment cabinet, gloves, and gown.

Preventing Needlestick Injuries

Take steps to avoid needlestick injuries when you administer I.V. drugs and when you handle certain preparations, such as immune globulin intravenous, which is made from human plasma and therefore may contain infectious agents such as viruses. Needleless administration systems have been developed to decrease the risk of needlestick injuries and exposure to such viruses as HIV.

Other Uses for I.V. Access

In addition to drug delivery, I.V. access is also used for infusing hydrating fluids, blood products, and total parenteral nutrition (TPN).

Parenteral Fluids

Parenteral fluids may be infused to maintain I.V. access, treat certain medical conditions (such as normal saline for hyperparathyroidism), or restore fluid volume in patients with hypovolemic shock or burns. (See *Selected water and electrolyte solutions,* page xxx.)

Blood Products

Blood products include whole blood, packed red blood cells, platelets, and plasma. Learn your facility's protocols and the techniques required for infusing them. Before you infuse blood, verify the prescriber's order and that the patient has appropriate I.V. access, typically an 18G or 20G catheter (smaller for children). Ensure that no solution other than normal saline is infusing in the I.V. line to be used. Two other critical steps are verifying the patient's ABO blood and Rh types and verifying his identity to ensure that the right product is given to the right patient. (See *Understanding blood types and Rh factor,* page xxxi.) Observe the patient continuously during the first 10 to 15 minutes because the majority of anaphylactic and ABO incompatibility reactions occur during that time. Blood infusions usually last no more than 4 hours because of the risk of septicemia.

SELECTED WATER AND ELECTROLYTE SOLUTIONS

The table below provides electrolyte contents for some common solutions you may administer in your clinical practice.

I.V. Solution	Electrolyte Contents
0.5% dextrose in water	No electrolytes
Dextrose 2.5% with ½ strength lactated Ringer's injection	1.4 mEq/L of calcium 54 to 55 mEq/L of chloride 14 mEq/L of lactate 2 mEq/L of potassium 65 mEq/L of sodium
Dextrose 5% with lactated Ringer's injection	2.7 to 3 mEq/L of calcium 109 to 112 mEq/L of chloride 28 mEq/L of lactate 4 mEq/L of potassium 130 mEq/L of sodium
Lactated Ringer's injection	2.7 to 3 mEq/L of calcium 109 to 110 mEq/L of chloride 28 mEq/L of lactate 4 mEq/L of potassium 130 mEq/L of sodium
⅙ M sodium lactate	167 mEq/L of lactate 167 mEq/L of sodium
0.45% sodium chloride	77 mEq/L of chloride 77 mEq/L of sodium
0.9% sodium chloride	154 mEq/L of chloride 154 mEq/L of sodium
3% sodium chloride	513 mEq/L of chloride 513 mEq/L of sodium
5% sodium chloride	855 mEq/L of chloride 855 mEq/L of sodium

Total Parenteral Nutrition

Also called I.V. hyperalimentation, TPN provides nutrition for patients unable to eat, digest, or absorb sufficient nutrients. TPN is typically administered by a central venous catheter, usually a subclavian catheter; however, PICC lines or tunneled catheters may

UNDERSTANDING BLOOD TYPES AND Rh FACTOR

Verification of ABO blood and Rh types is vital if you'll be giving blood products. Administering the wrong blood type or Rh factor could set off an immune response that results in the destruction of red blood cells (RBCs). Understanding the role that antigens and antibodies play in blood typing will help you understand the importance of transfusing the correct blood product.

Antigens are glycoproteins or glycolipids found on the membrane surface of RBCs. Specific antigens on the RBC designate an individual's ABO blood type. The four major blood types are A, B, AB, and O. Individuals inherit antigens and blood types from their parents. Within a few months of birth, a child develops antibodies against the antigens he doesn't have. The antigens and antibodies for the specific blood types are as follows:

Type	Antigen	Antibody
A	A	Anti-B
B	B	Anti-A
AB	A and B	None
O	None	Anti-A and Anti-B

Each patient should ideally receive his own specific blood type. However, in an emergency, type O blood can be given to anyone because it contains no A or B antigens. For this reason, people with type O blood are called *universal donors.* Conversely, persons with type AB blood, which has both antigens, can receive any blood type and are called *universal recipients.*

Antigens are also a component of the Rh factor; one of them—the D antigen—is of particular significance. Patients with the D antigen are considered Rh-positive, whereas patients who lack it are Rh-negative. Antibodies to the D antigen don't develop automatically; they can form if a person has received a transfusion or delivered a child with the antigen. If a person with antibodies to the D antigen receives a transfusion of Rh-positive blood, he can develop a transfusion reaction that results in RBC destruction.

also be used. Administer TPN as a continuous infusion, using an infusion pump. Monitor the patient for adverse reactions, including infection, sepsis, and venous thrombosis from the I.V. access; hyperglycemia if the patient can't metabolize the glucose in the TPN fast enough; or hypoglycemia if the infusion is stopped abruptly.

I.V. Drug Therapy and the Nursing Process

The nursing process helps guide you as you develop, implement, and evaluate your care, and it ensures that you'll deliver safe, consistent, effective I.V. drug therapy. It consists of five steps: assessment, nursing diagnosis, planning, implementation, and evaluation. In addition to these steps, you're responsible for documenting all aspects of your care before, during, and after drug administration.

Assessment

The first step in the nursing process, assessment involves gathering information essential to guide your patient's drug therapy. This information includes the patient's drug history, present drug use, allergies, medical history, and physical examination findings. Assessment is an ongoing process that serves as a baseline against which to compare any changes in your patient's condition; it's also the basis for developing and individualizing the patient's plan of care.

Drug History

The patient's drug history is critical in your planning of drug-related care. Ask about his previous use of OTC and prescription drugs as well as herbal remedies. For each drug, determine:
• the reason the patient took it
• the prescribed dosage
• the administration route
• the frequency of administration
• the duration of the drug therapy
• any adverse reactions the patient may have experienced and how he handled them.

If the patient received previous I.V. therapy, ask him the type of vascular access that was used and how he tolerated the therapy.

Also, determine if the patient has a history of drug abuse or addiction; if he has, find out the administration route he used. Depending on his physical and emotional state, you may need to obtain the drug history from other sources, such as family members, friends, or other caregivers, and from the medical record.

Present Drug Use

Ask about the patient's current use of OTC and prescription drugs as well as herbal remedies. As you did in the drug history, find out the specific details for each drug (dosage, route, frequency, and reason for taking). Also ask the patient if he thinks the drug has been effective and when he took the last dose.

If the patient uses herbal remedies, explore them because herbs may interact with certain drugs. Also ask about the patient's use of recreational drugs, such as alcohol and tobacco, as well as illegal drugs, such as marijuana and heroin. Again, be sure to ascertain the administration route he used. If the patient acknowledges use of these drugs, be alert for possible drug interactions. This information may also provide you with insight about the patient's response—or lack of response—to his current drug treatment plan.

Try to find out if the patient has any other problems that might affect his compliance with the drug treatment plan, and intervene appropriately. For instance, a patient who is unemployed and has no health insurance may fail to fill a needed prescription. In such a case, contact an appropriate individual in your facility who may be able to help the patient obtain financial assistance.

Be sure to ask if the patient's drug treatment plan requires special monitoring or follow-up laboratory tests. For example, patients who take antihypertensives need to have their blood pressure checked routinely, and those who take warfarin must have their prothrombin time tested regularly. Other patients must undergo periodic blood tests to assess hepatic and renal function. Ask whether the patient has followed this part of his treatment plan, and ask him if he knows the results of the latest monitoring or laboratory tests.

Allergies
Find out if the patient is allergic to any drugs or foods. If he is, determine the type of drug or food that triggers a reaction, the first time he had a reaction, the characteristics of the reaction, and other related information. Keep in mind that some patients consider annoying symptoms, such as indigestion, an allergic reaction. Be sure to document a true allergy according to your facility's policy to ensure that the patient doesn't receive that drug or a related one. Also document food allergies because they may lead to drug interactions or adverse drug reactions. For example, sulfite is a food additive as well as a drug additive, so a patient with an allergy to sulfite-containing foods is likely to react to sulfite-containing drugs.

Medical History
While reviewing your patient's medical history, determine if he has any acute or chronic conditions that may interfere with his drug therapy. Certain disorders involving major body systems, such as

the cardiovascular, GI, hepatic, and renal systems, may affect a drug's absorption, transport, metabolism, or excretion and interfere with its action; they also may increase the risk of adverse reactions and toxicity. For each disorder identified, try to determine when the condition was diagnosed, what drugs were prescribed, and who prescribed them. This information can help you determine whether the patient is receiving incompatible drugs and whether more than one prescriber is managing his drug therapy.

Ask a female patient if she is or may be pregnant or if she's breast-feeding. Many drugs are safe to use during pregnancy, but others may harm the fetus. Also, some drugs appear in breast milk. If your patient is or might be pregnant, check the FDA's pregnancy risk category for the prescribed drug and notify the prescriber if it may pose a risk to the fetus. If the patient is breast-feeding, find out if the drug appears in breast milk and intervene appropriately.

In addition, ask about any preexisting conditions or procedures that may have implications for the I.V. site selection, such as a history of lymphatic or superior vena caval obstruction, lymph node dissection, mastectomy, or radiation therapy to the upper torso, or the presence of an internal arteriovenous fistula for hemodialysis.

Physical Examination Findings

As part of the physical examination, note the patient's age and weight. Be aware that age determines the dosage of certain drugs, such as sedatives and hypnotics, whereas weight determines the dosage of others, including some I.V. antibiotics and anticoagulants. As you perform the physical examination, note any abnormal findings that may point to organ or body system dysfunction. For example, if you detect liver enlargement and ascites, the patient may have impaired hepatic function, which can affect the metabolism of a drug he's taking and lead to harmful adverse or toxic effects. Also note whether an organ or a body system appears to be responding to drug treatment. For example, if a patient has been taking an antibiotic to treat chronic bronchitis, thoroughly evaluate his respiratory status to measure his progress. And be sure to assess the patient for possible adverse reactions to the drugs he's taking.

Also assess the condition of potential vascular access sites, and evaluate their suitability for I.V. drug administration.

Assess the patient's neurologic function to ensure that he can understand his drug regimen and carry out required tasks, such as performing a finger stick to obtain blood for glucose measurement. If a patient can't understand essential drug information, you'll need to identify a family member or another person willing to help.

Nursing Diagnosis

Based on information derived from the assessment and physical examination findings, the nursing diagnoses are statements of actual or potential problems that a nurse is licensed to treat or manage alone or in collaboration with other members of the health care team. The diagnoses are worded according to guidelines established by the North American Nursing Diagnosis Association.

One of the most common nursing diagnoses related to drug therapy is *knowledge deficit,* which indicates that the patient doesn't have sufficient understanding of his drug regimen. However, adverse reactions are the basis for most nursing diagnoses related to drug administration. For example, a patient receiving an opioid analgesic might have a nursing diagnosis of *constipation* related to decreased intestinal motility or *ineffective breathing pattern* related to respiratory depression. Many antiarrhythmics cause orthostatic hypotension and thus may place an elderly patient at *high risk for injury* related to possible syncope. Broad-spectrum antibiotics, such as penicillin G, may lead to the overgrowth of *Clostridium difficile,* a bacterium that is normally present in the intestines. This overgrowth, in turn, may lead to pseudomembranous enterocolitis, characterized by abdominal pain and severe diarrhea. The nursing diagnoses in such a case might include *risk for infection* related to bacterial overgrowth, *alteration in comfort* related to abdominal pain, and *fluid balance deficit* related to diarrhea.

Planning

During the planning phase, you'll establish expected outcomes—or goals—for the patient and then develop specific nursing interventions to achieve them. Expected outcomes are observable or measurable goals that should occur as a result of nursing interventions and sometimes medical interventions. Developed in collaboration with the patient, the outcomes should be realistic and objective and should clearly communicate to other nurses the direction of the plan of care. They should be written as behaviors or responses for the patient, not the nurse, to achieve and should include a time frame for measuring the patient's progress. An example of a typical expected outcome is: "The patient will accurately demonstrate self-administration of insulin before discharge." Based on each outcome statement you create, you'll develop appropriate nursing interventions, which may include drug administration techniques, patient teaching, monitoring of vital signs, calculation of drug dosages based on weight, and recording of intake and output.

Implementation

As you implement nursing interventions, be sure to stringently follow the classic rule of drug administration: administer the right dose of the right drug by the right route to the right patient at the right time. Also, keep in mind that you have a legal and professional responsibility to follow institutional policy regarding standing orders, prescription renewal, and the use of nursing judgment. During the implementation phase, you'll also begin to evaluate the patient's expected outcomes and nursing interventions and make necessary changes to the plan of care.

Evaluation

Evaluation is an ongoing process rather than a single step in the nursing process. During this phase, you evaluate each expected outcome to determine whether or not it has been achieved and whether the original plan of care is working or needs to be modified. In evaluating a patient's drug treatment plan, you should determine whether or not the drug is controlling the signs and symptoms for which it was prescribed. You should also evaluate the patient for psychological or physiologic responses to the drug, especially adverse reactions. This constant monitoring allows you to make appropriate and timely suggestions for changes to the plan of care, such as dosage adjustments or changes in delivery routes, until each expected outcome has been achieved.

Documentation

You're responsible for documenting all your actions related to the patient's drug therapy, from the assessment phase to evaluation. Each time you give a drug, document the drug name, dose, time given, and your evaluation of its effect. Also document the condition of the I.V. insertion site, including the presence (be specific) or absence of any I.V.-related complications, specific interventions that were required, and the patient's response. When you give drugs that require additional nursing judgment, such as those prescribed on an as-needed basis, document the rationale for giving the drug and follow-up assessment or interventions for each dose.

If you decide to withhold a prescribed drug based on your nursing judgment, document your action and the rationale for it, and notify the prescriber in a timely manner. Whenever you notify a prescriber about a significant finding related to drug therapy, such as an adverse reaction, document the date and time, the person you contacted, what you discussed, and how you intervened.

abatacept
Orencia

Class and Category
Chemical: Human cytotoxic T-lymphocyte–associated antigen 4
Therapeutic: T-cell activation blocker
Pregnancy category: C

Indications and Dosages
▶ *To reduce signs and symptoms, induce major clinical response, slow the progression of structural damage, and improve physical function in patients with moderate to severe active rheumatoid arthritis, as monotherapy or as adjunct with disease-modifying anti-rheumatic drug (DMARD) therapy other than tumor necrosis factor (TNF) antagonists*
I.V. INFUSION

Adults. 30-min infusion of 500 mg for patients weighing less than 60 kg; 750 mg for patients weighing 60 to 100 kg; and 1,000 mg for patients weighing more than 100 kg. Repeat in 2 and 4 wk and then every 4 wk thereafter.

▶ *To reduce signs and symptoms in patients with moderate to severe active polyarticular juvenile idiopathic arthritis, as monotherapy or as adjunct with methotrexate therapy*
I.V. INFUSION

Children ages 6 to 17. 30-min infusion of 10 mg/kg for patients weighing less than 75 kg; 750 mg for patients weighing 75 to 100 kg; and 1,000 mg for patients weighing more than 100 kg. Repeat in 2 and 4 wk and then every 4 wk thereafter. *Maximum:* 1,000 mg.

Route	Onset	Peak	Duration
I.V.	Unknown	60 days	Unknown

Contraindications
Hypersensitivity to abatacept and its components

Interactions
DRUGS
live vaccines: Effects of vaccine may be blunted
TNF antagonists: Increased risk of serious infections

Mechanism of Action
Inhibits T-cell activation by binding to CD80 and CD86, blocking their interaction with CD28. Interaction with CD28 normally provides a co-stimulatory signal needed for T-cell activation. Without this signal, T cells aren't activated, which slows the structural damage in rheumatoid arthritis and improves physical function.

Adverse Reactions
CNS: Dizziness, headache
CV: Hypertension, hypotension
EENT: Nasopharyngitis, rhinitis, sinusitis
GI: Diverticulitis, nausea
GU: Acute pyelonephritis, UTI
MS: Back or limb pain
RESP: Bronchitis, cough, dyspnea, upper respiratory tract infection, pneumonia, wheezing
SKIN: Cellulites, flushing, pruritus, rash, urticaria
Other: Anaphylaxis, abatacept antibody formation, herpes simplex or localized infection, influenza, malignancies

Nursing Considerations
- Before starting abatacept, screen patient for latent tuberculosis, as ordered. If it's detected, expect to delay abatacept therapy until after effective tuberculosis treatment has been given.
- Use cautiously in patients with a history of recurrent infections or medical conditions that increase the risk of infection.
- Be aware that drug may be given with other DMARDs. Expect to avoid giving abatacept with TNF antagonists because of an increased risk of infection or with anakinra because combined effects are unknown.
- Reconstitute each abatacept vial with 10 ml of sterile water for injection using only the silicone-free disposable syringe provided and an 18G to 21G needle. If drug is accidentally reconstituted with siliconized syringe, discard the solution. To minimize foaming during reconstitution, rotate the vial by swirling it gently until contents are dissolved. Don't shake the vial. Once the powder is dissolved completely, vent the vial with a needle to dissipate any foam before withdrawal.
- Further dilute to 100 ml by withdrawing a volume equal to the volume of reconstituted drug from a 100-ml infusion bag or bottle of 0.9% sodium chloride solution. For example, for two

vials, remove 20 ml; for three vials, remove 30 ml, and for four vials, remove 40 ml. Slowly add the reconstituted solution from each vial prepared using the same silicone-free disposable syringe provided with each vial. Gently mix.

• Give each abatacept dose over 30 minutes using an infusion set and a sterile, non-pyrogenic, low–protein-binding filter. Discard any unused solution after 24 hours. Don't infuse abatacept concurrently in the same intravenous line with other drugs.

• Monitor patient closely for infusion-related reactions, such as dizziness, headache, and hypertension, especially during the first hour of the infusion. Notify prescriber if they occur.

• **WARNING** Watch closely for hypersensitivity reactions, changes in blood pressure, dyspnea, nausea, flushing, urticaria, cough, pruritus, rash, and wheezing. Although reactions are rarely life-threatening, notify prescriber and prepare to stop infusion and provide supportive care if needed.

• If patient has COPD, assess him often for respiratory dusfunction during abatacept therapy because adverse respiratory reactions are more likely in patients with COPD.

• Notify prescriber and expect to stop drug if patient develops a serious infection during abatacept therapy.

• Avoid giving live vaccines during and within 3 months after abatacept therapy because abatacept may decrease the vaccine's effectiveness.

PATIENT TEACHING

• Review signs and symptoms of a possible allergic reaction, including rash and dyspnea. Urge patient to report any such symptoms immediately.

• Urge patient to immediately report signs of infection, such as cough, fever, chills, dyspnea, or headache.

• Explain that patient should receive no live vaccines during and for 3 months after abatacept therapy.

• If patient has COPD, caution about the increased risk of adverse respiratory effects. Tell him to notify prescriber immediately if they occur.

abciximab

ReoPro

Class and Category

Chemical: Fab fragment of chimeric 7E3 antibody
Therapeutic: Platelet aggregation inhibitor

Pregnancy category: C

Indications and Dosages

▶ *To prevent acute myocardial ischemic complications after percutaneous transluminal coronary angioplasty (PTCA) in patients at high risk for abrupt closure of treated coronary artery*

I.V. INFUSION, I.V. INJECTION

Adults. 250 mcg/kg bolus 10 to 60 min before PTCA. *Maintenance:* 0.125 mcg/kg/min by continuous infusion for 12 hr. *Maximum:* 10 mcg/min.

▶ *To treat unstable angina in patients who haven't responded to conventional therapy and are scheduled to have PTCA within 24 hr*

I.V. INFUSION, I.V. INJECTION

Adults. 250 mcg/kg bolus; then 10 mcg/min by continuous infusion over 18 to 24 hr, concluding 1 hr after PTCA.

Route	Onset	Peak	Duration
I.V.	Unknown	Unknown	48 hr

Mechanism of Action

Binds to glycoprotein IIb/IIIa receptor sites on surface of activated platelets. Circulating fibrinogen can bind to these receptor sites and link platelets together, forming a clot that eventually blocks a coronary artery. By binding to receptor sites, abciximab prevents normal binding of fibrinogen and other factors and inhibits platelet aggregation.

Incompatibilities

Don't mix abciximab with other drugs. Give it through a separate I.V. line whenever possible.

Contraindications

Active internal bleeding, arteriovenous malformation or aneurysm, bleeding disorders, CVA in past 2 years or that caused significant neurologic deficit at any time, GI or GU bleeding in past 6 weeks, hypersensitivity to abciximab, intracranial neoplasm, I.V. dextran therapy before or during PTCA, oral anticoagulant therapy in past 7 days unless PT is less than 1.2 times the control, severe uncontrolled hypertension, surgery in past 6 weeks, thrombocytopenia, vasculitis

Interactions

DRUGS

cefamandole, cefoperazone, cefotetan, dipyridamole, heparin, NSAIDs, oral anticoagulants, thrombolytic drugs, ticlopidine: Increased risk of bleeding

Adverse Reactions

CNS: Confusion, dizziness, hyperesthesia

CV: Atrial fibrillation or flutter, bradycardia, embolism, hypotension, peripheral edema, pseudoaneurysm, supraventricular tachycardia, third-degree AV block, thrombophlebitis, weak pulse

GI: Dysphagia, hematemesis, nausea, vomiting

GU: Dysuria, hematuria, renal dysfunction, urinary frequency, urinary incontinence, urine retention

HEME: Anemia, bleeding, leukocytosis, thrombocytopenia

RESP: Bronchitis, bronchospasm, crackles, dyspnea, pleural effusion, pneumonia, pulmonary edema, pulmonary embolism, wheezing

SKIN: Pruritus, rash, urticaria

Other: Development of human antichimeric antibodies

Nursing Considerations

- Be aware that abciximab may be used with heparin and aspirin therapy.
- Obtain PT, APTT, and platelet count before initiating therapy.
- Inspect abciximab for particles; don't use if opaque particles are present. Don't shake container.
- Administer I.V. bolus over at least 1 minute, using a sterile, nonpyrogenic, low protein-binding 0.2- to 0.22-micron filter.
- For continuous I.V. infusion, withdraw 4.5 ml from 2-mg/ml solution and inject prescribed amount into 250-ml bag of normal saline solution or D_5W, using an in-line sterile, nonpyrogenic, low protein-binding 0.2- to 0.22-micron filter. Discard unused portion.
- Infuse prescribed amount, using a continuous infusion pump.
- Avoid I.M. injections, venipunctures, and use of indwelling urinary catheters, NG tubes, and automatic blood pressure cuffs during abciximab therapy to prevent bleeding. If appropriate, insert an intermittent I.V. access device to obtain blood samples.
- Monitor for GI, GU, and retroperitoneal bleeding and for bleeding at all puncture sites.
- **WARNING** If hemorrhage occurs, prepare to discontinue infusion immediately. Expect to treat severe thrombocytopenia with platelet transfusions if needed.
- Monitor for hypersensitivity reactions, such as rash, pruritus, wheezing, and dysphagia from laryngeal edema. If such reactions occur, discontinue infusion and notify prescriber immedi-

ately. If anaphylaxis occurs, administer epinephrine, antihistamines, and corticosteroids, as prescribed.

- Monitor PT, APTT, and activated clotting time during and after therapy.
- Obtain platelet count 2 to 4 hours after initial bolus and every 24 hours thereafter during abciximab therapy as ordered. Expect platelet function to return to normal within 48 hours of conclusion of therapy.
- Monitor vital signs and continuous ECG tracings during therapy.
- Store drug at 2° to 8° C (36° to 46° F). Protect from freezing.

PATIENT TEACHING

- Teach patient about possible adverse reactions associated with abciximab, including bleeding and hypersensitivity reactions, such as rash, urticaria, and dyspnea.
- Tell patient to prevent injury from falls by maintaining bed rest and from bleeding by keeping limb immobile while catheter sheath is in place.

acetazolamide sodium
acetazolamide

Acetazolam (CAN), Ak-Zol, Apo-Acetazolamide (CAN), Dazamide, Diamox, Diamox Sequels, Storzolamide

Class and Category

Chemical: Sulfonamide derivative
Therapeutic: Anticonvulsant, antiglaucoma agent, diuretic
Pregnancy category: C

Indications and Dosages

▶ *As short-term therapy to treat secondary glaucoma and preoperatively to treat acute congestive (angle-closure) glaucoma*

I.V. INJECTION, TABLETS

Adults. 250 mg I.V. or P.O. b.i.d. or every 4 hr; or 500 mg I.V. or P.O. initially, followed by 125 to 250 mg every 4 hr for severe acute glaucoma. To initially lower intraocular pressure rapidly, 500 mg I.V.; may repeat in 2 to 4 hr in acute cases, depending on patient response. Oral therapy usually starts after initial I.V. dose.

S.R. CAPSULES

Adults. 1 S.R. capsule (500 mg) b.i.d.

I.V. INJECTION

Children. 5 to 10 mg/kg/dose every 6 hr.

S.R. CAPSULES, TABLETS
Children. 10 to 15 mg/kg daily in divided doses every 6 to 8 hr.
▶ *To treat chronic simple (open-angle) glaucoma*
I.V. INJECTION, E.R. CAPSULES, TABLETS
Adults. 250 to 1,000 mg daily (in divided doses for dosages above 250 mg).
▶ *To induce diuresis in heart failure*
I.V. INJECTION, TABLETS
Adults. *Initial:* 250 to 375 mg or 5 mg/kg daily in morning.
Maintenance: 250 to 375 mg or 5 mg/kg on alternate days or for 2 days, followed by a drug-free day.
▶ *To treat drug-induced edema*
I.V. INJECTION, TABLETS
Adults. 250 to 375 mg daily for 1 to 2 days.
I.V. INJECTION, TABLETS
Children. 5 mg/kg/dose daily in morning.
▶ *To treat seizures, including generalized tonic-clonic, absence, and mixed seizures, and myoclonic jerk patterns*
I.V. INJECTION, TABLETS
Adults and children. 8 to 30 mg/kg daily in divided doses. *Optimal:* 375 to 1,000 mg daily; when used with other anticonvulsants, 250 mg daily.

Route	Onset	Peak	Duration
I.V.*	2 min	15 min	4 to 5 hr

Mechanism of Action

Inhibits the enyzme carbonic anhydrase, which normally appears in the eyes' ciliary processes, brain's choroid plexes, and kidneys' proximal tubule cells. In the eyes, enzyme inhibition decreases aqueous humor secretion, which lowers intraocular pressure. In the brain, inhibition may delay abnormal, intermittent, and excessive discharge from neurons that cause seizures. In the kidneys, it increases bicarbonate excretion, which carries out water, potassium, and sodium, thus inducing diuresis and metabolic acidosis. This acidosis counteracts respiratory alkalosis.

Contraindications

Chronic noncongestive angle-closure glaucoma; cirrhosis; hyperchloremic acidosis; hypersensitivity to acetazolamide; hypokale-

---

* Effects on intraocular pressure.

mia; hyponatremia; severe pulmonary obstruction; severe renal, hepatic, or adrenocortical impairment

Interactions
DRUGS

amphetamines, methenamine, phenobarbital, procainamide, quinidine: Decreased excretion and possibly toxicity of these drugs
corticosteroids: Increased risk of hypokalemia
cyclosporine: Increased blood cyclosporine level, possibly nephrotoxicity or neurotoxicity
diflunisal: Possibly significantly decreased intraocular pressure
lithium: Increased excretion and decreased effectiveness of lithium
primidone: Decreased blood and urine primidone levels
salicylates: Increased risk of salicylate toxicity

Adverse Reactions
CNS: Ataxia, confusion, depression, disorientation, dizziness, drowsiness, fatigue, fever, flaccid paralysis, headache, lassitude, malaise, nervousness, paresthesia, seizures, tremor, weakness
EENT: Altered taste, tinnitus, transient myopia
GI: Anorexia, constipation, diarrhea, hepatic dysfunction, melena, nausea, vomiting
GU: Crystalluria, decreased libido, glycosuria, hematuria, impotence, nephrotoxicity, phosphaturia, polyuria, renal calculi, renal colic, urinary frequency
HEME: Agranulocytosis, hemolytic anemia, leukopenia, pancytopenia, thrombocytopenia, thrombocytopenic purpura
SKIN: Photosensitivity, pruritus, rash, Stevens-Johnson syndrome, urticaria
Other: Acidosis, hyperuricemia, hypokalemia, weight loss

Nursing Considerations
- Be aware that I.V. acetazolamide may be used if patient cannot take oral drugs. I.M. injection is painful.
- Be aware that acetazolamide may increase the risk of hepatic encephalopathy in patients with hepatic cirrhosis.
- Reconstitute each 500-mg vial with at least 5 ml sterile water for injection. Use within 24 hours; drug has no preservative.
- Monitor blood test results during acetazolamide therapy to detect electrolyte imbalances.
- Monitor blood and urine glucose levels in patients with diabetes mellitus because acetazolamide may lead to elevated levels.
- Monitor patients with a history of calcium-containing calculi for drug-induced calculi.

- Monitor patients with gout or respiratory impairment for exacerbation of these conditions.
- Monitor fluid intake and output every 8 hours and body weight daily to detect excessive fluid and weight loss.

PATIENT TEACHING
- Instruct patient to take acetazolamide exactly as prescribed. Tell him to take a missed dose as soon as he remembers but not to take a double dose.
- Inform patient that tablets may be crushed and suspended in chocolate or other sweet syrup. Or, one tablet may be dissolved in 10 ml of hot water and added to 10 ml of honey or syrup.
- Advise patient to avoid potentially hazardous activities if dizziness or drowsiness occurs.
- Urge patient who takes high doses of salicylates to notify prescriber immediately if signs of salicylate toxicity, such as anorexia, tachypnea, and lethargy, occur.

acetylcysteine
Mucomyst, Mucosil

Class and Category
Chemical: N-acetyl derivative of cysteine
Therapeutic: Antidote (for acetaminophen overdose), mucolytic
Pregnancy category: B

Indications and Dosages
▶ *To treat acetaminophen overdose*
I.V. INFUSION
Adults and children. 300 mg/kg over 21 hr as follows: 150 mg/kg in 200 ml 5% dextrose over 60 min; followed by 50 mg/kg in 500 ml 5% dextrose over 4 hr; followed by 100 mg/kg in 1,000 ml 5% dextrose over 16 hr.
DOSAGE ADJUSTMENT Total volume adjusted individually for patients weighing less than 40 kg (88 lb) and for those who need fluid restriction.

Incompatibilities
Don't give acetylcysteine with nebulization equipment if drug may contact iron, copper, or rubber. Don't give drug with amphotericin B, ampicillin sodium, chlortetracycline, chymotrypsin, erythromycin, hydrogen peroxide, iodized oil, oxytetracycline, tetracycline, or trypsin.

Mechanism of Action
Decreases viscosity of pulmonary secretions by breaking disulfide links that bind glycoproteins in mucus. Reduces liver damage from acetaminophen overdose. Usually, acetaminophen's toxic metabolites bind with glutathione in the liver, which detoxifies them. When acetaminophen overdose depletes glutathione stores, toxic metabolites bind with protein in liver cells, killing them. Acetylcysteine maintains or restores levels of glutathione or acts as its substitute, which reduces liver damage from acetaminophen overdose.

Contraindications
Hypersensitivity to acetylcysteine; no contraindications when used as antidote

Interactions
DRUGS
activated charcoal: Possibly adsorption and decreased effectiveness of acetylcysteine
nitroglycerin: Increased effects of nitroglycerin and possibly significant hypotension and headache

Adverse Reactions
CNS: Chills, dizziness, drowsiness, fever, headache
CV: Hypertension, hypotension, tachycardia
EENT: Rhinorrhea, stomatitis, tooth damage
GI: Anorexia, constipation, hepatotoxicity, nausea, vomiting
RESP: Bronchospasm, chest tightness, hemoptysis
SKIN: Clammy skin, pruritus, rash, urticaria
Other: Angioedema

Nursing Considerations
• Be aware that acetylcysteine should be used cautiously in patients with asthma or a history of bronchospasm because drug may adversely affect respiratory function.
• To avoid fluid overload and possibly fatal hyponatremia or seizures, adjust total volume, as ordered, for patients who weigh less than 40 kg and for those who need fluid restriction.
• If needed, dilute 20% instillation or inhalation solution with normal saline solution or sterile water. The 10% solution may be used undiluted.
• To treat acetaminophen overdose, dilute 20% oral solution with cola or other soft drink to a concentration of 5%, and use within 1 hour. Acetylcysteine is most effective if given within

24 hours of acetaminophen ingestion. For specific supportive treatment of acetaminophen overdose, contact a regional poison center at 1-800-222-1222, or call a special hotline offering assistance to health professionals at 1-800-525-6115.

• If patient vomits loading dose or any maintenance dose within 1 hour of administration, repeat dose as prescribed.

• Keep in mind that a suicidal patient may not provide reliable information about vomiting. Watch such a patient to ensure that he receives all of prescribed dose.

• During treatment for acetaminophen overdose, monitor patient for signs of hepatotoxicity, such as prolonged bleeding time, altered coagulation, and easy bruising.

• Be aware that acetylcysteine may have a disagreeable odor, which disappears as treatment progresses.

• Because nebulization causes sticky residue on face and in mouth, have patient wash his face and rinse his mouth at the end of each treatment.

• Be aware that an open vial of solution may turn light purple; this change doesn't alter effectiveness.

• Refrigerate opened vials, and discard them after 96 hours.

• Assess type, frequency, and characteristics of patient's cough. Particularly note sputum. If cough doesn't clear secretions, prepare to perform mechanical suctioning.

• Monitor patient for tachycardia.

PATIENT TEACHING

• Instruct patient to notify prescriber immediately about nausea, rash, or vomiting.

• Warn patient about acetylcysteine's unpleasant smell; reassure him that it subsides as treatment progresses.

• To decrease mucus viscosity, encourage patient to consume 2 to 3 L of fluid daily unless contraindicated by another condition.

acyclovir sodium

Zovirax

Class and Category

Chemical: Synthetic purine nucleoside analogue
Therapeutic: Antiviral
Pregnancy category: B

Indications and Dosages

▶ *To treat an initial episode of severe genital herpes infection*

I.V. INFUSION

Adults and children age 12 and over. 5 mg/kg every 8 hr for 5 days. *Maximum:* 20 mg/kg every 8 hr.

Infants and children up to age 12. 250 mg/m^2 every 8 hr for 5 days. *Maximum:* 20 mg/kg every 8 hr.

▶ *To treat mucocutaneous herpes simplex (HSV-1 and HSV-2) infections in immunocompromised patients*

I.V. INFUSION

Adults and children age 12 and over. 5 mg/kg every 8 hr for 7 days. *Maximum:* 20 mg/kg every 8 hr.

Infants and children up to age 12. 10 mg/kg every 8 hr for 7 days. *Maximum:* 20 mg/kg every 8 hr.

▶ *To treat herpes simplex encephalitis*

I.V. INFUSION

Adults and children age 12 and over. 10 mg/kg every 8 hr for 10 days. *Maximum:* 20 mg/kg every 8 hr.

Children ages 3 months to 12 years. 20 mg/kg every 8 hr for 10 days. *Maximum:* 20 mg/kg every 8 hr.

▶ *To treat herpes zoster caused by varicella zoster virus in immuno-compromised patients*

I.V. INFUSION

Adults and children age 12 and over. 10 mg/kg every 8 hr for 7 days. *Maximum:* 20 mg/kg every 8 hr.

Children up to age 12. 20 mg/kg every 8 hr for 7 days. *Maximum:* 20 mg/kg every 8 hr.

▶ *To treat neonatal herpes simplex infections*

I.V. INFUSION

Infants up to age 3 months. 10 mg/kg every 8 hr for 10 days. *Maximum:* 20 mg/kg every 8 hr.

DOSAGE ADJUSTMENT Dosing interval increased to every 12 hr if patient's creatinine clearance is 25 to 50 ml/min/1.73 m^2 or to every 24 hr if creatinine clearance is 10 to 25 ml/min/1.73 m^2. Dosage reduced by 50% and dosing interval increased to every 24 hr if patient's creatinine clearance is 10 ml/min/1.73 m^2 or less. Hemodialysis patients require an extra dose after each hemodialysis session. Dosage for obese patients should be based on ideal body weight.

Incompatibilities

Don't mix acyclovir sodium with biological or colloidal solutions, such as blood products or protein-containing solutions. Don't mix with parabens because a precipitate may form.

Mechanism of Action
Prevents viral DNA replication of herpes simplex types 1 and 2 and varicella zoster virus. Infected cells selectively take up acyclovir, which is ultimately converted by virus-induced enzyme thymidine kinase to acyclovir triphosphate. Acyclovir triphosphate stops replication of viral DNA by incorporation into and termination of the growing DNA chain, and by inhibition and inactivation of the viral DNA polymerase, an enzyme used in the viral DNA replication process.

Contraindications
Hypersensitivity to acyclovir or valacyclovir

Interactions
DRUGS
nephrotoxic drugs (such as aminoglycosides, penicillin, tacrolimus): Increased risk of nephrotoxicity
probenecid: Increased and prolonged blood acyclovir level
zidovudine: Increased lethargy and fatigue

Adverse Reactions
CNS: Agitation, coma, confusion, delirium, dizziness, fever, hallucinations, light-headedness, obtundation, psychosis, seizures, somnolence, tiredness, tremor, weakness
GI: Anorexia, diarrhea, elevated liver function test results, nausea, thirst, vomiting
GU: Elevated BUN and serum creatinine levels, hematuria, renal failure
HEME: Anemia, leukocytosis, leukopenia, neutropenia, neutrophilia, thrombotic thrombocytic purpura or hemolytic-uremic syndrome, thrombocytopenia, thrombocytosis
SKIN: Pruritus, rash, urticaria
Other: Injection site edema, pain, or redness

Nursing Considerations
- For initial drug reconstitution, add 10 or 20 ml of sterile water for injection to each 500-mg or 1-g vial of acyclovir, respectively, to yield a concentration of 50 mg/ml. Shake well. Don't mix with bacteriostatic water for injection containing parabens to avoid precipitation.
- **WARNING** Don't mix acyclovir with bacteriostatic water for injection containing benzyl alcohol because neonates and immature infants may develop a fatal toxic syndrome character-

ized by CNS, respiratory, circulatory, and renal impairment and metabolic acidosis.

- Use reconstituted acyclovir within 12 hours when stored at room temperature of 15° to 25° C (59° to 77° F). If a precipitate forms during refrigeration, allow reconstituted acyclovir to warm to room temperature to dissolve the precipitate.
- Further dilute reconstituted acyclovir with 60 to 150 ml of standard electrolyte or dextrose solution to a concentration of 7 mg/ml or less. Concentrations greater than 10 mg/ml may produce phlebitis or inflammation at injection site if extravasation occurs.
- Use final solution within 24 hours when stored at 15° to 25° C.
- Obtain baseline BUN and serum creatinine levels before and during therapy, as ordered.
- **WARNING** Give acyclovir at a constant rate over at least 1 hour. Be aware that rapid delivery may cause renal tubular damage and acute renal failure.
- Expect to hydrate patient during acyclovir administration to avoid precipitation of drug in renal tubules; maximum urinary concentrations are reached within 2 hours.
- Monitor patient's BUN and serum creatinine levels, and assess input and output of patients who are dehydrated, are using other nephrotoxic drugs, or have preexisting impaired renal function because acyclovir increases the risk of nephrotoxicity. Be aware that drug may precipitate in renal tubules if maximum solubility of free acyclovir (2.5 mg/ml at 37° C in water) is exceeded.
- Evaluate for altered LOC, confusion, and psychosis in patients with neurologic abnormalities or a prior neurologic reaction to cytotoxic drugs and in immunocompromised and elderly patients because of potential for neuropsychiatric toxicity.
- Be aware that immunocompromised patients receiving acyclovir may be at risk for thrombotic thrombocytopenic purpura/hemolytic-uremic syndrome. Monitor such patients for signs and symptoms, including petechiae, fever, confusion, hematuria, and acute renal failure.
- Be aware that acyclovir therapy may need to be prolonged in an immunocompromised patient because lesions take longer to heal.
- Notify prescriber if patient doesn't improve within a few days of beginning acyclovir therapy.
- Before reconstituting drug, store it at 15° to 25° C (59° to 77° F).

PATIENT TEACHING
• Inform patient that acyclovir won't prevent transmission of herpes simplex virus to sexual partners or cure the condition but that condom use may help prevent transmission. Instruct patient to avoid sexual activity if he or his partner has signs or symptoms of genital herpes. In addition, explain that he may be contagious even before the first sign of a herpetic lesion appears.
• To decrease irritation to genital area, encourage patient to wear loose-fitting clothes during acyclovir therapy and to keep this area clean and dry.

adenosine
Adenocard, Adenoscan

Class and Category
Chemical: Monophosphorylated adenine riboside
Therapeutic: Antiarrhythmic
Pregnancy category: C

Indications and Dosages
▶ *To convert paroxysmal supraventricular tachycardia (PSVT) to normal sinus rhythm*
I.V. INJECTION
Adults and children weighing 50 kg (110 lb) or more. *Initial:* 6 mg by rapid peripheral I.V. bolus over 1 to 2 sec. If PSVT continues after 1 to 2 min, 12 mg given as rapid bolus and repeated in 1 to 2 min if needed.
WARNING Don't give single doses of more than 12 mg.
Children weighing less than 50 kg. *Initial:* 0.05 to 0.1 mg/kg as rapid central or peripheral I.V. bolus followed by saline flush. If PSVT continues after 1 to 2 min, additional bolus injections are given, incrementally increasing dose by 0.05 to 0.1 mg/kg. Follow each bolus with saline flush. Injections continue until PSVT converts to normal sinus rhythm or until patient reaches maximum single dose of 0.3 mg/kg.

Route	Onset	Peak	Duration
I.V.	Immediate	Immediate	Unknown

Incompatibilities
Don't mix adenosine with other drugs.

Mechanism of Action

Slows conduction time through the AV node and can interrupt reentry pathways through the AV node to restore normal sinus rhythm.

Contraindications

Atrial fibrillation or flutter; hypersensitivity to adenosine; second- or third-degree heart block or sick sinus syndrome, except in patients with a functioning artificial pacemaker; ventricular tachycardia

Interactions

DRUGS

carbamazepine: Increased heart block
digoxin, verapamil: Possibly increased depressant effect on SA or AV node
dipyridamole: Increased effects of adenosine
methylxanthines, such as theophylline: Antagonized effects of adenosine

FOODS

caffeine: Antagonized effects of adenosine

Adverse Reactions

CNS: Apprehension, dizziness, headache, heaviness in arms, light-headedness, nervousness, paresthesia, seizures
CV: Atrial fibrillation, bradycardia, chest pain or pressure, heart block, hypertension, hypotension, MI, palpitations, prolonged asystole, sinus exit block or pause, torsades de pointes, transient hypertension, ventricular fibrillation, ventricular tachycardia
EENT: Blurred vision, metallic taste, throat tightness
GI: Nausea, vomiting
MS: Jaw, neck, and back pain
RESP: Bronchoconstriction, bronchospasm, dyspnea, hyperventilation, respiratory arrest
SKIN: Diaphoresis, facial flushing
Other: Injection site reaction

Nursing Considerations

- Before use, inspect adenosine for crystals. If solution isn't clear, don't give it.
- Give adenosine by rapid I.V. bolus over 1 to 2 seconds. Slower administration can cause systemic vasodilation and reflex tachycardia.

- Expect prescriber to inject adenosine directly into a vein, if appropriate, to ensure that it reaches systemic circulation. If administered into an I.V. line, give as close to insertion site as possible and follow with rapid saline flush.
- Monitor heart rate and rhythm, blood pressure, and respiratory status frequently during adenosine therapy.
- Be aware that at the time of conversion to normal sinus rhythm, arrhythmias (such as PVCs, premature atrial contractions, sinus bradycardia, sinus tachycardia, and AV block) may occur for a few seconds but don't require intervention.
- **WARNING** Discontinue use and notify prescriber immediately if severe respiratory difficulties develop.
- Store adenosine at room temperature. Discard unused portion.

PATIENT TEACHING

- Instruct patient to report chest pain, palpitations, difficulty breathing, or severe headache during adenosine therapy.
- Warn patient that he may temporarily experience mild reactions, such as flushing, nausea, and dizziness.

alatrofloxacin mesylate
Trovan I.V.
trovafloxacin mesylate
Trovan

Class and Category
Chemical: Fluoroquinolone
Therapeutic: Antibacterial
Pregnancy category: C

Indications and Dosages
▶ *To treat life-threatening nosocomial pneumonia*
I.V. INFUSION, TABLETS
Adults. 300 mg I.V. every 24 hr, followed by 200 mg P.O. every 24 hr when patient is stabilized, for 10 to 14 days.
▶ *To treat life-threatening community-acquired pneumonia*
I.V. INFUSION, TABLETS
Adults. 200 mg I.V. every 24 hr, followed by 200 mg P.O. every 24 hr when patient is stabilized, for 7 to 14 days; or 200 mg P.O. every 24 hr for 7 to 14 days.
▶ *To treat complicated, life-threatening intra-abdominal infections, including postsurgical, gynecologic, and pelvic infections*

I.V. INFUSION, TABLETS
Adults. 300 mg I.V. every 24 hr, followed by 200 mg P.O. every 24 hr when patient is stabilized, for 7 to 14 days.
▶ *To treat complicated, life- or limb-threatening skin and soft-tissue infections, including diabetic foot infections*
I.V. INFUSION, TABLETS
Adults. 200 mg I.V. every 24 hr, followed by 200 mg P.O. every 24 hr when patient is stabilized, for 10 to 14 days; or 200 mg P.O. every 24 hr for 10 to 14 days.
DOSAGE ADJUSTMENT For patients with mild to moderate cirrhosis, 300-mg dosage reduced to 200 mg and 200-mg dosage reduced to 100 mg.

Mechanism of Action

Interferes with DNA gyrase, the enzyme necessary for DNA replication in aerobic and anaerobic bacteria. May be active against pathogens that are resistant to such antibiotics as penicillins, cephalosporins, aminoglycosides, macrolides, and tetracyclines.

Incompatibilities

Don't mix alatrofloxacin with or infuse it simultaneously through the same I.V. line as other drugs or any solutions containing multivalent cations, such as magnesium. Don't dilute alatrofloxacin with normal saline solution or lactated Ringer's solution.

Contraindications

Hypersensitivity to alatrofloxacin, quinolone antibiotics, trovafloxacin, or their components

Interactions
DRUGS
aluminum-, citric acid–, magnesium-, or sodium citrate–containing antacids; iron; morphine sulfate; sucralfate: Decreased absorption of oral trovafloxacin

Adverse Reactions
CNS: Dizziness, headache, light-headedness, seizures
CV: Hypotension
EENT: Hoarseness, throat tightness
GI: Abdominal pain, acute hepatic failure (evidenced by anorexia, dark urine, dysphagia, fatigue, jaundice, pale stools, and vomiting)

GU: Vaginitis
RESP: Dyspnea
SKIN: Erythema, photosensitivity, pruritus, rash, urticaria
Other: Angioedema, infusion site pain

Nursing Considerations

- Using aseptic technique, withdraw appropriate amount of ala-trofloxacin concentrate from vial and dilute further with appro-priate I.V. solution to a final concentration of 1 to 2 mg/ml. Compatible I.V. solutions are D₅W, 0.45 normal saline, D₅/0.45 normal saline, D₅/0.2 normal saline, and D₅/lactated Ringer's solutions.
- If you're using the same I.V. line to administer other drugs se-quentially, flush line with a compatible solution before and af-ter administering alatrofloxacin. Though it can't be used to di-lute alatrofloxacin, normal saline solution can be used to flush I.V. line.
- Refrigerate diluted solution up to 7 days or store at room tem-perature for 3 days in glass bottles or polyvinyl chloride I.V. containers.
- **WARNING** Infuse alatrofloxacin over 60 minutes; rapid or bolus I.V. injection may cause hypotension.
- Periodically assess patient's liver function test results. Results may be elevated for up to 21 days after alatrofloxacin adminis-tration.
- **WARNING** Be aware that alatrofloxacin may cause severe liver damage, which may lead to death or need for liver transplantation. Expect alatrofloxacin therapy to last no longer than 2 weeks because more prolonged therapy in-creases the risk of liver damage. Alatrofloxacin is reserved for hospitalized patients who have life- or limb-threatening in-fections.
- Protect vial from light before use. Store at room temperature; don't freeze.

PATIENT TEACHING
- Instruct patient to report rash; urticaria; trouble swallowing; swelling of lips, face, or tongue; hoarseness; throat tightness; abdominal pain; or nausea and vomiting.
- Advise patient to avoid potentially hazardous activities if he ex-periences dizziness or lightheadedness.
- Instruct patient to avoid exposure to direct sunlight and ultra-violet light (such as tanning beds).

alefacept
Amevive

Class and Category
Chemical: Recombinant leukocyte function–related antigen-3 immunoglobulin GI fusion protein
Therapeutic: Immunosuppresant
Pregnancy category: B

Indications and Dosages
▶ *To treat moderate to severe chronic plaque psoriasis in patients who are candidates for systemic therapy or phototherapy*
I.V. INJECTION
Adults. *Initial:* 7.5 mg every wk for 12 wk. After at least 12 wk in which drug isn't given, a second 12-wk course may be given, if needed and if patient's CD4 and T-lymphocyte counts are within normal ranges.

Mechanism of Action
Binds to the lymphocyte antigen and CD2 and inhibits LFA-3/CD2 interaction to interfere with T-lymphocyte activation. Alefacept also reduces the subsets of CD2+ T lymphocytes. Because activation of T lymphocytes plays a role in the pathophysiology of chronic plaque psoriasis, interference with lymphocytic activity helps to prevent plaque formation.

Incompatibilities
Don't add other drugs to solutions containing alefacept.

Contraindications
Breast-feeding, hypersensitivity to alefacept or its components

Interactions
DRUGS
None reported.

Adverse Reactions
CNS: Chills, dizziness, headache
CV: Coronary artery disease, MI
EENT: Pharyngitis
GI: Nausea
HEME: Lymphopenia
MS: Myalgia
RESP: Increased cough

SKIN: Pruritus, urticaria
Other: Angioedema, injection site pain or inflammation, infection, malignancies

Nursing Considerations

- Use alefacept cautiously in patients at high risk for cancer because this drug increases the risk. Know that alefacept isn't recommended for use in patients with a history of a systemic malignancy.
- Also use cautiously in patients with chronic infection or a history of recurrent infections. Drug may increase risk of infection because of its immunosuppressive action.
- Obtain a CD4+ and T-cell count before starting drug therapy, as ordered. If counts are below normal, expect to delay therapy. After therapy starts, monitor patient's CD4+ and T-cell counts weekly throughout therapy. If levels drop below 250 cells/mm^3, notify prescriber because drug will need to be withheld. If counts remain below 250 cells/mm^3 for 1 month, therapy should be stopped.
- Reconstitute drug with 0.6 ml of the supplied diluent (sterile water for injection) before administration. With the needle pointed at the side wall of the vial, slowly inject the diluent into the alefacept vial. Expect some foaming. To prevent excessive foaming, don't shake or vigorously agitate vial. Instead, swirl vial gently during dissolution, which usually takes less than 2 minutes.
- Give drug as soon as possible after reconstitution. Discard solution if not used within 4 hours.
- Don't filter reconstituted solution during preparation or administration.
- For I.V. use, prepare two syringes containing 3 ml normal saline solution to be used for flushing before and after giving drug. Then prime the winged infusion set with 3 ml normal saline solution and insert into vein. Attach the filled syringe to the infusion set and administer solution over no more than 5 seconds. Finish by flushing the set with 3 ml normal saline solution.
- Be aware that alefacept shouldn't be started in a patient with a serious infection. Monitor patient closely during and after therapy for signs and symptoms of infection. If these occur, report them to the prescriber immediately and start treatment, as prescribed, to reduce the risk of serious infection. If infection becomes serious, expect drug to be discontinued.
- Monitor patient for allergic reactions. If these occur, stop drug

and notify prescriber immediately.

PATIENT TEACHING
• Advise patient that weekly blood tests will be needed to monitor his WBC during alefacept therapy.
• Teach patient the signs and symptoms of infection and common warning signs of malignancy. Emphasize the need to comply with follow-up visits and promptly report to prescriber any unusual or sudden evidence of malignancy or infection.
• Inform female patient to notify prescriber if she becomes pregnant during alefacept therapy or 8 weeks afterward.

alglucerase
Ceredase

Class and Category
Chemical: Glucocerebrosidase beta-glucosidase
Therapeutic: Enzyme replacement
Pregnancy category: C

Indications and Dosages
▶ *To treat chronic nonneuropathic Gaucher's disease in patients with moderate to severe anemia, thrombocytopenia with bleeding tendencies, bone disease, or significant hepatomegaly or splenomegaly*
I.V. INFUSION
Adults and children age 2 and over. Highly individualized. 2.5 units/kg up to 60 units/kg infused over 1 to 2 hr, usually every 2 wk.
DOSAGE ADJUSTMENT Highly individualized dosage based on body size and disease severity. Some patients may need infusion once every other day; others may need it once every 4 wk. Maintenance dosage progressively reduced every 3 to 6 mo to as low as 1 units/kg.

Route	Onset	Peak	Duration
I.V.	Up to 60 min	Unknown	Variable

Mechanism of Action
Catalyzes hydrolysis of glucocerebroside to glucose and ceramide in membrane lipids. Gaucher's disease results from deficiency of the enzyme beta-glucocerebrosidase and causes the lipid glucocerebroside to accumulate in tissue macrophages.

Contraindications
Hypersensitivity to alglucerase

Adverse Reactions
CNS: Chills, dizziness, fatigue, fever, headache
CV: Transient peripheral edema, vasomotor irritability
EENT: Oral ulcerations
GI: Abdominal discomfort, diarrhea, nausea, vomiting
MS: Backache
Other: I.V. site burning, itching, or swelling

Nursing Considerations
- If patient is hypersensitive to alglucerase, expect to give antihistamines before starting alglucerase therapy.
- On day of dose, use aseptic technique to dilute alglucerase with normal saline solution to final volume of no more than 200 ml.
- Don't shake drug; doing so could inactivate it.
- Don't use alglucerase if it's discolored or contains precipitate.
- Be aware that drug doesn't contain preservatives. Discard unused portion.
- Infuse alglucerase with in-line I.V. particle filter.

PATIENT TEACHING
- Tell patient that he may experience flulike symptoms with each dose of alglucerase.
- Instruct patient to report headache, hot flashes, nausea, and other adverse reactions.
- Inform patient that alglucerase is derived from pooled human placental tissue and poses a slight risk of viral contamination.
- Advise patient to keep appointments for scheduled doses of alglucerase.

allopurinol sodium
Aloprim

Class and Category
Chemical: Hypoxanthine derivative, xanthine oxidase inhibitor
Therapeutic: Antihyperuricemic
Pregnancy category: C

Indications and Dosages
▶ *To treat increased serum and urine uric acid levels in patients with leukemia, lymphoma, and solid tumors when chemotherapy has increased those levels and patient can't tolerate oral therapy*

I.V. INFUSION

Adults. 200 to 400 mg/m^2 every day as a single infusion or in equal divided infusions every 6, 8, or 12 hr. *Maximum:* 600 mg every day.

Children. 200 mg/m^2 every day as a single infusion or in equally divided infusions every 6, 8, or 12 hr.

DOSAGE ADJUSTMENT Dosage adjusted to 200 mg daily if creatinine clearance is 10 to 20 ml/min/1.73 m^2, to 100 mg daily if creatinine clearance is 3 to 10 ml/min/1.73 m^2, or to 100 mg every other day if creatinine clearance falls below 3 ml/min/1.73 m^2.

Mechanism of Action

Inhibits uric acid production by inhibiting xanthine oxidase, the enzyme responsible for converting hypoxanthine and xanthine to uric acid. Allopurinol is metabolized to oxipurinol, which also inhibits xanthine oxidase.

Incompatibilities

Don't combine allopurinol in solution with amikacin, amphotericin B, carmustine, cefotaxime sodium, chlorpromazine hydrochloride, cimetidine hydrochloride, clindamycin phosphate, cytarabine, dacarbazine, daunorubicin hydrochloride, diphenhydramine hydrochloride, doxorubicin hydrochloride, doxycycline hyclate, droperidol, floxuridine, gentamicin sulfate, haloperidol lactate, hydroxyzine hydrochloride, idarubicin hydrochloride, imipenem and cilastatin sodium, mechlorethamine hydrochloride, meperidine hydrochloride, methylprednisolone sodium succinate, metoclopramide hydrochloride, minocycline hydrochloride, nalbuphine hydrochloride, netilmicin sulfate, ondansetron hydrochloride, prochlorperazine edisylate, promethazine hydrochloride, sodium bicarbonate, streptozocin, tobramycin sulfate, vinorelbine tartrate.

Contraindications

Hypersensitivity to allopurinol

Interactions

DRUGS

ACE inhibitors: Increased risk of hypersensitivity reactions
amoxicillin, ampicillin: Increased risk of rash
azathioprine, mercaptopurine: Inactivation of these drugs

chlorpropamide: Increased risk of hypoglycemia in patients with renal insufficiency

cyclophosphamide, other cytotoxic drugs: Enhanced bone marrow suppression

dicumarol: Increased half-life and anticoagulant action of dicumarol

thiazide diuretics: Possibly increased risk of allopurinol toxicity

uricosuric drugs: Increased urinary excretion of uric acid

vitamin C (large doses): Possibly urine acidification and increased risk of renal calculus formation

Adverse Reactions

CNS: Chills, coma, drowsiness, fever, headache, mental status changes, neuritis, paresthesia, peripheral neuropathy, seizures, somnolence

CV: Arrhythmias, cardiopulmonary arrest, hypertension, hypotension, vasculitis

EENT: Epistaxis, loss of taste

GI: Abdominal pain, diarrhea, elevated liver function test results, GI bleeding, granulomatous hepatitis, hepatic necrosis, hepatomegaly, intestinal obstruction, nausea, vomiting

GU: Exacerbation of renal calculi, hematuria, renal failure, UTI

HEME: Anemia, bone marrow depression, eosinophilia, leukocytosis, leukopenia, neutropenia, thrombocytopenia

MS: Arthralgia, exacerbation of gout, myopathy

SKIN: Alopecia; ecchymosis; jaundice; maculopapular, scaly, or exfoliative rash (sometimes fatal); pruritus; urticaria

Other: Septic shock

Nursing Considerations

- As ordered, obtain and review results of baseline CBC, uric acid levels, and renal and hepatic function studies before starting allopurinol therapy. Continue to monitor test results during therapy.
- Reconstitute and dilute to 6 mg/ml or less. To reconstitute, add 25 ml sterile water for injection to 30-ml vial of allopurinol powder. Dilute to desired concentration with normal saline solution or D$_5$W.
- Don't use if solution is discolored or contains particles.
- Store prepared solution at 20° to 25° C (68° to 77° F); don't refrigerate. Administer within 10 hours of reconstitution.
- Expect allopurinol therapy to begin 24 to 48 hours before start of chemotherapy.

- **WARNING** Discontinue allopurinol and notify prescriber immediately at first sign of a hypersensitivity reaction, such as a rash, which may precede more severe reactions.
- To decrease the risk of calculus formation, maintain fluid intake of up to 3 L daily and monitor patient for output of 2 L daily. Also, don't give patient vitamin C.

PATIENT TEACHING
- Instruct patient receiving allopurinol to drink at least 10 large glasses of water daily.
- Advise patient to report unusual bleeding or bruising, fever, chills, gout attack, numbness, and tingling.
- Inform patient that acute gout attacks may occur more frequently early in allopurinol treatment and that results may not be noticeable for 2 weeks or longer.
- Instruct patient not to drive or perform potentially hazardous tasks if allopurinol causes drowsiness.

alpha₁-proteinase inhibitor (human)
Prolastin, Zemaira

Class and Category
Chemical: Plasma protein
Therapeutic: Enzyme replacement
Pregnancy category: C

Indications and Dosages
▶ *To treat congenital alpha₁-antitrypsin deficiency in patients with signs of panacinar emphysema (Prolastin); to augment and maintain patients with emphysema who are deficient in alpha₁-proteinase inhibitor*

I.V. INFUSION
Adults. 60 mg/kg infused over 30 min for Prolastin and 15 min for Zemaira at a rate of at least 0.08 ml/kg/min once weekly.

Mechanism of Action
Replaces the enzyme alpha₁-antitrypsin, which normally inhibits the proteolytic enzyme elastase in patients with alpha₁-antitrypsin deficiency. Without alpha₁-proteinase inhibitor, elastase attacks and destroys alveolar membranes and causes emphysema.

Contraindications
Hypersensitivity to alpha₁-proteinase inhibitor, its components, or

other alpha₁-proteinase products; selective immunoglobulin A (IgA) deficiency in patients with anti-IgA antibodies

Interactions
ACTIVITIES

smoking: Inactivation of alpha₁-proteinase inhibitor

Adverse Reactions
CNS: Asthenia, dizziness, fever, headache, paresthesia
EENT: Sinusitis
HEME: Mild, transient leukocytosis
RESP: Exacerbation of existing COPD, upper respiratory tract infection
SKIN: Pruritus
Other: Flulike symptoms, infusion site pain

Nursing Considerations
- Use alpha₁-proteinase inhibitor cautiously in patients at risk for circulatory overload because drug is a colloid solution that increases plasma volume.
- Before reconstituting, remove alpha₁-proteinase inhibitor and diluent from refrigerator and let it warm to room temperature.
- To reconstitute, remove caps from vials and cleanse rubber stoppers with antiseptic solution. After stoppers are dry, remove protective cover from diluent end of transfer device and insert into center of upright diluent vial. Then remove protective cover from drug end of transfer device, invert the diluent vial with attached transfer device, and, using minimal force, insert drug end of transfer device into center of rubber stopper of upright drug vial. Make sure flange of transfer device rests on stopper surface so that diluent flows into drug vial.
- During diluent transfer, wet lyophilized cake completely by gently tilting the drug vial. Don't allow air inlet filter to face downward. (Take care not to lose the vacuum because this will prolong reconstitution.) Once diluent transfer is complete, pull transfer device along with attached diluent vial out of drug vial and discard. Gently swirl drug vial until powder is completely dissolved. Avoid shaking because doing so may cause drug to foam and degrade.
- If you need more than one vial of alpha₁-proteinase inhibitor, use aseptic technique to transfer reconstituted solution from each vial into a sterile I.V. administration container.
- Within 3 hours of reconstitution, administer at room temperature as an I.V. infusion using the large-volume 5-micron conical

filter provided. Place filter between distal end of I.V. administration set and infusion set, and infuse at 0.08 ml/kg/min or as determined by patient response and comfort. Expect the infusion to take about 15 minutes per vial.

- **WARNING** Alpha₁-proteinase inhibitor is made from human plasma and may contain infectious agents, such as viruses. Ensure that patient is immunized against hepatitis B before giving drug. If time doesn't allow for antibody formation, give a single dose of hepatitis B immune globulin with hepatitis B vaccine, as prescribed.
- Monitor patient for delayed fever, which may occur up to 12 hours after therapy. Fever usually resolves within 24 hours.

PATIENT TEACHING

- Tell patient to immediately report early evidence of an allergic reaction, such as chest tightness, difficult breathing, faintness, hives, wheezing, and any other unusual symptoms.
- Advise patient to notify prescriber if signs or symptoms of viral infection (chills, drowsiness, fever, and runny nose, followed 2 weeks later by joint pain and a rash) occur after receiving drug.
- Stress the importance of receiving weekly doses to maintain an adequate antielastase barrier in the lungs. Explain that treatment must continue for life.
- Warn patient not to smoke.

alteplase, recombinant
(tissue plasminogen activator, recombinant)
Activase, Activase rt-PA (CAN)

Class and Category
Chemical: Purified glycoprotein
Therapeutic: Thrombolytic
Pregnancy category: C

Indications and Dosages
▶ *To treat acute MI*
ACCELERATED I.V. INFUSION
Adults weighing more than 67 kg (148 lb). 15-mg bolus, followed by 50 mg infused over next 30 min and then by 35 mg infused over next 60 min.
Adults weighing 67 kg or less. 15-mg bolus, followed by 0.75 mg/kg (up to 50 mg) infused over next 30 min and then

0.5 mg/kg (up to 35 mg) infused over next 60 min.

I.V. INFUSION

Adults weighing more than 65 kg (143 lb). 100 mg infused over 3 hr as follows: 6 to 10 mg by bolus over first 1 to 2 min, 50 to 54 mg over remainder of first hr, 20 mg over second hr, and 20 mg over third hr.

Adults weighing 65 kg or less. 1.25 mg/kg infused over 3 hr on similar administration schedule for those weighing more than 65 kg.

▶ *To treat acute ischemic CVA*

I.V. INFUSION

Adults. 0.9 mg/kg infused over 60 min, with 10% of total dose given as bolus over first min. *Maximum:* 90 mg.

WARNING To avoid acute bleeding complications, expect to treat patient for acute ischemic CVA within 3 hr after onset of CVA symptoms and only after computed tomography or other diagnostic imaging method rules out intracranial hemorrhage.

▶ *To treat pulmonary embolism*

I.V. INFUSION

Adults. 100 mg infused over 2 hr.

Route	Onset	Peak	Duration
I.V.	Immediate	20 to 120 min	4 hr

Mechanism of Action

Binds to fibrin in a thrombus and converts trapped plasminogen to plasmin. Plasmin breaks down fibrin, fibrinogen, and other clotting factors, which dissolves the thrombus.

Incompatibilities

Don't add other drugs to solution that contains alteplase or infuse other drugs through same I.V. line.

Contraindications

For all indications: Active internal bleeding, arteriovenous malformation or aneurysm, bleeding diathesis, intracranial neoplasm, severe uncontrolled hypertension

For acute MI and pulmonary embolism only: History of CVA, intracranial or intraspinal surgery or trauma in past 2 months

For acute ischemic CVA only: Recent head trauma, recent intracranial surgery, recent previous CVA, seizure activity at onset of

CVA, subarachnoid hemorrhage, suspicion or history of intracranial hemorrhage

Interactions

DRUGS

drugs that alter platelet function (such as abciximab, acetylsalicylic acid, and dipyridamole), heparin, vitamin K antagonists: Increased risk of bleeding

Adverse Reactions

CNS: Cerebral edema, cerebral herniation, CVA, fever, seizures
CV: Arrhythmias (including bradycardia and electromechanical dissociation), cardiac arrest, cardiac tamponade, cardiogenic shock, cholesterol embolism, coronary thrombolysis, heart failure, hypotension, mitral insufficiency, myocardial reinfarction or rupture, pericardial effusion, pericarditis, venous thrombosis and embolism
EENT: Epistaxis, gingival bleeding, laryngeal edema
GI: GI bleeding, nausea, retroperitoneal bleeding, vomiting
GU: GU bleeding
RESP: Pleural effusion, pulmonary edema, pulmonary reembolization
SKIN: Bleeding at puncture sites, ecchymosis, rash, urticaria
Other: Anaphylaxis

Nursing Considerations

- If possible, obtain appropriate coagulation tests, such as PT, APTT, platelet count, and fibrin-fibrinogen degradation product titer, as ordered, before initiating alteplase therapy. Monitor coagulation test results during and after therapy.
- Immediately before using alteplase, reconstitute it only with sterile water for injection provided by manufacturer. Swirl gently to dissolve powder; don't shake.
- Be aware that 50-mg vials have a vacuum and should not be used if vacuum isn't present.
- Use a large-bore (18G) needle when reconstituting 50-mg vial and the transfer device provided when reconstituting 100-mg vial to direct the flow of sterile water for injection.
- When using transfer device, hold vial of alteplase upside down while pushing down onto transfer device connected to sterile water for injection. Then invert the vials to allow the sterile water for injection to flow into the alteplase.
- Store reconstituted solution at 2° to 30° C (36° to 86° F). Use reconstituted solution within 8 hours or discard.

- Use normal saline solution or D$_5$W immediately before drug administration if further dilution to a concentration of 0.5 mg/ml is desired. Mix by gently swirling or slowly inverting polyvinyl chloride bag or glass vial.
- Monitor for bleeding, especially at arterial puncture sites.
- Monitor blood pressure and heart rate and rhythm frequently during and after alteplase therapy.
- **WARNING** Alteplase therapy may cause arrhythmias from sudden reperfusion of the myocardium. Monitor continuous ECG for arrhythmias during drug therapy.
- Minimize bleeding from noncompressible sites by avoiding internal jugular and subclavian venous puncture sites. Avoid I.M. injection.
- Use a small-gauge (23G or smaller) needle for venipunctures. Use a distal arm vessel for venipunctures and for arterial punctures if needed. Apply pressure for 30 minutes after an arterial puncture, then apply a pressure dressing. Evaluate site frequently for signs of bleeding.
- Discontinue alteplase infusion immediately if serious bleeding occurs.
- After administering alteplase, apply pressure for at least 30 minutes and then apply a pressure dressing.
- Protect alteplase from excessive exposure to light.

PATIENT TEACHING
- Instruct patient beginning alteplase therapy to immediately report bleeding, including bleeding from the nose or gums.
- Advise patient to limit physical activity during alteplase administration to reduce the risk of injury and bleeding.

amikacin sulfate
Amikin

Class and Category
Chemical: Aminoglycoside
Therapeutic: Antibiotic
Pregnancy category: D

Indications and Dosages
▶ *To treat serious gram-negative bacterial infections (including septicemia; neonatal sepsis; respiratory tract, bone, joint, CNS, skin, soft-tissue, intra-abdominal, burn, and postoperative infections; and serious, complicated, and recurrent UTI) caused by* Acinetobacter, Entero-

bacter, Escherichia coli, Klebsiella, Proteus, Providencia, Pseudomonas, *and* Serratia; *and staphylococcal infections when penicillin is contraindicated*

I.V. INFUSION

Adults and children. 15 mg/kg daily in equal doses at equally spaced intervals (7.5 mg/kg every 12 hr or 5 mg/kg every 8 hr) for 7 to 10 days. *Maximum:* 1,500 mg daily.

Neonates. *Loading dose:* 10 mg/kg. *Maintenance:* 7.5 mg/kg every 12 hr for 7 to 10 days.

DOSAGE ADJUSTMENT For patients with impaired renal function, loading dose of 7.5 mg/kg daily, followed by maintenance dosage based on creatinine clearance and serum creatinine level and given every 12 hr. For morbidly obese patients, dosage not to exceed 1.5 g daily.

▶ *To treat uncomplicated UTI*

I.V. INFUSION

Adults. 250 mg b.i.d. for 7 to 10 days.

Route	Onset	Peak	Duration
I.V.	Immediate	Unknown	Unknown

Mechanism of Action

Binds to negatively charged sites on bacteria's outer cell membrane, disrupting cell integrity. Amikacin also binds to bacterial ribosomal subunits and inhibits protein synthesis. Both actions lead to cell death.

Incompatibilities

Don't mix or infuse amikacin with other drugs.

Contraindications

Hypersensitivity to amikacin or other aminoglycosides

Interactions

DRUGS

cephalosporins, enflurane, methoxyflurane, vancomycin: Increased nephrotoxic effects

general anesthetics: Increased risk of neuromuscular blockade

loop diuretics: Increased risk of *ototoxicity*

neuromuscular blockers: Possibly increased neuromuscular blockade and prolonged respiratory depression

penicillins: Possibly inactivation of or synergistic effects with amikacin

Adverse Reactions

CNS: Drowsiness, headache, loss of balance, neuromuscular blockade, tremor, vertigo
EENT: Hearing loss, ototoxicity, tinnitus
GI: Nausea, vomiting
GU: Azotemia, dysuria, nephrotoxicity, oliguria or polyuria, proteinuria
MS: Acute muscle paralysis; arthralgia; muscle fatigue, spasms, and weakness
RESP: Apnea
Other: Hyperkalemia

Nursing Considerations

• Expect to obtain results of culture and sensitivity tests before amikacin therapy begins.
• Prepare amikacin by adding contents of 500-mg vial to 100 to 200 ml of sterile diluent, such as normal saline solution or D₅W. Adjust amount of diluent proportionately for pediatric patients. Then infuse drug over 30 to 60 minutes.
• Don't use dark-colored solution. Solution color should range from colorless to light straw or pale yellow.
• Use 0.25- and 5-mg/ml I.V. solutions within 24 hours when stored at room temperature if they've been mixed with D₅W, D₅/normal saline, normal saline, lactated Ringer's, or other solutions noted in manufacturer's insert. These solutions remain potent for 60 days if stored at 4° C (39° F) and for 30 days if frozen at −15° C (5° F).
• Monitor patient for evidence of ototoxicity, such as tinnitus and vertigo, especially during high-dosage or prolonged amikacin therapy.
• **WARNING** Because amikacin may produce nephrotoxic effects, assess renal function before and daily during therapy, as ordered. To minimize renal tubule irritation, maintain patient hydration during therapy.
• Be aware that amikacin may exacerbate muscle weakness in such conditions as myasthenia gravis and Parkinson's disease.
• Measure serum amikacin concentrations as ordered, usually 30 to 90 minutes after injection (for peak concentration) and just before administering the next dose (for trough concentration).
• Be aware that amikacin may be administered by I.M. injection into a large muscle mass at same dosages used for I.V. administration.

PATIENT TEACHING
• Inform patient that daily laboratory tests are necessary during amikacin treatment.
• Instruct patient to report ringing in ears, hearing changes, headache, nausea, vomiting, and changes in urination.

aminocaproic acid
Amicar

Class and Category
Chemical: Aminohexanoic acid
Therapeutic: Antifibrinolytic, antihemorrhagic
Pregnancy category: C

Indications and Dosages
▶ *To treat excessive bleeding caused by fibrinolysis*
I.V. INJECTION
Adults. 4 to 5 g in 250 ml of diluent over 1 hr, followed by continuous infusion of 1 g/hr in 50 ml of diluent. Continue for 8 hr or until bleeding stops.

Route	Onset	Peak	Duration
I.V.	Immediate	Unknown	Under 3 hr

Mechanism of Action
Inhibits the breakdown of blood clots by interfering with plasminogen activator substances and producing antiplasmin activity.

Contraindications
Hypersensitivity to aminocaproic acid; signs of active intravascular clotting, as in disseminated intravascular coagulation; upper urinary tract bleeding

Interactions
DRUGS
activated prothrombin, prothrombin complex concentrates: Increased risk of thrombosis
estrogens, oral contraceptives: Increased risk of hypercoagulation

Adverse Reactions
CNS: CVA, delirium, dizziness, hallucinations, headache, malaise, weakness

CV: Bradycardia, cardiomyopathy, edema, elevated serum CK level, hypotension, ischemia, thrombophlebitis
EENT: Nasal congestion, tinnitus
GI: Abdominal cramps and pain, diarrhea, elevated AST level, nausea, vomiting
GU: Elevated BUN level, intrarenal obstruction, renal failure
HEME: Agranulocytosis, leukopenia, thrombocytopenia
MS: Myopathy, rhabdomyolysis
RESP: Dyspnea, pulmonary embolism
SKIN: Pruritus, rash
Other: Anaphylaxis, elevated serum aldolase level

Nursing Considerations
- Mix aminocaproic acid solution with sterile water for injection, normal saline solution, D₅W, or Ringer's solution.
- **WARNING** Avoid rapid administration because of increased risks of hypotension and bradycardia.
- Monitor neurologic status for drug-induced changes. Note that increased clotting may lead to CVA.
- Be aware that dosage adjustment may be needed for patient with impaired renal function.
- Store between 15° and 30° C (59° and 86° F).

PATIENT TEACHING
- Inform patient that he will be closely monitored during aminocaproic acid therapy and will have blood drawn for laboratory tests before, during, and after treatment.

aminophylline
(theophylline ethylenediamine)

Class and Category
Chemical: Xanthine
Therapeutic: Bronchodilator
Pregnancy category: C

Indications and Dosages
▶ *To relieve acute bronchospasm*
I.V. INFUSION
Adults (nonsmokers) not taking theophylline products. *Initial:* 6 mg/kg (equal to 4.7 mg/kg anhydrous theophylline), not to exceed 25 mg/min. *Maintenance:* 0.7 mg/kg/hr for first 12 hr; then 0.5 mg/kg/hr.
Children ages 9 to 16 not taking theophylline products. *Ini-*

tial: 6 mg/kg (equal to 4.7 mg/kg anhydrous theophylline), not to exceed 25 mg/min. *Maintenance:* 1 mg/kg/hr for first 12 hr; then 0.8 mg/kg/hr.

Children ages 6 months to 9 years and young adult smokers not taking theophylline products. *Initial:* 6 mg/kg (equal to 4.7 mg/kg anhydrous theophylline), not to exceed 25 mg/min. *Maintenance:* 1.2 mg/kg/hr for first 12 hr; then 1 mg/kg/hr.

Adults and children taking theophylline products. *Initial:* If possible, determine the time, amount, administration route, and form of last dose. Loading dose is based on principle that each 0.63 mg/kg (0.5 mg/kg anhydrous theophylline) administered as a loading dose raises serum theophylline level by 1 mcg/ml. Defer loading dose if serum theophylline level can be readily obtained. If this isn't possible and patient has no obvious signs of theophylline toxicity, prescriber may order 3.1 mg/kg (2.5 mg/kg anhydrous theophylline), which may increase serum theophylline level by about 5 mcg/ml. *Maintenance:* For adults (nonsmokers), 0.7 mg/kg/hr for first 12 hr, and then 0.5 mg/kg/hr. For children ages 9 to 16, 1 mg/kg/hr for first 12 hr, and then 0.8 mg/kg/hr. For children ages 6 months to 9 years and young adult smokers, 1.2 mg/kg/hr for first 12 hr, and then 1 mg/kg/hr.

DOSAGE ADJUSTMENT For elderly patients and those with cor pulmonale, dosage reduced to 0.6 mg/kg for 12 hr, then to 0.3 mg/kg. For patients with heart failure and hepatic disease, dosage reduced to 0.5 mg/kg for 12 hr, and then to 0.1 to 0.2 mg/kg.

Route	Onset	Peak	Duration
I.V.	Immediate	Unknown	4 to 8 hr

Mechanism of Action

Inhibits phosphodiesterase enzymes, causing bronchodilation. Normally, these enzymes inactivate cAMP and cGMP, which are responsible for bronchial smooth-muscle relaxation. Other mechanisms of action may include translocation of calcium, prostaglandin antagonism, stimulation of catecholamines, inhibition of cGMP metabolism, and adenosine receptor antagonism.

Incompatibilities

Don't add other drugs to prepared bag or bottle of aminophylline. Don't mix aminophylline in same syringe as doxapram. Avoid administering amiodarone, ciprofloxacin, diltiazem, dobutamine, hydralazine, or ondansetron into the Y port of a continuous infusion of aminophylline.

Contraindications

Active peptic ulcer disease, hypersensitivity to aminophylline, underlying seizure disorder

Interactions

DRUGS

activated charcoal, aminoglutethimide, barbiturates, ketoconazole, rifampin, sulfinpyrazone, sympathomimetics: Decreased blood theophylline level

allopurinol, calcium channel blockers, cimetidine, corticosteroids, disulfiram, ephedrine, influenza virus vaccine, interferon, macrolides, mexiletine, nonselective beta blockers, oral contraceptives, quinolones, thiabendazole: Increased blood theophylline level

benzodiazepines: Antagonized sedative effects of benzodiazepines

beta agonists: Increased effects of aminophylline and beta agonist

carbamazepine, isoniazid, loop diuretics: Increased or decreased blood theophylline level

halothane: Increased risk of cardiotoxicity

hydantoins: Decreased blood hydantoin level

ketamine: Increased risk of seizures

lithium: Decreased blood lithium level

neuromuscular blockers: Reversed neuromuscular blockade

propofol: Antagonized sedative effects of propofol

tetracyclines: Enhanced adverse effects of theophylline

FOODS

high-carbohydrate, low-protein diet: Decreased theophylline elimination and prolonged aminophylline half-life

low-carbohydrate, high-protein diet; charcoal-broiled beef: Increased theophylline elimination and shortened aminophylline half-life

ACTIVITIES

alcohol abuse: Increased effects of aminophylline

smoking (at least 1 pack daily): Decreased effects of aminophylline

Adverse Reactions

CNS: Dizziness, fever, headache, insomnia, irritability, restlessness, seizures

CV: Arrhythmias (including sinus tachycardia and life-threatening ventricular arrhythmias), hypotension, palpitations

ENDO: Hyperglycemia, syndrome of inappropriate ADH secretion

GI: Anorexia, diarrhea, epigastric pain, heavy feeling in stomach, hematemesis, indigestion, nausea, vomiting

GU: Diuresis, proteinuria, urine retention in men with prostate enlargement
MS: Muscle twitching
RESP: Respiratory arrest, tachypnea
SKIN: Alopecia, exfoliative dermatitis, flushing, rash, urticaria

Nursing Considerations
• Dilute aminophylline with D_5W, normal saline solution, or a dextrose and sodium chloride combination.
• **WARNING** Because aminophylline has a narrow therapeutic window (10 to 20 mcg/ml), closely monitor serum theophylline level and observe for signs of toxicity, such as tachycardia, tachypnea, nausea, vomiting, restlessness, and seizures. Keep in mind that acetaminophen, furosemide, phenylbutazone, probenecid, theobromine, coffee, tea, soft drinks, and chocolate can produce an inaccurate serum theophylline level.
• To determine peak serum theophylline level, draw blood sample 15 to 30 minutes after administering I.V. loading dose.
• Store between 15° and 30° C (59° and 86° F). Don't freeze; protect from light.
PATIENT TEACHING
• Advise patient to avoid excessive intake of caffeine (in coffee, tea, soft drinks, and chocolate), which can falsely elevate theophylline level.
• Inform patient that blood tests may be needed to monitor the effects of aminophylline.

amiodarone hydrochloride
Cordarone, Pacerone

Class and Category
Chemical: Iodinated benzofuran derivative
Therapeutic: Class III antiarrhythmic
Pregnancy category: D

Indications and Dosages
▶ *To treat life-threatening, recurrent ventricular fibrillation and hemodynamically unstable ventricular tachycardia when these arrhythmias don't respond to other drugs or when patient can't tolerate other drugs*
I.V. INFUSION
Adults. *Loading:* 150 mg over 10 min (15 mg/min) followed by 360 mg infused over 6 hr (1 mg/min). *Maintenance:* 540 mg in-

fused over 18 hr (0.5 mg/min); then after the first 24 hr, 720 mg infused over 24 hr (0.5 mg/min), continued up to 96 hr or until rhythm is stable. Change to oral form as soon as possible.

Route	Onset	Peak	Duration
I.V.	Hours to 3 days	1 to 3 wk	Weeks to months

Mechanism of Action
Acts on cardiac cell membranes, prolonging repolarization and the refractory period and raising ventricular fibrillation threshold. Drug relaxes vascular smooth muscles, mainly in coronary circulation, and improves myocardial blood flow. It relaxes peripheral vascular smooth muscles, decreasing peripheral vascular resistance and myocardial oxygen consumption.

Incompatibilities
Amiodarone is incompatible with heparin. To prevent precipitation, don't add amiodarone admixed with D_5W to aminophylline 4 mg/ml, cefamandole nafate, cefazolin sodium, or mezlocillin sodium, and don't mix amiodarone 3 mg/ml with sodium bicarbonate.

Contraindications
Bradycardia that causes syncope (unless pacemaker is present), cardiogenic shock, hypersensitivity to amiodarone or its components, hypokalemia, hypomagnesemia, SA node dysfunction, second- and third-degree AV block (unless pacemaker is present)

Interactions
DRUGS
anticoagulants: Increased anticoagulant response, which can result in serious bleeding
azole antifungals, fluoroquinolones, macrolide antibiotics: Increased risk of prolonged QT interval and life-threatening arrhythmias
beta blockers: Increased serum levels of beta blockers with increased risk of AV block, hypotension, and bradycardia
calcium channel blockers: Increased serum levels of these drugs and increased risk of AV block, bradycardia, and hypotension
cholestyramine, phenytoin, rifampin, St. John's wort: Decreased serum amiodarone level
cimetidine: Increased serum amiodarone level
clopidogrel: Possibly decreased inhibition of platelet aggregation
cyclosporine: Increased serum cyclosporine level

dextromethorphan, methotrexate, phenytoin: Increased serum levels of these drugs and increased risk of toxicity if amiodarone is taken orally for more than 2 weeks

digoxin: Increased serum digoxin level and risk of digitalis toxicity

diltiazem, propranolol, verapamil: Increased risk of hemodynamic and electrophysiologic abnormalities

disopyramide: Increased serum disopyramide level with QT-interval prolongation and increased risk of arrhythmias

fentanyl: Increased serum fentanyl level with increased risk of bradycardia, decreased cardiac output, and hypotension

flecainide: Increased serum flecainide level

HMG-CoA reductase inhibitors, such as atorvastatin and simvastatin: Possibly increased risk of myopathy and rhabdomyolysis

hydantoins: Increased serum hydantoin level with long-term use and reduced serum amiodarone level

lidocaine: Increased serum lidocaine level and increased risk of seizures and bradycardia

loratadine, trazodone: Increased risk of QT-interval prolongation and torsades de pointes

potassium- and magnesium-depleting drugs: Increased risk of hypokalemia and hypomagnesemia

procainamide: Increased serum procainamide or N-acetylprocainamide level

quinidine: Increased serum quinidine level with risk of life-threatening arrhythmias

ritonavir: Increased serum amiodarone level with increased risk of cardiotoxicity

theophylline: Increased serum theophylline level; increased risk of theophylline toxicity

warfarin: Increased PT and risk of bleeding

FOODS

grapefruit juice: Increased serum amiodarone level

Adverse Reactions

CNS: Abnormal gait, ataxia, confusion, delirium, disorientation, dizziness, fatigue, fever, hallucinations, headache, insomnia, involuntary motor activity, lack of coordination, malaise, paresthesia, peripheral neuropathy, pseudotumor cerebri, sleep disturbances, tremor

CV: Arrhythmias (including bradycardia, electromechanical dissociation, torsades de pointes, and ventricular tachycardia or fibrillation), cardiac arrest, cardiogenic shock, edema, heart failure, hypotension, vasculitis

EENT: Abnormal salivation, abnormal taste and smell, blurred vision, corneal microdeposits, dry eyes, halo vision, lens opacities, macular degeneration, optic neuritis, optic neuropathy, papilledema, permanent blindness, photophobia, scotoma

ENDO: Hyperthyroidism, hypothyroidism, syndrome of inappropriate antidiuretic hormone secretion, thyroid cancer, thyrotoxicosis

GI: Abdominal pain, anorexia, cirrhosis, constipation, diarrhea, elevated liver function test results, hepatitis, nausea, pancreatitis, vomiting

GU: Acute renal failure, decreased libido, epididymitis, impotence, renal impairment or insufficiency

HEME: Agranulocytosis, aplastic or hemolytic anemia, coagulation abnormalities, neutropenia, pancytopenia, spontaneous bruising, thrombocytopenia

MS: Muscle weakness, myopathy, rhabdomyolysis

RESP: Acute respiratory distress syndrome; bronchospasm; infiltrates that lead to dyspnea, cough, hemoptysis, hypoxia, pulmonary alveolar hemorrhage, pulmonary fibrosis, pulmonary interstitial pneumonitis, crackles, and wheezing; pleuritis; pneumonia; respiratory arrest or failure

SKIN: Alopecia, bluish gray pigmentation, erythema multiforme, exfoliative dermatitis, flushing, photosensitivity, pruritus, rash, skin cancer, Stevens-Johnson syndrome, toxic epidermal necrolysis

Other: Anaphylactic shock, angioedema

Nursing Considerations

- **WARNING** Be aware that I.V. amiodarone may cause or worsen pulmonary disorders that may develop days to weeks after therapy and progress to respiratory failure or even death.
- Monitor vital signs and oxygen levels often during and after giving amiodarone. Keep emergency equipment and drugs nearby.
- **WARNING** Monitor continuous ECG; check for increased PR and QRS intervals, arrhythmias, and heart rate below 60 beats/min because amiodarone toxicity may cause or worsen arrhythmias.
- Monitor serum amiodarone level, which normally ranges from 1.0 to 2.5 mcg/ml.
- Assess liver enzyme and thyroid hormone levels; drug inhibits conversion of T_4 to T_3 and may cause drug-induced hyperthyroidism that may in turn lead to thyrotoxicosis and arrhythmia breakthrough or increased severity of arrhythmia.

PATIENT TEACHING
- Explain that frequent monitoring and laboratory tests will be needed during treatment.
- Advise patient to report swollen hands and feet, wheezing, dyspnea, cough, nausea, vomiting, dark urine, fatigue, yellow skin or sclerae, stomach pain, light-headedness, fainting, or a rapid, slow, pounding, or irregular heartbeat.
- Instruct patient to report abnormal bleeding or bruising.

ammonium chloride

Class and Category
Chemical: Ammonium ion
Therapeutic: Acidifier
Pregnancy category: C

Indications and Dosages
▶ *To treat hypochloremia and metabolic alkalosis*
I.V. INFUSION
Adults. Individualized based on serum bicarbonate level. *Usual:* 100 to 200 mEq added to 500 or 1,000 ml of normal saline solution, infused at 5 ml/min or less (about 3 hr for an infusion of 1,000 ml).

Route	Onset	Peak	Duration
I.V.	1 to 3 min	3 to 6 hr	Unknown

Mechanism of Action
Is converted to urea and hydrochloric acid in the liver. During conversion, the drug is dissociated into ammonium and chloride ions, and hydrogen ions are released. These ions enter into the blood and extracellular fluid, where hydrogen reacts with bicarbonate ions to form water and carbon dioxide. This process decreases bicarbonate ions and increases chloride ions in the blood and extracellular fluid, which decreases blood and urine pH and corrects alkalosis.

Incompatibilities
Don't mix ammonium chloride with alkalies and their carbonates, codeine, lead or silver salts, levorphanol, methadone, or strong oxidizing agents such as potassium chlorate.

Contraindications
Hypersensitivity to ammonium chloride or its components,

markedly impaired renal or hepatic function, metabolic alkalosis caused by vomiting of hydrochloric acid and accompanied by sodium loss caused by sodium bicarbonate excretion in urine

Interactions

DRUGS

amphetamines, salicylates, sulfonylureas, tricyclic antidepressants: Decreased therapeutic blood ammonium level

chlorpropamide: Increased effects of ammonium

Adverse Reactions

CNS: Fever, headache

CV: Phlebitis or thrombosis extending from injection site

GI: Indigestion, nausea, severe hepatic dysfunction, vomiting

RESP: Hyperventilation

SKIN: Extravasation

Other: Injection site infection, irritation, or pain; hypovolemia; severe metabolic acidosis (with large doses)

Nursing Considerations

- Before using ammonium chloride solution, warm it to room temperature by placing infusion in warm water to dissolve crystals.
- During I.V. administration, keep sodium bicarbonate or sodium lactate nearby to treat overdose.
- Infuse ammonium chloride slowly to avoid I.V. site pain and irritation.
- **WARNING** Watch for evidence of ammonia toxicity, including arrhythmias, such as bradycardia; coma; irregular breathing; pallor; retching; seizures; diaphoresis; and twitching.
- Monitor for signs of metabolic acidosis, such as increased respirations, increased serum pH, restlessness, and diaphoresis.
- Monitor serum bicarbonate level and results of urinalysis and renal and liver function tests as appropriate.
- Store drug below 40° C (104° F). Don't freeze.

PATIENT TEACHING

- Tell patient who's taking ammonium chloride to consume more potassium-rich foods, such as bananas, oranges, cantaloupe, spinach, dried fruit, and potatoes.

amobarbital sodium

Amytal

Class, Category, and Schedule

Chemical: Barbiturate

Therapeutic: Anticonvulsant, sedative-hypnotic
Pregnancy category: D
Controlled substance schedule: II

Indications and Dosages

▶ *To produce sedation*
I.V. INJECTION
Adults. 30 to 50 mg b.i.d. or t.i.d. and may range from 15 to 120 mg b.i.d or t.i.d. *Maximum:* 1,000 mg/dose.
Children over age 6. 65 to 500 mg/dose for preoperative sedation.

▶ *To induce a hypnotic state*
I.V. INJECTION
Adults. 65 to 200 mg/dose. *Maximum:* 1,000 mg/dose.
Children age 6 and over. 65 to 500 mg/dose.

▶ *To manage seizures*
I.V. INJECTION
Adults. *Usual:* 65 to 500 mg up to a maximum of 1,000 mg. Dosage for acute seizures determined by patient's response. Doses of 200 to 500 mg are typically required to control seizures.
Children age 6 and over. 65 to 500 mg.
Children up to age 6. 3 to 5 mg/kg/dose.

WARNING Use I.V. route only when other routes aren't appropriate. Inject slowly—at a rate of 50 mg/min or less—to prevent sudden respiratory depression, apnea, laryngospasm, or hypotension.

Route	Onset	Peak	Duration
I.V.	Unknown	Unknown	10 to 12 hr

Mechanism of Action

Nonselectively acts on the CNS to depress the sensory cortex, decrease motor activity, alter cerebellar function, and produce drowsiness, sedation, and hypnosis. Appears to reduce wakefulness and alertness by acting in the thalamus, where it depresses the reticular activating system and interferes with impulse transmission from the periphery to the cortex. Produces CNS depressant effects ranging from mild sedation and anxiety reduction to anesthesia and coma.

Incompatibilities

Don't mix amobarbital in solution with other drugs.

Contraindications

Alcoholism, history of porphyria, history of sedative or barbiturate addiction, hypersensitivity to barbiturates, renal or hepatic disease, severe respiratory disease, sleep apnea, suicidal tendency, uncontrolled pain

Interactions

DRUGS

acetaminophen: Increased blood acetaminophen level and risk of hepatotoxicity

antihistamines, CNS depressants, phenothiazines, tranquilizers: Increased CNS depression

beta blockers, carbamazepine, clonazepam, corticosteroids, digitoxin, doxycycline, estrogens, griseofulvin, metronidazole, oral anticoagulants, oral contraceptives, phenylbutazones, quinidine, theophyllines, tricyclic antidepressants: Decreased blood levels and effects of these drugs

chloramphenicol: Inhibited amobarbital metabolism; enhanced chloramphenicol metabolism

MAO inhibitors: Increased blood level and sedative effects of amobarbital

methoxyflurane: Increased nephrotoxicity

phenytoin: Altered effects of phenytoin

rifampin: Decreased blood level and effects of amobarbital

valproic acid: Increased amobarbital effects

ACTIVITIES

alcohol use: Increased blood level of amobarbital and additive CNS depressant effects

Adverse Reactions

CNS: Agitation, anxiety, ataxia, CNS depression, confusion, dizziness, hallucinations, hangover, headache, hyperkinesia, insomnia, nightmares, nervousness, paradoxical stimulation, psychiatric disturbance, somnolence, syncope, vertigo

CV: Bradycardia, hypotension, shock

EENT: Laryngospasm

GI: Constipation, diarrhea, epigastric pain, nausea, vomiting

RESP: Apnea, bronchospasm, hypoventilation, respiratory depression

SKIN: Exfoliative dermatitis, rash, Stevens-Johnson syndrome, urticaria

Other: Angioedema, gangrene of arm or leg from accidental injection into artery, injection site tissue damage and necrosis, physical and psychological dependence, potentially fatal withdrawal syndrome, tolerance

Nursing Considerations

- Be aware that amobarbital shouldn't be given during third trimester of pregnancy because repeated use can cause dependence in neonate. It also shouldn't be given to breast-feeding women because it may cause CNS depression in infants.
- Prepare amobarbital using sterile water for injection.
- Closely monitor blood pressure, pulse, and respirations during administration. Keep emergency equipment and drugs nearby in case respiratory depression or adverse hemodynamic effects occur. Be aware that patients with cardiovascular disease are at increased risk for adverse circulatory reactions, particularly when drug is administered too fast, and that those with pulmonary diseases associated with obstruction or dyspnea are at increased risk for ventilatory depression. Anticipate the risk of hypotension, even when giving drug at recommended rate.
- Monitor for hypersensitivity reactions, such as bronchospasm, difficulty breathing, facial edema, and urticaria, especially in patients with a history of asthma, angioedema, or urticaria.
- **WARNING** Don't administer solution after 30 minutes of exposure to air. Solution quickly becomes unstable because amobarbital sodium hydrolyzes in solution.
- **WARNING** To prevent tissue damage and necrosis at peripheral insertion sites, monitor closely for signs of extravasation. Be aware that accidental arterial injection may cause gangrene of arm or leg.
- Anticipate that amobarbital's CNS effects may exacerbate major depression, suicidal tendencies, or other mental disorders.
- Closely monitor debilitated or elderly patients, as appropriate, because they're more likely to experience such adverse CNS reactions as confusion, depression, and excitement. Take safety precautions.
- Be aware that amobarbital may cause paradoxical stimulation (excitement, euphoria, restlessness) in patients with acute pain and in children.
- Evaluate for signs of intensified or prolonged hypnotic effect in patients with shock or uremia.
- Assess hyperthyroid patients for exacerbated symptoms, such as increased nervousness and palpitations, due to amobarbital use.
- Be aware that barbituate-induced respiratory depression may cause complications in patients with severe anemia.
- Be aware that drug may trigger signs and symptoms in patients with acute intermittent porphyria.

- To prevent withdrawal symptoms, such as diaphoresis, insomnia, irritability, nightmares, and tremors, expect to taper amobarbital dosage gradually after long-term use, especially for epileptic patients.

PATIENT TEACHING
- Instruct patient to report severe dizziness, persistent drowsiness, rash, or skin lesions during amobarbital therapy.

amphotericin B
Amphocin, Fungizone Intravenous
amphotericin B cholesteryl sulfate complex
Amphotec
amphotericin B lipid complex
Abelcet
amphotericin B liposomal complex
AmBisome

Class and Category
Chemical: Amphoteric polyene macrolide
Therapeutic: Antifungal
Pregnancy category: B

Indications and Dosages
▶ *To treat severe fungal infections, using amphotericin B*
I.V. INFUSION
Adults and adolescents. *Initial:* 1-mg test dose in 20 ml of D_5W infused over 20 to 30 min; if test dose is tolerated, administer 0.25 to 0.3 mg/kg daily prepared as a 0.1-mg/ml infusion and given over 2 to 6 hr. Increased in 5- to 10-mg increments up to 50 mg daily, based on patient tolerance and infection severity, not to exceed a total daily dose of 1.5 mg/kg. *Maximum:* 50 mg daily infused over 2 to 6 hr.
Children. *Initial:* 0.25 mg/kg daily in D_5W infused over 6 hr; then increased in 0.125- to 0.25-mg/kg increments daily or every other day as tolerated. *Maximum:* 1 mg/kg or 30 mg/m^2 of body surface daily.
▶ *To treat aspergillosis, using amphotericin B cholesteryl sulfate complex*
I.V. INFUSION
Adults and children. Test dose of 1.6 to 8.3 mg in 10 ml of D_5W infused over 15 to 30 min; if test dose is tolerated, then 3 to 4 mg/kg once daily infused at 1 mg/kg/hr.

▶ *To treat invasive amphotericin B–resistant fungal infections, using amphotericin B lipid complex*

I.V. INFUSION

Adults and children. 5 mg/kg daily infused at 2.5 mg/kg/hr.

▶ *To treat severe aspergillosis, candidiasis, or cryptococcosis, using amphotericin B liposomal complex*

I.V. INFUSION

Adults and children. 3 to 5 mg/kg daily infused over 2 hr. Infusion time may be decreased to 1 hr if tolerated, or increased if patient experiences discomfort.

▶ *To treat leishmaniasis, using amphotericin B liposomal complex*

I.V. INFUSION

Immunocompetent adults and children. 3 mg/kg daily infused over 2 hr on days 1 through 5 and on days 14 and 21. Infusion time may be decreased to 1 hr if tolerated, or increased if patient experiences discomfort.

Immunocompromised adults and children. 4 mg/kg daily infused over 2 hr on days 1 through 5 and on days 10, 17, 24, 31, and 38. Infusion time may be decreased to 1 hr if tolerated, or increased if patient experiences discomfort.

▶ *To treat presumed fungal infections in patients with febrile neutropenia, using amphotericin B lipid complex*

I.V. INFUSION

Adults and children. 3 mg/kg daily infused over 2 hr. Infusion time may be decreased to 1 hr if tolerated, or increased if patient experiences discomfort.

Route	Onset	Peak	Duration
I.V.	Immediate	Unknown	Unknown

Mechanism of Action

Binds to sterols in fungal cell plasma membranes, which changes membrane permeability and allows loss of potassium and small molecules from cells. This action results in cell impairment or death.

Incompatibilities

Don't reconstitute amphotericin B with diluents other than those recommended because solutions containing sodium chloride or bacteriostatic agents (such as benzyl alcohol) may cause drug precipitation.

Contraindications

Hypersensitivity to amphotericin B or its components

Interactions

DRUGS

antineoplastics: Increased risk of bronchospasm, hypotension, and nephrotoxicity

corticosteroids, corticotropin: Increased risk of hypokalemia and subsequent cardiac dysfunction

cyclosporine, nephrotoxic drugs: Increased risk of nephrotoxicity

digitalis glycosides: Possibly hypokalemia and more severe digitalis toxicity

flucytosine: Possibly increased flucytosine toxicity

leukocyte transfusion: Possibly dyspnea, hypoxemia, and pulmonary infiltrates

skeletal muscle relaxants: Possibly hypokalemia and subsequent increased muscle relaxation

zidovudine: Possibly myelotoxicity and nephrotoxicity

Adverse Reactions

CNS: Chills, fever, headache, tiredness, weakness

CV: Chest pain, hypotension, irregular heartbeat

EENT: Pharyngitis

GI: Abdominal pain, anorexia, diarrhea, dysphagia, hepatic failure, indigestion, nausea, vomiting

GU: Decreased or increased urine output, impaired renal function

HEME: Anemia, leukopenia, thrombocytopenia, unusual bleeding or bruising

MS: Arthralgia, muscle spasms, myalgia

RESP: Apnea, dyspnea, hypoxia, pulmonary edema, tachypnea

SKIN: Flushing, jaundice, maculopapular rash, pruritus and redness especially around ears, urticaria

Other: Anaphylaxis, hypocalcemia, hypokalemia, hypomagnesemia, infusion site pain and thrombophlebitis

Nursing Considerations

- To prepare amphotericin B, add 10 ml of sterile water for injection (without a bacteriostatic agent) to vial containing 50 mg of amphotericin B. For I.V. infusion, dilute the solution containing 5 mg/ml to 0.1 mg/ml by adding 1 ml (5 mg) of solution to 49 ml of D$_5$W with a pH above 4.2.
- Before using D$_5$W to dilute amphotericin B solution, aseptically determine injection's pH. If pH is below 4.2, follow manufacturer's instructions for buffering it.

- Because reconstituted amphotericin B is a colloidal suspension, avoid using an in-line membrane filter or use one with a mean pore diameter of more than 1 micron to prevent significant drug removal.

- To prepare amphotericin B cholesteryl sulfate complex, reconstitute it with sterile water for injection. Using a sterile syringe and a 20G needle, rapidly add 10 or 20 ml of sterile water for injection to a 50- or 100-mg vial, respectively, to obtain a solution containing 5 mg of amphotericin B per milliliter. Then shake gently by hand, rotating vial until all solids are dissolved. The fluid may be clear or opalescent. For infusion, further dilute reconstituted solution to about 0.6 mg/ml. Don't filter the solution. Flush existing line with D_5W or use a separate line. Don't use an in-line filter.

- To prepare amphotericin B lipid complex, shake vial gently until you see no yellow sediment. Using an 18G needle, withdraw prescribed dose from required number of vials into one or more 20-ml syringes. Replace needle with 5-micron filter needle that's supplied with each vial. Empty syringe contents into bag of D_5W so that final concentration is 1 mg/ml. Expect to use a concentration of 2 mg/ml for pediatric patients and patients with cardiovascular disease. Before infusion, shake bag until contents are mixed thoroughly. Flush existing line with D_5W or use a separate line. Don't use an in-line filter. If infusion exceeds 2 hours, shake infusion bag every 2 hours.

- To prepare amphotericin B liposomal complex, add 12 ml sterile water for injection (without a bacteriostatic agent) to each 50-mg vial to achieve a concentration of 4 mg amphotericin B per milliliter. Immediately shake vial vigorously for at least 30 seconds until all particles completely disperse. Withdraw prescribed dose of amphotericin B liposomal complex suspension. Then use a 5-micron filter to inject it into D_5W to provide a final concentration of 1 to 2 mg/ml. Expect to use a lower concentration (0.2 to 0.5 mg/ml) for infants and young children. Flush existing line with D_5W or use a separate line. You may use an in-line filter with a mean pore diameter of at least 1 micron.

- To help minimize fever and shaking chills, expect to administer an antipyretic, an antihistamine, meperidine, or a corticosteroid just before infusing amphotericin B.

- Assess I.V. insertion site regularly to detect extravasation of amphotericin B, which may cause severe local irritation. To minimize local thrombophlebitis, plan to add heparin to infusion or to administer amphotericin on alternate days, which also may help prevent anorexia. Alternate-day dose shouldn't exceed 1.5 mg/kg.

• Monitor renal function closely because of risk of renal impairment. Plan to assess serum creatinine level every other day while amphotericin B dosage is increasing and then at least twice weekly during continued therapy. If serum creatinine or BUN level increases significantly, expect to discontinue amphotericin B until renal function improves. Be aware that a cumulative dose of more than 4 g may cause irreversible renal dysfunction.

• Expect to monitor CBC and platelet count weekly throughout therapy to detect adverse hematologic effects. Also monitor serum calcium, magnesium, and potassium levels twice weekly throughout therapy to detect abnormalities.

• Before drug reconstitution, store amphotericin B at 2° to 8° C (36° to 46° F), and protect from light. Use reconstituted amphotericin B within 24 hours if stored at room temperature or within 1 week if refrigerated. Use immediately if solution was reconstituted and diluted in D_5W.

• Before drug reconstitution, store amphotericin B cholesteryl sulfate complex at 15° to 30° C (59° to 86° F) unless otherwise specified. After reconstitution, store at 2° to 8° C (36° to 46° F). Use reconstituted amphotericin B cholesteryl sulfate complex within 24 hours.

• Before drug dilution, store amphotericin B lipid complex at 2° to 8° C, and protect from light. Use amphotericin B lipid complex within 6 hours if stored at room temperature or within 48 hours if stored at 2° to 8° C. Don't freeze.

• Before drug reconstitution, store amphotericin B liposomal complex at 2° to 8° C. Use reconstituted amphotericin B liposomal complex within 24 hours if stored at 2° to 8° C. Begin infusion of diluted drug within 6 hours. Don't freeze.

PATIENT TEACHING

• Instruct patient to report pain or discomfort at I.V. insertion site of amphotericin.

• Advise patient to report adverse reactions immediately, especially shortness of breath, chest pain, or wheezing.

ampicillin sodium
Ampicin (CAN), Omnipen-N, Polycillin-N, Totacillin-N

Class and Category
Chemical: Semisynthetic aminopenicillin
Therapeutic: Antibiotic
Pregnancy category: B

Indications and Dosages
▶ *To treat GI and GU infections (other than gonorrhea) caused by susceptible strains of* Shigella, Salmonella typhi *and other species,* Escherichia coli, Proteus mirabilis, *and enterococci*
I.V. INFUSION
Adults and children weighing 20 kg (44 lb) or more.
500 mg P.O. every 6 hr or 250 to 500 mg I.V. every 6 hr.
Children weighing less than 20 kg. 50 to 100 mg/kg daily in divided doses P.O. every 6 hr or 12.5 mg/kg I.V. every 6 hr.
▶ *To treat gonorrhea caused by susceptible strains of non–penicillinase-producing* Neisseria gonorrhoeaea
I.V. INFUSION
Adults and children weighing 45 kg (99 lb) or more. 500 mg every 6 hr.
Children weighing less than 40 kg (88 lb). 50 mg/kg daily in divided doses every 6 to 8 hr.
▶ *To treat respiratory tract infections caused by susceptible strains of non–penicillinase-producing* Haemophilus influenzae, *staphylococci, and streptococci, including* Streptococcus pneumoniae
I.V. INFUSION
Adults and children weighing 40 kg or more. 250 to 500 mg I.V. every 6 to 8 hr.
Children weighing less than 40 kg. 25 to 50 mg/kg daily I.V. in divided doses every 6 to 8 hr.
Children weighing less than 20 kg. 12.5 mg/kg I.V. every 6 hr.
▶ *To treat septicemia*
I.V. INFUSION
Adults. 8 to 14 g I.V. daily in divided doses every 3 to 4 hr for at least 3 days; then I.M.
Children. 150 to 200 mg/kg daily I.V. in divided doses every 3 to 4 hr for at least 3 days; then I.M.
▶ *To prevent bacterial endocarditis from dental, oral, or upper respiratory tract procedures*
I.V. INFUSION
Adults. 2 g within 30 min of procedure.
Children. 50 mg/kg within 30 min of procedure.

▶ *To treat bacterial meningitis caused by susceptible strains of* Neisseria meningitidis
I.V. INFUSION
Adults. 8 to 14 g daily or 150 to 200 mg/kg daily I.V. in equally divided doses every 3 to 4 hr for at least 3 days; then I.M. at same dosage and schedule.
Children. 100 to 200 mg/kg daily I.V. in equally divided doses every 3 to 4 hr for at least 3 days; then I.M. at same dosage and schedule.
▶ *To treat listeriosis*
I.V. INFUSION
Adults and children weighing 20 kg or more. 50 mg/kg every 6 hr.
Children weighing less than 20 kg. 12.5 mg/kg every 6 hr.

Route	Onset	Peak	Duration
I.V.	Immediate	Unknown	Unknown

Mechanism of Action
Inhibits bacterial cell wall synthesis. The rigid, cross-linked cell wall is assembled in several steps. Ampicillin exerts its effects on susceptible bacteria in the final stage of the cross-linking process by binding with and inactivating penicillin-binding proteins (enzymes responsible for linking the cell wall strands). This action causes bacterial cell lysis and death.

Incompatibilities
Don't mix ampicillin and any aminoglycoside in the same I.V. bag, bottle, or tubing; otherwise, both drugs will be inactivated. If patient must receive both drugs, administer them in separate sites at least 1 hour apart.

Contraindications
Hypersensitivity to any penicillin, infection caused by penicillinase-producing organism

Interactions
DRUGS
allopurinol: Increased risk of rash, particularly with hyperuricemia
aminoglycosides: Possibly inactivated action of aminoglycoside and ampicillin when given together
heparin, oral anticoagulants: Increased risk of bleeding

oral contraceptives: Possibly reduced contraceptive effectiveness and breakthrough bleeding

probenecid: Possibly increased serum ampicillin level and ampicillin toxicity

tetracyclines: Possibly impaired action of ampicillin

Adverse Reactions

CNS: Chills, fatigue, fever, headache, malaise

CV: Chest pain, edema, thrombophlebitis

EENT: Epistaxis, glossitis, laryngeal stridor, mucocutaneous candidiasis, stomatitis, throat tightness

GI: Abdominal distention, diarrhea, enterocolitis, flatulence, gastritis, nausea, pseudomembranous colitis, vomiting

GU: Dysuria, urine retention, vaginal candidiasis

HEME: Agranulocytosis, anemia, eosinophilia, leukopenia, thrombocytopenia, thrombocytopenic purpura

SKIN: Erythema multiforme; erythematous, mildly pruritic maculopapular rash or other types of rash; exfoliative dermatitis; pruritus; urticaria

Other: Anaphylaxis, facial edema, injection site pain

Nursing Considerations

• Avoid giving ampicillin to patients with mononucleosis because of increased risk of rash.

• Expect to give ampicillin for 48 to 72 hours after patient becomes asymptomatic. For streptococcal infection, expect to give ampicillin for at least 10 days after cultures show streptococcal eradication to reduce risk of rheumatic fever or glomerulonephritis.

• To dilute ampicillin for intermittent infusion, add 5 ml of sterile water or bacteriostatic water for injection to each 125-, 250-, or 500-mg vial or 7.4 to 10 ml of diluent to each 1- or 2-g vial. Infuse in suitable diluent at less than 30 mg/ml.

• **WARNING** Infuse I.V. solution for 3 to 5 minutes for each 125 or 500 mg or 10 to 15 minutes for each 1 or 2 g. More rapid infusion may cause seizures.

• Monitor patient closely for anaphylaxis, which may be life-threatening. Patients at greatest risk are those with a history of multiple allergies, hypersensitivity to cephalosporins, or a history of asthma, hay fever, or urticaria.

• Notify prescriber if patient has evidence of superinfection; expect to stop drug and provide appropriate treatment.

• **WARNING** In an anaphylactic reaction, stop drug, notify pre-

scriber immediately, and provide immediate treatment with epinephrine, airway management, oxygen, and I.V. corticosteroids, as needed.
• If long-term or high-dose ampicillin therapy is required, closely monitor results of renal and liver function tests and CBCs.
PATIENT TEACHING
• Review signs of allergic reaction; if they occur, tell patient to contact prescriber immediately.

ampicillin sodium and sulbactam sodium

Unasyn

Class and Category

Chemical: Aminopenicillin, beta-lactamase inhibitor
Therapeutic: Broad-spectrum antibiotic
Pregnancy category: B

Indications and Dosages

▶ *To treat skin and soft-tissue infections caused by beta-lactamase–producing strains of* Staphylococcus aureus, Escherichia coli, Klebsiella *species (including* K. pneumoniae*),* Proteus mirabilis, Bacteroides fragilis, Enterobacter *species, and* Acinetobacter calcoaceticus; *intra-abdominal infections caused by beta-lactamase–producing strains of* E. coli, Klebsiella *species (including* K. pneumoniae*),* Bacteroides *species (including* B. fragilis*), and* Enterobacter *species; gynecologic infections caused by beta-lactamase–producing strains of* E. coli *and* Bacteroides *species (including* B. fragilis*)*

I.V. INFUSION

Adults and children age 12 and over weighing 40 kg (88 lb) or more. 1.5 (1 g of ampicillin and 0.5 g of sulbactam) to 3 g (2 g of ampicillin and 1 g of sulbactam) every 6 hr, up to a maximum of 8 g of ampicillin and 4 g of sulbactam daily.

Children age 1 and over weighing less than 40 kg. 300 mg/kg (200 mg of ampicillin and 100 mg of sulbactam) daily in divided doses every 6 hr.

DOSAGE ADJUSTMENT Dosing frequency reduced to every 6 to 8 hr for patients with creatinine clearance of 30 ml/min/1.73 m^2 or more, to every 12 hr for patients with creatinine clearance of 15 to 29 ml/min/1.73 m^2, and to every 24 hr for patients with creatinine clearance of 5 to 14 ml/min/1.73 m^2.

Route	Onset	Peak	Duration
I.V.	Immediate	Unknown	Unknown

Mechanism of Action

Inhibits bacterial cell wall synthesis. The rigid, cross-linked cell wall is assembled in several steps. The drug exerts its effects on susceptible bacteria in the final stage of the cross-linking process by binding with and inactivating penicillin-binding proteins (enzymes responsible for linking the cell wall strands). This action causes bacterial cell lysis and death. When ampicillin is administered alone, beta-lactamases may degrade it, making it ineffective. When combined with sulbactam, degradation can't occur. So sulbactam extends ampicillin's bactericidal effects to beta-lactamase–producing bacteria.

Incompatibilities

To prevent mutual inactivation, don't mix ampicillin sodium and sulbactam sodium in the same I.V. bag, bottle, or tubing with an aminoglycoside. If patient must receive both drugs, administer them in separate sites at least 1 hour apart.

Contraindications

Hypersensitivity to ampicillin sodium and sulbactam sodium, its components, or any penicillin

Interactions

DRUGS

allopurinol: Increased risk of rash, particularly in hyperuricemic patient

aminoglycosides: Possibly inactivation of both drugs when given together

heparin, oral anticoagulants: Increased risk of bleeding

oral contraceptives: Possibly reduced contraceptive effectiveness and breakthrough bleeding

probenecid: Possibly increased blood ampicillin level and risk of ampicillin toxicity

tetracyclines: Possibly impaired action of ampicillin sodium and sulbactam sodium

Adverse Reactions

CNS: Chills, fatigue, fever, headache, malaise

CV: Chest pain, edema, thrombophlebitis

EENT: Black "hairy" tongue, epistaxis, glossitis, laryngeal stridor, mucocutaneous candidiasis, stomatitis, throat tightness

GI: Abdominal distention, diarrhea, enterocolitis, flatulence, gastritis, nausea, pseudomembranous colitis, vomiting
GU: Dysuria, urine retention, vaginal candidiasis
HEME: Agranulocytosis, anemia, eosinophilia, leukopenia, thrombocytopenia, thrombocytopenic purpura
SKIN: Erythema multiforme; erythematous, mildly pruritic maculopapular rash or other rash; exfoliative dermatitis; mucosal bleeding; pruritus; urticaria
Other: Anaphylaxis, facial edema

Nursing Considerations

- Avoid administering ampicillin sodium and sulbactam sodium to patients with mononucleosis because of increased risk of a rash.
- Add 3.2 ml of sterile water for injection to each 1.5-g vial or 6.4 ml to each 3-g vial. This provides a total concentration of 375 mg/ml (250 mg/ml of ampicillin and 125 mg/ml of sulbactam). Using a suitable diluent and the concentrations recommended in manufacturer's insert (including sterile water for injection, lactated Ringer's, or $D_5/0.45$ normal saline solution), further dilute to a final concentration of 3 to 45 mg/ml (2 to 30 mg/ml of ampicillin and 1 to 15 mg/ml of sulbactam).
- Let solution stand to allow foaming to dissipate; inspect for complete solubility before administering.
- Administer I.V. dose by slow injection over 10 to 15 minutes or by infusion over 15 to 30 minutes when diluted further.
- Monitor patient closely for anaphylaxis, which may be life-threatening. Patients at greatest risk are those with a history of hypersensitivity to penicillin, multiple allergies, hypersensitivity to cephalosporins, or a history of asthma, hay fever, or urticaria.
- **WARNING** If drug triggers an anaphylactic reaction, discontinue drug, notify prescriber immediately, and provide appropriate therapy. Anaphylaxis requires immediate treatment with epinephrine as well as airway management and administration of oxygen and I.V. corticosteroids, as needed.
- Monitor patient closely for diarrhea, which may signal pseudomembranous colitis. If diarrhea occurs, notify prescriber. If pseudomembranous colitis is diagnosed, expect to discontinue drug and, possibly, administer fluids, electrolytes, protein, and antibiotic effective against *Clostridium difficile*.
- Keep in mind that each 1.5-g dose of ampicillin and sulbactam contains 5 mEq of sodium; take this into account when calculating patient's daily sodium intake.

- Be aware that drug's potency varies, depending on amount and type of diluent used and how solution is stored. For example, dilution with normnal saline solution for a final concentration of 45 mg/ml (30/15 mg/ml) retains potency for 8 hours when stored at 25° C (77° F) and for 48 hours when stored at 4° C (39° F). A dilution with normal saline solution for a final concentration of 30 mg/ml (20/10 mg/ml) retains potency for 72 hours when stored at 4° C. See manufacturer's insert for further details.

PATIENT TEACHING
- Instruct patient receiving ampicillin sodium and sulbactam sodium to immediately report diarrhea and any sudden or unusual symptoms, such as shortness of breath, wheezing, rash, chest pain, or facial swelling.

anidulafungin
Eraxis

Class and Category
Chemical: Semi-synthetic echinocandin
Therapeutic: Antifungal
Pregnancy category: C

Indications and Dosages
▶ *To treat candidemia and other forms of* Candida *infection, such as intra-abdominal abscess and peritonitis*
I.V. INFUSION
Adults. 200 mg on day 1, followed by 100 mg daily, continued for at least 14 days after the last positive culture.
▶ *To treat esophageal candidiasis*
I.V. INFUSION
Adults. 100 mg on day 1, followed by 50 mg daily for at least 14 days and for at least 7 days following resolution of symptoms.

Contraindications
Hypersensitivity to anidulafungin, its components, or other echinocandins

---

Mechanism of Action
Inhibits glucan synthase, an enzyme needed for formation of 1,3-beta-D glucan, a substance essential for construction of the fungal cell wall. Because the fungus cannot exist without a cell wall, the infection resolves.

Interactions
DRUGS
None reported.

Adverse Reactions
CNS: Headache, dizziness, seizures
CV: Artial fibrillation, deep vein thrombosis, hypertension, hypotension, right bundle branch block, sinus arrhythmia, ventricular extrasystoles
ENDO: Hyperglycemia
GI: Diarrhea, elevated liver enzymes, dyspepsia, heptic necrosis, nausea
HEME: Leukopenia, neutropenia, thrombocytopenia
RESP: Dyspnea
SKIN: Flushing, pruritus, rash, urticaria
Other: Angioneurotic edema, hypercalcemia, hypokalemia, hyperkalemia, hypernatremia, hypomagnesemia

Nursing Considerations
- Reconstitute each 50-mg vial with 15 ml of supplied diluent (20% dehydrated alcohol in water for injection) to reach 3.33 mg/ml. Use within 24 hours after reconstitution.
- Further dilute reconstituted solution with 5% dextrose or normal saline solution. For 50-mg dose, dilute with 100 ml; for 100-mg dose, dilute with 250 ml; and for 200-mg dose, dilute with 500 ml.
- Give as an intravenous infusion at no more than 1.1 mg/minute.
- Monitor liver function, as ordered. If abnormalities occur or hepatic function worsens, notify prescriber and expect to stop drug.

PATIENT TEACHING
- Inform patient that anidulafungin therapy will last 2 or more weeks. If the patient has esophageal candidiasis, explain that therapy will last at least 1 week after symptoms resolve. If the patient has an abdominal abscess or peritonitis, explain that therapy will last 2 weeks after culture is negative.
- Tell patient to promptly report any histamine-related symptoms, such as rash, pruritus, or urticaria.

anistreplase
(anisoylated plasminogen-streptokinase activator complex)
Eminase

Class and Category
Chemical: p-Anisoylated derivative of the Lys-plasminogen-streptokinase activator complex
Therapeutic: Thrombolytic enzyme
Pregnancy category: C

Indications and Dosages
▶ *To treat acute MI (to lyse thrombi obstructing coronary arteries, reduce infarct size, improve ventricular function, and reduce mortality)*
I.V. INFUSION
Adults. 30 units injected over 2 to 5 min.

Route	Onset	Peak	Duration
I.V.	Immediate	20 min to 2 hr	4 to 6 hr

Mechanism of Action
Indirectly promotes the conversion of plasminogen to plasmin, an enzyme that breaks down fibrin clots, fibrinogen, and other plasma proteins, including procoagulant factors V and VIII.

Incompatibilities
Don't add other drugs to anistreplase solution or infuse other drugs through same I.V. line.

Contraindications
Active internal bleeding, arteriovenous malformation or aneurysm, bleeding diathesis, history of CVA, hypersensitivity to anistreplase or streptokinase, intracranial neoplasm, intracranial or intraspinal surgery or trauma within past 2 months, severe uncontrolled hypertension

Interactions
DRUGS
aspirin, dipyridamole, and other drugs that alter platelet function; heparin; vitamin K antagonists: Possibly increased risk of bleeding if administered before anistreplase

Adverse Reactions
CNS: Dizziness, fever, headache, intracranial hemorrhage
CV: Ankle edema, arrhythmias (especially accelerated idioventricular rhythm, conduction disorders, premature ventricular beats, sinus bradycardia, ventricular fibrillation, ventricular tachycardia), hypotension, vasculitis

EENT: Epistaxis
GI: Abdominal pain or swelling, constipation, GI bleeding, nausea, vomiting
GU: Hematuria, proteinuria, vaginal bleeding
HEME: Bleeding tendency, eosinophilia, mild to severe hemorrhage
MS: Arthralgia, back pain, joint stiffness, myalgia
RESP: Bronchospasm, dyspnea, hemoptysis
SKIN: Flushing, pruritus, rash, urticaria
Other: Anaphylaxis, angioedema

Nursing Considerations

- Obtain appropriate coagulation studies (such as PT, APTT, platelet count, and fibrin-fibrinogen degradation product titer) before initiating anistreplase treatment, if possible.
- To reconstitute anistreplase, slowly direct 5 ml of sterile water for injection or sodium chloride for injection against side of vial. Then gently roll vial to mix dry powder and fluid and minimize foaming. Don't shake vial. The resulting solution should be colorless to pale yellow and transparent.
- Before administering solution, inspect it for particles and discoloration. If present, discard and reconstitute drug from a new vial. Then withdraw entire contents of vial. Don't dilute reconstituted solution further before administration; don't add it to I.V. fluid. Don't add other drugs to vial or syringe that contains anistreplase. Discard drug if it isn't administered within 30 minutes of reconstitution.
- For maximum effectiveness, expect to administer anistreplase as soon as possible after onset of MI symptoms.
- Closely monitor all puncture sites, such as catheter insertion and needle puncture sites, for bleeding.
- Monitor the following patients for evidence of bleeding or hemorrhage because they're at increased risk during anistreplase therapy: those with acute pericarditis (risk of hemopericardium, possibly leading to cardiac tamponade); cerebrovascular disease; hemorrhagic ophthalmic conditions; history of major surgery, GI or GU bleeding, or trauma within past 10 days; hypertension; mitral stenosis with atrial fibrillation (risk of embolism); pregnancy; septic thrombophlebitis; severe hepatic or renal disease; or subacute bacterial endocarditis.
- Avoid giving I.M. injections and handling patient unnecessarily during anistreplase therapy. Perform venipuncture only when necessary, using a 23G or smaller needle.

- If the patient needs an arterial puncture after anistreplase administration, use an arm vessel that allows easy manual compression. Apply pressure for 30 minutes. Then apply a pressure dressing and check puncture site frequently for bleeding.
- Use continuous cardiac monitoring because arrhythmias may occur during reperfusion. Keep antiarrhythmics on hand during anistreplase therapy, and manage arrhythmias according to facility policy.
- Keep epinephrine, glucocorticoids, and antihistamines nearby to treat anaphylaxis.
- Know that anistreplase may be less effective if given more than 5 days after previous anistreplase or streptokinase administration. This occurs because patient may have developed antistreptokinase antibodies, which make him more resistant to the drug and make drug therapy less effective. Elevated serum antistreptokinase antibody levels and reduced drug effectiveness can persist for 5 days to 12 months.
- Store drug between 2° and 8° C (36° and 46° F).

PATIENT TEACHING
- Instruct patient receiving anistreplase to report adverse reactions immediately, especially bleeding, dizziness, and chest pain.

antihemophilic factor
antihemophilic factor (recombinant), plasma/albumin-free method (rAHF-PFM)
Advate
antihemophilic factor (human)
Alphanate
antihemophilic factor–von Willebrand factor complex (human, dried, pasteurized)
Humate-P

Class and Category
Chemical: Recombinant protein
Therapeutic: Antihemophilic factor
Pregnancy category: C

Indications and Dosages
▶ *To prevent and control bleeding episodes in patients with hemophilia A and patients with factor VIII inhibitors not exceeding 10 Bethesda Units/ml*

I.V. INJECTION

Adults and children. Highly individualized. *For early hemarthrosis, muscle bleeding episode, or mild oral bleeding episode:* Dose administered to achieve peak post-infusion factor VIII activity in blood (determined by multiplying dose administered/kg body weight by 2) between 20% and 40% of normal with infusions every 12 to 24 hr for 1 to 3 days until bleeding episode resolved. *For more extensive hemarthrosis, muscle bleeding episode, or hematoma:* Dose administered to achieve peak post-infusion factor VIII activity in blood between 30% and 60% of normal with infusions every 12 to 24 hr for 3 or more days until pain and disability are resolved. *For life-threatening bleeding episodes:* Dose administered to achieve peak post-infusion factor VIII activity in blood between 60% and 100% with infusions every 8 to 24 hr until bleeding episode stops.

▶ *To prevent and control perioperative bleeding in patients with hemophilia A*

I.V. INJECTION

Adults and children. Highly individualized. *For minor surgery, including tooth extraction:* Dose administered to achieve peak post-infusion factor VIII activity in blood (determined by multiplying dose administered/kg body weight by 2) between 60% and 100% of normal, given as a single bolus infusion within 1 hr of operation, with optional additional dose every 12 to 24 hr, as needed. *For major surgery:* Dose administered to achieve peak post-infusion factor VIII activity in blood between 80% and 100% preoperatively and postoperatively with infusions every 8 to 24 hr.

▶ *To prevent or treat bleeding in hemophilia A*

I.V. INJECTION (HUMATE-P)

Adults. Highly individualized. *For mild hemorrhage, such as early joint or muscle bleeding or severe epistaxis:* Loading dose of 15 international units/kg to achieve factor VIII:C plasma level about 30% of normal, with half the loading dose repeated once or twice daily for 1 to 2 days as needed. *For moderate hemorrhage, such as advanced joint or muscle bleeding; neck, tongue, or pharyngeal hematoma without airway compromise; tooth extraction; or severe abdominal pain:* Loading dose of 25 international units/kg to achieve factor VIII:C plasma level about 50% of normal, followed by 15 international units/kg every 8 to 12 hr for first 1 to 2 days to keep factor VIII:C plasma level at 30% of normal, and then 15 international units/kg once or twice daily for total of up to 7 days or until adequate wound healing. *For life-threatening hemorrhage, as may occur*

*in major surgery; GI bleeding; neck, tongue, or pharyngeal hematoma
with potential for airway compromise; intracranial, intra-abdominal, or
intrathoracic bleeding; or fractures:* Loading dose of 40 to 50 international units/kg, followed by 20 to 25 international units/kg every
8 hr to keep factor VIII:C plasma level at 80% to 100% of normal for 7 days, followed by 20 to 25 international units/kg once
or twice daily for another 7 days to keep factor VIII:C level at
30% to 50% of normal.

▶ *To treat spontaneous and trauma-induced bleeding episodes and
prevent excessive bleeding during and after surgery in patients with von
Willebrand disease when use of desmopressin is inadequate*
I.V. INJECTION (HUMATE-P)
Adults and children. 40 to 80 international units/kg every 8 to
12 hr as needed.

▶ *To prevent excessive bleeding during and after surgery in patients
with von Willebrand disease*
I.V. INJECTION (HUMATE-P)
Adults and children. Highly individualized. *For emergency surgery:* Loading dose of 50 to 60 international units/kg, followed by
half the loading dose every 6 to 12 hr as needed. *For planned surgery:* Individualized loading dose based on patient's need 1 to 2 hr
before surgery, followed by half the loading dose every 6 to 12 hr
for at least 12 hr (oral surgery), 48 hr (minor surgery), or 72 hr
(major surgery).

Route	Onset	Peak	Duration
I.V.	Immediate	5 min	Unknown

Mechanism of Action
Provides supplemental factor VIII, the coagulation factor needed for blood to
clot that is missing in patients with hemophilia A and diminished in patients
with factor VIII inhibitors. After blood clots, bleeding stops.

Contraindications
Life-threatening, immediate hypersensitivity reactions, including
anaphylaxis, with previous use of drug or exposure to mouse or
hamster proteins

Interactions
DRUGS
None reported.

Adverse Reactions
CNS: Dizziness, fever, headache, rigidity
CV: Chest pain
EENT: Taste perversion
GI: Abdominal pain, diarrhea, nausea
HEME: Bleeding tendency, decreased coagulation factor VIII, decreased hematocrit, hematoma, hemolytic anemia
MS: Joint swelling, lower limb edema
RESP: Dyspnea
SKIN: Diaphoresis, pruritus
Other: Anaphylaxis, catheter-related infection, hot flashes

Nursing Considerations
- Check to confirm that clotting defect is factor VIII deficiency before administering antihemophilic factor because drug isn't effective in treating other coagulation factor deficiencies.
- Reconstitute Advate or Alphanate using sterile water for injection. Bring both drug and diluent to room temperature; then clean stoppers with antiseptic solution and allow to dry. Remove protective covering from one end of double-ended needle and insert through center of diluent stopper. Remove protective covering from other end of double-ended needle. Invert diluent bottle over upright drug bottle; then rapidly insert free end of needle through drug stopper at center. The vacuum in bottle will draw in the diluent. Then disconnect the two bottles by removing needle from diluent bottle stopper, and remove the needle from drug bottle. Swirl gently until all drug is dissolved. Avoid shaking to prevent foaming and degradation of drug. Administer in a separate line within 3 hours of reconstitution.
- Reconsititute Humate-P following manufacturer illustrations and guidelines in package insert.
- Take patient's pulse before and periodically during drug administration. If rate increases significantly, reduce administration rate or temporarily halt the injection to allow pulse rate to return to basline before resuming administration.
- To administer Advate or Alphanate, use only plastic material because protein in drug will adhere to glass. Attach filter needle to syringe and draw back plunger to draw air into syringe. Insert needle into reconstituted drug vial. Inject air into bottle and then withdraw drug from vial. Remove and discard filter needle from syringe, attach a suitable needle, and inject I.V. bolus at no greater than 10 ml/min over no more than 5 min.
- To administer Humate-P, slowly inject I.V. bolus at no more

than 4 ml/min using a venipuncture or other suitable intravenous injection set.

- Monitor patient's plasma factor VIII level (and von Willebrand factor:ristocetin cofactor if patient has von Willebrand disease) during and after treatment to ensure an adequate level has been reached and is being maintained, as ordered.
- Monitor patient for anaphylaxis, and have emergency equipment nearby.
- After giving drug, monitor patient for formation of neutralizing antibodies to factor VIII, a complication of treating hemophilia A that may cause continued bleeding. Obtain laboratory analysis to detect the neutralizing antibodies, as ordered.
- Monitor patients with blood types A, B, and AB for hemolysis when giving large doses.

PATIENT TEACHING
- Teach patient and caregivers how to administer drug at home in an emergency situation.
- Instruct patient to stop drug and seek emergency help immediately if he has an acute allergic reaction, such as hives, chest tightness, wheezing, low blood pressure, or fainting during or after drug administration.

antithrombin III, human
(AT-III, heparin co-factor I)
ATnativ, Thrombate III

Class and Category
Chemical: Alpha$_2$-globulin
Therapeutic: Anticoagulant, antithrombotic
Pregnancy category: C

Indications and Dosages
▶ *To treat patients with hereditary antithrombin III (AT-III) deficiency who are undergoing surgery or obstetric procedures or who have thromboembolism*

I.V. INJECTION

Adults and children. *Initial:* Individualized dosage (based on weight, degree of AT-III deficiency, and desired level of AT-III to be achieved) sufficient to increase AT-III activity to 120% of normal, administered at 50 to 100 international units/min. *Maintenance:* Individualized dosage sufficient to keep AT-III activity at 80% or more of normal, administered every 24 hr for 2 to

8 days, depending on patient's condition and history and prescriber's judgment. A pregnant, immobilized, or postsurgical patient may need more prolonged therapy.

Route	Onset	Peak	Duration
I.V.	Immediate	Unknown	4 days

Mechanism of Action
Inhibits blood coagulation by inactivating thrombin; activated forms of factors IX, X, XI, and XII; and plasmin.

Incompatibilities
Don't mix AT-III with other drugs or solutions.

Interactions
DRUGS
heparin: Enhanced anticoagulant effect

Adverse Reactions
CNS: Chills, dizziness, fever, light-headedness
CV: Chest pain or tightness, hypotension, vasodilation
EENT: Unpleasant taste
GI: Abdominal cramps, bowel fullness, nausea
GU: Diuresis
HEME: Hematoma
RESP: Dyspnea
SKIN: Oozing lesions, urticaria

Nursing Considerations
• Reconstitute AT-III with 10 ml sterile water for injection (provided by manufacturer) or alternate solution, such as normal saline solution or D_5W injection. Don't shake the vial. Let solution come to room temperature before administration. If desired, dilute reconstituted solution further, using same diluent.
• **WARNING** Don't use diluent that contains benzyl alcohol to reconstitute AT-III for a neonate. This can cause a fatal toxic syndrome characterized by metabolic acidosis, CNS depression, respiratory problems, renal failure, hypotension, seizures, and intracranial hemorrhage.
• Don't refrigerate reconstituted solution. Use it within 3 hours and discard unused solution.
• If after 30 minutes the initial dose doesn't increase AT-III activ-

ity to 120% of normal, expect prescriber to increase dosage.
• If patient requires a dosage increase, monitor AT-III activity more frequently and expect to adjust dosage accordingly.
• Expect to reduce heparin dosage to prevent bleeding during AT-III therapy.
• If mild adverse reactions occur, decrease infusion rate, as prescribed. If severe reactions occur, discontinue infusion, as prescribed, until they subside.
• Evaluate serum AT-III level twice a day until dosage is stabilized. After that, evaluate level once daily, immediately before administering a dose.
• Store drug between 2° and 8° C (36° and 46° F).

PATIENT TEACHING
• Inform patient that blood will be drawn periodically during AT-III therapy to guide dosage adjustments.

argatroban

Acova

Class and Category

Chemical: N2-substituted derivative of arginine
Therapeutic: Anticoagulant
Pregnancy category: B

Indications and Dosages

▶ *To prevent or treat thrombosis in patients with heparin-induced thrombocytopenia*

I.V. INFUSION

Adults. 2 mcg/kg/min as a continuous infusion. *Maximum:* 10 mcg/kg/min.

DOSAGE ADJUSTMENT Dosage adjusted as prescribed to maintain a therapeutic APTT of 1.5 to 3 times the initial baseline value, not to exceed 100 sec. Initial dosage reduced to 0.5 mcg/kg/min for patients with moderate hepatic impairment.

Route	Onset	Peak	Duration
I.V.	Immediate	3 to 4 hr	Unknown

Mechanism of Action

Forms a tight bond with thrombin, neutralizing this enzyme's actions, even when the enzyme is trapped within clots. Thrombin causes fibrinogen to convert to fibrin, which is essential for clot formation.

Incompatibilities

Don't mix argatroban with other drugs.

Contraindications

Active major bleeding, hypersensitivity to argatroban or its components

Interactions

DRUGS

alteplase, antineoplastic drugs, antiplatelets, antithymocyte globulin, heparin, NSAIDs, reteplase, salicylates, streptokinase, strontium chloride Sr 89, warfarin: Increased risk of bleeding

porfimer: Possibly decreased efficacy of porfimer photodynamic therapy

Adverse Reactions

CNS: Cerebrovascular bleeding, fever, headache

CV: Atrial fibrillation, cardiac arrest, hypotension, unstable angina, ventricular tachycardia

GI: Abdominal pain, anorexia, diarrhea, elevated liver function test results, GI bleeding, nausea, vomiting

GU: Elevated BUN and serum creatinine levels, hematuria (microscopic), UTI

HEME: Hypoprothrombinemia

RESP: Cough, dyspnea, hemoptysis, pneumonia

SKIN: Bleeding at puncture site, rash

Other: Sepsis

Nursing Considerations

- Using normal saline solution, D_5W, or lactated Ringer's solution, dilute argatroban to 1 mg/ml before administration.
- Use diluted solution within 24 hours if it has been stored at 15° to 30° C (59° to 86° F), protected from direct sunlight, and kept in ambient indoor light. Use solution within 48 hours if it has been stored between 2° and 8° C (36° and 46° F) and kept in the dark.
- **WARNING** Monitor patients with thrombocytopenia or those receiving daily doses of salicylates greater than 6 g for signs and symptoms of bleeding because they're at increased risk of bleeding from hypoprothrombinemia.
- **WARNING** Expect to perform blood coagulation tests before and 2 hours after start of therapy because of the major risk of bleeding associated with argatroban. Be aware that coagulopathy must be ruled out before therapy starts.
- Monitor the following patients for evidence of bleeding because

they're at increased risk during argatroban therapy: actively menstruating females; patients with known vascular or organ abnormalities, such as severe uncontrolled hypertension, advanced renal disease, infective endocarditis, dissecting aortic aneurysm, diverticulitis, hemophilia, hepatic disease (especially if associated with a deficiency of vitamin K–dependent clotting factors), inflammatory bowel disease, or peptic ulcer disease; and those who have recently had a CVA, major surgery (including eye, brain, or spinal cord surgery), large vessel puncture or organ biopsy, lumbar puncture, spinal anesthesia, or major bleeding (including intracranial, GI, intraocular, retroperitoneal, or pulmonary bleeding).

• Whenever possible, avoid I.M. injections in patients receiving argatroban to decrease the risk of bleeding.

• Be aware that thrombin times may not be helpful for monitoring argatroban activity because all thrombin-dependent coagulation tests are affected by the drug.

• Monitor APTT periodically, as ordered, during treatment to verify therapeutic drug levels.

• Expect drug dosage to be tapered before discontinuation to prevent the risk of rebound hypercoagulopathy; drug's effects last for only a short time once drug is discontinued.

• Store unopened vials between 15° and 30° C (59° and 86° F); protect from freezing and light.

PATIENT TEACHING

• Explain to a patient receiving argatroban that heparin-induced thrombocytopenia is an antigen-antibody immunologic response that isn't related to the dosage of heparin he may have received.

• Inform patient that argatroban is a blood thinner that is administered in the hospital by infusion into a vein. Explain that he'll be switched to another drug before discharge if he requires long-term anticoagulation.

• Advise patient to immediately report unusual or unexplained bleeding, such as blood in urine, easy bruising, nosebleeds, tarry stools, and vaginal bleeding.

• Instruct patient to be careful to avoid injury while receiving argatroban. For example, suggest that he brush his teeth gently, using a soft-bristled toothbrush, and take special care when flossing.

• Inform patient that the risk of bleeding associated with argatroban lasts for only a short time once drug is discontinued.

atenolol

Apo-Atenol (CAN), Novo-Atenol (CAN), Tenormin

Class and Category

Chemical: Beta-adrenergic blocker (beta$_1$ and at high doses beta$_2$)
Therapeutic: Antianginal, antihypertensive
Pregnancy category: D

Indications and Dosages

▶ *To treat acute MI*

I.V. INFUSION, TABLETS

Adults. *Initial:* 5 mg I.V. slowly over 5 min, followed by another 5 mg I.V. 10 min later. After an additional 10 min (if tolerated), 50 mg P.O., followed by another 50 mg P.O. 12 hr later. *Maintenance:* 50 mg P.O. b.i.d. or 100 mg P.O. daily for 6 to 9 days or until discharge from hospital.

DOSAGE ADJUSTMENT Dosage reduced to 50 mg daily P.O. for patients with creatinine clearance of of 15 to 35 ml/min/1.73 m^2 and to 25 mg daily for patients with creatinine clearance of less than 15 ml/min/1.73 m^2.

Route	Onset	Peak	Duration
I.V.	Immediate	5 min	12 hr
P.O.	1 hr	2 to 4 hr	24 hr

Mechanism of Action

Inhibits stimulation of beta$_1$-receptor sites, located primarily in the heart, causing a decrease in cardiac excitability, cardiac output, and myocardial oxygen demand. At high doses, atenolol inhibits stimulation of beta$_2$ receptors in the lungs, which may cause bronchoconstriction.

Contraindications

Cardiogenic shock, heart block greater than first degree, hypersensitivity to beta blockers, overt heart failure, sinus bradycardia

Interactions

DRUGS

calcium channel blockers (such as verapamil and diltiazem): Possibly symptomatic bradycardia and conduction abnormalities
catecholamine-depleting drugs (such as reserpine): Additive antihypertensive effect
clonidine: Rebound hypertension

Adverse Reactions

CNS: Depression, disorientation, dizziness, drowsiness, emotional lability, fatigue, fever, lethargy, light-headedness, short-term memory loss, vertigo

CV: Arrhythmias, including bradycardia and heart block; cardiogenic shock; cold arms and legs; heart failure; mesenteric artery thrombosis; mitral insufficiency; myocardial reinfarction; orthostatic hypotension; Raynaud's phenomenon

EENT: Dry eyes, laryngospasm, pharyngitis

GI: Diarrhea, ischemic colitis, nausea

GU: Renal failure

HEME: Agranulocytosis

MS: Leg pain

RESP: Bronchospasm, dyspnea, pulmonary emboli, respiratory distress, wheezing

SKIN: Erythematous rash

Other: Allergic reaction

Nursing Considerations

- Be aware that although its exact mechanism of action is unknown, atenolol improves survival rate in patients with a known or suspected acute MI.
- Dilute atenolol with dextrose, sodium chloride, or dextrose and sodium chloride solution.
- Inspect solution for particles or discoloration before administration.
- During I.V. atenolol therapy, monitor vital signs and cardiac rhythm closely.
- Expect to administer digoxin, a diuretic, or both at first sign of heart failure, and monitor patient closely. If heart failure continues, expect to discontinue atenolol.
- Closely monitor patient with hyperthyroidism because atenolol may mask some signs of thyrotoxicosis. Avoid abrupt withdrawal of atenolol, which may precipitate thyrotoxicosis.
- Assess diabetic patients for signs of hypoglycemia other than tachycardia (such as dizziness and sweating) because atenolol may mask tachycardia caused by hypoglycemia. Unlike other beta-adrenergic blockers, atenolol doesn't mask other signs of hypoglycemia, cause hypoglycemia, or delay the return of blood glucose to a normal level.
- Monitor patients with heart failure controlled by digitalis glycosides or diuretics for exacerbation of heart failure.
- Monitor for adverse effects, such as symptomatic bradycardia or hypotension, in patients with conduction abnormalities or left

ventricular dysfunction who are receiving verapamil or diltiazem.

- Monitor for signs of reduced peripheral circulation, such as cold hands and feet, in patients with Raynaud's syndrome or other peripheral vascular disease.
- Because atenolol is excreted by the kidneys, monitor patients with impaired renal function for increased atenolol effects.
- Discard atenolol solution if it isn't used within 48 hours.
- Stop atenolol therapy and notify prescriber if patient develops bradycardia, hypotension, or another serious adverse reaction.
- If patient also receives clonidine, expect to discontinue atenolol several days before gradually withdrawing clonidine. Then expect to restart atenolol therapy several days after clonidine has been discontinued.
- Store drug between 20° and 25° C (68° and 77° F); protect from freezing and light.

PATIENT TEACHING
- Instruct patient not to stop taking atenolol abruptly because angina could worsen and an MI or arrhythmia might occur.
- While patient is being weaned from atenolol, tell him to perform minimal physical activity to prevent chest pain.
- Inform patient that atenolol may alter his blood glucose level and mask symptoms of hypoglycemia.
- Advise patient to report evidence of an adverse reaction, such as trouble breathing, shortness of breath, dizziness, or a rash.

atracurium besylate

Tracrium

Class and Category
Chemical: Biquaternary ammonium ester
Therapeutic: Skeletal muscle relaxant
Pregnancy category: C

Indications and Dosages
▶ *To facilitate endotracheal intubation and induce skeletal muscle relaxation for surgery or mechanical ventilation as adjunct to anesthesia*
I.V. INFUSION, I.V. INJECTION
Adults and children age 2 and over. *Initial:* 0.4 to 0.5 mg/kg by I.V. bolus for nearly complete neuromuscular blockade. *Maintenance:* 0.08 to 0.1 mg/kg 20 to 45 min after initial dose during prolonged surgery. Maintenance doses may be given every 15 to

25 min for patients under balanced anesthesia. Patients having extended surgical procedures may need an infusion of 9 to 10 mcg/kg/min after an initial I.V. bolus to counteract the spontaneous return of neuromuscular function. Thereafter, 5 to 10 mcg/kg/min is given as a constant infusion.

Children ages 1 month to 2 years receiving halothane anesthesia. *Initial:* 0.3 to 0.4 mg/kg. Frequent maintenance doses may be required.

Route	Onset	Peak	Duration
I.V.	2 to 2.5 min	3 to 5 min	35 to 70 min

Mechanism of Action
Inhibits nerve impulse transmission by competing with acetylcholine for cholinergic receptors on motor end plate.

Incompatibilities
Don't mix atracurium in same syringe or administer it through same I.V. needle as an alkaline solution, such as a barbiturate injection. Don't mix atracurium with lactated Ringer's injection.

Contraindications
Hypersensitivity to atracurium, its components, or benzyl alcohol

Interactions
DRUGS

aminoglycosides, enflurane, furosemide, halothane, isoflurane, lithium, magnesium salts, polymyxin antibiotics, procainamide, quinidine, thiazide diuretics: Possibly enhanced or prolonged atracurium effects
opioid analgesics: Possibly additive histamine release and increased risk and severity of bradycardia and hypotension

Adverse Reactions
CNS: Seizures
CV: Bradycardia, hypertension, hypotension, tachycardia
MS: Inadequate or prolonged neuromuscular blockade
RESP: Apnea, bronchospasm, dyspnea, laryngospasm, wheezing
SKIN: Flushing, rash, urticaria
Other: Anaphylaxis, injection site reaction

Nursing Considerations
• Anticipate using lower doses of atracurium for patients with neuromuscular disease, severe electrolyte disorders, or carcinomatosis because of the risk of enhanced neuromuscular block-

ade and difficulties with reversal. Lower doses may also be used for patients at risk for adverse reactions related to histamine release.

- Keep atropine nearby to treat atracurium-induced bradycardia.
- For I.V. infusion, dilute atracurium with normnal saline solution, D_5W, or D_5 in normal saline solution. To prepare a solution that yields 200 mcg of atracurium/ml, add 2 ml of atracurium to 98 ml of diluent. To prepare a solution that yields 500 mcg/ml, add 5 ml of atracurium to 95 ml of diluent.
- Store prepared solution in refrigerator or at room temperature for up to 24 hours. Discard unused portion after 24 hours.
- Closely monitor blood pressure of patients with hypotension.
- Monitor patient closely for adverse reactions, especially those related to histamine release. Be aware that atracurium is more likely than other neuromuscular blockers to cause flushing.
- Before use, store undiluted atracurium at 2° to 8° C (36° to 46° F); don't freeze. Use drug within 14 days if stored at room temperature, even if it's refrigerated later.

PATIENT TEACHING
- Explain purpose of atracurium treatment to patient.

atropine
AtroPen
atropine sulfate

Class and Category
Chemical: Belladonna alkaloid
Therapeutic: Anticholinergic, antimuscarinic
Pregnancy category: C

Indications and Dosages
▶ *To reduce respiratory tract secretions related to anesthesia*
I.V. INJECTION
Adults. 0.4 to 0.6 mg preoperatively.
Children. 0.01 mg/kg up to total of 0.4 mg preoperatively, repeated every 4 to 6 hr, p.r.n.
▶ *To correct bradycardia*
I.V. INJECTION
Adults. 0.4 to 1 mg. If no response to first dose, repeat once after 5 min.
Children. 0.01 to 0.02 mg/kg with a minimum dose of 0.1 mg and a maximum dose of 0.5 mg. If no response to first dose, repeat once after 5 min.

▶ *To treat cholinesterase inhibitor (such as neostigmine, pilocarpine, and methacholine) toxicity*

I.V. INJECTION

Adults. 2 to 4 mg. Then 2 mg every 5 to 10 min until muscarinic signs (bradycardia, vasodilation, and pupil dilation) disappear or signs of atropine intoxication develop.

I.V. INJECTION

Children. 1 mg. Then 0.5 to 1 mg every 5 to 10 min until muscarinic signs disappear or signs of atropine intoxication develop.

▶ *To treat mushroom (muscarine) toxicity*

I.V. INJECTION

Adults. 1 to 2 mg every hr until respiratory signs and symptoms subside.

▶ *To treat pesticide (organophosphate) toxicity*

I.V. INJECTION

Adults. 1 to 2 mg, repeated in 20 to 30 min as soon as cyanosis has cleared. Then dosage continued until definite improvement is maintained, possibly for 2 or more days.

Route	Onset	Peak	Duration
I.V.	Immediate	2 to 4 min	Brief

Mechanism of Action

Inhibits acetylcholine's muscarinic action at the neuroeffector junctions of smooth muscles, cardiac muscles, exocrine glands, SA and AV nodes, and the urinary bladder. In small doses, atropine inhibits salivary and bronchial secretions and diaphoresis. In moderate doses, it increases impulse conduction through the AV node and increases heart rate. In large doses, it decreases GI and urinary tract motility and gastric acid secretion.

Contraindications

Angle-closure glaucoma, asthma, GI obstructive disease (achalasia, pyloric obstruction, pyloroduodenal stenosis), hepatic disease, hypersensitivity to atropine or its components, ileus, intestinal atony, myasthenia gravis, myocardial ischemia, obstructive uropathy, renal disease, severe ulcerative colitis, tachycardia, toxic megacolon, unstable cardiovascular status in acute hemorrhage

Interactions

DRUGS

adsorbent antidiarrheals, antacids: Decreased atropine absorption

amantadine, anticholinergics, antidyskinetics, glutethimide, meperidine,

muscle relaxants, phenothiazines, tricyclic antidepressants and other drugs with anticholinergic properties, including antiarrhythmics (disopyramide, procainamide, quinidine), antihistamines, buclizine, meclizine: Increased atropine effects
antimyasthenics: Reduced intestinal motility
cyclopropane: Risk of ventricular arrhythmias
haloperidol: Decreased antipsychotic effect
ketoconazole: Decreased ketoconazole absorption
metoclopramide: Decreased effect on GI motility
opioid analgesics: Increased risk of ileus, severe constipation, and urine retention
potassium chloride, especially wax-matrix forms: Possibly GI ulcers
urinary alkalizers (calcium or magnesium antacids, carbonic anhydrase inhibitors, citrates, sodium bicarbonate): Delayed excretion and increased risk of adverse atropine effects

Adverse Reactions

CNS: Agitation, amnesia, anxiety, ataxia, Babinski's or Chaddock's reflex, behavioral changes, CNS stimulation (with high doses), coma, confusion, decreased concentration, decreased tendon reflexes, delirium, dizziness, drowsiness, fever, hallucinations, headache, hyperreflexia, insomnia, lethargy, mania, mental disorders, nervousness, paranoia, restlessness, seizures, somnolence, stupor, syncope, vertigo, weakness
CV: Arrhythmias, bradycardia (with low doses), cardiac dilation, chest pain, hypertension, hypotension, left ventricular failure, MI, palpitations, tachycardia (with high doses), weak or impalpable peripheral pulses
EENT: Acute angle-closure glaucoma, altered taste, blepharitis, blindness, blurred vision, conjunctivitis, cyclophoria, cycloplegia, decreased visual acuity or accommodation, dry eyes or conjunctiva, dry mucous membranes, dry mouth, eye irritation, eyelid crusting, heterophoria, increased intraocular pressure, keratoconjunctivitis, lacrimation, laryngitis, laryngospasm, mydriasis, nasal congestion, oral lesions, photophobia, pupils poorly reactive to light, strabismus, tongue chewing
GI: Abdominal distention, abdominal pain, bloating, constipation, decreased bowel sounds or food absorption, delayed gastric emptying, dysphagia, heartburn, ileus, nausea, vomiting
GU: Bladder distention, enuresis, impotence, urinary hesitancy, urinary urgency, urine retention
MS: Dysarthria, hypertonia, muscle twitching
RESP: Bradypnea, dyspnea, inspiratory stridor, pulmonary

edema, respiratory failure, shallow breathing, subcostal recession, tachypnea

SKIN: Cold skin, cyanosis, decreased sweating, dermatitis, flushing, rash, urticaria

Other: Anaphylaxis, dehydration, injection site reaction, polydipsia, sensations of warmth

Nursing Considerations

- Avoid using high-dose atropine sulfate therapy in patients with ulcerative colitis because of risk of toxic megacolon or in patients with hiatal hernia and reflux esophagitis because of risk of esophagitis
- WARNING Assess for symptoms of toxic doses of atropine, such as excitement, agitation, drowsiness, and confusion, which are likely to affect elderly patients even with low doses. If these symptoms occur, take safety precautions to prevent patient injury.
- Assess bowel and bladder elimination. Notify prescriber about diarrhea, constipation, urinary hesitancy, or urine retention.

PATIENT TEACHING

- Advise patient to notify prescriber if he has persistent or severe diarrhea, constipation, or difficulty urinating.

azathioprine sodium

Imuran

azathioprine

Imuran

Class and Category

Chemical: Purine analogue
Therapeutic: Antimetabolite, immunosuppressant
Pregnancy category: D

Indications and Dosages

▶ *To prevent kidney transplant rejection*

I.V. INFUSION, TABLETS

Adults and children. *Initial:* 3 to 5 mg/kg daily I.V. or P.O. as a single dose on or 1 to 3 days before day of transplant, followed by 3 to 5 mg/kg daily I.V. after surgery until P.O. dose is tolerated. *Maintenance:* 1 to 3 mg/kg daily P.O.

DOSAGE ADJUSTMENT Dosage reduced for patients with oliguria (such as from tubular necrosis) after transplantation because their drug or metabolite excretion may be delayed.

Route	Onset	Peak	Duration
I.V., P.O.	4 to 8 wk	Unknown	Several days

Mechanism of Action
May prevent proliferation and differentiation of activated B and T cells by interfering with purine (protein) and nucleic acid (DNA and RNA) synthesis.

Contraindications
Hypersensitivity to azathioprine

Interactions
DRUGS
ACE inhibitors, drugs that affect bone marrow and cell development in bone marrow (such as co-trimoxazole): Possibly severe leukopenia
allopurinol: Possibly increased therapeutic and adverse effects of azathioprine
anticoagulants: Possibly decreased anticoagulant action
cyclosporine: Possibly decreased blood cyclosporine level
methotrexate: Possibly increased blood level of azathioprine metabolite 6-mercaptopurine, which can lead to cell death
neuromuscular blockers: Possibly decreased or reversed action of neuromuscular blocker

Adverse Reactions
CNS: Fever, malaise
GI: Abdominal pain, diarrhea, hepatotoxicity (elevated liver function test results), nausea, pancreatitis, steatorrhea, vomiting
HEME: Leukopenia, macrocytic anemia, pancytopenia, thrombocytopenia
MS: Arthralgia, myalgia
SKIN: Alopecia, rash
Other: Infection, lymphomas and other neoplasms

Nursing Considerations
• Before I.V. administration, add 20 ml of sterile water for injection to azathioprine vial and swirl it until clear solution forms. The resulting drug concentration is 100 mg and can be diluted further, usually in normal saline solutin or D₅W, as prescribed. Calculate infusion rate based on final volume to be infused. Then administer over 30 to 60 minutes or as prescribed (from 5 minutes to 8 hours).
• Obtain results of baseline laboratory tests, including WBC, RBC, and platelet counts. Then expect to monitor results once a

week during first month of therapy, twice a month during second and third months of therapy, and once a month or more frequently thereafter.

• Be aware that hematologic reactions typically are dose-related and may occur late in therapy, especially in patients with transplant rejection.

• **WARNING** If WBC count decreases rapidly or remains significantly and consistently low, expect to reduce dosage or discontinue use of azathioprine.

• Periodically monitor liver function test results to detect early signs of hepatotoxicity.

• If patient develops thrombocytopenia, take bleeding precautions, such as avoiding I.M. injections and venipunctures, applying ice to areas of trauma, and checking I.V. infusion sites every 2 hours for bleeding.

• If patient also receives an oral anticoagulant, monitor his PT.

• Know that azathioprine therapy increases the risk of viral, fungal, bacterial, and protozoal infections. Monitor for signs of infection, such as fever, chills, sore throat, and mouth sores. Expect to administer aggressive antibiotic, antiviral, or other drug therapy and to reduce azathioprine dosage.

• Minimize risk of infection. If patient has severe leukopenia, take neutropenic precautions, such as placing him in a private room, limiting visitors, and screening visitors for communicable illnesses.

• If oral azathioprine causes GI upset, administer it in divided doses or with meals.

• Store parenteral form and tablets at 15° to 25° C (59° to 77° F). Keep in a dry place and protect from light.

PATIENT TEACHING

• Advise patient to take oral azathioprine with food or meals to minimize GI upset.

• **WARNING** Teach patient to recognize and report signs of infection, such as sore throat and fever.

• Teach patient how to reduce the risk of bleeding and how to maintain safety so that he doesn't fall.

azithromycin
Zithromax

Class and Category
Chemical: Azalide (subclass of macrolide)

Therapeutic: Antibiotic
Pregnancy category: B

Indications and Dosages

▶ *To treat community-acquired pneumonia*
I.V. INFUSION
Adults and adolescents age 16 or over. 500 mg I.V. as a single dose daily for at least 2 days, followed by 500 mg P.O. as a single dose daily until patient completes 7 to 10 days of therapy.
▶ *To prevent* Mycobacterium avium *complex in patients with advanced HIV infection*
I.V. INFUSION
Adults. 1.2 g once weekly, as indicated.
▶ *To treat pelvic inflammatory disease*
I.V. INFUSION
Adults. 500 mg I.V. as a single dose daily for 1 to 2 days, followed by 250 mg P.O. as a single dose daily until patient completes 7 days of therapy.

Mechanism of Action

Binds to a ribosomal subunit of susceptible bacteria, blocking peptide translocation and inhibiting RNA-dependent protein synthesis. Drug concentrates in phagocytes, macrophages, and fibroblasts, which release it slowly and may help move it to infection sites.

Incompatibilities

Don't add I.V. substances, additives, or drugs to azithromycin I.V. solution, and don't infuse them through the same I.V. line as azithromycin.

Contraindications

Hypersensitivity to azithromycin, to erythromycin, or to ketolide or macrolide antibiotics

Interactions

DRUGS
antacids that contain aluminum or magnesium: Possibly decreased peak blood azithromycin level, but extent of absorption is unchanged
carbamazepine, cyclosporine, phenytoin, terfenadine (drugs metabolized by cytochrome P-450 system): Possibly increased blood levels of these drugs

digoxin: Possibly increased blood digoxin level

dihydroergotamine, ergotamine: Possibly severe peripheral vasospasm and abnormal sensations (acute ergot toxicity)

HMG-CoA reductase inhibitors: Increased risk of severe myopathy or rhabdomyolysis

pimozide: Possibly sudden death

theophylline: Possibly increased blood theophylline level

triazolam: Possibly decreased excretion and increased therapeutic effects of triazolam

warfarin: Possibly increased anticoagulation

FOODS

food: Dramatically increased absorption rate of azithromycin

Adverse Reactions

CNS: Dizziness, fatigue, headache, somnolence, vertigo

CV: Chest pain, elevated serum CK level, palpitations, prolonged QT interval, torsades de pointes

EENT: Hearing loss, mucocutaneous candidiasis, tinnitus

ENDO: Hyperglycemia

GI: Abdominal pain, diarrhea, elevated liver function test results, nausea, pseudomembranous colitis, vomiting

GU: Elevated BUN and serum creatinine levels, nephritis, vaginal candidiasis

HEME: Leukopenia, neutropenia, thrombocytopenia

SKIN: Jaundice, photosensitivity, rash, Stevens-Johnson syndrome, toxic epidermal necrolysis, urticaria

Other: Allergic reaction, angioedema, elevated serum phosphorus level, hyperkalemia, infusion site reaction (such as pain and redness), superinfection

Nursing Considerations

- Obtain culture and sensitivity test results, if possible, before starting therapy.
- Use azithromycin cautiously in patients with hepatic dysfunction (because drug is metabolize in the liver) or renal dysfunction (because effects are unknown in this group).
- **WARNING** Don't give drug by I.V. bolus because it may cause erythema, pain, swelling, tenderness, or other reaction at the site. Infuse over 60 minutes or longer, as prescribed (typically 1 mg/ml over 3 hours or 2 mg/ml over 1 hour.)
- If hepatic function is impaired, monitor liver function studies because azithromycin is eliminated mainly by the liver.
- Assess patient for bacterial or fungal superinfection, which may

occur with prolonged or repeated therapy. If it occurs, expect to give another antibiotic or antifungal.

- Monitor bowel elimination; if needed, obtain stool culture to rule out pseudomembranous colitis. If it occurs, expect to stop azithromycin and give fluid, electrolytes, and antibiotics effective against *Clostridium difficile.*

PATIENT TEACHING
- Tell patient to immediately report evidence of allergic reactions, such as rash, itching, hives, chest tightness, and trouble breathing.
- Warn patient that abdominal pain and loose, watery stools may occur. If diarrhea persists or becomes severe, urge him to contact prescriber and replace fluids.
- Because azithromycin may destroy normal flora, teach patient to watch for and immediately report signs of superinfection, such as white patches in the mouth.

aztreonam

Azactam

Class and Category

Chemical: Monobactam
Therapeutic: Antibiotic
Pregnancy category: B

Indications and Dosages

▶ *To treat infections of the urinary tract, lower respiratory tract, skin, soft tissue, female reproductive tract; intra-abdominal infections; septicemia; and surgical abscesses caused by susceptible strains of gram-negative bacteria*

I.V. INFUSION, I.V. INJECTION

Adults. 0.5 to 2 g every 8 to 12 hr up to a maximum of 8 g daily. For life-threatening systemic infection, 2 g every 6 to 8 hr up to a maximum of 8 g daily.

Children ages 9 months to 16 years. 30 mg/kg every 6 to 8 hr up to 120 mg/kg daily; 50 mg/kg every 4 to 6 hr (for *Pseudomonas aeruginosa*).

DOSAGE ADJUSTMENT If creatinine clearance is 10 to 30 ml/min/1.73 m^2, initial dose is 1 to 2 g; then 50% of usual dose at usual interval. If creatinine clearance less than 10 ml/min/1.73 m^2, initial dose is 500 mg to 2 g; then 25% of the usual dose every 6, 8, or 12 hr.

Route	Onset	Peak	Duration
I.V. infusion, injection	Immediate	Immediate	Unknown

Mechanism of Action

Inhibits bacterial cell wall synthesis in susceptible aerobic gram-negative bacteria. These bacteria assemble rigid, cross-linked cell walls in several steps. Aztreonam affects the final cross-linking stage by inactivating penicillin-binding protein 3 (the enzyme that links cell wall strands), which causes cell lysis and death.

Incompatibilities

Don't mix aztreonam in same I.V. solution as cephradine, metronidazole, or nafcillin sodium. Don't mix it in same I.M. injection solution as local anesthetic.

Contraindications

Hypersensitivity to aztreonam or its components

Interactions

DRUGS

aminoglycosides (prolonged or high-dose therapy): Increased risk of nephrotoxicity and ototoxicity

cefoxitin, imipenem: Possibly antagonized action of aztreonam

furosemide, probenecid: Possibly increased blood aztreonam level

Adverse Reactions

CNS: Confusion, dizziness, fever, headache, insomnia, malaise, paresthesia, seizures, vertigo

CV: Chest pain, hypotension, transient ECG changes

EENT: Altered taste, diplopia, halitosis, mouth ulcers, mucocutaneous candidiasis, nasal congestion, sneezing, tinnitus, tongue numbness

GI: Abdominal cramps, diarrhea, elevated liver function test results, GI bleeding, hepatitis, nausea, pseudomembranous colitis, vomiting

GU: Breast tenderness, elevated serum creatinine level, vaginal candidiasis

HEME: Anemia, eosinophilia, leukocytosis, neutropenia, pancytopenia, positive Coombs' test, prolonged PT and APTT, thrombocytopenia, thrombocytosis

MS: Myalgia

RESP: Bronchospasm, dyspnea, wheezing

SKIN: Diaphoresis, erythema multiforme, exfoliative dermatitis, flushing, jaundice, petechiae, pruritus, purpura, rash, toxic epidermal necrolysis, urticaria
Other: Allergic reaction; injection site pain, phlebitis, swelling, or thrombophlebitis

Nursing Considerations

- Obtain culture and sensitivity test results, if possible, before initiating therapy. If patient is acutely ill, expect to begin therapy before results are available.
- Keep in mind that other antimicrobials may be used with aztreonam in seriously ill patients at risk for gram-positive infection.
- Expect to use I.V. route for patients who need single doses over 1 g and those with life-threatening systemic infections, such as septicemia or peritonitis.
- To reconstitute aztreonam for I.V. bolus injection, use sterile water for injection.
- Immediately after adding diluent to vial, shake it vigorously to mix. After obtaining correct dose, discard unused solution.
- Be aware that reconstituted solution may turn light pink on standing at room temperature. This doesn't affect drug potency.
- Administer I.V. bolus injection directly into I.V. tubing over 3 to 5 minutes.
- **WARNING** When preparing aztreonam for I.V. infusion, use at least 50 ml of appropriate infusion solution per gram of aztreonam. Further dilute drug in I.V. solution, such as normal saline, D_5W, D_5/normal saline, lactated Ringer's, or Ringer's solution.
- Know that I.V. infusion may be administered over 20 to 60 minutes.
- Flush I.V. tubing with solution, such as normal saline solution, before and after administering I.V. infusion to reduce risk of incompatibilities.
- If prescribed, mix aztreonam in same I.V. solution with other antibiotics (such as ampicillin sodium, cefazolin sodium, clindamycin phosphate, gentamicin sulfate, or tobramycin sulfate), or mix it with cloxacillin sodium and vancomycin hydrochloride in peritoneal dialysis solution.
- Prepare solution for I.M. injection using sterile or bacteriostatic water or sodium chloride for injection. Administer injection deep into large muscle, such as in dorsogluteal or ventrogluteal area.

- Assess patient for signs of bacterial or fungal superinfection, which may occur with prolonged or repeated therapy. If superinfection occurs, treat it as prescribed.
- Monitor bowel elimination; if needed, obtain stool culture to rule out pseudomembranous colitis. If this adverse reaction occurs, expect to discontinue aztreonam and administer fluid, electrolytes, and antibiotics that are effective against Clostridium difficile.
- Evaluate patient's renal and liver function test results, as ordered, if the patient has renal or hepatic impairment.
- Monitor renal function if patient is receiving an aminoglycoside because of the increased risk of nephrotoxicity.

PATIENT TEACHING

- Stress the importance of taking the full course of aztreonam exactly as prescribed, even if the patient feels better before finishing it.
- Teach patient to recognize and immediately report signs and symptoms of allergic reactions, such as chest tightness, difficulty breathing, hives, itching, and rash.
- Urge patient to report watery, bloody stools to prescriber immediately, even up to 2 months after drug therapy has ended.
- Because aztreonam may destroy normal flora, teach patient to watch for and immediately report signs of superinfection, such as white patches in mouth.

B

basiliximab
Simulect

Class and Category
Chemical: Chimeric (murine or human) monoclonal antibody
Therapeutic: Immunosuppressant
Pregnancy category: B

Indications and Dosages
▶ *To prevent acute kidney transplant rejection*
I.V. INFUSION, I.V. INJECTION
Adults and adolescents over age 15. 20 mg within 2 hr before
transplant, then 20 mg 4 days after transplant.
Children and adolescents ages 2 to 15. 12 mg/m^2 within 2 hr
before transplant; then 12 mg/m^2 4 days after transplant. *Maximum:* 20 mg/dose.

Route	Onset	Peak	Duration
I.V.	Unknown	Unknown	22 to 50 days

Mechanism of Action
Initiates immunosuppression by blocking interleukin-2 receptors located on
the surface of activated T cells. Normally, interleukin-2 is released by stimulated T lymphocytes, causing activation and differentiation of other T lymphocytes responsible for cell-mediated immunity.

Incompatibilities
Don't add or infuse any other drugs simultaneously through same
I.V. line as basiliximab.

Contraindications
Hypersensitivity to basiliximab or its components

Interactions
None known.

Adverse Reactions

CNS: Asthenia, dizziness, fever, headache, insomnia, tremor
CV: Hypertension, peripheral edema
EENT: Oral candidiasis, pharyngitis, rhinitis
ENDO: Hyperglycemia
GI: Abdominal pain, constipation, diarrhea, indigestion, nausea, vomiting
GU: Dysuria, increased urinary nitrogen level, UTI
HEME: Anemia
MS: Back pain, leg pain
RESP: Cough, dyspnea, upper respiratory tract infection
SKIN: Acne
Other: Hypercholesterolemia, hyperkalemia, hyperuricemia, hypocalcemia, hypokalemia, hypophosphatemia, impaired wound healing, metabolic acidosis, weight gain

Nursing Considerations

- To reconstitute basiliximab, add 5 ml sterile water for injection to powder and shake vial gently to dissolve. Further dilute with normal saline or D_5W for infusion to a volume of 50 ml. Gently invert infusion bag to avoid foaming; don't shake. Drug should appear clear to opalescent and colorless. Don't use if you detect particles.
- Give reconstituted drug as a bolus dose directly through a central or peripheral I.V. line, or give the diluted solution I.V. over 20 to 30 minutes. Be aware that bolus dose may cause nausea, vomiting, and a localized injection site reaction, including pain.
- Monitor blood pressure, heart rate, and respiratory status during drug administration and for a brief period thereafter.
- Expect togive drug with cyclosporine and corticosteroids.
- Don't store reconstituted drug at room temperature for longer than 4 hours; don't refrigerate it for longer than 24 hours.
- **WARNING** Be aware that patient may develop hypersensitivity reactions, including anaphylaxis, bronchospasm, dyspnea, hypotension, pruritus, rash, respiratory failure, sneezing, tachycardia, urticaria, and wheezing, on initial exposure or following re-exposure after several months. Notify prescriber immediately if such reactions occur.
- Store unreconstituted drug at 2° to 8° C (36° to 46° F).
PATIENT TEACHING
- Inform patient that second dose of basiliximab will be given 4 days after transplant and that she may also receive cyclosporine and corticosteroid therapy.

• Inform patient that because of drug's immunosuppressant effects, she may experience slower wound healing and be more susceptible to upper respiratory tract infections.

benzquinamide hydrochloride
Emete-Con

Class and Category
Chemical: Benzoquinolizine amide
Therapeutic: Antiemetic
Pregnancy category: Not rated

Indications and Dosages
▶ *To treat nausea and vomiting related to anesthesia or surgery*
I.V. OR I.M. INJECTION
Adults. 25 mg or 0.2 to 0.4 mg/kg by slow infusion (1 ml every 0.5 to 1 min) as a single dose, followed by I.M. doses. Or 50 mg or 0.5 to 1 mg/kg I.M., repeated in 1 hr; then every 3 to 4 hr, p.r.n.

Route	Onset	Peak	Duration
I.V.	15 min	Unknown	Unknown

Mechanism of Action
Exhibits antiemetic, antihistaminic, mild cholinergic, and sedative effects by unknown mechanism.

Contraindications
Hypersensitivity to benzquinamide or its components

Interactions
DRUGS
vasopressors: Increased hypertensive effects

Adverse Reactions
CNS: Chills, dizziness, drowsiness, excitement, fatigue, fever, headache, insomnia, nervousness, restlessness, tremor, weakness
CV: Atrial fibrillation, hypertension, hypotension, premature atrial or ventricular contractions
EENT: Blurred vision, dry mouth, increased salivation
GI: Anorexia, hiccups, nausea
MS: Muscle twitching

SKIN: Diaphoresis, flushing, rash, urticaria

Nursing Considerations

- **WARNING** Avoid I.V. route when administering benzquin-amide to patients with cardiovascular disease because sudden blood pressure increases and transient arrhythmias may occur. Use I.V. route only for patients without cardiovascular disease who aren't receiving a preanesthetic or cardiovascular drug.
- Reconstitute drug with 2.2 ml of sterile water or bacteriostatic water for injection containing benzyl alcohol or methylparaben and propylparaben to yield 2 ml of a 25-mg/ml solution.
- Take safety precautions to reduce the risk of injury from CNS depression.
- Store reconstituted drug at room temperature. Solution retains potency for 14 days.

PATIENT TEACHING

- Advise patient to stay in bed after receiving benzquinamide and to call for assistance to reduce the risk of injury.
- Instruct patient to report whether nausea and vomiting have been relieved.

benztropine mesylate

Apo-Benztropine (CAN), Cogentin, PMS Benztropine (CAN)

Class and Category

Chemical: Tertiary amine
Therapeutic: Antidyskinetic, central-acting anticholinergic
Pregnancy category: C

Indications and Dosages

▶ *As adjunct to treat all forms of Parkinson's disease*
I.V. INJECTION, TABLETS
Adults with Parkinson's disease. 1 to 2 mg daily (usual dose) with a range of 0.5 to 6 mg daily.
Adults with idiopathic Parkinson's disease. *Initial:* 0.5 to 1 mg at bedtime. *Maximum:* 4 to 6 mg daily.
Adults with postencephalitic Parkinson's disease. 2 mg daily in one or more doses; may begin with 0.5 mg at bedtime and increase as needed.

▶ *To control extrapyramidal symptoms (except tardive dyskinesia) caused by phenothiazines and other neuroleptic drugs*
I.V. OR I.M. INJECTION
Adults. 1 to 4 mg once or twice daily.

▶ *To treat acute dystonic reactions*
I.V. OR I.M. INJECTION
Adults. *Initial:* 1 to 2 ml (1 to 2 mg total dose) I.V. or I.M. *Maintenance:* 1 to 2 mg P.O. b.i.d. to prevent recurrence.

Route	Onset	Peak	Duration
I.V., I.M	15 min	Unknown	24 hr
P.O.	1 to 2 hr	Unknown	24 hr

Mechanism of Action

Blocks acetylcholine's action at cholinergic receptor sites. This action restores the normal balance of dopamine and acetylcholine in the brain, which relaxes muscle movement and decreases drooling, rigidity, and tremor. Benztropine also may inhibit dopamine reuptake and storage, which prolongs dopamine's action.

Contraindications

Achalasia, bladder neck obstruction, glaucoma, hypersensitivity to benztropine mesylate or its components, megacolon, myasthenia gravis, prostatic hypertrophy, pyloric or duodenal obstruction, stenosing peptic ulcer

Interactions

DRUGS
amantadine: Possibly increased adverse anticholinergic effects
digoxin: Possibly increased blood digoxin level
haloperidol: Possibly increased schizophrenic symptoms, decreased serum haloperidol level, and development of tardive dyskinesia
levodopa: Possibly decreased levodopa effectiveness
phenothiazines: Possibly reduced phenothiazine effects and increased psychiatric symptoms

Adverse Reactions

CNS: Agitation, confusion, delirium, delusions, depression, disorientation, dizziness, drowsiness, euphoria, excitement, fever, hallucinations, headache, light-headedness, listlessness, memory loss, nervousness, paranoia, psychosis, weakness
CV: Hypotension, mild bradycardia, orthostatic hypotension, palpitations, tachycardia
EENT: Angle-closure glaucoma, blurred vision, diplopia, dry mouth, increased intraocular pressure, mydriasis, suppurative parotitis

GI: Constipation, duodenal ulcer, epigastric distress, ileus, nausea, vomiting
GU: Dysuria, urinary hesitancy, urine retention
MS: Muscle spasms, muscle weakness
SKIN: Decreased sweating, dermatoses, flushing, rash, urticaria

Nursing Considerations

- Expect to administer I.V. or I.M. benztropine when patient needs more rapid response than oral drug can provide. Be aware that I.M. route is commonly used because it provides effects in about the same time as I.V. route. Watch for improvement a few minutes after administration. If parkinsonian symptoms reappear, expect to repeat dose.
- Know that therapy generally begins with a low dose followed by gradual increases of 0.5 mg every 5 or 6 days because benztropine has a cumulative action.
- Assess muscle rigidity and tremor as a baseline. Then monitor them frequently for improvement, which indicates the effectiveness of benztropine.
- Administer benztropine before or after meals based on patient's need and response. If the patient has increased salivary secretions, expect to administer benztropine after meals. If patient has dry mouth, plan to give drug before meals unless nausea develops.
- **WARNING** When administering benztropine to patient with drug-induced extrapyramidal reactions, be alert for exacerbation of psychiatric symptoms.
- Know that high-dose benztropine therapy may cause weakness and inability to move specific muscle groups. If this occurs, expect to reduce benztropine dosage.
- Store drug at 15° to 30° C (59° to 86° F). Don't freeze.

PATIENT TEACHING
- Warn patient that benztropine has a cumulative effect, increasing her risk of adverse reactions and overdose.
- Caution patient to avoid driving and similar activities until the effects of benztropineare known because drug may cause blurred vision, dizziness, and drowsiness.
- **WARNING** Because benztropine decreases sweating, urge patient to avoid extremely hot or humid conditions to reduce the risk of heatstroke and severe hyperthermia. This is especially important for elderly patients and those who abuse alcohol or have chronic illnesses or CNS disorders.
- Explain to the patient the need to have eye examinations and

intraocular pressure measurements periodically because ben-ztropine may cause angle-closure glaucoma and increase intraocular pressure.

betamethasone sodium phosphate

Betnesol (CAN), Celestone Phosphate, Selestoject

Class and Category

Chemical: Synthetic glucocorticoid
Therapeutic: Anti-inflammatory
Pregnancy category: C

Indications and Dosages

▶ *To treat conditions accompanied by severe inflammation and conditions requiring immunosuppression*

I.V. INJECTION (BETAMETHASONE SODIUM PHOSPHATE)

Adults. *Initial:* Variable (given in emergency situations or when oral therapy isn't possible). *Maximum:* 9 mg daily.

▶ *To treat bursitis, gouty arthritis, osteoarthritis, periostitis of cuboid, peritendinitis, rheumatoid arthritis, skin lesions, tenosynovitisintra-articular, intrabursal, or intradermal injection (betamethasone acetate-betamethasone sodium phosphate)*

Adults with bursitis, peritendinitis, or tenosynovitis. 1 ml by intrabursal or intra-articular injection. Three or four injections given every 1 to 2 wk.

Adults with osteoarthritis or rheumatoid arthritis. 0.5 to 2 ml, depending on joint size.

Adults with foot bursitis. 0.25 to 0.5 ml every 3 to 7 days.

Adults with foot tenosynovitis or periostitis of cuboid. 0.5 ml every 3 to 7 days.

Adults with acute gouty arthritis. 0.5 to 1 ml every 3 to 7 days.

Adults with skin lesions. 0.2 ml/cm^2 intradermally, up to 1 ml weekly.

DOSAGE ADJUSTMENT Dosage reduced for elderly patients and accompanied by periodic monitoring of blood pressure and blood glucose and electrolyte levels.

Route	Onset	Peak	Duration
I.V.	Rapid	Unknown	Unknown
Other	Unknown	Unknown	1 to 2 wk*

* For intra-arterial or intrasynovial injection; 1 week for intralesional injection in soft tissue.

Mechanism of Action

Binds to intracellular glucocorticoid receptors and suppresses inflammatory and immune responses by:

- inhibiting neutrophil and monocyte accumulation at inflammation site and suppressing their phagocytic and bactericidal activity
- stabilizing lysosomal membranes
- suppressing antigen response of macrophages and helper T cells
- inhibiting synthesis of inflammatory response mediators, such as cytokines, interleukins, and prostaglandins.

Contraindications

Live virus vaccination, systemic fungal infection

Interactions

DRUGS

anticholinesterase drugs: Possibly antagonized anticholinesterase effects in myasthenia gravis

barbiturates: Possibly decreased effects of betamethasone

cyclosporine: Possibly increased risk of cyclosporine toxicity

digitalis glycosides: Possibly increased risk of digitalis toxicity

estrogens: Possibly decreased excretion of betamethasone

hydantoins, rifampin: Possibly increased excretion and decreased therapeutic effects of betamethasone

insulin, oral antidiabetics: Possibly increased blood glucose level

isoniazid: Possibly decreased blood isoniazid level

ketoconazole: Possibly decreased excretion of betamethasone

oral anticoagulants: Possibly increased or decreased action of anticoagulants, requiring adjusted anticoagulant dosage

oral contraceptives: Possibly increased half-life and concentration and decreased excretion of betamethasone

potassium-wasting diuretics: Increased risk of hypokalemia

salicylates: Possibly decreased blood level and therapeutic effects of salicylates

somatrem: Possibly inhibition of somatrem's growth-promoting effects

theophyllines: Possibly changes in effects of both drugs

Adverse Reactions

CNS: Fatigue, headache, increased ICP with papilledema, insomnia, malaise, neuritis, paresthesia, seizures, steroid psychosis, syncope, vertigo

CV: Arrhythmias, ECG changes, fat embolism, heart failure, hypertension, thromboembolism, thrombophlebitis

EENT: Cataracts, exophthalmos, glaucoma, increased intraocular pressure

ENDO: Cushingoid symptoms (buffalo hump, central obesity, decreased carbohydrate tolerance, fat pad enlargement, moon face), fluid retention, growth suppression in children, hyperglycemia, negative nitrogen balance, secondary adrenocortical and pituitary unresponsiveness (in times of stress)

GI: Abdominal distention, increased appetite, nausea, pancreatitis, peptic ulcer (possibly with perforation), ulcerative esophagitis, vomiting

GU: Amenorrhea, glycosuria, menstrual irregularities

HEME: Leukocytosis

MS: Aseptic necrosis of femoral and humeral heads, loss of muscle mass, muscle weakness, osteoporosis, spontaneous pathologic and vertebral compression fractures, tendon rupture

RESP: Bronchospasm

SKIN: Acneiform lesions, allergic dermatitis, ecchymosis, facial erythema, hirsutism, impaired wound healing, increased sweating, petechiae, lupuslike lesions, purpura, rash, subcutaneous fat atrophy, thin and fragile skin, urticaria

Other: Anaphylaxis, angioedema, hypocalcemia, hypokalemia, sodium retention, suppressed reaction to skin tests, weight gain

Nursing Considerations

- If patient has spent time in the tropics or has unexplained diarrhea, make sure latent or active amebiasis has been ruled out before betamethasone therapy starts because drug may cause condition to worsen.
- **WARNING** Administer betamethasone with extreme caution in patients with known or suspected Strongylides (threadworm) infestation because drug-induced immunosuppression may lead to Strongylides hyperinfection and dissemination with widespread larval migration. Severe enterocolitis and life-threatening gram-negative septicemia may follow.
- Expect prescriber to order baseline ophthalmic examination before initiating therapy because prolonged betamethasone use may lead to increased intraocular pressure, glaucoma, and subsequent optic nerve damage. Use betamethasone cautiously in patients with ocular herpes simplex because corneal perforation may occur.
- Assess for signs of infection before administering betamethasone because drug may mask those signs. Because drug may cause

immunosuppression, new infection may develop during therapy. If so, expect to administer appropriate antibiotic.

- Review serum electrolyte levels, as ordered, before initiating therapy. Monitor these levels often during therapy to detect imbalances. Sodium and water retention and potassium and calcium depletion may occur with high-dose betamethasone therapy. If so, expect to restrict sodium intake and provide potassium and calcium supplements.

- Because betamethasone is linked to peptic ulcer formation, expect to administer it with an antacid or H_2-receptor blocker.

- **WARNING** Monitor ECG tracings for arrhythmias, and evaluate patient for anaphylactic reactions, such as angioedema and seizures, which have been associated with rapid I.V. administration of high-dose corticosteroids.

- **WARNING** During long-term betamethasone therapy, assess for signs of adrenal suppression and insufficiency (fatigue, hypotension, lassitude, nausea, vomiting, and weakness) when patient is exposed to stress. If she exhibits these signs, notify prescriber at once.

- Watch for evidence of steroid psychosis, such as delirium, clouded sensorium, euphoria, insomnia, mood swings, personality changes, and severe depression, which may develop 15 to 30 days after therapy begins. Be prepared to discontinue therapy. If this isn't possible, expect to give psychotropic drugs.

- After intra-articular injection, assess joint for marked increase in pain, local swelling, and more restricted movement. If patient also develops fever and malaise, suspect septic arthritis and notify prescriber immediately. Expect to assist with joint fluid aspiration to confirm septic arthritis.

- Monitor patient for cushingoid signs and symptoms, such as moon face, buffalo hump, central obesity, striae, acne, ecchymosis, and weight gain. Notify prescriber if they occur.

PATIENT TEACHING

- Reinforce signs of adrenal insufficiency and possible need for dosage increases during stress. Advise patient to notify prescriber immediately if signs of insufficiency occur or if she's exposed to stress.

- Instruct patient to avoid exposure to infections because drug can cause immunosuppression. Also teach patient to recognize and immediately report signs of infection.

- After intra-articular injection, advise patient not to overuse joint and to continue other treatments such as physical therapy.

biperiden lactate
Akineton Lactate

Class and Category
Chemical: Tertiary amine
Therapeutic: Anticholinergic, antidyskinetic
Pregnancy category: C

Indications and Dosages
▶ *To control extrapyramidal symptoms (except tardive dyskinesia) caused by phenothiazines and other neuroleptic drugs*
I.V. INJECTION
Adults. 2 mg repeated every 30 min until symptoms resolve or maximum of four consecutive doses in 24 hr is reached.

Route	Onset	Peak	Duration
I.V.	15 min	Unknown	1 to 8 hr

Mechanism of Action
Blocks acetylcholine's action at cholinergic receptor sites. This action restores a normal balance of dopamine and acetylcholine in the brain, which relaxes muscle movement and decreases rigidity and tremors. Biperiden also may inhibit dopamine reuptake and storage, which prolongs dopamine action.

Contraindications
Achalasia, angle-closure glaucoma, bladder neck obstruction, bowel obstruction, hypersensitivity to biperiden, myasthenia gravis, prostatic hypertrophy, pyloric or duodenal obstruction, stenosing peptic ulcer, toxic megacolon

Interactions
DRUGS
amantadine: Possibly increased adverse anticholinergic effects
digoxin: Possibly increased serum digoxin level
haloperidol: Possibly increased schizophrenic symptoms, decreased serum haloperidol level, and development of tardive dyskinesia
levodopa: Possibly decreased levodopa effectiveness
phenothiazines: Possibly reduced phenothiazine effects and increased psychiatric symptoms

Adverse Reactions
CNS: Agitation, confusion, delirium, delusions, depression, disori-

entation, dizziness, drowsiness, euphoria, excitement, fever, hallucinations, headache, light-headedness, listlessness, memory loss, nervousness, paranoia, psychosis, weakness

CV: Hypotension, mild bradycardia, orthostatic hypotension, palpitations, tachycardia

EENT: Angle-closure glaucoma, blurred vision, diplopia, dry mouth, increased intraocular pressure, mydriasis, photosensitivity, suppurative parotitis

GI: Constipation, ileus, nausea, vomiting

GU: Dysuria, urinary hesitancy, urine retention

MS: Muscle spasms, muscle weakness

SKIN: Decreased sweating, dermatoses, flushing, rash, urticaria

Nursing Considerations
- Expect to give I.V. biperiden when patient needs more rapid response than oral drug can provide. It also may be given I.M.
- Obtain baseline blood pressure and heart rate. Monitor patient for hypotension and other CV effects, and help patient change position as needed.
- Assess muscle rigidity and tremor at baseline, and monitor them often for improvement, which indicates drug effectiveness.
- Inspect solution for particles and discoloration before use.
- Administer I.V. biperiden slowly.
- **WARNING** Be alert for exacerbation of psychiatric symptoms during biperiden therapy.
- Store drug at 15° to 30° C (59° to 86° F) and protect from light. Don't freeze.

PATIENT TEACHING
- Teach patient about possible adverse effects of biperiden, including CNS effects. Advise her to report such symptoms as dizziness, depression, confusion, rash, vision changes, and eye pain to her prescriber.
- Instruct patient to avoid sudden position changes.
- Inform patient that she may experience increased eye sensitivity to light during biperiden therapy.

bivalirudin
Angiomax

Class and Category
Chemical: Hirudin analogue
Therapeutic: Anticoagulant
Pregnancy category: B

Indications and Dosages

▶ *As adjunct to provide anticoagulation and prevent thrombosis in patients with unstable angina who are having percutaneous transluminal coronary angioplasty or percutaneous coronary intervention; to provide anticoagulation and prevent thrombosis in patients with or at risk of heparin-induced thrombocytopenia or heparin-induced thrombocytopenia thrombosis syndrome who are having percutaneous coronary intervention*

I.V. INFUSION

Adults. *Initial:* Immediately before angioplasty, 0.75-mg/kg bolus followed by 1.75 mg/kg/hr as a continuous infusion for duration of procedure. Five minutes after bolus dose and while continuous infusion is running, additional 0.3-mg/kg dose may be given if needed. After procedure, 1.75 mg/kg/hr may be given for 4 hr by continuous infusion, followed by 0.2 mg/kg/hr for up to 20 hr if needed.

DOSAGE ADJUSTMENT Infusion dosage possibly reduced to 1 mg/kg/hr for patients with severe renal impairment (glomerular filtration rate of 10 to 29 ml/min) and to 0.25 mg/ kg/hr for dialysis-dependent patients.

Route	Onset	Peak	Duration
I.V.	Immediate	Unknown	1 hr after end of infusion

Mechanism of Action

Selectively binds to thrombin, including thrombin trapped in established clots. Without thrombin, fibrinogen can't convert to fibrin and clots can't form.

Incompatibilities

Don't mix any other drugs in same I.V. line before or during bivalirudin administration. Mixing with alteplase, amiodarone, amphotericin B, chlorpromazine HCL, diazepam, prochlorperazine edisylate, reteplase, streptokinase, and vancomycin HCL can result in haze, particulate formation, or precipitation.

Contraindications

Active major bleeding, hypersensitivity to bivalirudin or its components

Interactions

DRUGS

alteplase, antineoplastic drugs, antithymocyte globulin, heparin, NSAIDs, platelet inhibitors, reteplase, streptokinase, strontium chloride Sr 89, warfarin: Risk of bleeding

porfimer: Possibly decreased efficacy of porfimer photodynamic therapy

salicylates: Increased risk of hypoprothrombinemia and bleeding

Adverse Reactions

CNS: Headache, intracranial hemorrhage

CV: Hypotension, thrombosis

EENT: Bleeding from mouth, epistaxis

GI: Abdominal cramps, diarrhea, GI or retroperitoneal bleeding, nausea, vomiting

GU: Hematuria, vaginal bleeding

HEME: Severe bleeding, thrombocytopenia

MS: Back pain

RESP: Hemoptysis, hemothorax

SKIN: Ecchymosis

Other: Anaphylaxis, injection site bleeding, hematoma, or pain

Nursing Considerations

- To reconstitute bivalirudin, add 5 ml of sterile water for injection to each 250-mg vial and swirl gently until dissolved. For initial infusion, dilute each reconstituted vial in 50 ml of D_5W or normal saline solution to yield 5 mg/ml.
- For subsequent low-rate infusion, further dilute reconstituted drug in 500 ml of D_5W or normal saline solution to a final concentration of 0.5 mg/ml.
- Expect to give patient 300 to 325 mg of aspirin P.O. daily, as prescribed, during bivalirudin therapy.
- **WARNING** Expect to monitor blood coagulation tests before and regularly during therapy because bleeding is a major risk of bivalirudin therapy.
- **WARNING** Monitor patient often for evidence of bleeding because no antidote for bivalirudin is available. If life-threatening bleeding occurs, notify prescriber immediately, stop drug, and prepare to monitor APTT and other coagulation tests as ordered. Be aware that blood transfusions may be needed. Patients with an increased risk of bleeding include females with active menstruation; patients with vascular or organ abnormalities, such as severe uncontrolled hypertension, advanced renal disease, infective endocarditis, dissecting aortic aneurysm, diverticulitis, hemophilia, hepatic disease (especially from a deficiency in vitamin K–dependent clotting factors), inflammatory bowel disease, or peptic ulcer disease;

and those who have recently had a CVA, major surgery (including eye, brain, or spinal cord surgery), large vessel or lumbar puncture, organ biopsy, spinal anesthesia, or major bleeding (including intracranial, GI, intraocular, retroperitoneal, or pulmonary bleeding).

• If patient is receiving gamma brachytherapy, watch closely for evidence of thrombosis (weak or absent pulse, pallor, pain) because drug may increase the risk in these patients.

• If possible, avoid I.M. injections to decrease the risk of bleeding.

• Discard any unused portion of drug.

PATIENT TEACHING

• Inform patient that bivalirudin is a blood thinner used only in the hospital setting.

• Instruct patient to check her skin for bruising or red spots and to immediately report back or stomach pain, difficulty breathing, dizziness or fainting, and unusual bleeding, such as black or tarry stools, blood in urine, coughing up blood, heavy menstrual bleeding, or nosebleeds. Drug may need to be discontinued.

• Urge patient to avoid injury while receiving bivalirudin—for example, by brushing her teeth gently using a soft-bristled toothbrush.

• Caution patient not to take anti-inflammatory drugs, such as ibuprofen, naproxen, ketoprofen, aspirin, and aspirin-like products, or other blood thinners, such as warfarin, while receiving bivalirudin unless prescriber instructs her to do so.

bleomycin sulfate

Blenoxane

Class and Category

Chemical: Cytotoxic glycopeptide antibiotic mixture
Therapeutic: Antineoplastic antibiotic
Pregnancy category: D

Indications and Dosages

▶ *To treat squamous cell carcinoma of the head and neck (including mouth, tongue, tonsil, sinus, palate, lip, buccal mucosa, gingiva, epiglottis, nasopharynx, oropharynx, and larynx), skin, penis, cervix, and vulva; non-Hodgkin's lymphomas; and testicular carcinoma*

I.V. INJECTION

Adults and adolescents. 0.25 to 0.5 units/kg or 10 to 20 units/m^2 over at least 10 min once or twice a week.

▶ *To treat Hodgkin's disease*

I.V. INJECTION

Adults and adolescents. *Initial:* 0.25 to 0.5 units/kg or 10 to 20 units/m² over at least 10 min once or twice a week. *Maintenance:* 1 unit daily or 5 units weekly if 50% response occurs. Each dose should be administered over at least 10 min.

DOSAGE ADJUSTMENT Patients with Hodgkin's disease or non-Hodgkin's lymphoma are given a test dose of 2 units or less for the first two doses because of possible anaphylactoid reaction. For patients with impaired renal function (regardless of indication), dosage decreased to 50% of normal dose if serum creatinine level is 1.5 to 2 mg/dl; to 25% of normal dose if serum creatinine level is 2.5 to 4 mg/dl; to 20% of normal dose if serum creatinine level is 4 to 6 mg/dl; and to 5% to 10% of normal dose if serum creatinine level is 6 to 10 mg/dl.

Mechanism of Action

May inhibit cell's ability to replicate or reproduce by inhibiting DNA synthesis and, to a lesser extent, RNA and protein synthesis. Bleomycin is effective against both cycling and noncycling cells, but it appears to be most effective in the G_2 phase of cell division.

Incompatibilities

Don't mix bleomycin with D_5W or other solutions containing dextrose to avoid a loss in potency.

Contraindications

Hypersensitivity or a history of idiosyncratic reaction to bleomycin

Interactions

DRUGS

antineoplastics: Increased risk of pulmonary and mucosal toxicity and bone marrow depression

cisplatin: Increased risk of bleomycin toxicity due to bleomycin accumulation

digoxin: Decreased blood digoxin level

general anesthetics: Increased risk of pulmonary deterioration and fibrosis

live virus vaccines: Severe and possibly fatal infections

phenytoin: Decreased blood phenytoin level

vincristine: Increased therapeutic effect of bleomycin

Adverse Reactions

CNS: Chills, fever

CV: Pleuropericarditis, Raynaud's phenomenon, vascular toxicity (cerebral arteritis, CVA, MI, thrombotic microangiopathy), vasospasm (when used in combination with vinblastine for testicular cancer)

EENT: Stomatitis

GI: Anorexia, elevated liver function test results, hepatotoxicity, vomiting

GU: Cystitis, elevated BUN and serum creatinine levels, hematuria

HEME: Decreased hemoglobin level, leukopenia, thrombocytopenia

RESP: Pneumonitis progressing to pulmonary fibrosis, pulmonary toxicity (decreased diffusion capacity, lung volume, and vital capacity; dyspnea; crackles)

SKIN: Alopecia, erythema, hyperkeratosis, hyperpigmentation, mucocutaneous toxicity, nail changes, rash, skin tenderness, striae, vesiculation

Other: Idiosyncratic reaction (chills, fever, hypotension, confusion, faintness, wheezing), injection site phlebitis, tumor site pain, weight loss

Nursing Considerations

- Be aware that bleomycin should be administered only under the supervision of a qualified physician where appropriate diagnostic and treatment facilities are available.
- Follow facility protocols for preparation and handling of antineoplastic drugs and appropriate disposal of used equipment.
- Add 5 or 10 ml of sodium chloride for injection to a 15-unit or 30-unit vial of bleomycin.
- Store reconstituted bleomycin at room temperature and use within 24 hours.
- Be aware that premedication with acetaminophen, steroids, and diphenhydramine may be administered to reduce the risk of anaphylaxis and drug-induced fever.
- Expect pulmonary function tests and chest X-rays to be ordered before initiation of therapy to establish patient's baseline pulmonary status.
- **WARNING** Monitor patient's respiratory status, including auscultation and evaluation of breathing patterns during and after therapy, to assist with early detection of pulmonary toxicity. This complication occurs in about 10% of patients receiving bleomycin, especially elderly patients, those who have received cytotoxic drugs, those who are receiving bleomycin in combination with other antineoplastics, those

receiving oxygen therapy during and after surgery, smokers, and patients receiving a total dose greater than 400 units. Expect drug to be discontinued if pulmonary changes are detected. Be aware that pulmonary symptoms can occur up to 1 month after therapy ends.

- Be aware that patients who have been treated with radiation therapy are at increased risk for pulmonary and mucocutaneous toxicity and bone marrow depression.
- **WARNING** Be aware that patients with lymphoma may develop a severe idiosyncratic reaction (chills, fever, hypotension, confusion, faintness, and wheezing) similar to anaphylaxis, especially after first or second dose. This reaction may occur immediately or several hours after dose is given. Notify prescriber immediately if such a reaction occurs. Expect to give antihistamines, corticosteroids, pressor agents, and volume expanders, as prescribed.
- Obtain BUN and serum creatinine levels before starting therapy, and monitor patient for signs and symptoms of declining renal function during therapy, especially if patient has significant renal function impairment.
- Monitor for elevated liver function test results, which may indicate drug-induced hepatotoxicity.
- Monitor patient for signs of adverse skin and mucous membrane effects, which occur in 25% to 50% of patients undergoing bleomycin therapy, usually 2 or 3 weeks after administration of 150 to 200 units.
- Be aware that fraction of inspired oxygen (FIO_2) is maintained at 25%—approximately that of room air—during and after surgery to reduce the risk of pulmonary complications. Expect fluid replacement to be colloid rather than crystalloid.
- Store unreconstituted vials at 2° to 8° C (36° to 46° F).

PATIENT TEACHING
- Teach patient about adverse reactions related to bleomycin, and advise her to immediately report any that occur.
- Stress the need for periodic chest X-rays, which may be ordered every 1 to 2 weeks, to detect adverse pulmonary reactions.
- Advise patient to inform all health care providers, including dentists, that she is receiving bleomycin.
- Encourage patient to maintain good oral hygiene and adequate nutritional intake. If she develops stomatitis, suggest that she try eating bland, soft foods served cold or at room temperature to decrease irritation.

bretylium tosylate

Bretylate (CAN), Bretylol

Class and Category

Chemical: Bromobenzyl quaternary ammonium compound
Therapeutic: Class III antiarrhythmic
Pregnancy category: C

Indications and Dosages

▶ *To prevent and treat ventricular fibrillation and to treat life-threatening ventricular arrhythmias that don't respond to first-line antiarrhythmics, such as lidocaine*

I.V. INFUSION, I.V. INJECTION

Adults with immediate life-threatening ventricular arrhythmias. *Initial:* 5 mg/kg undiluted by rapid I.V. injection; if ventricular fibrillation persists, 10 mg/kg repeated as often as needed. *Continuous suppression:* 1 to 2 mg/min or 5 to 10 mg/kg of diluted I.V. solution infused over at least 8 min every 6 hr.

Adults with other ventricular arrhythmias. *Initial:* 5 to 10 mg/kg of diluted I.V. solution infused over at least 8 min and repeated every 1 to 2 hr if arrhythmia continues. *Maintenance:* 5 to 10 mg/kg diluted I.V. solution infused over at least 8 min every 6 hr, or 1 to 2 mg/min infused continuously.

DOSAGE ADJUSTMENT Dosing interval increased for patients with impaired renal function because bretylium is excreted primarily by kidneys.

Route	Onset	Peak	Duration
I.V.	5 to 10 min*	6 to 9 hr	6 to 24 hr

Contraindications

Digitalis toxicity, hypersensitivity to bretylium

Interactions

DRUGS

catecholamines (such as dopamine and norepinephrine): Increased vasopressor effects of catecholamines
digoxin: Possibly worsening of digitalis toxicity

Adverse Reactions

CNS: Anxiety, confusion, dizziness, emotional lability, fever, lethargy, light-headedness, paranoid psychosis, syncope, vertigo

---

* For suppression of ventricular fibrillation; 20 to 120 min for suppression of ventricular tachycardia.

Mechanism of Action

Bretylium prolongs the repolarization phase of the action potential and lengthens the effective refractory period, which helps stop reentry arrhythmias. It also acts on adrenergic nerve terminals. Initially, it causes norepinephrine release, increasing heart rate and blood pressure. Then it blocks norepinephrine release, as shown, decreasing heart rate and blood pressure. It also increases the ventricular threshold, making the ventricular myocardium less responsive to ectopic impulses and preventing ventricular fibrillation.

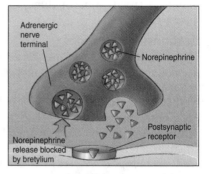

CV: Angina, arrhythmias (including bradycardia and more frequent PVCs), hypotension, orthostatic hypotension, transient hypertension
EENT: Mild conjunctivitis, nasal congestion
GI: Abdominal pain, diarrhea, hiccups, nausea, vomiting
GU: Renal dysfunction
RESP: Dyspnea
SKIN: Diaphoresis, erythematous macular rash, flushing
Other: Injection site pain

Nursing Considerations

- **WARNING** Monitor patients with severe aortic stenosis or pulmonary hypertension for signs of hypotension, a common effect of bretylium therapy.
- Be aware that bretylium is always diluted for I.V. administration *except* when used in life-threatening ventricular fibrillation. In this instance, use *undiluted* bretylium and administer it as quickly as possible.
- Dilute bretylium in a compatible I.V. solution, such as D_5W, D_5/normal saline solution, D_5/lactated Ringer's solution, normal saline solution, 5% sodium bicarbonate, 20% mannitol, 1/6 molar sodium lactate, lactated Ringer's solution, calcium chloride in D_5W, and potassium chloride in D_5W. Dilute to a concentration of at least 500 mg/50 ml.
- Be aware that bretylium is also available in 5% dextrose; this form should be used for I.V. infusion only.

- For I.V. infusion, dilute drug and give at 1 to 2 mg/minute, using an infusion pump or other appropriate rate control device.
- **WARNING** Be aware that patient may experience hypotension while supine. Have patient remain supine until tolerance develops. If her supine systolic blood pressure falls below 75 mm Hg, expect to administer dopamine or norepinephrine and monitor her blood pressure closely because vasopressor effects intensify when these drugs are given together.
- Be alert for transient hypertension and increased frequency of arrhythmias because bretylium initially triggers release of norepinephrine. Monitor patient's ECG tracings and blood pressure continuously, and notify prescriber of changes.
- Monitor serum bretylium level. Notify prescriber if level falls outside therapeutic range of 0.5 to 1.5 mcg/ml.
- Store drug at 15° to 30° C (59° to 86° F). Don't freeze.

PATIENT TEACHING
- Advise patient receiving bretylium to immediately report chest pain or pressure, pain at I.V. site, or rash.
- Warn patient that she may feel dizzy or light-headed even when lying down. Instruct her to remain supine and to ask for assistance when attempting to move or sit up. Tell her that this sensation usually subsides in a few days.

bumetanide
Bumex

Class and Category
Chemical: Sulfonamide derivative
Therapeutic: Loop diuretic
Pregnancy category: C

Indications and Dosages
▶ *To treat edema caused by heart failure, hepatic disease, and renal disease, including nephrotic syndrome*
I.V. INFUSION, I.V. INJECTION
Adults. 0.5 to 1 mg over 1 to 2 min; may repeat every 2 to 3 hr if necessary. *Maximum:* 10 mg daily.
DOSAGE ADJUSTMENT Continuous infusion (12 mg over 12 hr) may be more effective and less toxic than intermittent infusion in patients with severe chronic renal insufficiency.

Route	Onset	Peak	Duration
I.V.	In min	15 to 30 min	3.5 to 4 hr

Mechanism of Action
Inhibits the reabsorption of sodium, chloride, and water in the ascending limb of the loop of Henle, which promotes their excretion and reduces fluid volume.

Contraindications
Anuria, hepatic coma, hypersensitivity to bumetanide or its components, severe electrolyte depletion

Interactions
DRUGS

aminoglycosides: Increased risk of ototoxity

antihypertensives: Increased antihypertensive effect

indomethacin: Slowed increase in urine and sodium excretion, inhibited plasma renin activity

lithium: Decreased lithium renal clearance, increased risk of lithium toxicity

probenecid: Decreased sodium excretion

Adverse Reactions
CNS: Dizziness, encephalopathy, headache

CV: Chest pain, hypotension

EENT: Ototoxicity

ENDO: Hyperglycemia

GI: Nausea

GU: Azotemia, difficulty maintaining erection, elevated serum creatinine level, premature ejaculation

MS: Muscle spasms

Other: Hyperuricemia, hypocalcemia, hypochloremia, hypokalemia, hyponatremia, hypovolemia

Nursing Considerations
- **WARNING** Be aware that patients who are hypersensitive to sulfonamides may be hypersensitive to bumetanide. Monitor such patients closely when starting therapy.
- Expect to use parenteral route for patients with impaired GI absorption or those for whom oral route isn't practical. Switch to oral route, as prescribed, as soon as possible.
- Discard unused bumetanide parenteral solution 24 hours after preparation.
- Assess fluid and electrolyte balance closely because bumetanide is a potent diuretic (40 to 60 times more potent than furose-

mide). Monitor fluid intake and output once every 8 hours, evaluate serum electrolyte levels when ordered, and assess for imbalances.

• **WARNING** Be aware that high-dose or too-frequent administration can cause profound diuresis and water and electrolyte depletion, especially in elderly patients.

• Monitor serum potassium level regularly to check for hypokalemia, especially if patient takes a digitalis glycoside for heart failure or has hepatic cirrhosis, ascites, aldosteronism, potassium-losing nephropathy, diarrhea, or a history of ventricular arrhythmias.

• Assess for signs of ototoxicity, such as tinnitus, daily. Rarely, bumetanide may cause ototoxicity, especially with I.V. administration, high doses, and increased frequency of administration in a patient with renal impairment.

• Monitor results of renal function tests during bumetanide therapy to detect adverse reactions.

• Store drug at 15° to 30° C (59° to 86° F), and protect from light. Don't freeze.

PATIENT TEACHING

• Inform patient that fluid intake and output will be monitored during bumetanide therapy. Advise her to report signs and symptoms of electrolyte imbalance, such as dizziness, headache, and muscle spasms.

• Teach patient about adverse reactions, and tell her to report any that occur.

• Advise patient to avoid potentially hazardous activities until drug's CNS effects are known.

• Review potassium-rich foods, and encourage patient to include them in her daily diet.

• Inform diabetic patient that her blood glucose level will be monitored regularly; urge her to report signs or symptoms of hyperglycemia.

buprenorphine hydrochloride
Buprenex

Class, Category, and Schedule
Chemical: Opioid, thebaine derivative
Therapeutic: Narcotic analgesic
Pregnancy category: C
Controlled substance schedule: V

Indications and Dosages

▶ *To control moderate to severe pain*

I.V INJECTION

Adults and children age 12 and older. 0.3 mg every 6 hr or more, p.r.n. A second 0.3-mg dose given 30 to 60 min after first dose, if needed.

DOSAGE ADJUSTMENT I.V. dose reduced by half in elderly or debilitated patients and in those who have respiratory disease or also use another CNS depressant.

Children ages 2 to 12. 0.002 to 0.006 mg/kg every 4 to 6 hr, p.r.n.

Route	Onset	Peak	Duration
I.V.	Less than 15 min	Less than 1 hr	6 to 10 hr*

Mechanism of Action

May bind with CNS receptors to alter the perception of and emotional response to pain. Buprenorphine may act by displacing narcotic agonists from their binding sites and competitively inhibiting their actions.

Incompatibilities

Don't administer I.V. buprenorphine through the same I.V. line as diazepam or lorazepam.

Contraindications

Hypersensitivity to buprenorphine or its components

Interactions

DRUGS

CNS depressants, MAO inhibitors: Additive hypotensive and respiratory and CNS depressant effects of these drugs
narcotic analgesics: Reduced therapeutic effects if buprenorphine is given before another narcotic analgesic

Adverse Reactions

CNS: Dizziness, headache, sedation, vertigo
CV: Bradycardia, hypertension, hypotension
EENT: Miosis
GI: Nausea, vomiting
RESP: Bronchospasm, hypoventilation
SKIN: Diaphoresis, pruritus, rash, urticaria

---

* 4 to 5 hr in children ages 2 to 12.

Other: Anaphylaxis; angioedema; injection site pain, redness, and swelling

Nursing Considerations

• Use buprenorphine cautiously in patients with severe hepatic or renal impairment, myxedema, hypothyroidism, adrenal insufficiency, CNS depression, coma, toxic psychosis, prostatic hypertrophy, urethral stricture, acute alcoholism, alcohol withdrawal syndrome, kyphoscoliosis, or biliary tract dysfunction. Also use cautiously in patients who abuse drugs, have been opioid-dependent, or receive a drug that decreases hepatic clearance.

• Use drug cautiously in patients with head injury, intracranial lesions, or other conditions that could increase CSF pressure.

• **WARNING** Administer buprenorphine over at least 2 minutes. Be aware that rapid administration of other opioid analgesics has caused anaphylaxis, severe respiratory depression, hypotension, peripheral circulatory collapse, and cardiac arrest. Keep emergency equipment and drugs nearby.

• Inspect injection site for local reactions; don't use the same site twice.

• Monitor vital signs and response to drug often, especially after giving first dose.

PATIENT TEACHING

• Instruct patient to lie down during buprenorphine administration and for a period afterward to lessen drug's hypotensive effects (dizziness, light-headedness) and other adverse effects such as nausea and vomiting.

• Advise patient to change position slowly and to avoid rising quickly from a sitting or lying position.

• Advise patient to avoid potentially hazardous activities until drug's CNS effects are known.

butorphanol tartrate
Stadol

Class, Category, and Schedule
Chemical: Opioid
Therapeutic: Anesthesia adjunct, opioid analgesic
Pregnancy category: C
Controlled substance schedule: II

Indications and Dosages
▶ *To manage pain*

I.V. INJECTION

Adults. 0.5 to 2 mg (usually 1 mg) every 3 to 4 hr, p.r.n.

▶ *As adjunct to provide preoperative anesthesia*

I.V. INJECTION

Adults. Individualized; average of 2 mg 60 to 90 min before surgery.

▶ *As adjunct to provide anesthesia*

I.V. INJECTION

Adults. Individualized; average of 1 to 4 mg initially and then supplemental doses of 0.5 to 1 mg, p.r.n. Total usually required during surgery is 60 to 180 mcg/kg (0.06 to 0.18 mg/kg).

DOSAGE ADJUSTMENT Dosage reduced by half for elderly patients and those with impaired hepatic or renal function.

Route	Onset	Peak	Duration
I.V.	2 to 3 min	30 min	2 to 4 hr

Mechanism of Action

May bind with and stimulate mu and kappa opiate receptors in the spinal cord and higher levels in the CNS. In this way, butorphanol is believed to alter the perception of and emotional response to pain.

Contraindications

Acute respiratory depression, diarrhea due to poisoning, hypersensitivity to butorphanol or its components (including the preservative benzethonium chloride)

Interactions

DRUGS

CNS depressants: Additive CNS depression

ACTIVITIES

alcohol use: Additive CNS depression

Adverse Reactions

CNS: Anxiety, confusion, difficulty performing purposeful movements, difficulty speaking, dizziness, euphoria, floating feeling, headache, lethargy, nervousness, paresthesia, somnolence, syncope, tremor, vertigo

CV: Chest pain, hypotension, palpitations, tachycardia, vasodilation

EENT: Blurred vision, dry mouth, tinnitus

GI: Anorexia, constipation, epigastric pain, nausea, vomiting

RESP: Apnea, respiratory depression, shallow breathing

SKIN: Clammy skin, pruritus, sensation of warmth

Nursing Considerations

- Give butorphanol slowly, over several minutes. Be aware that rapid administration may cause anaphylaxis, severe respiratory depression, hypotension, peripheral circulatory collapse, and cardiac arrest. Keep emergency equipment and drugs nearby.
- Assess respiratory status closely, especially in patients having an acute asthma attack and those with chronic respiratory disease, hypothyroidism, or conditions that increase cerebrospinal fluid pressure, because drug causes respiratory depression. Pediatric, elderly, extremely ill, or debilitated patients and those who have recently taken or are currently taking drugs with respiratory depressant effects are also more sensitive to butorphanol's effects.
- Frequently monitor blood pressure after giving butorphanol. If severe hypertension develops (rare), stop drug at once and notify prescriber. If patient isn't opioid-dependent, expect to administer naloxone to reverse drug's effects.
- Monitor patient for evidence of drug-induced CNS depression or increased CSF pressure, such as altered LOC, restlessness, and irritability, in patients with a head injury, intracranial lesions, or other conditions that could cause these effects. Patients who are taking or have recently taken drugs that depress the CNS are also more susceptible to these effects. Take appropriate safety precautions.
- Because butorphanol can increase cardiac workload, use it with extreme caution in patients with acute MI, ventricular dysfunction, or coronary insufficiency.
- Be aware that butorphanol may induce or exacerbate arrhythmias or seizures in patients with a history of these conditions and may mask symptoms of acute abdominal conditions.
- Monitor patients with renal or hepatic impairment and those receiving a drug that decreases hepatic clearance for signs of increased butorphanol effects because drug is metabolized in the liver and excreted by the kidneys.
- Be aware that patients with a history of drug abuse (including acute alcoholism), emotional instability, or suicidal ideation or attempts are at increased risk for opioid abuse; however, the risk of drug dependence from butorphanol is lower than with some other opioid analgesics.
- Monitor patients with prostatic hypertrophy, renal function impairment, recent urinary tract surgery, or urethral stricture for signs of urine retention (such as trouble voiding or feeling that

the bladder isn't empty after voiding), peripheral edema, or weight gain.

• Store drug at 15° to 30° C (59° to 86° F), and protect from light. Don't freeze.

PATIENT TEACHING

• Instruct patient to lie down during butorphanol administration and for a period afterward to lessen drug's hypotensive effects (dizziness, light-headedness) and other adverse effects, such as nausea and vomiting.

• Advise patient to change position slowly and to avoid rising quickly from a sitting or lying position.

• Advise patient to avoid potentially hazardous activities until drug's CNS effects are known.

• Tell patient to avoid alcohol and other CNS depressants, including OTC drugs, during butorphanol therapy because of possible additive CNS depression.

calcitriol
(1,25-dihydroxycholecalciferol)
Calcijex

Class and Category
Chemical: Sterol derivative, vitamin D analogue
Therapeutic: Antihypocalcemic, antihypoparathyroid
Pregnancy category: C

Indications and Dosages
▶ *To treat hypoparathyroidism*
I.V. INJECTION
Adults. *Initial:* 1 to 2 mcg 3 times/wk given every other day. Each dose increased 0.5 to 1 mcg at 2- to 4-wk intervals, if needed.

Mechanism of Action
Binds to specific receptors of the intestinal mucosa to increase calcium absorption from the intestines. It also may regulate calcium ion transfer from bone to blood and stimulate calcium reabsorption in the distal renal tubules, making more calcium available in the body.

Contraindications
Hypercalcemia, vitamin D toxicity

Interactions
DRUGS
cholestyramine: Decreased calcitriol absorption
digitalis glycosides: Possibly arrhythmias
ketoconazole: Decreased blood calcitriol level
magnesium-containing antacids (I.V. form): Hypermagnesemia
mineral oil: Decreased blood calcitriol level (with prolonged use of mineral oil)
phenobarbital, phenytoin: Decreased synthesis and blood level of calcitriol
thiazide diuretics: Hypercalcemia

Adverse Reactions
SKIN: Erythema multiforme, lip swelling, pruritus, rash, urticaria
Other: Anaphylaxis

Nursing Considerations
• Make sure patient has adequate calcium intake.
• Store drug at room temperature and protect from heat and direct light.
• In high-dose or long-term calcitriol therapy, be alert for vitamin D toxicity. Early evidence includes abdominal or bone pain, constipation, dry mouth, headache, metallic taste, myalgia, nausea, somnolence, vomiting, and weakness. Late evidence includes albuminuria, anorexia, arrhythmias, azotemia, conjunctivitis (calcific), decreased libido, elevated AST and ALT levels, elevated BUN level, vascular calcification, hypercholesterolemia, hypertension, hyperthermia, irritability, mild acidosis, nephrocalcinosis, nocturia, pancreatitis, photophobia, polydipsia, polyuria, pruritus, rhinorrhea, and weight loss.

PATIENT TEACHING
• Warn against taking other forms of vitamin D with calcitriol.
• Advise patient to notify prescriber immediately if signs of toxicity, such as headache, irritability, nausea, photophobia, vomiting, weakness, and weight loss, develop.

calcium chloride
Calciject (CAN)

calcium gluceptate
Calcium Stanley (CAN)

calcium gluconate

Class and Category
Chemical: Elemental cation
Therapeutic: Antihypermagnesemic agent, antihypocalcemic agent, calcium replacement, cardiotonic agent
Pregnancy category: C

Indications and Dosages
▶ *To replace calcium in hypocalcemia*
I.V. INFUSION (CALCIUM CHLORIDE)
Adults. 0.5 to 1 g every 1 to 3 days, infused at less than 1 ml/min.
Children. 25 mg/kg given over several minutes.

I.V. INJECTION (CALCIUM GLUCEPTATE)
Adults and children. 1.1 to 4.4 g I.V. at a rate not to exceed 2 ml (36 mg)/min.
I.V. INJECTION (CALCIUM GLUCONATE)
Adults. 970 mg given slowly and repeated if needed until tetany is controlled.
Children. 200 to 500 mg as a single dose given slowly and repeated if needed until tetany is controlled.
▶ *As adjunct to treat magnesium intoxication*
I.V. INJECTION (CALCIUM CHLORIDE)
Adults. 500 mg promptly and repeated p.r.n., based on response.
▶ *As adjunct in cardiac resuscitation*
I.V. INJECTION (CALCIUM CHLORIDE)
Adults. 0.5 to 1 g.
Children. 0.2 ml/kg.
▶ *As adjunct in exchange transfusion*
I.V. INJECTION (CALCIUM GLUCONATE)
Adults. 1.35 mEq after each 100 ml of citrated blood is exchanged.
Neonates. 0.45 mEq after each 100 ml of citrated blood is exchanged.
I.V. INJECTION (CALCIUM GLUCEPTATE)
Neonates. 110 mg after each 100 ml of citrated blood is exchanged.

Mechanism of Action
Increases levels of intracellular and extracellular calcium, which is needed to maintain homeostasis, especially in the nervous and musculoskeletal systems. Also plays a role in normal cardiac and renal function, respiration, coagulation, and cell membrane and capillary permeability. Helps regulate the release and storage of neurotransmitters and hormones.

Incompatibilities
To avoid precipitation, don't administer I.V. calcium chloride, gluceptate, or gluconate through the same I.V. line as bicarbonates, carbonates, phosphates, sulfates, or tartrates. Don't mix with tetracyclines to avoid rendering tetracyclines inactive.

Contraindications
Hypercalcemia, hypersensitivity to calcium salts or their components, hypophosphatemia, renal calculi, ventricular fibrillation

Interactions
DRUGS

atenolol: Decreased blood atenolol level and beta blockade

calcitonin: Possibly antagonized effects of calcitonin in hypercalcemia treatment

calcium supplements, magnesium-containing preparations: Increased serum calcium or magnesium level, especially in patients with impaired renal function

cellulose sodium phosphate: Decreased effectiveness of cellulose sodium phosphate in preventing hypercalciuria

digitalis glycosides: Increased risk of arrhythmias

estrogens, oral contraceptives (estrogen-containing): Increased calcium absorption

etidronate: Decreased etidronate absorption

fluoroquinolones: Reduced fluoroquinolone absorption by calcium carbonate

gallium nitrate: Antagonized effects of gallium nitrate

iron salts: Decreased gastric absorption of iron

magnesium sulfate (parenteral): Neutralized effects of magnesium by parenteral calcium salts

neuromuscular blockers (except succinylcholine): Possibly reversal of neuromuscular blockade by parenteral calcium salts; enhanced or prolonged neuromuscular blockade induced by tubocurarine

norfloxacin: Decreased norfloxacin bioavailability

phenytoin: Decreased bioavailability of phenytoin and calcium

potassium phosphates, potassium and sodium phosphates: Increased risk of calcium deposition in soft tissue

sodium bicarbonate: Possibly milk-alkali syndrome

sodium fluoride: Reduced fluoride and calcium absorption

sodium polystyrene sulfonate: Possibly metabolic alkalosis if patient has renal impairment

tetracyclines: Decreased tetracycline absorption and blood level, leading to decreased anti-infective response

thiazide diuretics: Possibly hypercalcemia

verapamil: Reversed verapamil effects

vitamin A (more than 25,000 units/day): Possibly stimulation of bone loss, decreased effects of calcium supplementation, and hypercalcemia

vitamin D (high doses): Excessively increased calcium absorption
FOODS

caffeine: Possibly decreased calcium absorption
ACTIVITIES

alcohol use (excessive), smoking: Possibly decreased calcium absorption

Adverse Reactions
CNS: Paresthesia
CV: Hypotension, irregular heartbeat
GI: Nausea, vomiting
SKIN: Diaphoresis, flushing, or sensation of warmth
Other: Hypercalcemia; injection site burning, pain, rash, or redness

Nursing Considerations
- **WARNING** Be aware that calcium chloride injection contains three times as much calcium per milliliter as calcium gluconate injection.
- Warm solution to room temperature before administration.
- Don't use calcium gluceptate if you detect crystals.
- If you observe crystals in calcium gluconate, you can dissolve them by warming solution to 30° to 40° C (86° to 104° F).
- Administer I.V. calcium through an infusing I.V. solution, using a small-bore needle inserted into a large vein to minimize irritation. Give calcium slowly to prevent excess calcium from reaching the heart and causing adverse cardiovascular reactions. Adverse reactions often result from too-rapid administration. If ECG tracings are abnormal or patient reports injection site discomfort, expect to temporarily discontinue administration.
- Maintain patient in a recumbent position for 30 minutes after administration to prevent dizziness from hypotension.
- Assess regularly for extravasation because calcium causes necrosis. If infiltration occurs, discontinue I.V. calcium and notify prescriber immediately.
- Regularly monitor serum calcium level and evaluate therapeutic response by verifying the absence of Chvostek's and Trousseau's signs. Be aware that patients with dehydration, electrolyte imbalance, renal function impairment, or sarcoidosis are at increased risk for hypercalcemia. Patients with diarrhea or GI malabsorption may have increased fecal calcium excretion.
- Monitor vital signs and ECG tracings as appropriate. Calcium administration may cause a temporary increase in blood pressure, especially in elderly or hypertensive patients.
- Assess for arrhythmias in patients with cardiac disease, those receiving digitalis glycosides, and those with a history of ventricular fibrillation during cardiac resuscitation.
- Monitor for signs of calculi formation, such as pain radiating from the lumbar region, in patients with a history of renal calculi.

- Store calcium at 15° to 30° C (59° to 86° F), and protect from heat, moisture, and direct light. Don't freeze.

PATIENT TEACHING
- Instruct patient to immediately report pain at calcium injection site.
- Tell patient to avoid excessive use of tobacco and excessive consumption of alcoholic beverages and caffeine-containing products because these substances may decrease calcium absorption.
- Teach patient with hypocalcemia about the need for calcium and vitamin D intake as well as weight-bearing exercise.

capreomycin sulfate
Capastat

Class and Category
Chemical: Polypeptide antibiotic isolated from *Streptomyces capreolus*
Therapeutic: Antitubercular agent
Pregnancy category: C

Indications and Dosages
▶ *As adjunct to treat pulmonary tuberculosis caused by* Mycobacterium tuberculosis *when primary drugs have been ineffective or can't be used because of toxicity*

I.V. INFUSION
Adults. 1 g daily for 60 to 120 days, followed by 1 g two or three times weekly for 12 to 24 mo. *Maximum:* 20 mg/kg daily.

Mechanism of Action
May interfere with lipid and nucleic acid biosynthesis in actively growing tubercle bacilli.

Contraindications
Hypersensitivity to capreomycin or its components

Interactions
DRUGS
aminoglycosides (parenteral): Increased risk of ototoxicity, nephrotoxicity, and neuromuscular blockade
nephrotoxic drugs (such as amphotericin B): Increased risk of nephrotoxicity
neuromuscular blockers: Enhanced neuromuscular blockade
ototoxic drugs (such as quinidine): Increased risk of ototoxicity

polymyxins (parenteral): Increased risk of nephrotoxicity and neuro-muscular blockade

Adverse Reactions

CNS: Dizziness, vertigo
EENT: Ototoxicity
GI: Elevated liver function test results
GU: Nephrotoxicity
HEME: Leukocytosis, leukopenia
SKIN: Maculopapular rash, urticaria
Other: Injection site pain, induration, or bleeding

Nursing Considerations

- Expect capreomycin dosage to be decreased for patients with re-duced renal clearance.
- Reconstitute sterile capreomycin powder with 0.9% sodium chloride injection or sterile water for injection. Add 2, 2.15, 2.63, 3.3, or 4.3 ml of diluent to a 1-g vial of capreomycin to yield a concentration of 370, 350, 300, 250, or 200 mg/ml, re-spectively. Let stand for 2 to 3 minutes to allow for complete dissolution.
- Dilute reconstituted drug for I.V. injection with 100 ml of nor-mal saline solution. Administer over 60 minutes.
- Store reconstituted capreomycin at 2° to 8° C (36° to 46° F) for up to 24 hours. Be aware that a color change to pale straw color with subsequent darkening doesn't indicate loss of po-tency or development of toxicity.
- Monitor results of renal function tests and assess urine for sedi-ment to detect signs of renal injury or nephrotoxicity.
- Assess patient for changes in hearing. Ensure that he receives audiometric testing and vestibular function assessments regularly.
- Monitor patient closely for signs of a hypersensitivity reaction, such as urticaria and maculopapular rash, especially in patients with a history of hypersensitivity reactions to other drugs.

PATIENT TEACHING

- Advise patient receiving capreomycin to report excessive bleed-ing at injection site.
- Instruct patient to notify prescriber immediately if he develops hearing loss or ringing in ears.
- Explain the need for frequent laboratory tests to monitor renal function.
- Tell patient that tuberculosis therapy lasts for 12 to 24 months and that another drug will also be prescribed.

• Explain that noncompliance may decrease effectiveness and increase duration of treatment.

caspofungin acetate
Cancidas

Class and Category
Chemical: Echinocandins
Therapeutic: Antifungal
Pregnancy category: C

Indications and Dosages
▶ *To treat invasive aspergillosis in patients refractory to or intolerant of other therapies; to treat candidemia and candidal infections in intra-abdominal abscesses, peritonitis, and pleural space infections*
I.V. INFUSION
Adults. *Initial:* 70 mg on day 1, followed by 50 mg daily. *Maximum:* 70 mg daily.
▶ *To treat presumed fungal infections in febrile, neutropenic patients*
I.V. INFUSION
Adults. *Initial:* 70 mg on day 1, followed by 50 mg daily for at least 14 days, including at least 7 days after neutropenia and symptoms have resolved. Increased to 70 mg daily as needed. *Maximum:* 70 mg daily.
DOSAGE ADJUSTMENT Dosage reduced to 35 mg daily after initial 70-mg loading dose in moderate hepatic insufficiency.
▶ *To treat esophageal candidiasis*
I.V. INFUSION
Adults. 50 mg daily.
DOSAGE ADJUSTMENT Dosage reduced to 35 mg daily in moderate hepatic insufficiency.

Incompatibilities
Don't mix or infuse with other drugs. Don't admix with diluents that contain dextrose.

Contraindications
Hypersensitivity to caspofungin acetate or its components

Interactions
DRUGS
carbamazepine, dexamethasone, efavirenz, nelfinavir, nevirapine, phenytoin, rifampin: Possibly decreased blood caspofungin level
cyclosporine: Transient increases in ALT and AST levels
tacrolimus: Possibly decreased blood tacrolimus level

Mechanism of Action

Caspofungin acetate interferes with fungal cell membrane synthesis by inhibiting the synthesis of b (1,3)-D-glucan. A polypeptide, b (1,3)-D-glucan is the essential component of the fungal cell membrane that makes it rigid and protective. Without it, fungal cells rupture and die. This mechanism of action is most effective against susceptible filamentous fungi, such as *Aspergillus*.

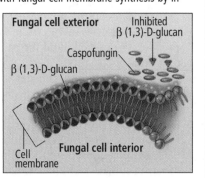

Adverse Reactions

CNS: Chills, dizziness, fever, headache, insomnia, paresthesia, tremor
CV: Edema, hypertension, hypotension, phlebitis, tachycardia, thrombophlebitis
GI: Abdominal pain, diarrhea, elevated liver function test results, hepatic dysfunction, jaundice, nausea, vomiting
GU: Elevated BUN or serum creatinine level, proteinuria, renal insufficiency
HEME: Decreased hemoglobin and hematocrit
MS: Back pain, myalgia
RESP: Bronchospasm, dyspnea, stridor, tachypnea
SKIN: Diaphoresis, erythema, flushing, pruritus, rash, sensation of warmth
Other: Decreased serum bicarbonate level, facial edema, hypercalcemia, hyperkalemia, hyperphosphatemia, hypokalemia, hypomagnesemia, infusion site reaction

Nursing Considerations

- To prepare 70-mg loading dose, let vial reach room temperature. Reconstitute by adding 10.5 ml of normal saline solution to vial. Dilute for administration by transferring 10 ml of reconstituted drug to 250 ml of normal saline solution.
- To prepare 70-mg loading dose from two 50-mg vials, add 10.5 ml of normal saline solution to each vial; then transfer 14 ml of prepared solution to 250 ml of normal saline solution.
- To prepare daily 50-mg infusion, let vial reach room tempera-

ture. Reconstitute by adding 10.5 ml of normal saline solution to vial. Dilute for administration by transferring only 10 ml of reconstituted drug to 250 ml of normal saline solution.

- To prepare daily 50-mg infusion at reduced volume, add 10 ml of reconstituted drug to 100 ml of normal saline solution.
- To prepare 35-mg daily dose for patient with moderate hepatic insufficiency, reconstitute 50-mg vial with 10.5 ml of normal saline solution. To dilute, transfer only 7 ml of reconstituted drug to 250 ml of normal saline solution or, if needed, to 100 ml of normal saline solution.
- When preparing powder for reconstitution, mix gently to obtain a clear solution. Don't use if solution is cloudy or contains precipitate. Discard unused solution after 24 hours.
- Infuse drug slowly over approximately 1 hour.
- Expect to increase daily dose to 70 mg, as prescribed, for patients not responding to carbamazepine, dexamethasone, efavirenz, nelfinavir, nevirapine, phenytoin, or rifampin.
- Watch for flushed skin, and assess patient often for unexplained temperature elevation.
- Assess for airway patency if patient develops excessive facial edema or respiratory stridor. Provide emergency airway management if complete obstruction occurs.
- Monitor patient's liver function test results, as ordered, and report abnormalities.

PATIENT TEACHING
- Urge patient to notify prescriber immediately if he has difficulty talking, swallowing, or breathing during caspofungin administration.

cefazolin sodium
Ancef

Class and Category
Chemical: First-generation cephalosporin,
7-aminocephalosporanic acid
Therapeutic: Antibiotic
Pregnancy category: B

Indications and Dosages
▶ *To treat respiratory tract infections caused by group A beta-hemolytic streptococci,* Haemophilus influenzae, Klebsiella *species,* Staphylococcus aureus, *and* Streptococcus pneumoniae; *skin and soft-tissue infections caused by* S. aureus, *group A beta-hemolytic and other strains*

of streptococci; biliary tract infections caused by Escherichia coli,
Klebsiella *species,* Proteus mirabilis, S. aureus, *and various strains of
streptococci; bone and joint infections caused by* S. aureus; *genital
infections, such as epididymitis and prostatitis, caused by* E. coli,
Klebsiella *species,* P. mirabilis, *and some strains of enterococci;
septicemia caused by* E. coli, Klebsiella *species,* P. mirabilis, S. aureus,
and S. pneumoniae; *and endocarditis caused by group A beta-hemolytic
streptococci and* S. aureus

I.V. INFUSION, I.V. INJECTION

Adults. For mild infections, 250 to 500 mg every 8 hr; for moderate to severe infections, 500 to 1,000 mg every 6 to 8 hr; and
for severe life-threatening infections, 1,000 to 1,500 mg every
6 hr. *Maximum:* 6 g daily.

Children. For mild to moderate infections, 25 to 50 mg/kg daily
divided equally and given t.i.d. or q.i.d.; for severe infections,
100 mg/kg daily divided equally and given t.i.d. or q.i.d.

▶ *To treat pneumococcal pneumonia*

I.V. INFUSION, I.V. INJECTION

Adults. 500 mg every 12 hr.

▶ *To treat acute uncomplicated UTI caused by* E. coli, Klebsiella
species, P. mirabilis, *and some strains of* Enterobacter *and*
Enterococcus

I.V. INFUSION, I.V. INJECTION

Adults. 1 g every 12 hr.

▶ *To provide surgical prophylaxis*

I.V. INFUSION, I.V. INJECTION

Adults. 1 g 30 to 60 min before surgery; 0.5 to 1 g during surgery if it lasts 2 hr or longer; 0.5 to 1 g every 6 to 8 hr for 24 hr
after surgery.

DOSAGE ADJUSTMENT After initial loading dose appropriate to infection's severity, dosage interval at least 8 hr for
adults with creatinine clearance of 35 to 54 ml/min/1.73 m^2;
dosage reduced by 50% and given every 12 hr for adults with
creatinine clearance of 11 to 34 ml/min/1.73 m^2; and dosage reduced by 50% and given every 18 to 24 hr for adults with creatinine clearance of 10 ml/min/1.73 m^2 or less. Dosage reduced
to 60% and given every 12 hr for children with creatinine
clearance of 40 to 70 ml/min/1.73 m^2; dosage reduced to 25%
and given every 12 hr for children with creatinine clearance of
20 to 40 ml/min/1.73 m^2; and dosage reduced to 10% and
given every 24 hr for children with creatinine clearance of 5 to
20 ml/min/1.73 m^2.

Mechanism of Action

Interferes with bacterial cell wall synthesis by inhibiting the final step in the cross-linking of peptidoglycan strands. Peptidoglycan makes cell membranes rigid and protective. Without it, bacterial cells rupture and die.

Incompatibilities

To prevent mutual inactivation, don't mix cefazolin with aminoglycosides. Also avoid mixing cefazolin with other drugs, including pentamidine isethionate.

Contraindications

Hypersensitivity to cephalosporins or their components

Interactions

DRUGS

aminoglycosides, loop diuretics: Additive nephrotoxicity
probenecid: Increased and prolonged blood cefazolin level

Adverse Reactions

CNS: Chills, fever, headache, seizures
CV: Edema
EENT: Hearing loss
GI: Abdominal cramps, diarrhea, elevated liver function test results, hepatic failure, hepatitis, hepatomegaly, nausea, oral candidiasis, pseudomembranous colitis, vomiting
GU: Elevated BUN and serum creatinine levels, nephrotoxicity, renal failure, vaginal candidiasis
HEME: Eosinophilia, hemolytic anemia, hypoprothrombinemia, neutropenia, thrombocytopenia, unusual bleeding
MS: Arthralgia
RESP: Dyspnea
SKIN: Ecchymosis, erythema, erythema multiforme, pruritus, rash, Stevens-Johnson syndrome
Other: Anaphylaxis; injection site pain, redness, and swelling; superinfection

Nursing Considerations

- Use cefazolin cautiously in patients with impaired renal function or a history of GI disease, particularly colitis. Also use drug cautiously in patients who are hypersensitive to penicillin because cross-sensitivity has occurred in about 10% of such patients.

- Obtain culture and sensitivity tests, as ordered, before therapy.
- **WARNING** To prevent unintentional overdose, cefazolin for injection USP and dextrose injection USP shouldn't be used in children who require less than the full adult dose.
- Reconstitute 500-mg vial of drug with 2 ml of sterile water for injection (or 1-g vial with 2.5 ml). Shake well until dissolved.
- For direct I.V. injection, further dilute reconstituted solution with at least 5 ml sterile water for injection. Inject slowly over 3 to 5 minutes in tubing of a flowing compatible I.V. solution.
- For intermittent I.V. infusion, reconstitute 500 to 1,000 mg in 50 to 100 ml of normal saline solution, D_5W, $D_{10}W$, D_5/lactated Ringer's, D_5/0.2 normal saline solution, D_5/0.45 normal saline solution, D_5/normal saline solution, lactated Ringer's injection, 5% or 10% invert sugar in sterile water for injection, 5% sodium bicarbonate (Ancef), or Ringer's injection.
- Store reconstituted cefazolin up to 24 hours at room temperature or 10 days under refrigeration.
- Monitor I.V. site for irritation, phlebitis, and extravasation.
- Monitor BUN and serum creatinine levels for early signs of nephrotoxicity. Also monitor fluid intake and output; decreasing urine output may indicate nephrotoxicity.
- Be aware that an allergic reaction may occur a few days after therapy starts.
- Monitor patient's bowel elimination; if needed, obtain a stool culture to test for pseudomembranous colitis. If it occurs, expect to stop cefazolin and give fluids, electrolytes, and antibiotics effective against *Clostridium difficile.*
- Watch for evidence of superinfection: cough, diarrhea, drainage, fever, malaise, pain, perineal itching, rash, redness, swelling.
- Assess for pharyngitis, ecchymosis, bleeding, and arthralgia; they may indicate a blood dyscrasia.

PATIENT TEACHING
- Instruct patient to complete the prescribed course of therapy.
- Urge patient to report watery, bloody stools to prescriber immediately, even up to 2 months after drug therapy has ended.

cefepime hydrochloride
Maxipime

Class and Category
Chemical: Fourth-generation cephalosporin, 7-aminocephalosporanic acid

Therapeutic: Antibiotic
Pregnancy category: B

Indications and Dosages

▶ *To treat mild to moderate UTI caused by* Escherichia coli,
Klebsiella pneumoniae, *or* Proteus mirabilis
I.V. INFUSION
Adults and children age 12 and over. 500 to 1,000 mg every
12 hr for 7 to 10 days.

▶ *To treat severe UTI caused by* E. coli *or* K. pneumoniae, *moderate
to severe skin and soft-tissue infections caused by* Staphylococcus
aureus *or* Streptococcus pyogenes
I.V. INFUSION
Adults and children age 12 and over. 2 g every 12 hr for
10 days.

▶ *To treat moderate to severe pneumonia caused by* Enterobacter
species, K. pneumoniae, Pseudomonas aeruginosa, *or* Streptococcus
pneumoniae
I.V. INFUSION
Adults and children age 12 and over. 1 to 2 g every 12 hr for
10 days.

▶ *To treat febrile neutropenia*
I.V. INFUSION
Adults and children age 12 and over. 2 g every 8 hr for
7 days or until neutropenia resolves.

▶ *To treat complicated intra-abdominal infections (together with
metronidazole) caused by alpha-hemolytic streptococci,* Bacteroides
fragilis, E. coli, Enterobacter *species,* K. pneumoniae, *or* P.
aeruginosa
I.V. INFUSION
Adults and children age 12 and over. 2 g every 12 hr for 7 to
10 days.

DOSAGE ADJUSTMENT Dosing interval increased from 12 to
24 hr and from 8 to 12 hr for patients with creatinine clearance
of 30 to 60 ml/min/1.73 m^2; dosing interval increased from 8 or
12 hr to 24 hr and dose decreased from 2 g every 12 hr to 1 g
every 24 hr (all other doses remain unchanged) for patients
with creatinine clearance of 11 to 29 ml/min/1.73 m^2; dosage
decreased from 500 mg every 12 hr to 250 mg every 24 hr, from
1,000 mg every 12 hr to 250 mg every 24 hr, from 2,000 mg
every 12 hr to 500 mg every 24 hr, and from 2 g every 8 hr to
1 g every 24 hr if creatinine clearance is less than 11 ml/min/
1.73 m^2.

Incompatibilities

Don't add cefepime to solutions that contain ampicillin in a concentration of more than 40 mg/ml. Don't add drug to solutions that contain aminophylline, gentamycin, metronidazole, netilmicin sulfate, tobramycin, or vancomycin.

Mechanism of Action

Interferes with bacterial cell wall synthesis by inhibiting the final step in the cross-linking of peptidoglycan strands. Peptidoglycan makes cell membranes rigid and protective. Without it, bacterial cells rupture and die.

Contraindications

Hypersensitivity to cephalosporins or their components

Interactions

DRUGS

aminoglycosides, loop diuretics: Increased risk of renal failure in patients with renal disease

Adverse Reactions

CNS: Chills, fever, headache, seizures

CV: Edema

EENT: Hearing loss

GI: Abdominal cramps, diarrhea, elevated liver function test results, hepatic failure, hepatomegaly, nausea, oral candidiasis, pseudomembranous colitis, vomiting

GU: Elevated BUN level, nephrotoxicity, renal failure, vaginal candidiasis

HEME: Eosinophilia, hemolytic anemia, hypoprothrombinemia, neutropenia, thrombocytopenia, unusual bleeding

MS: Arthralgia

RESP: Dyspnea

SKIN: Ecchymosis, erythema, erythema multiforme, pruritus, rash, Stevens-Johnson syndrome

Other: Anaphylaxis; injection site pain, redness, and swelling; superinfection

Nursing Considerations

- Use cefepime cautiously in patients with impaired renal function or a history of GI disease, particularly colitis. Also use cautiously in patients hypersensitive to penicillin because cross-sensitivity has occurred in about 10% of such patients.

- If possible, obtain culture and sensitivity test results, as ordered, before giving drug.
- For I.V. infusion, reconstitute according to manufacturer's guidelines. Administer over 30 minutes.
- Be aware that an allergic reaction may occur a few days after therapy starts.
- Monitor BUN and serum creatinine levels for early signs of nephrotoxicity. Also monitor fluid intake and output; decreasing urine output may indicate nephrotoxicity. Be aware that unadjusted dosages of cefepime in renally impaired patients may cause myoclonus and seizures.
- Assess bowel pattern daily; severe diarrhea may indicate pseudomembranous colitis.
- Assess for signs of superinfection, such as perineal itching, fever, malaise, redness, pain, swelling, drainage, rash, diarrhea, and cough or sputum changes.
- Assess for pharyngitis, ecchymosis, bleeding, and arthralgia; they may indicate a blood dyscrasia.

PATIENT TEACHING
- Tell patient to immediately report severe diarrhea to the prescriber.

cefmetazole sodium
Zefazone

Class and Category
Chemical: Second-generation cephalosporin, 7-aminocephalosporanic acid
Therapeutic: Antibiotic
Pregnancy category: B

Indications and Dosages
▶ *To treat UTI caused by* Escherichia coli; *lower respiratory tract infections, such as bronchitis and pneumonia, caused by* E. coli, Haemophilus influenzae, Staphylococcus aureus, *or* Streptococcus pneumoniae; *skin and soft-tissue infections caused by* Bacteroides fragilis, B. melaninogenicus, E. coli, Klebsiella oxytoca, Klebsiella pneumoniae, Morganella morganii, Proteus mirabilis, Proteus vulgaris, S. aureus, Staphylococcus epidermidis, Streptococcus agalactiae, *or* Streptococcus pyogenes; *and intra-abdominal infections caused by* B. fragilis, Clostridium perfringens, E. coli, K. oxytoca, *or* K. pneumoniae

I.V. INFUSION

Adults. 2 g every 6 to 12 hr for 5 to 14 days.

DOSAGE ADJUSTMENT Dosage reduced to 1 to 2 g every 12 hr for patients with creatinine clearance of 50 to 90 ml/min/ 1.73 m^2; 1 to 2 g every 16 hr for patients with creatinine clearance of 30 to 49 ml/min/1.73 m^2; 1 to 2 g every 24 hr for patients with creatinine clearance of 10 to 29 ml/min/1.73 m^2; and 1 to 2 g every 48 hr for patients with creatinine clearance of less than 10 ml/min/1.73 m^2.

▶ *To provide surgical prophylaxis for vaginal hysterectomy*

I.V. INFUSION

Adults. 2 g as a single dose given 30 to 90 min before surgery, or 1 g given 30 to 90 min before surgery and repeated 8 and 16 hr later.

▶ *To provide surgical prophylaxis for abdominal hysterectomy and for high-risk cholecystectomy*

I.V. INFUSION

Adults. 1 g given 30 to 90 min before surgery and repeated 8 and 16 hr later.

▶ *To provide surgical prophylaxis for cesarean section*

I.V. INFUSION

Adults. 2 g as a single dose after cord is clamped or 1 g after cord is clamped and then repeated 8 and 16 hr later.

▶ *To provide surgical prophylaxis for colorectal surgery*

I.V. INFUSION

Adults. 2 g as a single dose 30 to 90 min before surgery, or 2 g given 30 to 90 min before surgery and repeated 8 and 16 hr later.

Mechanism of Action

Interferes with bacterial cell wall synthesis by inhibiting the final step in the cross-linking of peptidoglycan strands. Peptidoglycan makes cell membranes rigid and protective. Without it, bacterial cells rupture and die.

Contraindications

Hypersensitivity to cephalosporins or their components

Interactions

DRUGS

aminoglycosides, loop diuretics: Increased risk of nephrotoxicity
anticoagulants: Possibly increased anticoagulant effect
probenecid: Increased and prolonged blood cefmetazole level

ACTIVITIES

alcohol use: Possibly disulfiram-like reaction

Adverse Reactions

CNS: Chills, fever, headache, seizures

CV: Edema

EENT: Hearing loss, oral candidiasis

GI: Abdominal cramps, diarrhea, elevated liver function test results, hepatic failure, hepatomegaly, nausea, pseudomembranous colitis, vomiting

GU: Elevated BUN level, nephrotoxicity, renal failure, vaginal candidiasis

HEME: Eosinophilia, hemolytic anemia, hypoprothrombinemia, neutropenia, thrombocytopenia, unusual bleeding

MS: Arthralgia

RESP: Dyspnea

SKIN: Ecchymosis, erythema, erythema multiforme, pruritus, rash, Stevens-Johnson syndrome

Other: Anaphylaxis, infusion site thrombophlebitis, superinfection

Nursing Considerations

- If possible, obtain culture and sensitivity test results, as ordered, before giving cefmetazole.
- Reconstitute drug with sterile water for injection, bacteriostatic water for injection, or 0.9% sodium chloride for injection.
- Store reconstituted solution for up to 24 hours at room temperature or for up to 7 days when refrigerated. Solution may also be frozen at −20° C (−4° F) or less for up to 6 weeks.
- Dilute primary solution as needed to 1 to 20 mg/ml in D_5W, normal saline solution, lactated Ringer's solution, or 1% lidocaine solution without epinephrine. Diluted solution remains potent for 24 hours if stored at room temperature, for 7 days if refrigerated, and for 6 weeks if frozen.
- Monitor for signs of an allergic reaction, such as difficulty breathing or a rash, especially in patients who are hypersensitive to penicillin, because cross-sensitivity has occurred in about 10% of such patients.
- Monitor BUN and serum creatinine levels to detect early signs of nephrotoxicity, especially in patients with impaired renal function. Also monitor fluid intake and output; decreasing urine output may indicate nephrotoxicity.
- Assess bowel pattern daily; severe diarrhea may indicate pseudomembranous colitis. Patients with a history of GI disease, particularly colitis, are at increased risk.

- Assess for signs of superinfection, such as perineal itching, fever, malaise, redness, pain, swelling, drainage, rash, diarrhea, and cough or sputum changes.
- Assess for pharyngitis, ecchymosis, bleeding, and arthralgia, which may indicate a blood dyscrasia. Monitor PT and bleeding time as ordered.
- Don't refreeze thawed solutions.

PATIENT TEACHING
- Advise patient receiving cefmetazole to immediately report severe diarrhea or signs or symptopms of blood dyscrasia or superinfection. Inform him that yogurt or buttermilk can help decrease diarrhea.
- Instruct patient to avoid alcohol during therapy and for at least 3 days after taking last dose.
- Review with patient other possibly serious adverse reactions, including difficulty breathing, rash, and chest tightness, and tell him to report any that occur.

cefonicid sodium
Monocid

Class and Category
Chemical: Second-generation cephalosporin, 7-aminocephalosporanic acid
Therapeutic: Antibiotic
Pregnancy category: B

Indications and Dosages
▶ *To treat lower respiratory tract infection caused by* Escherichia coli, Haemophilus influenzae, Klebsiella pneumoniae, *or* Streptococcus pneumoniae; *UTI caused by* E. coli, K. pneumoniae, Morganella morganii, Proteus mirabilis, Proteus vulgaris, *or* Providencia rettgeri; *skin and soft-tissue infections caused by* Staphylococcus aureus, Staphylococcus epidermidis, Streptococcus agalactiae, *or* Streptococcus pyogenes; *septicemia caused by* E. coli *or* S. pneumoniae; *and bone and joint infections caused by* S. aureus
I.V. INFUSION, I.V. INJECTION
Adults. For mild to moderate infection, 1 g every 24 hr; for severe or life-threatening infection, 2 g every 24 hr.
▶ *To treat uncomplicated UTI*
I.V. INFUSION, I.V. INJECTION
Adults. 500 mg every 24 hr.
DOSAGE ADJUSTMENT Initial dose reduced to 75 mg/kg in

patients with impaired renal function. Then, if creatinine clearance is 60 to 79 ml/min/1.73 m^2, dosage reduced to 10 to 25 mg/kg every 24 hr; if clearance is 40 to 59 ml/min/1.73 m^2, reduced to 8 to 20 mg/kg every 24 hr; if clearance is 20 to 39 ml/min/1.73 m^2, reduced to 4 to 15 mg/kg every 24 hr; if clearance is 10 to 19 ml/min/1.73 m^2, reduced to 4 to 15 mg/kg every 48 hr; if clearance is 5 to 9 ml/min/1.73 m^2, reduced to 4 to 15 mg/kg every 3 to 5 days; if clearance is less than 5 ml/minute/1.73 m^2, reduced to 3 to 4 mg/kg every 3 to 5 days.

▶ *To provide surgical prophylaxis*
I.V. INFUSION, I.V. INJECTION
Adults. 1 g 60 min before surgery. Dose repeated once daily, if needed, for 2 days after prosthetic arthroplasty or open-heart surgery.

Mechanism of Action

Interferes with bacterial cell wall synthesis by inhibiting the final step in the cross-linking of peptidoglycan strands. Peptidoglycan makes cell membranes rigid and protective. Without it, bacterial cells rupture and die.

Incompatibilities

To prevent mutual inactivation, don't mix cefonicid with aminoglycosides.

Contraindications

Hypersensitivity to cephalosporins or their components

Interactions

DRUGS
aminoglycosides, loop diuretics: Increased risk of nephrotoxicity
probenecid: Increased and prolonged blood cefonicid level

Adverse Reactions

CNS: Chills, fever, headache, seizures
CV: Edema
EENT: Hearing loss, oral candidiasis
GI: Abdominal cramps, diarrhea, elevated liver function test results, hepatic failure, hepatomegaly, nausea, pseudomembranous colitis, vomiting
GU: Elevated BUN level, nephrotoxicity, renal failure, vaginal candidiasis

HEME: Eosinophilia, hemolytic anemia, hypoprothrombinemia, neutropenia, thrombocytopenia, unusual bleeding
MS: Arthralgia
RESP: Dyspnea
SKIN: Ecchymosis, erythema, erythema multiforme, pruritus, rash, Stevens-Johnson syndrome
Other: Anaphylaxis, infusion site thrombophlebitis, superinfection

Nursing Considerations

- If possible, obtain culture and sensitivity test results, as ordered, before giving cefonicid.
- Reconstitute each 500-mg vial of drug with 2 ml of sterile water for injection (or each 1-g vial with 2.5 ml).
- For I.V. infusion, dilute further in 50 to 100 ml of compatible solution, such as D_5W, $D_{10}W$, $D_5/0.2$ normnal saline solution, $D_5/0.45$ normal saline solution, or D_5/normal saline solution.
- Be aware that 1 g of cefonicid/18 ml of sterile water for injection is an isotonic solution.
- Store reconstituted solution at room temperature for up to 24 hours or under refrigeration for up to 72 hours.
- Administer I.V. injection slowly over 3 to 5 minutes through tubing of a flowing compatible I.V. solution.
- Monitor patient for evidence of allergic reaction, such as difficulty breathing or a rash, especially in patients who are hypersensitive to penicillin, because cross-sensitivity has occurred in about 10% of such patients.
- Monitor BUN and serum creatinine levels to detect early signs of nephrotoxicity, especially in patients with impaired renal function. Also monitor fluid intake and output; decreasing urine output may indicate nephrotoxicity.
- Assess bowel pattern daily; severe diarrhea may indicate pseudomembranous colitis. Patients with a history of GI disease, particularly colitis, are at increased risk.
- Assess for signs of superinfection, such as perineal itching, fever, malaise, redness, pain, swelling, drainage, rash, diarrhea, and cough or sputum changes.
- Assess for pharyngitis, ecchymosis, bleeding, and arthralgia, which may indicate a blood dyscrasia. Monitor PT and bleeding time as ordered.
- Before reconstituting drug, store it at 2° to 8° C (36° to 46° F). Protect from light.

PATIENT TEACHING
- Advise patient receiving cefonicid to immediately report severe

diarrhea or signs of blood dyscrasia or superinfection. Inform him that yogurt or buttermilk can help decrease diarrhea.
• Review with patient other possibly serious adverse reactions, including difficulty breathing, rash, and chest tightness, and tell him to report any that occur.

cefoperazone sodium
Cefobid

Class and Category
Chemical: Third-generation cephalosporin, 7-aminocephalosporanic acid
Therapeutic: Antibiotic
Pregnancy category: B

Indications and Dosages
▶ *To treat respiratory tract infection caused by* Enterobacter *species,* Escherichia coli, Haemophilus influenzae, Klebsiella pneumoniae, Proteus mirabilis, Pseudomonas aeruginosa, Staphylococcus aureus, Streptococcus pneumoniae, Streptococcus pyogenes, *or other streptococci (excluding enterococci); UTI caused by* E. coli *or* P. aeruginosa; *uncomplicated gonorrhea caused by* Neisseria gonorrhoeae; *gynecologic infections caused by anaerobic gram-positive cocci,* Bacteroides *species,* Clostridium *species,* E. coli, Staphylococcus epidermidis, *or* Streptococcus agalactiae; *bacterial septicemia caused by* E. coli, Klebsiella *species,* S. aureus, Serratia marcescens, *or streptococci; skin and soft-tissue infections caused by* P. aeruginosa, S. aureus, *or* S. pyogenes; *and intra-abdominal infections caused by anaerobic gram-negative bacilli,* E. coli, *or* P. aeruginosa
I.V. INFUSION
Adults. 1 to 2 g every 12 hr. For severe infections or those caused by less sensitive organisms, 6 to 12 g daily divided into equal doses and given b.i.d., t.i.d., or q.i.d. *Maximum:* 12 g daily.

Mechanism of Action
Interferes with bacterial cell wall synthesis by inhibiting the final step in the cross-linking of peptidoglycan strands. Peptidoglycan makes cell membranes rigid and protective. Without it, bacterial cells rupture and die.

Incompatibilities
To prevent mutual inactivation, don't mix cefoperazone with

aminoglycosides. Also avoid mixing cefoperazone with other drugs, including pentamidine isethionate.

Contraindications
Hypersensitivity to cephalosporins or their components

Interactions
DRUGS
aminoglycosides, loop diuretics: Increased risk of nephrotoxicity
oral anticoagulants, other drugs that affect blood clotting: Increased anticoagulant effect
ACTIVITIES
alcohol use: Disulfiram-like reaction from acetaldehyde accumulation

Adverse Reactions
CNS: Chills, fever, headache, seizures
CV: Edema
EENT: Hearing loss, oral candidiasis
GI: Abdominal cramps, diarrhea, elevated liver function test results, hepatic failure, hepatomegaly, nausea, pseudomembranous colitis, vomiting
GU: Elevated BUN level, nephrotoxicity, renal failure, vaginal candidiasis
HEME: Eosinophilia, hemolytic anemia, hypoprothrombinemia, neutropenia, thrombocytopenia, unusual bleeding
MS: Arthralgia
RESP: Dyspnea
SKIN: Ecchymosis, erythema, erythema multiforme, pruritus, rash, Stevens-Johnson syndrome
Other: Anaphylaxis, infusion site thrombophlebitis, superinfection

Nursing Considerations
- Expect cefoperazone dosage to be reduced for patients with combined renal and hepatic function impairment. Monitor serum drug levels in patients with impaired hepatic function or biliary obstruction who are receiving more than 4 g/day; dosage may need to be reduced.
- If possible, obtain culture and sensitivity test results, as ordered, before giving drug.
- Reconstitute cefoperazone for injection with required amount of diluent; then dilute further in compatible solution, such as D_5W, $D_{10}W$, D_5/lactated Ringer's solution, D_5/0.2 normal saline solution, D_5/normal saline soluiton, lactated Ringer's solution,

normal saline solution, Normosol M and D₅W, or Normosol R. (See manufacturer's guidelines for details.)

- After drug reconstitution, let foam dissipate and inspect solution to ensure complete dissolution.
- Store reconstituted solution of cefoperazone for injection at room temperature for 24 hours.
- Be aware that cefoperazone also comes in a minibag (cefoperazone injection) with a concentration of 1 or 2 g/50 ml. Before use, store minibag at −25° to −10° C (−13° to 14° F). Thaw at room temperature of 25° C (77° F) or under refrigeration at 5° C (41° F). Don't thaw with warm bath or microwave. Make sure that all ice crystals have melted before use.
- After thawing minibag, use it within 48 hours if stored at room temperature or within 14 days if refrigerated. Don't refreeze. Discard solution if it's cloudy or contains precipitate.
- To prevent air embolism, don't administer minibags (cefoperazone injection) using I.V. lines with series connections.
- Give drug as intermittent infusion over 15 to 30 minutes or as continuous infusion. Direct bolus injection isn't recommended.
- Monitor BUN and serum creatinine levels to detect early signs of nephrotoxicity. Also monitor fluid intake and output; decreasing urine output may indicate nephrotoxicity.
- Monitor for signs of an allergic reaction, such as difficulty breathing or a rash, especially in patients who are hypersensitive to penicillin, because cross-sensitivity has occurred in about 10% of such patients.
- Assess bowel pattern daily; severe diarrhea may indicate pseudomembranous colitis. Patients with a history of GI disease, particularly colitis, are at increased risk.
- Assess for pharyngitis, ecchymosis, bleeding, and arthralgia, which may indicate a blood dyscrasia. Monitor PT and bleeding time as ordered. Be prepared to administer vitamin K, if ordered, to treat hypoprothrombinemia.
- Assess for signs of superinfection, such as perineal itching, fever, malaise, redness, pain, swelling, drainage, rash, diarrhea, and cough or sputum changes.
- Before reconstituting cefoperazone for injection, store at 15° to 30° C (59° to 86° F). Protect from light.

PATIENT TEACHING

- Ask patient to avoid alcohol during cefoperazone therapy and for at least 3 days after taking the last dose.
- Instruct patient to immediately report severe diarrhea or signs

of blood dyscrasia or superinfection. Inform him that yogurt or buttermilk can help decrease diarrhea.
• Review with patient other possibly serious adverse reactions, including difficulty breathing, rash, and chest tightness, and tell him to report any that occur.

cefotaxime sodium

Claforan

Class and Category

Chemical: Third-generation cephalosporin, 7-aminocephalosporanic acid
Therapeutic: Antibiotic
Pregnancy category: B

Indications and Dosages

▶ *To provide perioperative prophylaxis*
I.V. INFUSION, I.V. INJECTION
Adults and children weighing more than 50 kg (110 lb). 1 g 30 to 90 min before surgery.
▶ *To provide perioperative prophylaxis related to cesarean section*
I.V. INFUSION, I.V. INJECTION
Adults. 1 g as soon as cord is clamped, then 1 g every 6 hr for up to two doses.
▶ *To treat disseminated gonorrhea*
I.V. INFUSION, I.V. INJECTION
Adults and children weighing more than 50 kg. 1 g every 8 hr.
▶ *To treat uncomplicated infections caused by susceptible organisms*
I.V. INFUSION, I.V. INJECTION
Adults and children weighing more than 50 kg. 1 g every 12 hr.
Children ages 1 month to 12 years weighing less than 50 kg. 50 to 180 mg/kg/day in four to six divided doses.
Children ages 1 to 4 weeks. 50 mg/kg I.V. every 8 hr.
Children age 1 week and younger. 50 mg/kg I.V. every 12 hr.
▶ *To treat moderate to severe infections caused by susceptible organisms*
I.V. INFUSION, I.V. INJECTION
Adults and children weighing more than 50 kg. 1 to 2 g every 8 hr.
Children ages 1 month to 12 years weighing less than 50 kg. 50 to 180 mg/kg daily in four to six divided doses. More

serious infections, including meningitis, warrant higher dosages.

Children ages 1 to 4 weeks. 50 mg/kg I.V. every 8 hr.

Children age 1 week and younger. 50 mg/kg I.V. every 12 hr.

▶ *To treat septicemia and other infections that commonly require antibiotics in higher doses than those used to treat moderate to severe infections*

I.V. INFUSION, I.V. INJECTION

Adults and children weighing more than 50 kg. 2 g every 6 to 8 hr.

▶ *To treat life-threatening infections caused by susceptible organisms*

I.V. INFUSION, I.V. INJECTION

Adults and children weighing more than 50 kg. 2 g every 4 hr. *Maximum:* 12 g/day.

Children ages 1 month to 12 years weighing less than 50 kg. 50 to 180 mg/kg/day in four to six divided doses.

Children ages 1 to 4 weeks. 50 mg/kg every 8 hr.

Children age 1 week and younger. 50 mg/kg every 12 hr.

DOSAGE ADJUSTMENT Dosage reduced by 50% for patients with creatinine clearance less than 20 ml/min/1.73 m^2.

Mechanism of Action

Interferes with bacterial cell wall synthesis by inhibiting the cross-linking of peptidoglycan strands. Peptidoglycan makes cell membranes rigid and protective. Without it, bacterial cells rupture and die.

Incompatibilities

To prevent mutual inactivation, don't mix cefotaxime with aminoglycosides. Also avoid mixing cefotaxime with other drugs, including pentamidine isethionate.

Contraindications

Hypersensitivity to cephalosporins or their components

Interactions

DRUGS

aminoglycosides, loop diuretics: Increased risk of nephrotoxicity

probenecid: Increased and prolonged blood cefotaxime level

Adverse Reactions

CNS: Chills, fever, headache, seizures

CV: Edema

EENT: Hearing loss

GI: Abdominal cramps, diarrhea, elevated liver function test results, hepatic failure, hepatomegaly, nausea, oral candidiasis, pseudomembranous colitis, vomiting

GU: Elevated BUN level, nephrotoxicity, renal failure, vaginal candidiasis

HEME: Eosinophilia, hemolytic anemia, hypoprothrombinemia, neutropenia, thrombocytopenia, unusual bleeding

MS: Arthralgia

RESP: Dyspnea

SKIN: Ecchymosis, erythema, erythema multiforme, pruritus, rash, Stevens-Johnson syndrome, toxic epidermal necrolysis

Other: Anaphylaxis; injection site pain, redness, and swelling; superinfection

Nursing Considerations

- Use cefotaxime cautiously in patients with impaired renal function, a history of GI disease (especially colitis), or hypersensitivity to penicillin; cross-sensitivity has occurred in about 10% of such patients.
- If possible, obtain culture and sensitivity test results, as ordered, before giving drug.
- For I.V. use, reconstitute each 0.5-, 1-, or 2-g vial with 10 ml of sterile water for injection. Shake to dissolve.
- For intermittent I.V. infusion, further dilute in 50 to 100 ml of D$_5$W or normal saline solution.
- **WARNING** When preparing drug for a neonate, don't use diluent that contains benzyl alcohol; it could cause a fatal toxic syndrome.
- Give cefotaxime by I.V. injection over 3 to 5 minutes through tubing of a flowing compatible I.V. solution. Temporarily stop other solutions being given through same I.V. site.
- Discard unused drug after 24 hours if stored at room temperature, 5 days if refrigerated.
- Protect cefotaxime powder and solution from light and heat.
- Monitor I.V. sites for signs of phlebitis or extravasation. Rotate I.V. sites every 72 hours.
- Monitor BUN and serum creatinine levels and fluid intake and output for signs of nephrotoxicity.
- Be aware that an allergic reaction may occur a few days after therapy starts.
- Monitor patient's bowel elimination; if needed, obtain a stool culture to test for pseudomembranous colitis. If it occurs, expect to stop cefotaxime and give fluids, electrolytes, and antibiotics effective against *Clostridium difficile*.

- Assess patient for pharyngitis, ecchymosis, bleeding, and arthralgia, which may indicate a blood dyscrasia. Monitor CBC, PT, and bleeding time, as ordered.
- Monitor patient closely for superinfection. If signs appear, notify prescriber and expect to stop drug and give appropriate care.

PATIENT TEACHING

- Urge patient to report watery, bloody stools to prescriber immediately, even up to 2 months after drug therapy has ended.

cefoxitin sodium
Mefoxin

Class and Category
Chemical: Second-generation cephalosporin, 7-aminocephalosporanic acid
Therapeutic: Antibiotic
Pregnancy category: B

Indications and Dosages
▶ *To provide surgical prophylaxis*
I.V. INFUSION, I.V. INJECTION
Adults. 2 g 30 to 60 min before surgery and then 2 g every 6 hr after first dose for up to 24 hr.
Children age 3 months or over. 30 to 40 mg/kg 30 to 60 min before surgery and then every 6 hr after first dose for up to 24 hr.
▶ *To provide surgical prophylaxis for cesarean section*
I.V. INFUSION, I.V. INJECTION
Adults. 2 g as a single dose as soon as cord is clamped or 2 g as soon as cord is clamped followed by 2 g 4 and 8 hr after initial dose.
▶ *To provide surgical prophylaxis for transurethral prostatectomy*
I.V. INFUSION, I.V. INJECTION
Adults. 1 g 30 to 60 min before surgery and then 1 g every 8 hr for up to 5 days.
▶ *To treat infection, including septicemia, gynecologic infection, intra-abdominal infection, UTI, and infection of the lower respiratory tract, skin, soft tissue, bones, and joints caused by anaerobes (including* Bacteroides *species,* Clostridium *species,* Fusobacterium *species,* Peptococcus niger, *and* Peptostreptococcus *species), gram-negative organisms (including* Escherichia coli, Haemophilus influenzae *[and ampicillin-resistant strains],* Klebsiella, *and* Proteus *species), and gram-positive organisms (including* Staphylococcus aureus *[penicillinase- and*

non–penicillinase-producing strains], Staphylococcus epidermidis, Streptococcus agalactiae, Streptococcus pneumoniae, *and* Streptococcus pyogenes*)*

I.V. INFUSION, I.V. INJECTION

Adults. For uncomplicated infections, 1 g every 6 to 8 hr; for moderate to severe infections, 1 g every 4 hr or 2 g every 6 to 8 hr; for infections that commonly require high-dose antibiotics (such as gas gangrene), 2 g every 4 hr or 3 g every 6 hr.

Children age 3 months or over. 80 to 160 mg/kg/day in equal doses and given every 4 to 6 hr (with higher dosages used for more severe infections). *Maximum:* 12 g/day.

DOSAGE ADJUSTMENT Dosage reduced to 1 to 2 g every 8 to 12 hr if creatinine clearance is 30 to 50 ml/min/1.73 m^2; to 1 to 2 g every 12 to 24 hr if clearance is 10 to 29 ml/min/1.73 m^2; to 0.5 to 1 g every 12 to 24 hr if clearance is 5 to 9 ml/min/1.73 m^2; and to 0.5 to 1 g every 24 to 48 hr if clearance is less than 5 ml/min/1.73 m^2.

Mechanism of Action

Interferes with bacterial cell wall synthesis by inhibiting the final step in the cross-linking of peptidoglycan strands. Peptidoglycan makes cell membranes rigid and protective. Without it, bacterial cells rupture and die.

Incompatibilities

To prevent mutual inactivation, don't mix cefoxitin with aminoglycosides. Also avoid mixing cefoxitin with other drugs, including pentamidine isethionate.

Contraindications

Hypersensitivity to cephalosporins or their components

Interactions

DRUGS

aminoglycosides, loop diuretics: Increased risk of nephrotoxicity

Adverse Reactions

CNS: Chills, fever, headache, seizures
CV: Edema
EENT: Hearing loss
GI: Abdominal cramps, diarrhea, elevated liver function test results, hepatic failure, hepatomegaly, nausea, oral candidiasis, pseudomembranous colitis, vomiting

GU: Elevated BUN level, nephrotoxicity, renal failure, vaginal candidiasis

HEME: Eosinophilia, hemolytic anemia, hypoprothrombinemia, neutropenia, thrombocytopenia, unusual bleeding

MS: Arthralgia

RESP: Dyspnea

SKIN: Ecchymosis, erythema, erythema multiforme, flushing, pruritus, rash, Stevens-Johnson syndrome, urticaria

Other: Anaphylaxis; injection site pain, redness, and swelling; superinfection

Nursing Considerations

- Use cefoxitin cautiously in patients hypersensitive to penicillin; cross-sensitivity has occurred in about 10% of such patients. Also use cautiously in patients with a history of GI disease, particularly colitis, because of an increased risk of pseudomembranous colitis.
- If possible, obtain culture and sensitivity test results, as ordered, before giving drug.
- For I.V. use, reconstitute 1 g with 10 ml of sterile water for injection or 2 g with 10 to 20 ml of diluent.
- For I.V. injection, administer slowly over 3 to 5 minutes through tubing of a flowing compatible I.V. solution.
- For intermittent infusion, further dilute with 50 to 100 ml of D$_5$W or normal saline solution.
- For continuous high-dose infusion, add cefoxitin to I.V. solutions of D$_5$W, normal saline solution, or D$_5$/normal saline solution.
- Discard unused drug after 24 hours if stored at room temperature or after 1 week if refrigerated.
- Be aware that powder or solution may darken during storage, a change that doesn't reflect altered potency.
- Be aware that an allergic reaction may occur a few days after therapy starts.
- Monitor BUN and serum creatinine levels for early signs of nephrotoxicity. Also monitor fluid intake and output; decreasing urine output may indicate nephrotoxicity.
- Assess bowel pattern daily; severe diarrhea may indicate pseudomembranous colitis.
- Assess for pharyngitis, ecchymosis, bleeding, and arthralgia; they may indicate a blood dyscrasia.

PATIENT TEACHING

- Tell patient to immediately report severe diarrhea to prescriber.

ceftazidime

Ceptaz, Fortaz, Tazicef, Tazidime

Class and Category

Chemical: Third-generation cephalosporin,
7-aminocephalosporanic acid
Therapeutic: Antibiotic
Pregnancy category: B

Indications and Dosages

▶ *To treat infection caused by gram-negative organisms (including* Acinetobacter, Citrobacter, Enterobacter, Escherichia coli, Haemophilus influenzae, Klebsiella, Neisseria, Proteus mirabilis, Proteus vulgaris, Pseudomonas aeruginosa, Salmonella, Serratia, *and* Shigella*), gram-positive organisms (including* Streptococcus agalactiae, Streptococcus pneumoniae, *and* Streptococcus pyogenes *[group B streptococci]), as well as* Staphylococcus aureus *(penicillinase- and non–penicillinase-producing strains)*

I.V. INFUSION

Adults and children age 12 and over. 1 g every 8 to 12 hr.

I.V. INFUSION

Children ages 1 month to 12 years. 30 to 50 mg/kg every 8 hr.

Neonates up to age 1 month. 30 mg/kg every 12 hr. *Maximum:* 6 g/day.

▶ *To treat uncomplicated UTI*

I.V. INFUSION

Adults and children age 12 and over. 250 mg every 12 hr.

▶ *To treat complicated UTI*

I.V. INFUSION

Adults and children age 12 and over. 500 mg every 8 to 12 hr.

▶ *To treat uncomplicated pneumonia and mild skin and soft-tissue infection*

I.V. INFUSION

Adults and children age 12 and over. 0.5 to 1 g every 8 hr.

▶ *To treat bone and joint infection*

I.V. INFUSION

Adults and children age 12 and over. 2 g every 12 hr.

▶ *To treat serious gynecologic and intra-abdominal infection, meningitis, and life-threatening infection, especially in immunocompromised patients*

I.V. INFUSION
Adults and children age 12 and over. 2 g every 8 hr.
▶ *To treat pseudomonal lung infection in patients with cystic fibrosis and normal renal function*
I.V. INFUSION
Adults and children age 1 month and over. 30 to 50 mg/kg every 8 hr. *Maximum:* 6 g daily.
Neonates up to age 1 month. 30 mg/kg every 12 hr.
DOSAGE ADJUSTMENT Dosage reduced to 1 g every 12 hr if creatinine clearance is 31 to 50 ml/min/1.73 m^2; to 1 g every 24 hr if clearance is 16 to 30 ml/min/1.73 m^2; to 0.5 g every 24 hr if clearance is 6 to 15 ml/min/1.73 m^2; and to 0.5 g every 48 hr if clearance is less than 6 ml/min/1.73 m^2.

Mechanism of Action
Interferes with bacterial cell wall synthesis by inhibiting the cross-linking of peptidoglycan strands. Peptidoglycan makes the cell membrane rigid and protective. Without it, bacterial cells rupture and die.

Incompatibilities
Don't mix ceftazidime with aminoglycosides to prevent mutual inactivation. Vancomycin is physically incompatible with ceftazidime (precipitate may form); flush I.V. line between these drugs if given through same tubing. Avoid mixing ceftazidime with other drugs, including pentamidine isethionate.

Contraindications
Hypersensitivity to cephalosporins or their components

Interactions
DRUGS
aminoglycosides, loop diuretics: Increased risk of nephrotoxicity
estrogen/progesterone oral contraceptives: Decreased contraceptive effectiveness

Adverse Reactions
CNS: Chills, fever, headache, seizures
CV: Edema
EENT: Hearing loss
GI: Abdominal cramps, diarrhea, elevated liver function test results, hepatic failure, hepatomegaly, nausea, oral candidiasis, pseudomembranous colitis, vomiting

GU: Elevated BUN level, nephrotoxicity, renal failure, vaginal candidiasis
HEME: Eosinophilia, hemolytic anemia, hypoprothrombinemia, neutropenia, thrombocytopenia, unusual bleeding
MS: Arthralgia
RESP: Dyspnea
SKIN: Ecchymosis, erythema, erythema multiforme, pruritus, rash, Stevens-Johnson syndrome
Other: Anaphylaxis; injection site pain, redness, and swelling; superinfection

Nursing Considerations

• Use ceftazidime cautiously in patients hypersensitive to penicillin because cross-sensitivity occurs in about 10% of them. Watch for allergic reactions a few days after therapy starts.
• Use cautiously in patients with a history of GI disease, particularly colitis, because risk of pseudomembranous colitis is increased.
• Know that ceftazidime L-arginine (Ceptaz) is not recommended for children under age 12.
• If possible, obtain culture and sensitivity test results, as ordered, before giving drug.
• Protect ceftazidime powder and reconstituted drug from heat and light; both tend to darken during storage.
• If pharmacy delivers frozen solution, thaw it at room temperature, not in water bath or microwave. Store thawed solution for up to 12 hours at room temperature or 7 days in refrigerator; don't refreeze.
• **WARNING** When preparing drug for neonates or immature infants, don't use diluents containing benzyl alcohol because they are linked to a fatal toxic syndrome.
• For I.V. bolus, reconstitute 1 to 2 g with 10 ml sterile water for injection, D_5W, or sodium chloride for injection. Shake to dissolve. Administer I.V. injection slowly over 3 to 5 minutes through tubing of a flowing compatible I.V. fluid.
• For intermittent infusion, further dilute in 50 to 100 ml of D_5W or normal saline solution. Avoid using sodium bicarbonate injection as a diluent because drug is least stable in it. During ceftazidime administration, temporarily stop other solutions being given at the same I.V. site.
• Rotate I.V. sites every 72 hours. Assess for phlebitis and extravasation.
• Monitor patient's bowel elimination; if needed, obtain a stool

culture to test for pseudomembranous colitis. If it occurs, expect to stop ceftazidime and give fluids, electrolytes, and antibiotics effective against *Clostridium difficile.*

- Monitor CBC, hematocrit, and serum AST, ALT, bilirubin, LD, and alkaline phosphatase levels during long-term therapy.
- Monitor PT, as ordered, in at-risk patients, such as those with renal or hepatic impairment or poor nutritional state and those receiving anticoagulant or prolonged antibiotic therapy. Notify prescriber if PT decreases, and expect to give vitamin K.
- Assess for perineal itching, fever, malaise, redness, swelling, rash, and change in cough or sputum; they may indicate a superinfection.
- Watch for pharyngitis, ecchymosis, bleeding, and arthralgia (possible blood dyscrasia). Monitor PT and bleeding time.

PATIENT TEACHING
- Urge patient to report watery, bloody stools to prescriber immediately, even up to 2 months after drug therapy has ended.
- Instruct patient to report evidence of blood dyscrasia or superinfection.

ceftizoxime sodium

Cefizox

Class and Category

Chemical: Third-generation cephalosporin, 7-aminocephalosporanic acid
Therapeutic: Antibiotic
Pregnancy category: B

Indications and Dosages

▶ *To treat mild to moderate infection of the lower respiratory tract, skin, soft tissue, bones, and joints; septicemia; meningitis; and intra-abdominal infections caused by anaerobes (such as* Bacteroides *species,* Peptococcus, *and* Peptostreptococcus)*, gram-negative organisms (including* Escherichia coli, Haemophilus influenzae, Klebsiella, *and* Proteus mirabilis)*, and gram-positive organisms (including* Enterobacter *species,* Serratia *species,* Staphylococcus aureus, Staphylococcus epidermidis, Streptococcus agalactiae, Streptococcus pneumoniae, *and* Streptococcus pyogenes)

I.V. INFUSION, I.V. INJECTION

Adults and children age 12 and over. 1 to 2 g every 8 to 12 hr.

▶ *To treat severe or refractory infections of the type listed above*

I.V. INFUSION, I.V. INJECTION
Adults and children age 12 and over. 1 g every 8 hr or 2 g
every 8 to 12 hr.

▶ *To treat life-threatening infections of the type listed above*
I.V. INFUSION, I.V. INJECTION
Adults and children age 12 and over. 3 to 4 g every 8 hr or,
if required, up to 2 g every 4 hr.

▶ *To treat bacterial infection in children*
I.V. INFUSION, I.V. INJECTION
Children age 6 months and over. 50 mg/kg every 6 to 8 hr.

▶ *To treat uncomplicated UTI*
I.V. INFUSION, I.V. INJECTION
Adults. 500 mg every 12 hr.

▶ *To treat pelvic inflammatory disease*
I.V. INFUSION, I.V. INJECTION
Adults. 2 g every 8 hr.

DOSAGE ADJUSTMENT If creatinine clearance is 50 to
79 ml/min/1.73 m², dosage reduced to 0.5 g every 8 hr for less
severe infections and 0.75 to 1.5 g every 8 hr for life-threatening infections. If creatinine clearance is 5 to 49 ml/min/1.73 m²,
dosage reduced to 0.25 to 0.5 g every 12 hr for less severe infections and 0.5 to 1 g every 12 hr for life-threatening infections. If creatinine clearance is 4 ml/min/1.73 m² or less, dosage reduced to 0.5 g every 48 hr or 0.25 g every 24 hr for less
severe infections and 0.5 to 1 g every 48 hr or 0.5 g every 24 hr
for life-threatening infections.

Mechanism of Action

Interferes with bacterial cell wall synthesis by inhibiting the final step in the
cross-linking of peptidoglycan strands. Peptidoglycan makes the cell membrane rigid and protective. Without it, bacterial cells rupture and die.

Incompatibilities

Don't mix ceftizoxime with aminoglycosides to prevent mutual
inactivation.

Contraindications

Hypersensitivity to cephalosporins or their components

Interactions

DRUGS
aminoglycosides, loop diuretics: Increased risk of nephrotoxicity

probenecid: Increased and prolonged blood ceftizoxime level

Adverse Reactions

CNS: Chills, fever, headache, seizures

CV: Edema

EENT: Hearing loss

GI: Abdominal cramps, diarrhea, elevated liver function test results, hepatic failure, hepatomegaly, nausea, oral candidiasis, pseudomembranous colitis, vomiting

GU: Elevated BUN level, nephrotoxicity, renal failure, vaginal candidiasis

HEME: Eosinophilia, hemolytic anemia, hypoprothrombinemia, neutropenia, thrombocytopenia, unusual bleeding

MS: Arthralgia

RESP: Dyspnea

SKIN: Ecchymosis, erythema, erythema multiforme, pruritus, rash, Stevens-Johnson syndrome

Other: Anaphylaxis; infusion site pain, redness, and swelling; superinfection

Nursing Considerations

- If possible, obtain culture and sensitivity test results, as ordered, before giving ceftizoxime.
- Reconstitute ceftizoxime for injection with sterile water for injection as follows: for 500-mg vial, add 5 ml; for 1-g vial, add 10 ml; and for 2-g vial, add 20 ml. Shake well. Dilute reconstituted solution further with 50 to 100 ml of a compatible solution, such as normal saline solution or D_5W, before I.V. infusion.
- Be aware that reconstituted drug may be stored for 24 hours at room temperature or 96 hours if refrigerated.
- Administer I.V. injection slowly over 3 to 5 minutes through tubing of a flowing compatible I.V. fluid.
- Be aware that ceftizoxime also comes in a minibag (ceftizoxime injection) with a concentration of 1 or 2 g/50 ml. Before using minibag, store it at –25° to –10° C (–13° to 14° F). Thaw it at room temperature or in refrigerator.
- Discard minibag after 48 hours if stored at room temperature or after 28 days if refrigerated. Don't refreeze. Don't use solution if it contains precipitate or is cloudy.
- To prevent air embolism, don't administer minibag using I.V. lines with series connections.
- Assess I.V. site for extravasation and phlebitis.
- Monitor BUN and serum creatinine levels to detect early signs

of nephrotoxicity, especially in patients with impaired renal function. Also monitor fluid intake and output; decreasing urine output may indicate nephrotoxicity.

- Assess bowel elimination pattern daily; severe diarrhea may indicate pseudomembranous colitis. Patients with a history of GI disease, particularly colitis, are at increased risk.
- Monitor for signs of an allergic reaction, such as difficulty breathing or a rash, especially in patients who are hypersensitive to penicillin, because cross-sensitivity has occurred in about 10% of such patients. Be aware that an allergic reaction may occur a few days after therapy starts.
- Assess CBC, hematocrit, and serum AST, ALT, bilirubin, LD, and alkaline phosphatase levels during long-term therapy.
- Assess for pharyngitis, ecchymosis, bleeding, and arthralgia, which may indicate a blood dyscrasia. Monitor PT and bleeding time as ordered.
- Assess patient for evidence of superinfection, such as perineal itching, fever, redness, swelling, rash, and change in cough or sputum.
- Before reconstituting drug, store it at 15° to 30° C (59° to 86° F).

PATIENT TEACHING
- Advise patient receiving ceftizoxime to immediately report severe diarrhea or signs of blood dyscrasias or superinfection. Inform him that yogurt and buttermilk can help maintain intestinal flora and decrease diarrhea.
- Review with patient other possibly serious adverse reactions, such as difficulty breathing, rash, and chest tightness, and tell him to report any that occur.

ceftriaxone sodium
Rocephin

Class and Category
Chemical: Third-generation cephalosporin, 7-aminocephalosporanic acid
Therapeutic: Antibiotic
Pregnancy category: B

Indications and Dosages
▶ *To treat infection of the lower respiratory tract, skin, soft tissue, urinary tract, bones, and joints; sinusitis; intra-abdominal infections; and septicemia caused by anaerobes (including* Bacteroides bivius,

Bacteroides fragilis, Bacteroides melaninogenicus, *and* Peptostreptococcus *species), gram-negative organisms (including* Citrobacter *species,* Enterobacter aerogenes, Escherichia coli, Haemophilus influenzae, Klebsiella *species,* Neisseria *species,* Proteus mirabilis, Proteus vulgaris, Providencia *species,* Salmonella *species,* Serratia marcescens, Shigella, *and some strains of* Pseudomonas aeruginosa*), and gram-positive organisms (including* Staphylococcus aureus, Streptococcus pneumoniae, *and* Streptococcus pyogenes*)*

I.V. INFUSION

Adults. 1 to 2 g once daily or in equally divided doses b.i.d. *Maximum:* 4 g daily.

Children. 50 to 75 mg/kg daily in divided doses every 12 hr. *Maximum:* 2 g daily.

▶ *To treat meningitis*

I.V. INFUSION

Children. *Initial:* 100 mg/kg on first day; then 100 mg/kg once daily or in divided doses every 12 hr for 7 to 14 days. *Maximum:* 4 g daily.

▶ *To treat disseminated gonoccocal infection and pelvic inflammatory disease*

I.V. INFUSION

Adults: 1 g every 24 hr.

▶ *To treat gonococcal meningitis and endocarditis*

I.V. INFUSION

Adults. 1 to 2 g every 12 hr for 10 to 14 days (meningitis) or for 4 wk or longer (endocarditis).

▶ *To provide surgical prophylaxis*

I.V. INFUSION

Adults. 1 g 30 min to 2 hr before surgery.

Mechanism of Action

Interferes with bacterial cell wall synthesis by inhibiting the final step in the cross-linking of peptidoglycan strands. Peptidoglycan makes the cell membrane rigid and protective. Without it, bacterial cells rupture and die.

Incompatibilities

Don't admix ceftriaxone with pentamidine isethionate, labetalol, or other antibiotics, such as aminoglycosides, because of potential for incompatibility, such as substantial mutual inactivation. Also, don't mix with calcium-containing solutions or products because a potentially fatal (especially in newborns) ceftriaxone-calcium salt could precipitate in the lungs and kidneys.

Contraindications
Hypersensitivity to cephalosporins or their components

Interactions
DRUGS
aminoglycosides, loop diuretics: Increased risk of nephrotoxicity

Adverse Reactions
CNS: Chills, fever, headache, seizures
CV: Edema
EENT: Hearing loss
GI: Abdominal cramps, diarrhea, elevated liver function test re-
sults, hepatic failure, hepatomegaly, nausea, oral candidiasis,
pseudolithiasis, pseudomembranous colitis, vomiting
GU: Elevated BUN level, nephrotoxicity, renal failure, vaginal
candidiasis
HEME: Eosinophilia, hemolytic anemia, hypoprothrombinemia,
neutropenia, thrombocytopenia, unusual bleeding
MS: Arthralgia
RESP: Allergic pneumonitis, dyspnea
SKIN: Ecchymosis, erythema, erythema multiforme, pruritus,
rash, Stevens-Johnson syndrome
Other: Anaphylaxis; injection site pain, redness, and swelling; su-
perinfection

Nursing Considerations
- Use ceftriaxone cautiously in patients who are hypersensitive to
  penicillins because cross-sensitivity has occurred in about 10%
  of such patients.
- If possible, obtain culture and sensitivity results, as ordered, before giving drug.
- Protect powder from light.
- For I.V. use, reconstitute with an appropriate diluent, such as
  sterile water for injection or sodium chloride for injection, as
  follows: 250-mg vial, add 2.4 ml; 500-mg vial, add 4.8 ml; 1-g
  vial, add 9.6 ml; and 2-g vial, add 19.2 ml to yield 100 mg/ml.
  For piggyback bottles, reconstitute with 10 ml of diluent indicated above for 1-g bottle and 20 ml for 2-g bottle. After reconstitution, further dilute to 50 to 100 ml with diluent indicated
  above and infuse over 30 minutes.
- **WARNING** Do not administer calcium-containing solutions
  or products within 48 hours of ceftriaxone because a potentially fatal ceftriaxone-calcium salt could precipitate in the

lungs or kidneys.

- Monitor patient's BUN and serum creatinine levels to detect early signs of nephrotoxicity. Also, monitor fluid intake and output; decreasing urine output may indicate nephrotoxicity.
- Monitor patient for allergic reactions a few days after therapy starts.
- Assess patient's CBC, hematocrit, and serum AST, ALT, bilirubin, LD, and alkaline phosphatase levels during long-term ceftriaxone therapy.
- Monitor patient's bowel elimination; if needed, obtain a stool culture to test for pseudomembranous colitis. If it occurs, expect to stop ceftriaxone and give fluids, electrolytes, and antibiotics effective against *Clostridium difficile.*
- Assess patient for perineal itching, fever, malaise, redness, swelling, rash, and change in cough or sputum; they may indicate a superinfection.
- Assess patient for pharyngitis, ecchymosis, bleeding, and arthralgia; they may indicate a blood dyscrasia.

PATIENT TEACHING
- Tell patient to immediately report evidence of blood dyscrasia or superinfection to prescriber.
- Encourage patient to report watery, bloody stools to prescriber immediately, even up to 2 months after drug therapy has ended.

cefuroxime sodium
Zinacef

Class and Category
Chemical: Second-generation cephalosporin, 7-aminocephalosporanic acid
Therapeutic: Antibiotic
Pregnancy category: B

Indications and Dosages
▶ *To treat disseminated gonococcal infection and uncomplicated pneumonia*
I.V. INFUSION, I.V. INJECTION
Adults. 750 mg every 8 hr.
▶ *To treat bone and joint infection*
I.V. INFUSION, I.V. INJECTION
Adults. 1.5 g every 8 hr.
Children over age 3 months. 50 to 150 mg/kg/day in divided

doses every 8 hr. *Maximum:* Adult dose.

▶ *To treat bacterial meningitis*
I.V. INFUSION
Adults. 1.5 to 3 g every 8 hr.
Children over age 1 month. 50 to 80 mg/kg every 6 to 8 hr.
Neonates up to age 1 month. 33.3 to 50 mg/kg every 8 to 12 hr.

▶ *To treat moderate infection other than those listed above*
I.V. INFUSION, I.V. INJECTION
Adults. 750 mg every 8 hr for 5 to 10 days.
I.V. INFUSION, I.V. INJECTION
Children over age 3 months. 50 mg/kg daily in equally divided doses every 6 to 8 hr.

▶ *To treat severe or complicated infection other than those listed above*
I.V. INFUSION, I.V. INJECTION
Adults. 1.5 g every 8 hr.
Children over age 3 months. 100 mg/kg daily in equally divided doses every 6 to 8 hr.

▶ *To treat life-threatening infections other than those listed above*
I.V. INFUSION, I.V. INJECTION
Adults. 1.5 g every 6 hr.

▶ *To provide perioperative prophylaxis*
I.V. INFUSION, I.V. INJECTION
Adults. 1.5 g 30 to 60 min before surgery (at induction of anesthesia for open-heart surgery), and then 0.75 g every 8 hr thereafter (1.5 g every 12 hr for a total of 6 g with open-heart surgery).

DOSAGE ADJUSTMENT Parenteral dosage reduced to 0.75 g every 12 hr if creatinine clearance is 10 to 20 ml/min/1.73 m^2 or to 0.75 g every 24 hr if less than 10 ml/min/1.73 m^2.

Mechanism of Action

Interferes with bacterial cell wall synthesis by inhibiting the final step in the cross-linking of peptidoglycan strands. Peptidoglycan makes the cell membrane rigid and protective. Without it, bacterial cells rupture and die.

Incompatibilities

Don't admix parenteral cefuroxime with other antibiotics, such as aminoglycosides, because of potential for incompatibility, such as substantial mutual inactivation. If they're administered concurrently, don't mix them in the same I.V. bag or bottle.

Contraindications

Hypersensitivity to cephalosporins or their components

Interactions

DRUGS

aminoglycosides, loop diuretics: Increased risk of nephrotoxicity
antacids, H$_2$-receptor antagonists, omeprazole: Decreased cefuroxime axetil absorption
probenecid: Increased and prolonged blood cefuroxime level

Adverse Reactions

CNS: Chills, fever, headache, seizures
CV: Edema
EENT: Hearing loss, oral candidiasis
GI: Abdominal cramps, diarrhea, elevated liver function test results, hepatic failure, hepatomegaly, nausea, pseudomembranous colitis, vomiting
GU: Elevated BUN level, nephrotoxicity, renal failure, vaginal candidiasis
HEME: Eosinophilia, hemolytic anemia, hypoprothrombinemia, neutropenia, thrombocytopenia, unusual bleeding
MS: Arthralgia
RESP: Dyspnea
SKIN: Ecchymosis, erythema, erythema multiforme, pruritus, rash, Stevens-Johnson syndrome
Other: Anaphylaxis; injection site edema, pain, and redness; superinfection

Nursing Considerations

• Use cefuroxime cautiously in patients hypersensitive to penicillin because cross-sensitivity has occurred in about 10% of such patients.
• If possible, obtain culture and sensitivity results, as ordered, before giving drug.
• For I.V. use, reconstitute following manufacturer's instructions according to type of preparation available. Solution ranges in color from light yellow to amber.
• If using a container of frozen parenteral solution, thaw at room temperature or under refrigeration before administration; make sure all ice crystals have melted. Don't force thawing by microwave irradiation.
• Store reconstituted parenteral drug up to 24 hours at room temperature or 96 hours refrigerated. Thawed solutions may be stable 24 hours at room temperature or 28 days refrigerated.

- Administer I.V. injection over 3 to 5 minutes through tubing of a flowing compatible I.V. fluid.
- Monitor I.V. site for extravasation and phlebitis.
- Monitor patient's BUN and serum creatinine levels and fluid intake and output to detect signs of nephrotoxicity. Monitor patients with renal impairment closely because they may have greater toxic reactions to cefuroxime.
- Monitor patient for allergic reactions continuing up to a few days after therapy starts. Patients with a history of some form of allergy, especially to drugs, are at increased risk for an allergic reaction.
- Monitor patient's bowel elimination; if needed, obtain a stool culture to test for pseudomembranous colitis. If it occurs, expect to stop cefuroxime and give fluids, electrolytes, and antibiotics effective against *Clostridium difficile.*
- Assess patient for pharyngitis, ecchymosis, bleeding, and arthralgia, which may indicate a blood dyscrasia.
- Monitor PT and bleeding time, as ordered. Be prepared to administer vitamin K, if ordered, to treat hypothrombinemia.

PATIENT TEACHING
- Instruct patient to shake oral suspension well before measuring each dose and to use an accurate liquid-measuring device for each dose.
- Advise patient using single-dose packets of oral suspension to empty the contents of one packet into a glass and add at least 10 ml (2 tsp) of cold water; apple, grape, or orange juice; or lemonade. Tell him to stir well and consume entire mixture at once.
- Inform patient that yogurt and buttermilk help maintain intestinal flora and can decrease diarrhea during therapy.
- Instruct patient to immediately report to prescriber evidence of blood dyscrasia.
- Urge patient to report watery, bloody stools to prescriber immediately, even up to 2 months after drug therapy has ended.

cephapirin sodium
Cefadyl

Class and Category
Chemical: First-generation cephalosporin, 7-aminocephalosporanic acid
Therapeutic: Antibiotic

Pregnancy category: B

Indications and Dosages

▶ *To treat respiratory tract infection, skin and soft-tissue infections, UTI, septicemia, endocarditis, and osteomyelitis caused by gram-negative organisms (including* Escherichia coli, Haemophilus influenzae, Klebsiella *species, and* Proteus mirabilis*) and gram-positive organisms (including group A beta-hemolytic streptococci,* Streptococcus pneumoniae, *and staphylococci, including coagulase-positive, coagulase-negative, and penicillinase-producing—but not methicillin-resistant—strains of* Staphylococcus aureus*)*

I.V. INFUSION, I.V. INJECTION

Adults. 0.5 to 1 g every 4 to 6 hr. *Maximum:* 12 g daily.

Children over age 3 months. 40 to 80 mg/kg/day divided into four equal doses and given every 6 hr. *Maximum:* 12 g daily.

▶ *To provide surgical prophylaxis*

I.V. INFUSION, I.V. INJECTION

Adults. 1 to 2 g 30 to 60 min before surgery, 1 to 2 g during long procedure, and 1 to 2 g every 6 hr after surgery for 24 hr.

DOSAGE ADJUSTMENT For open-heart surgery or prosthetic arthroplasty, prophylaxis continued for 3 to 5 days after procedure, if needed.

Mechanism of Action

Interferes with bacterial cell wall synthesis by inhibiting the final step in the cross-linking of peptidoglycan strands. Peptidoglycan makes the cell membrane rigid and protective. Without it, bacterial cells rupture and die.

Contraindications

Hypersensitivity to cephalosporins or their components

Interactions

DRUGS

aminoglycosides, loop diuretics: Increased risk of nephrotoxicity

probenecid: Increased and prolonged blood cephapirin level

Adverse Reactions

CNS: Chills, fever, headache, seizures

CV: Edema

EENT: Hearing loss

GI: Abdominal cramps, diarrhea, elevated liver function test results, hepatic failure, hepatomegaly, nausea, oral candidiasis, pseudomembranous colitis, vomiting

GU: Elevated BUN level, nephrotoxicity, renal failure, vaginal candidiasis

HEME: Eosinophilia, hemolytic anemia, hypoprothrombinemia, neutropenia, thrombocytopenia, unusual bleeding

MS: Arthralgia

RESP: Dyspnea

SKIN: Ecchymosis, erythema, erythema multiforme, pruritus, rash, Stevens-Johnson syndrome

Other: Anaphylaxis; infusion site pain, redness, and swelling; superinfection

Nursing Considerations

- If possible, obtain culture and sensitivity test results, as ordered, before giving cephapirin.
- For I.V. injection, reconstitute 1 g with 10 ml or more of appropriate diluent, such as sterile water for injection. Administer I.V. injection slowly over 3 to 5 minutes through tubing of a flowing compatible I.V. fluid.
- For I.V. infusion, dilute further in 50 ml of D_5W or normal saline solution and infuse over 15 to 30 minutes. Stop primary I.V. solution during cephapirin administration.
- Store reconstituted drug for 12 to 48 hours (depending on diluent used) at room temperature or for 10 days in refrigerator.
- Don't administer a cloudy solution.
- Assess I.V. site for extravasation and phlebitis.
- Monitor BUN and serum creatinine levels to detect early signs of nephrotoxicity, especially in patients with impaired renal function. Also monitor fluid intake and output; decreasing urine output may indicate nephrotoxicity.
- Monitor for signs of an allergic reaction, such as difficulty breathing or a rash, especially in patients who are hypersensitive to penicillin, because cross-sensitivity has occurred in about 10% of such patients. Be aware that an allergic reaction may occur a few days after therapy starts.
- Assess CBC, hematocrit, and serum AST, ALT, bilirubin, LD, and alkaline phosphatase levels during long-term therapy.
- Assess bowel elimination pattern daily; severe diarrhea may indicate pseudomembranous colitis. Patients with a history of GI disease, particularly colitis, are at increased risk.
- Assess for pharyngitis, ecchymosis, bleeding, and arthralgia, which may indicate a blood dyscrasia. Monitor PT and bleeding time, as ordered.
- Assess patient for a furry tongue, perineal itching, and loose,

foul-smelling stools, any of which may indicate a super-infection.

- Before reconstituting cephapirin for injection, store it at 15° to 30° C (59° to 86° F).

PATIENT TEACHING

- Instruct patient receiving cephapirin to immediately report severe diarrhea or signs of blood dyscrasias or superinfection. Inform him that yogurt and buttermilk can help maintain intestinal flora and decrease diarrhea during therapy.
- Review with patient other possibly serious adverse reactions, such as difficulty breathing, rash, and chest tightness, and tell him to report any that occur.

chloramphenicol sodium succinate
Chloromycetin

Class and Category
Chemical: Dichloroacetic acid derivative
Therapeutic: Antibiotic
Pregnancy category: Not rated

Indications and Dosages
▶ *To treat serious infection for which less potentially dangerous drugs are ineffective or contraindicated*
I.V. INFUSION
Adults. 12.5 mg/kg every 6 hr. *Maximum:* 4 g daily.
Children. 12.5 mg/kg every 6 hr.
Full-term infants age 2 weeks and over. 12.5 mg/kg every 6 hr or 25 mg/kg every 12 hr.
Preterm and full-term infants up to age 2 weeks. 6.25 mg/kg every 6 hr.
▶ *To treat bacteremia or meningitis*
I.V. INFUSION
Children. 50 to 100 mg/kg daily in divided doses every 6 hr.
DOSAGE ADJUSTMENT Dosage limited to 25 mg/kg daily for infants and children with immature metabolic processes.

Mechanism of Action
Produces a bacteriostatic effect on susceptible organisms by inhibiting protein synthesis, thereby preventing amino acids from being transferred to growing polypeptide chains.

Contraindications
Hypersensitivity to chloramphenicol or its components

Interactions
DRUGS

alfentanil: Prolonged alfentanil effect

barbiturates: Increased blood barbiturate level; decreased blood chloramphenicol level

blood-dyscrasia–causing drugs (such as captropil and cephalosporins), bone marrow depressants (including colchicine and methotrexate): Increased bone marrow depression

chlorpropamide, tolbutamide: Increased hypoglycemic effects of these drugs

clindamycin, erythromycin, lincomycin: Decreased antibacterial effects of these drugs

cyclophosphamide: Decreased or delayed activation of cyclophosphamide, increased bone marrow depression

hepatic enzyme inducers (including rifampin): Decreased blood chloramphenicol level

hydantoins: Increased blood hydantoin level, possibly resulting in toxicity, including increased bone marrow depression; decreased blood chloramphenicol level

iron salts: Increased serum iron level

oral anticoagulants: Enhanced anticoagulant effect

oral contraceptives containing estrogen: Decreased contraceptive effect with prolonged chloramphenicol use

penicillins: Decreased penicillin activity, synergistic effects with treatment of certain microorganisms

vitamin B_{12}: Antagonized hematopoietic response to vitamin B_{12}

Adverse Reactions
CNS: Confusion, delirium, depression, fever, headache, peripheral neuropathy

CV: Gray syndrome in neonates

EENT: Glossitis, optic neuritis, stomatitis

GI: Diarrhea, nausea, vomiting

HEME: Aplastic anemia, bone marrow depression, granulocytopenia, hypoplastic anemia, leukopenia, reticulocytopenia, thrombocytopenia

SKIN: Macular or vesicular rash, urticaria

Other: Anaphylaxis, angioedema

Nursing Considerations
• **WARNING** Keep in mind that chloramphenicol should never

be used to treat minor infections or for prophylaxis because of the many serious toxicities associated with its use.

• Be aware that patients with impaired or immature renal function (especially neonates and infants) may require reduced dosage. Monitor chloramphenicol concentrations, as ordered.

• Prepare a 10% solution by adding 10 ml of sterile water for injection or D_5W to each 1-g vial of chloramphenicol. Administer over at least 1 minute.

• Know that diluted I.V. solution is stable for 24 to 48 hours when stored at room temperature or refrigerated (depending on manufacturer's recommendation). Don't use if it's cloudy.

• Monitor CBC as ordered for signs of blood dyscrasias, including leukopenia and thrombocytopenia.

• Assess for fever, sore throat, tiredness, unusual bleeding, or ecchymosis, which may indicate a blood dyscrasia.

• Perform neurologic assessments regularly, looking for signs and symptoms of peripheral neuropathy.

• **WARNING** If early signs of gray syndrome (failure to feed, pallor, cyanosis, abdominal distention, irregular respirations, and vasomotor collapse) appear, notify prescriber and be prepared to stop drug immediately.

• Be aware that chloramphenicol may increase bone marrow depression in patients receiving radiation therapy.

• Be aware that administering chloramphenicol at term or during labor puts neonate at risk for gray syndrome and administering drug to breast-feeding woman may have toxic effects on infant.

• Before reconstituting chloramphenicol, store it at 15° to 25° C (59° to 77° F).

PATIENT TEACHING

• Instruct patient receiving chloramphenicol to immediately report signs of blood dyscrasias.

• **WARNING** Advise patient to be alert for signs and symptoms of potentially fatal, irreversible bone marrow depression, which leads to aplastic anemia and is characterized by fever, pallor, pharyngitis, severe fatigue and weakness, and unusual bleeding or bruising. Bone marrow depression may occur weeks to months after therapy ends and seems unrelated to administration route. Stress the importance of prescribed follow-up care.

• Urge patient to use a soft-bristled toothbrush and to avoid using toothpicks or dental floss because of increased risk of infection and gingival bleeding due to drug's effects on blood counts.

chlordiazepoxide hydrochloride
Librium

Class, Category, and Schedule
Chemical: Benzodiazepine
Therapeutic: Antianxiety agent
Pregnancy category: Not rated
Controlled substance schedule: IV

Indications and Dosages
▶ *To provide short-term management of severe anxiety*
I.V. INJECTION
Adults. *Initial:* 50 to 100 mg. Then 25 to 50 mg t.i.d. or q.i.d., p.r.n. *Maximum:* 300 mg daily.
▶ *To provide short-term treatment of acute alcohol withdrawal*
I.V. INJECTION
Adults. *Initial:* 50 to 100 mg. Repeated in 2 to 4 hr, followed by individualized oral dosage if needed to control symptoms. *Maximum:* 300 mg daily.
DOSAGE ADJUSTMENT Dosage reduced to 25 to 50 mg for elderly or debilitated patients and for children age 12 and older.

Mechanism of Action
May potentiate the effects of gamma-aminobutyric acid (GABA) and other in-hibitory neurotransmitters by binding to specific benzodiazepine receptors in the limbic and cortical areas of the CNS. By binding to these receptors, chlor-diazepoxide increases GABA's inhibitory effects and blocks cortical and limbic arousal, which helps control emotional behavior. It also helps relieve symp-toms of alcohol withdrawal by causing CNS depression.

Contraindications
Hypersensitivity to chlordiazepoxide or its components

Interactions
DRUGS
cimetidine, disulfiram, fluoxetine, isoniazid, ketoconazole, metoprolol, oral contraceptives, propoxyphene, propranolol, valproic acid: Increased blood chlordiazepoxide level
CNS depressants: Increased CNS effects
digoxin: Increased blood digoxin level and risk of digitalis toxicity
levodopa: Decreased efficacy of levodopa's antiparkinsonian effects

neuromuscular blockers: Potentiated, counteracted, or diminished effects of neuromuscular blockers

phenytoin: Possibly increased phenytoin toxicity

probenecid: Shortened onset of action or prolonged effect of chlordiazepoxide

rifampin: Decreased chlordiazepoxide effects

theophyllines: Antagonized sedative effects of chlordiazepoxide

ACTIVITIES

alcohol use: Increased CNS effects

Adverse Reactions

CNS: Ataxia, confusion, depression, drowsiness

CV: ECG changes, hypotension, tachycardia

GI: Hepatic dysfunction

HEME: Agranulocytosis

SKIN: Jaundice

Other: Infusion site pain, redness, and swelling

Nursing Considerations

- **WARNING** Be aware that prolonged use of therapeutic doses of chlordiazepoxide can lead to dependence.
- Reconstitute ampule contents with 5 ml of sterile water for injection or sodium chloride for injection. Agitate gently until completely dissolved. Administer slowly over 1 minute immediately after reconstitution. Discard unused portions.
- **WARNING** Don't use supplied diluent (provided for I.M. use) to prepare drug for I.V. use because air bubbles form on the surface.
- Be aware that rapid I.V. administration may cause apnea, hypotension, bradycardia, and cardiac arrest. Keep emergency equipment and drugs nearby. Observe patient for 5 hours or longer, as needed.
- Monitor patients with porphyria for signs of an exacerbation, such as fever, photosensitivity, abdominal pain, and neuropathy.
- Monitor patient for adverse reactions, especially if he has hypoalbuminemia, which increases drug's sedative effects.
- Observe for signs of phlebitis or thrombophlebitis after I.V. administration.
- Monitor patients with impaired hepatic or renal function for signs of increased CNS effects due to slowed chlordiazepoxide metabolism or excretion because drug is metabolized by liver and excreted by kidneys.
- Monitor a hyperactive, aggressive child or any patient with a history of psychiatric disorders for paradoxical reactions, such as

excitement, stimulation, and acute rage, during first 2 weeks of therapy.
- Before reconstituting chlordiazepoxide, store it at 15° to 30° C (59° to 86° F).

PATIENT TEACHING
- Caution patient about possible drowsiness, and advise him to avoid activities requiring alertness until chlordiazepoxide's full CNS effects are known.

chlorothiazide
Diuril
chlorothiazide sodium
Diuril

Class and Category
Chemical: Sulfonamide derivative
Therapeutic: Antihypertensive, diuretic
Pregnancy category: B

Indications and Dosages
▶ *To produce diuresis*
I.V. INFUSION, I.V. INJECTION
Adults. 250 mg every 6 to 12 hr.

Route	Onset	Peak	Duration
I.V.	15 min	4 hr	6 to 12 hr

Contraindications
Anuria; hepatic coma; hypersensitivity to chlorothiazide, its components, sulfonamides, or related thiazide diuretics; renal failure

Interactions
DRUGS
allopurinol: Increased risk of allopurinol hypersensitivity
amiodarone: Increased risk of arrhythmias from hypokalemia
amphotericin B, glucocorticoids: Intensified electrolyte depletion
anesthetics: Potentiated effects of anesthetics
anticholinergics: Increased chlorothiazide absorption
anticoagulants, methenamines, sulfonylureas: Decreased effects of these drugs
antihypertensives: Increased antihypertensive effect
antineoplastics: Prolonged antineoplastic-induced leukopenia
calcium: Possibly increased blood calcium level

Mechanism of Action

A thiazide diuretic, chlorothiazide inhibits sodium (Na+) reabsorption and promotes movement of Na+, chloride (Cl−), and water (H$_2$O) from blood in peritubular capillaries into the nephron's distal convoluted tubule, as shown. Initially, chlorothiazide may reduce blood pressure by decreasing extracellular fluid volume, plasma volume, and cardiac output. It also directly dilates arteries. After several weeks, extracellular fluid volume, plasma volume, and cardiac output return to normal. Peripheral vascular resistance remains decreased.

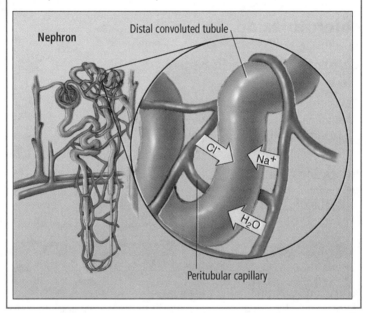

cholestyramine, colestipol: Decreased chlorothiazide absorption
diazoxide: Hyperglycemia, hypotension
digitalis glycosides: Increased risk of digitalis-induced arrhythmias
dopamine: Increased diuretic effect of both drugs
lithium: Increased risk of lithium toxicity
loop diuretics: Synergistic effects, resulting in profound diuresis and serious electrolyte imbalances
methyldopa: Potential development of hemolytic anemia
neuromuscular blockers: Increased neuromuscular blockade
NSAIDs: Possibly reduced diuretic effect of chlorothiazide
sympathomimetics: Possibly inhibited antihypertensive effect of chlorothiazide
vitamin D: Enhanced vitamin D action

Adverse Reactions

CNS: Dizziness, headache, paresthesia, restlessness, vertigo, weakness
CV: Orthostatic hypotension
ENDO: Hyperglycemia
GI: Abdominal cramps, anorexia, constipation, diarrhea, gastric irritation, nausea, pancreatitis, vomiting
GU: Glycosuria, hematuria, impotence, interstitial nephritis, renal dysfunction or failure
HEME: Agranulocytosis, aplastic anemia, hemolytic anemia, leukopenia, thrombocytopenia
MS: Muscle spasms
SKIN: Jaundice, photosensitivity, purpura, rash, urticaria
Other: Anaphylactic reactions, hypercalcemia, hyperuricemia, hypochloremic alkalosis, hypokalemia, hypomagnesemia, hyponatremia, hypovolemia

Nursing Considerations

- Don't give parenteral form of chlorothiazide by I.M. or subcutaneous route.
- For I.V. use, reconstitute with at least 18 ml of sterile water for injection. Discard unused solution after 24 hours. Reconstituted solution is compatible with dextrose solution or normal saline solution for infusion.
- Watch I.V. site closely. If extravasation occurs, stop infusion and tell prescriber at once.
- Weigh patient daily to assess fluid loss and drug effectiveness. Also, check blood pressure often if used to treat hypertension; antihypertensive effect may not appear for days.
- Assess patient for electrolyte imbalances.
- Monitor renal function closely, especially in elderly patients, because the risk of toxicity increases with renal impairment.

PATIENT TEACHING
- Encourage patient to eat a high-potassium diet.
- Instruct patient to rise slowly to minimize effects of orthostatic hypotension.
- Tell patient to immediately notify prescriber about weakness, cramps, nausea, vomiting, restlessness, excessive thirst, drowsiness, tiredness, increased heart rate, diarrhea, sudden joint pain, or dizziness.
- Inform patient with diabetes mellitus that his blood glucose will be monitored and that his oral antidiabetic dosage may need to be increased.

chlorpromazine hydrochloride

Largactil (CAN), Thorazine

Class and Category

Chemical: Propylamine derivative of phenothiazine
Therapeutic: Antiemetic, antipsychotic, tranquilizer
Pregnancy category: Not rated

Indications and Dosages

▶ *To provide intraoperative control of nausea and vomiting*
I.V. INJECTION
Adults. 25 mg diluted to 1 mg/ml with sodium chloride for injection and given at a rate not to exceed 2 mg every 2 min. *Maximum:* 25 mg.
Children age 6 months and over. 0.275 mg/kg diluted to at least 1 mg/ml with sodium chloride for injection and given at a rate not to exceed 1 mg every 2 min. *Maximum:* 75 mg/day for children ages 5 to 12 years or weighing 50 to 100 lb; 40 mg daily for children up to age 5 years or weighing up to 50 lb.

▶ *To treat intractable hiccups*
I.V. INFUSION
Adults. 25 to 50 mg diluted in 500 to 1,000 ml of normal saline solution and administered at 1 mg/min with patient in supine position.

▶ *To treat tetanus (usually as adjunct to barbiturates)*
I.V. INFUSION
Adults. 25 to 50 mg diluted to at least 1 mg/ml and given at no more than 1 mg/min.
Children age 6 months and over. 0.55 mg/kg every 6 to 8 hr, diluted to at least 1 mg/ml and given at no more than 1 mg/ 2 min. *Maximum:* 75 mg daily for children ages 5 to 12 or weighing 50 to 100 lb; 40 mg daily for children up to age 5 or weighing up to 50 lb.

DOSAGE ADJUSTMENT Dosage possibly reduced for patients who have hepatic dysfunction. Dosage reduced to one-third to one-half the normal adult dosage for elderly or debilitated patients.

Incompatibilities

Don't mix chlorpromazine with thiopental, atropine, or solutions that don't have a pH of 4 to 5 because a precipitate will form. Don't mix chlorpromazine injection in same syringe with other drugs.

Mechanism of Action

Depresses areas of the brain that control activity and aggression, including the cerebral cortex, hypothalamus, and limbic system, by an unknown mechanism. Chlorpromazine prevents nausea and vomiting by inhibiting or blocking dopamine receptors in the medullary chemoreceptor trigger zone and peripherally by blocking the vagus nerve in the GI tract. It may relieve anxiety by causing indirect reduction in arousal and increased filtering of internal stimuli to the reticular activating system in the brain stem.

Contraindications

Comatose states; hypersensitivity to chlorpromazine, phenothiazines, or their components; use of large amounts of CNS depressants

Interactions

DRUGS

amphetamines: Decreased amphetamine effectiveness, decreased antipsychotic effectiveness of chlorpromazine

barbiturates: Decreased plasma level and, possibly, effectiveness of chlorpromazine

CNS depressants: Prolonged and intensified CNS depression

metrizamide: Possibly lowered seizure threshold

oral anticoagulants: Decreased anticoagulant effect

phenytoin: Interference with phenytoin metabolism, increased risk of phenytoin toxicity

propranolol: Increased plasma levels of both drugs

thiazide diuretics: Possibly increased orthostatic hypotension

ACTIVITIES

alcohol use: Prolonged and intensified CNS depression

Adverse Reactions

CNS: Drowsiness, extrapyramidal reactions (dystonia, fever, motor restlessness, pseudoparkinsonism, and tardive dyskinesia), neuroleptic malignant syndrome, seizures

CV: ECG changes, such as nonspecific, usually reversible Q- and T-wave changes; orthostatic hypotension; tachycardia

EENT: Blurred vision, dry mouth, nasal congestion, ocular changes (fine particle deposits in lens and cornea) with long-term therapy

ENDO: Gynecomastia, hyperglycemia, hypoglycemia, lactation, moderate breast engorgement

GI: Constipation, ileus, nausea

GU: Amenorrhea, ejaculation disorders, impotence, priapism, urine retention

HEME: Agranulocytosis, aplastic anemia, eosinophilia, hemolytic anemia, leukopenia, pancytopenia, thrombocytopenic purpura
SKIN: Exfoliative dermatitis, jaundice, photosensitivity, tissue necrosis, urticaria

Nursing Considerations

- Protect chlorpromazine solution from light. Solution should be clear and colorless to pale yellow. Discard markedly discolored solution.
- Don't inject drug subcutaneously because it can cause severe tissue necrosis.
- Wear gloves when working with liquid or injectable form because parenteral solution may cause contact dermatitis.
- For I.V. injection, dilute chlorpromazine with sodium chloride for injection to a concentration that yields 1 mg/ml before administration.
- **WARNING** Be aware that chlorpromazine contains benzyl alcohol, which can cause a fatal toxic syndrome in neonates or immature infants, characterized by CNS, respiratory, circulatory, and renal impairment and metabolic acidosis. Dosage has not been established for infants younger than age 6 months.
- **WARNING** Be alert for possible suppressed cough reflex, which increases patient's risk of aspirating vomitus.
- **WARNING** If neuroleptic malignant syndrome (hyperpyrexia, muscle rigidity, altered mental status, autonomic instability) develops, notify prescriber immediately and expect to discontinue drug and begin intensive medical treatment. Monitor carefully for recurrence if patient resumes antipsychotic therapy.
- Monitor patients (especially children) with chronic respiratory disorders (such as severe asthma or emphysema) or acute respiratory tract infections for exacerbations of these conditions caused by chlorpromazine's CNS depressant effects. Be aware that patients with cardiovascular, hepatic, or renal disease are at increased risk for developing hypotension, heart failure, and arrhythmias.
- Monitor patients with a history of hepatic encephalopathy from cirrhosis for increased sensitivity to drug's CNS effects.
- Because of chlorpromazine's anticholinergic effects, monitor patients with a history of or predisposition to glaucoma for evidence of this disorder, such as eye pain, vision changes, or nausea and vomiting from increased intraocular pressure.

- Be aware that drug should be used cautiously in those who are exposed to organophosphorus insecticides.
- Monitor patients who have been exposed to extreme heat for heatstroke due to drug-induced suppression of temperature regulation. Symptoms include tachycardia, fever, and confusion.
- Be aware that pediatric and elderly patients are at increased risk for developing hypotension amd extrapyramidal reactions, especially if they're acutely ill or debilitated.
- Before reconstituting chlorpromazine, store it at 15° to 30° C (59° to 86° F).

PATIENT TEACHING
- Because chlorpromazine may cause drowsiness, dizziness, and blurred vision (especially during the first few days of therapy), advise patient to avoid potentially hazardous activities until drug's CNS effects are known.
- Advise patient, especially if elderly, to rise slowly from a supine or seated position to avoid dizziness, light-headedness, and fainting.
- Urge patient to avoid alcohol because of possible additive effects and hypotension.
- Inform patient that drug may reduce body's response to heat and cold; advise him to avoid temperature extremes, as in very cold or hot showers.
- If patient reports dry mouth, suggest sugarless chewing gum, hard candy, and fluids.
- Urge patient to report sudden sore throat or other signs of infection.

cidofovir
Vistide

Class and Category
Chemical: Synthetic purine nucleotide analogue
Therapeutic: Antiviral
Pregnancy category: C

Indications and Dosages
I.V. INFUSION
▶ *To treat cytomegalovirus (CMV) retinitis in patients with AIDS*
Adults. Induction dose of 5 mg/kg infused over 1 hr once every wk for 2 wk. *Maintenance:* 5 mg/kg infused over 1 hr once every 2 wk. Probenecid should be given before and after each cidofovir dose.

DOSAGE ADJUSTMENT Maintenance dosage reduced to 3 mg/kg if serum creatinine level increases by 0.3 or 0.4 mg/dl above baseline.

Mechanism of Action
Ultimately converted by pyrimidine nucleoside monophosphate kinase and other cellular enzymes to cidofovir diphosphate. Cidofovir diphosphate suppresses cytomegalovirus (CMV) replication by incorporation into and termination of the growing DNA chain, and by selective inhibition and inactivation of viral DNA polymerase, an enzyme used in the viral DNA replication process.

Incompatibilities
Don't add other drugs or supplements to cidofovir solutions.

Contraindications
Concurrent administration within 7 days of other nephrotoxic drugs; direct intraocular injection; hypersensitivity to cidofovir or severe hypersensitivity to probenecid or other sulfa-containing drugs; serum creatinine level greater than 1.5 mg/dl, calculated creatinine clearance less than or equal to 55 ml/min/1.73 m^2, or urine protein level greater than or equal to 100 mg/dl (proteinuria greater than or equal to 2+)

Interactions
DRUGS
nephrotoxic drugs (such as aminoglycosides, amphotericin B, foscarnet, NSAIDs, and pentamidine): Increased risk of nephrotoxicity

Adverse Reactions
CNS: Asthenia, fever, headache
EENT: Iritis, ocular hypotony, uveitis, vision changes
GI: Anorexia, diarrhea, nausea, vomiting
GU: Elevated serum creatinine level, nephrotoxicity, proteinuria
HEME: Neutropenia
Other: Decreased serum sodium bicarbonate levels, metabolic acidosis

Nursing Considerations
- **WARNING** Be aware that cidofovir is for I.V. infusion only and is not for direct intraocular injection.
- Monitor serum creatinine and urine protein levels within 48 hours of an upcoming cidofovir dose, as ordered. Expect

maintenance dosage to be decreased if serum creatinine level increases by 0.3 or 0.4 mg/dl above baseline. Expect therapy to stop if serum creatinine level increases by at least 0.5 mg/dl above baseline or if patient develops proteinuria of 3+ or more.

- Monitor WBC count with differential before cidofovir dose to detect drug-induced neutropenia. Also, assess patient for signs of neutropenia, including fever, chills, and sore throat.
- Expect to administer 2 g of probenecid 3 hours before each dose of cidofovir and 1 g 2 hours and 8 hours after each dose— for a total of 4 g—to minimize the risk of nephrotoxicity.
- Give at least 1 L of normal saline solution over 1 to 2 hours immediately before giving cidofovir. Another infusion of 1 L of normal saline solution over 1 to 3 hours may be prescribed for patients who can tolerate the extra fluid, to be started when cidofovir infusion starts or immediately afterward.
- Be aware that adverse reactions can vary when cidofovir is given in combination therapy. Review information for all drugs given as part of a specific regimen, including drug interactions and adverse effects.
- Be aware that an antiemetic may be prescribed to help reduce nausea from probenecid. Also, be prepared to administer prophylactic or therapeutic antihistamines or acetaminophen if patient develops an allergic or hypersensitivity reaction.
- Be aware that cidofovir has mutagenic properties. Follow facility protocol for preparation and handling of such drugs and for appropriate disposal of used equipment. Thoroughly wash any skin exposed to cidofovir with soap and water.
- Inspect each vial of cidofovir before administration; discard it if you detect particles or discoloration. Dilute each dose of cidofovir with 100 ml of normal saline solution. Give within 24 hours. Diluted solutions not used immediately may be stored at 2° to 8° C (36° to 46° F) but must be used within the original 24-hour period. Allow refrigerated solution to return to room temperature before giving it.
- Administer cidofovir at a constant rate over a 1-hour period, using an infusion pump.
- Assess patient for changes in vision, such as decreased vision, which may indicate decreased intraocular pressure. Ensure that patient's intraocular pressure is measured periodically.

PATIENT TEACHING
- Instruct patient to eat some food before each dose of probenecid to help reduce drug-related nausea and vomiting.

- Stress the need to take the full course of probenecid with each dose of cidofovir to decrease the risk of adverse reactions.
- Advise patient to comply with follow-up ophthalmic exams to assess drug effectiveness and monitor for adverse reactions. Inform patient that CMV retinitis may continue to progress during and following treatment.
- Inform patient who is also receiving zidovudine that a dosage adjustment or temporary discontinuation of zidovudine may be needed on the day of cidofovir therapy.
- If patient develops neutropenia, urge him to avoid sports and other activities that increase the risk of accidental injury. Also advise him to take measures to avoid infection, such as maintaining good oral hygiene (for example, by using a soft-bristled toothbrush) and washing hands before touching eyes or nose.

cimetidine hydrochloride

Novo-Cimetine (CAN), Tagamet

Class and Category

Chemical: Imidazole derivative
Therapeutic: Antiulcer agent, gastric acid secretion inhibitor, H_2-receptor antagonist
Pregnancy category: B

Indications and Dosages

▶ *To treat and prevent recurrence of duodenal ulcer*
I.V. INJECTION
Adults. *Initial:* 300 mg every 6 to 8 hr. Dosage increased, if needed, by increasing frequency. *Maximum:* 2,400 mg daily.
▶ *To treat active, benign gastric ulcer*
I.V. INJECTION
Adults and adolescents. *Initial:* 300 mg every 6 to 8 hr. Dosage increased, if needed, by increasing frequency. *Maximum:* 2,400 mg/day.
▶ *To treat pathologic hypersecretory conditions, such as Zollinger-Ellison syndrome*
I.V. INJECTION
Adults and adolescents. *Initial:* 300 mg every 6 to 8 hr. Dosage increased, if needed, by increasing frequency. *Maximum:* 2,400 mg daily.
▶ *To prevent stress-related upper GI bleeding during hospitalization*
I.V. INFUSION
Adults. 50 mg/hr by continuous infusion for 7 days.

Route	Onset	Peak	Duration
I.V.	Unknown	Unknown	4 to 5 hr

Mechanism of Action
Blocks histamine's action at H_2-receptor sites on the stomach's parietal cells. This action reduces gastric fluid volume and acidity. Cimetidine also decreases the amount of gastric acid that's secreted in response to food, caffeine, insulin, betazole, or pentagastrin.

Incompatibilities
Don't mix cimetidine in same I.V. solution with aminophylline or barbiturates. Don't mix drug in same syringe with pentobarbital sodium.

Contraindications
Hypersensitivity to cimetidine or its components

Interactions
DRUGS

antacids, anticholinergics, metoclopramide: Decreased cimetidine absorption

benzodiazepines, calcium channel blockers, carbamazepine, chloroquine, labetalol, lidocaine, metoprolol, metronidazole, moricizine, pentoxifylline, phenytoin, propafenone, propranolol, quinidine, quinine, sulfonylureas, tacrine, theophyllines, triamterene, tricyclic antidepressants, valproic acid, warfarin: Reduced metabolism and increased blood levels and effects of these drugs, possibly toxicity from these drugs

carmustine: Increased carmustine myelotoxicity

digoxin, fluconazole: Possibly decreased blood levels of these drugs

ferrous salts, indomethacin, ketoconazole, tetracyclines: Decreased effects of these drugs

flecainide: Increased flecainide effects

fluorouracil: Increased blood fluorouracil level after long-term cimetidine use

ketoconazole: Decreased blood ketoconazole level

opioid analgesics: Increased toxic effects of opioid analgesics

oral anticoagulants: Increased anticoagulant effect

procainamide: Increased blood procainamide level

succinylcholine: Increased neuromuscular blockade

tocainide: Decreased tocainide effects

FOODS

caffeine: Decreased caffeine metabolism and increased blood level

ACTIVITIES
alcohol use: Possibly increased blood alcohol level

Adverse Reactions

CNS: Confusion, dizziness, hallucinations, headache, peripheral neuropathy, somnolence
ENDO: Mild gynecomastia if used longer than 1 month
GI: Mild and transient diarrhea
GU: Impotence, transiently elevated serum creatinine level
SKIN: Rash

Nursing Considerations

• Don't use cimetidine if solution is discolored or contains precipitate.
• For I.V. injection, dilute cimetidine in normal saline solution to a total volume of 20 ml. Inject drug over 5 minutes or more.
• Use diluted solution within 48 hours when stored at room temperature.
• **WARNING** Be aware that rapid delivery of cimetidine can increase the risk of arrhythmias and hypotension.
• For intermittent I.V. infusion, dilute drug in at least 50 ml of D_5W or other compatible I.V. solution. Infuse over 15 to 20 minutes.
• Be especially alert for confusion in elderly or debilitated patients who receive cimetidine.
• Before using cimetidine, store it at 15° to 30° C (59° to 86° F).
PATIENT TEACHING
• Advise patient to avoid alcohol during cimetidine therapy to prevent interactions.
• Caution patient that cigarette smoking increases gastric acid secretion and can worsen gastric disease.

ciprofloxacin

Cipro I.V.

Class and Category

Chemical: Fluoroquinolone derivative
Therapeutic: Antibiotic
Pregnancy category: C

Indications and Dosages

▶ *To prevent inhalation anthrax after exposure or to treat inhalation anthrax*

I.V. INFUSION
Adults and adolescents. 400 mg every 12 hr for 60 days.
Children. 10 mg/kg every 12 hr for 60 days. *Maximum:*
400 mg/dose or 800 mg daily.

▶ *To treat acute sinusitis caused by gram-negative organisms (including* Campylobacter jejuni, Citrobacter diversus, Citrobacter freundii, Enterobacter cloacae, Escherichia coli, Haemophilus influenzae, Haemophilus parainfluenzae, Klebsiella pneumoniae, Morganella morganii, Neisseria gonorrhoeae, Proteus mirabilis, Proteus vulgaris, Providencia rettgeri, Providencia stuartii, Pseudomonas aeruginosa, Serratia marcescens, Shigella flexneri, *and* Shigella sonnei*) and gram-positive organisms (including* Enterococcus faecalis, Staphylococcus aureus, Staphylococcus epidermidis, *and* Streptococcus pneumoniae*)*
I.V. INFUSION
Adults. For mild to moderate infection, 400 mg every 12 hr.
▶ *To treat bone and joint infections caused by susceptible organisms listed above*
I.V. INFUSION
Adults. For mild to moderate infection, 400 mg every 12 hr for 4 to 6 wk. For severe or complicated infection, 400 mg every 8 hr.
▶ *To treat skin and soft-tissue infection caused by susceptible organisms listed above*
I.V. INFUSION
Adults. For mild to moderate infection, 400 mg every 12 hr. For severe or complicated infections, 400 mg every 8 hr.
▶ *To treat chronic bacterial prostatitis caused by susceptible organisms listed above*
I.V. INFUSION
Adults. 400 mg every 12 hr.
▶ *To treat UTIs caused by susceptible organisms listed above*
I.V. INFUSION
Adults. For mild to moderate infection, 200 mg every 12 hr. For severe or complicated infection, 400 mg every 12 hr.
▶ *To treat lower respiratory tract infections caused by susceptible organisms listed above*
I.V. INFUSION
Adults. For mild to moderate infection, 400 mg every 12 hr. For severe or complicated infection, 400 mg every 8 hr.
▶ *To treat intra-abdominal infections caused by susceptible organisms listed above*

I.V. INFUSION
Adults. 400 mg every 8 hr along with parenteral metronidazole.
▶ *To treat mild to severe nosocomial pneumonia caused by susceptible organisms listed above*
I.V. INFUSION
Adults. 400 mg every 8 hr.
▶ *To treat typhoid fever caused by* Salmonella typhi *or infectious diarrhea caused by* C. jejuni, E. coli, S. flexneri, *or* S. sonnei
DOSAGE ADJUSTMENT Dosage reduced to 250 to 500 mg every 12 hr in patients with creatinine clearance of 30 to 50 ml/min/1.73 m^2; and to 250 to 500 mg P.O. or 200 to 400 mg I.V. every 18 hr in patients with creatinine clearance of 5 to 29 ml/min/1.73 m^2.

Mechanism of Action
Inhibits the enzyme DNA gyrase, which is responsible for the unwinding and supercoiling of bacterial DNA before it replicates, and causes bacterial cells to die.

Incompatibilities
Don't administer parenteral ciprofloxacin with aminophylline, amoxicillin, cefepime, clindamycin, dexamethasone, floxacillin, furosemide, heparin, or phenytoin.

Contraindications
Hypersensitivity to ciprofloxacin, quinolones, or their components; concurrent therapy with tizanidine

Interactions
DRUGS
antacids, didanosine, iron supplements, sucralfate, zinc- or iron-containing multivitamins: Decreased ciprofloxacin absorption
cyclosporine: Elevated serum creatinine and cyclosporine levels
glyburide: Severe hypoglycemia
methylxanthines, theophylline, tizanidine: Increased blood levels of these drugs leading possibly to increased toxicity
NSAIDs (except acetylsalicylic acid): Increased risk of seizures with high doses of ciprofloxacin
oral anticoagulants: Enhanced anticoagulant effects
phenytoin: Increased or decreased blood phenytoin level
probenecid: Increased blood level of ciprofloxacin and, possibly, toxicity

FOODS

caffeine: Increased caffeine effects

dairy products: Delayed drug absorption

Adverse Reactions

CNS: Agitation, anxiety, cerebral thrombosis, confusion, dizziness, headache, insomnia, light-headedness, migraine, nightmares, paranoia, peripheral neuropathy, restlessness, seizures, syncope, toxic psychosis

CV: Angina, atrial flutter, cardiopulmonary arrest, cardiovascular collapse, hypertension, MI, orthostatic hypotension, palpitations, phlebitis, tachycardia, torsades de pointes, vasculitis, ventricular ectopy

EENT: Oral candidiasis

GI: Abdominal pain, constipation, diarrhea, elevated liver function test results, flatulence, GI bleeding, hepatic failure or necrosis, hepatitis, indigestion, intestinal perforation, jaundice, nausea, necrosis pancreatitis, pseudomembranous colitis, vomiting

GU: Crystalluria, hematuria, increased serum creatinine level, interstitial nephritis, nephrotoxicity, renal calculi, renal failure, urine retention, vaginal candidiasis

HEME: Agranulocytosis, bone marrow depression, hemolytic anemia, lymphadenopathy, pancytopenia

MS: Tendon rupture

RESP: Bronchospasm, pulmonary embolism, respiratory arrest

SKIN: Erythema multiforme, exfoliative dermatitis, photosensitivity, rash, Stevens-Johnson syndrome, toxic epidermal necrolysis, urticaria

Other: Acidosis, anaphylaxis, angioedema, serum sickness–like reaction

Nursing Considerations

- Obtain culture and sensitivity test results, as ordered, before giving ciprofloxacin.
- Use drug cautiously in patients with CNS disorders and in patients who may have increased susceptibility to drug's effect on the QT interval, such as those taking class IA or III antiarrhythmics and those with uncorrected hypokalemia or a history of prolonged QT interval.
- Dilute I.V. ciprofloxacin concentrate to 1 to 2 mg/ml using D_5W or sodium chloride for injection. Don't dilute solutions that come from the manufacturer in D_5W before I.V. infusion. Infuse slowly over 1 hour.

- Store reconstituted solution for up to 14 days at room temperature or refrigerated.
- Be aware that patient should be well hydrated during therapy to help prevent alkaline urine, which may lead to crystalluria and nephrotoxicity.
- Assess patient's hepatic, renal, and hematologic functions periodically, as ordered, for patients receiving prolonged therapy.
- Monitor patient closely for diarrhea, which may reflect pseudomembranous colitis. If signs and symptoms develop, notify prescriber and expect to obtain a stool specimen to check for pseudomembranous colitis, to withhold ciprofloxacin, and to treat diarrhea with fluids, electrolytes, and antibiotics effective against *Clostridium difficile.*
- Assess patient for evidence of peripheral neuropathy. Notify prescriber and expect to stop drug if patient complains of pain, burning, tingling, numbness, or weakness in extremities or if physical examination reveals deficits in light touch, pain, temperature, position sense, vibratory sensation, or motor strength.
- Monitor patients (especially children, elderly patients, and patients receiving corticosteroids) for evidence of tendon rupture, such as pain, inflammation, and swelling at the site. Be aware that tendon rupture may occur during or after ciprofloxacin therapy. Notify prescriber about suspected tendon rupture, and have patient rest and refrain from exercise until tendon rupture has been ruled out. If present, expect to provide supportive care as ordered.
- Assess patient routinely for signs of rash or other hypersensitivity reaction, even after patient has received several doses. Stop drug and notify prescriber immediately at first sign of rash, jaundice, or any other suggestion of hypersensitivity. Be prepared to provide supportive emergency care.

PATIENT TEACHING
- Encourage patient to drink plenty of fluids during therapy to help prevent crystalluria.
- Urge patient to avoid caffeinated products because caffeine may accumulate in the body during ciprofloxacin therapy and cause excessive stimulation.
- Instruct patient to notify prescriber at first sign of allergy, such as rash.
- Urge patient to avoid hazardous activities until CNS effects of drug are known.
- Advise patient to notify prescriber about changes in limb sensa-

tion or movement, pain, inflammation, or swelling over a joint.
- Urge patient to report watery, bloody stools to prescriber immediately, even up to 2 months after drug therapy has ended.
- Tell patient to notify prescriber at first sign of rash or other hypersensitivity reaction.

cisplatin
Platinol (CAN), Platinol-AQ

Class and Category
Chemical: Inorganic metal complex
Therapeutic: Alkylating-like antineoplastic
Pregnancy category: D

Indications and Dosages
▶ *To treat metastatic testicular tumors*
I.V. INFUSION
Adults. 20 mg/m² daily for 5 days every 21-day cycle. *Maximum:* 120 mg/m² for each course.
▶ *To treat metastatic ovarian tumors*
I.V. INFUSION
Adults also receiving cyclophosphamide sequentially. 75 to 100 mg/m² per cycle every 4 wk. *Maximum:* 120 mg/m² for each course.
Adults not receiving cyclophosphamide. 100 mg/m² per cycle every 4 wk. *Maximum:* 120 mg/m² for each course.
Adults also receiving paclitaxel. 75 mg/m² every 3 wk for six courses. *Maximum:* 120 mg/m² for each course.
▶ *To treat advanced bladder cancer*
I.V. INFUSION
Adults: 50 to 70 mg/m² per cycle every 3 or 4 wk. *Maximum:* 120 mg/m² for each course.

Mechanism of Action
May bind to DNA within the cell, thus interfering with DNA function and synthesis. May also have a smaller effect on RNA synthesis. Cisplatin's actions are cell-cycle-phase–nonspecific.

Incompatibilities
Don't use needles or I.V. sets containing aluminum to give cisplatin because precipitate could form and potency be decreased.

Contraindications

Hearing impairment, hypersensitivity to cisplatin or other platinum-containing drugs, myelosuppression

Interactions

DRUGS

antihistamines, buclizine, cyclizine, loxapine, meclizine, phenothiazines, thioxanthenes, trimethobenzamide: Possibly masked ototoxicity effects
bleomycin: Increased risk of bleomycin toxicity
blood-dyscrasia–causing drugs (including ACE inhibitors, cephalosporins, and NSAIDs): Increased leukopenic and thrombocytopenic effects of cisplatin
bone marrow depressants (such as amphotericin B, colchicine, and paclitaxel): Increased effects of these drugs
nephrotoxic drugs (such as acyclovir, aminoglycosides, and penicillamine): Potentiated risk of nephrotoxicity
ototoxic drugs (such as capreomycin, furosemide, and NSAIDs): Increased risk of ototoxicity
vaccines, killed virus: Possibly decreased antibody response to vaccine
vaccines, live virus: Possibly increased adverse effects of vaccine virus, life-threatening infection, and decreased antibody response to vaccine

Adverse Reactions

CNS: Neurotoxicity
EENT: Optic neuritis, ototoxicity, papilledema, stomatitis, vision changes
ENDO: Syndrome of inappropriate ADH secretion
GI: Anorexia, nausea, vomiting
GU: Nephrotoxicity, uric acid nephropathy
HEME: Anemia, hemolytic anemia, leukopenia, thrombocytopenia
SKIN: Extravasation
Other: Anaphylaxis, hyperuricemia, hypocalcemia, hypomagnesemia

Nursing Considerations

- Be aware that cisplatin should be administered only under the supervision of a qualified physician or nurse in settings where appropriate diagnostic and treatment facilities are available.
- **WARNING** Make sure that emergency equipment and drugs, such as antihistamines, epinephrine, and I.V. corticosteroids, are available in case of anaphylaxis.
- Follow facility protocols for preparation and handling of antineoplastic drugs and appropriate disposal of used equipment.

- **WARNING** To decrease the risk of inadvertent overdose, contact prescriber if cumulative cisplatin dose for each cycle exceeds 100 mg/m².
- Monitor creatinine clearance, serum uric acid, and BUN levels, as ordered, before initiating cisplatin therapy and before each subsequent course to detect early signs of nephrotoxicity. Expect dosage to be reduced for patients with impaired renal function.
- Monitor CBC, including hematocrit, platelet count, and WBC count with differential, before and periodically during therapy.
- Monitor serum electrolyte levels, including magnesium, sodium, potassium, and calcium levels, before initiating therapy and before each subsequent course. Be aware that tetany associated with hypocalcemia and hypomagnesemia has been reported.
- Hydrate patient, as ordered, with 1 to 2 L of fluid 8 to 12 hours before cisplatin administration.
- **WARNING** Wear gloves when handling cisplatin. If cisplatin comes in contact with skin or mucosa, immediately and thoroughly wash skin with soap and water and flush mucosa with water.
- Dilute prescribed dose of cisplatin with 2 L of D_5/0.45 normal saline solution or D_5/0.3 normal saline solution that contains 37.5 g of mannitol.
- **WARNING** Don't expose cisplatin to needles or administration sets containing aluminum because a precipitate will form and drug potency will be decreased.
- Anticipate dosage reduction if patient is also receiving radiation therapy or a drug that depresses bone marrow.
- Reconstitute cisplatin for injection (available in Canada only) by adding 10 or 50 ml of sterile water for injection to 10- or 50-mg vial, respectively. Further dilute using D_5/0.45 normal saline solution or D_5/0.3 normal saline solution. Diluted solution is stable for 20 hours at 27° C (80° F). Protect from light if not used within 6 hours of removal from vial.
- Administer an antiemetic, as prescribed, before initiation of cisplatin therapy. Infuse cisplatin as prescribed. Protect from light if diluted cisplatin is not administered within 6 hours.
- Be prepared to hydrate patient for 24 hours after cisplatin administration, and assess for adequate urine output.
- Observe patient for signs of leukopenia or infection, including fever, chills, pharyngitis, tiredness or weakness, and unusual bleeding or ecchymosis.

- Perform neurologic assessment to check for signs of neurotoxicity, such as paresthesia of the hands and feet, loss of taste or motor function, seizures, muscle spasms, and areflexia. Expect to discontinue cisplatin therapy if neurotoxicity occurs.
- Monitor serum uric acid level, especially in patients with a history of gout or urate calculi. Be aware that allopurinol may be prescribed to help prevent uric acid nephropathy. Expect antigout drug dosage to be adjusted if blood uric acid level is elevated from cisplatin therapy.
- Assess for signs of extravasation at I.V. infusion site, such as redness, swelling, or pain. Be aware that concentrations greater than 0.5 mg/ml put the patient at increased risk for tissue cellulitis, fibrosis, and necrosis.
- Be aware that effects of radiation therapy or bone marrow depressants may be increased when these treatments are administered concurrently with cisplatin. Patients with a history of bone marrow depression, chickenpox (including recent exposure), or herpes zoster are at increased risk for severe generalized disease.
- Monitor patient for signs and symptoms of syndrome of inappropriate ADH secretion, including dizziness, confusion, agitation, and tiredness or weakness.
- Expect subsequent courses of cisplatin therapy to be initiated after an appropriate time interval when serum creatinine level is below 1.5 mg/dl or BUN level is below 25 mg/dl (or both); platelet count is above or equal to $100,000/mm^3$; WBC count is greater than or equal to $4,000/mm^3$; and audiometric testing indicates hearing is within normal limits.
- Store cisplatin injection at 15° to 25° C (59° to 77° F); don't refrigerate.
- Store cisplatin for injection (available in Canada only) at 15° to 30° C (59° to 86° F), and protect from light.

PATIENT TEACHING

- Instruct patient receiving cisplatin to immediately report unusual bruising or bleeding; black, tarry stools; blood in urine or stools; pinpoint red spots on skin; numbness or tingling in fingers or toes; and ringing in ears or hearing loss.
- Urge patient not to receive live or killed virus vaccines during cisplatin therapy and for 3 months to 1 year after completion of therapy, unless approved by prescriber. Instruct him to avoid people who have received such vaccines or to wear a protective mask when he's around them.

- Caution patient to avoid sports and other activities that increase the risk of accidental injury. Also advise him to take measures to avoid infection, such as maintaining good oral hygiene (for example, by using soft-bristled toothbrush) and washing hands before touching eyes or nose.
- Stress the importance of keeping scheduled follow-up appointments and undergoing prescribed diagnostic tests, such as neurologic function studies and audiometric testing, before each course of cisplatin to monitor for adverse drug effects.
- Suggest that patient with stomatitis eat soft, bland foods served cold or at room temperature to decrease irritation.

clindamycin phosphate
Cleocin, Dalacin C Phosphate (CAN)

Class and Category
Chemical: Lincosamide
Therapeutic: Antibacterial and antiprotozoal antibiotic
Pregnancy category: B

Indications and Dosages
▶ *To treat serious respiratory tract infection caused by anaerobes such as occur with anaerobic pneumonitis, empyema, and lung abscess and those caused by pneumococci, staphylococci, and streptococci; serious skin and soft-tissue infections caused by anaerobes, staphylococci, and streptococci; septicemia caused by anaerobes; intra-abdominal infections caused by anaerobes such as occur with intra-abdominal abscess and peritonitis; infections of the female pelvis and genital tract caused by anaerobes such as occur with endometritis, nongonococcal tubo-ovarian abscess, pelvic cellulitis, and postsurgical vaginal cuff infection; bone and joint infections caused by* Staphylococcus aureus; *as adjunct therapy in chronic bone and joint infections*

I.V. INFUSION

Adults and adolescents age 16 and over. For serious infections, 600 to 1,200 mg daily in equally divided doses b.i.d. to q.i.d.; for severe infections, 1,200 to 2,700 mg daily in equally divided doses b.i.d. to q.i.d.; for life-threatening infections, 4,800 mg daily in equally divided doses b.i.d. to q.i.d.
Children ages 1 month to 16 years. 20 to 40 mg/kg/day in equally divided doses t.i.d. or q.i.d. based on severity of infection.
Neonates younger than age 1 month. 15 to 20 mg/kg daily in equally divided doses t.i.d. or q.i.d. based on severity of infection.

Mechanism of Action

Inhibits protein synthesis in susceptible bacteria by binding to the 50S subunits of bacterial ribosomes and preventing peptide bond formation, which causes bacterial cells to die.

Incompatibilities

Don't administer clindamycin with aminophylline, ampicillin, barbiturates, calcium gluconate, magnesium sulfate, or phenytoin because these drugs are physically incompatible.

Contraindications

Hypersensitivity to clindamycin or lincomycin

Interactions

DRUGS

chloramphenicol, erythromycin: Possibly antagonized effects of clindamycin

neuromuscular blockers: Increased neuromuscular blockade

Adverse Reactions

CNS: Fatigue, headache
CV: Hypotension
EENT: Glossitis, metallic or unpleasant taste, stomatitis
GI: Abdominal pain, diarrhea, esophagitis, nausea, pseudomembranous colitis, vomiting
HEME: Agranulocytosis, eosinophilia, leukopenia, neutropenia, thrombocytopenic purpura
SKIN: Pruritus, rash, urticaria
Other: Anaphylaxis, infusion site thrombophlebitis, superinfection

Nursing Considerations

- Expect to obtain a specimen for culture and sensitivity testing before giving first dose of clindamycin.
- Give I.V. dose by infusion only; don't give bolus dose. Dilute 300 mg of clindamycin in 50 ml of diluent and give over 10 minutes. Dilute 600 mg of clindamycin in 100 ml of diluent and give over 20 minutes. Dilute 900 mg of clindamycin in 100 ml of diluent and give over 30 minutes.
- Store diluted parenteral solution up to 24 hours at room temperature.
- **WARNING** When preparing clindamycin for neonates or premature infants, don't use drug containing benzyl alcohol because it may cause a fatal toxic syndrome of CNS, respiratory,

circulatory, and renal impairment and metabolic acidosis.

- Be aware that drug should be used cautiously in patients with atopy, significant allergies, or a history of asthma.
- Check I.V. site frequently for phlebitis and irritation.
- Monitor results of liver function tests, CBC, and platelet counts during prolonged therapy.
- Monitor serum drug levels, as ordered, in patients with impaired hepatic or renal function who are receiving high doses. A dosage adjustment may be necessary.
- Observe patient for evidence of superinfection, such as vaginal itching and sore mouth, and for signs of pseudomembranous colitis, which may occur 2 to 9 days after therapy begins. Patients with a history of GI disease, particularly colitis or regional enteritis, are at increased risk for colitis. Be aware that antibiotic-related diarrhea and colitis are more common and may be more severe and less well tolerated in elderly patients.
- Before diluting drug, store it at 15° to 30° C (59° to 86° F).

PATIENT TEACHING

- Advise patient receiving clindamycin to immediately report signs or symptoms of colitis (severe diarrhea and abdominal cramps) or superinfection (an inflamed mouth or vagina), as well as rash or lesions.

coagulation factor VIIa (recombinant)
NovoSeven, NovoSeven RT

Class and Category
Chemical: Vitamin K–dependent glycoprotein
Therapeutic: Antihemophilic, hemostatic
Pregnancy category: C

Indications and Dosages
▶ *To treat bleeding episodes in pagtients with hemophilia A or B or with inhibitors to factor VIII or factor IX*
I.V. INJECTION
Adults. 90 mcg/kg injected over 2 to 5 minutes every 2 hr until hemostasis achieved; then every 3 to 6 hr, as needed.
▶ *To prevent bleeding in surgical intervention or invasive procedure in hemophilia A or B patients with inhibitors to factor VIII or factor IX*
I.V. INJECTION
Adults. 90 mcg/kg injected over 2 to 5 minutes immediately before surgery or procedure; then every 2 hr throughout surgery or

procedure. After minor surgery, 90 mcg/kg injected over 2 to 5 minutes every 2 hr for 48 hr; then 90 mcg/kg injected over 2 to 5 minutes every 2 to 6 hr until healing has occurred. After major surgery, 90 mcg/kg over 2 to 5 minutes every 2 hr for 5 days; then 90 mcg/kg over 2 to 5 minutes every 4 hr until healing has occurred.

▶ *To treat or prevent bleeding episodes in patients with congenital factor VII deficiency*
I.V. INFUSION
Adults. 15 to 30 mcg/kg over 2 to 5 minutes every 4 to 6 hr until hemostasis occurs.

▶ *To treat patients with acquired hemophilia*
I.V. INFUSION
Adults. 70 to 90 mcg/kg over 2 to 5 minutes every 2 to 3 hr until hemostasis occurs.

Mechanism of Action

Factor VIIa activates the extrinsic pathway of coagulation by forming complexes with tissue factor to activate factors IX and X. Activated factor X complexes with other factors to convert prothrombin to thrombin. Thrombin then converts fibrinogen to fibrin which leads to the formation of a hemostatic plug to produce local hemostais. This process may also occur on the surface of activated platelets.

Contraindications

Hypersensitivity to recombinant coagulation factor VIIa; its components; or to mouse, hamster or bovine proteins.

Interactions
DRUGS
activated and nonactivated prothrombin complex concentrates: Increased risk of thrombosis

Adverse Reactions
CNS: Fever, headache
CV: Acute MI, bradyarrhythmia, chest tightness or pain, edema, hypertension, hypotension, supraventricular tachycardia, thrombosis
EENT: Epistaxis
GI: Nausea, vomiting
HEMA: Disseminated intravascular coagulation, hemorrhage
MS: Arthralgia

RESP: Wheezing
SKIN: Pruritis, purpura, rash, urticaria
Other: Anaphylaxis, injection site reaction

Nursing Considerations

- Be aware that patients with disseminated intravascular coagulation, advanced atherosclerotic disease, crush injury, septicemia, or receiving concomitant treatment with activated or nonactivated prothrombin complex concentrate are at increased risk for a thrombotic event such as myocardial ischemia or infarction and cerebral ischemia or infarction.
- Monitor factor VII–deficient patients' PT and factor VII coagulant activity before and after administration of drug. If factor VIIa activity fails to reach the expected level, the PT is not corrected or bleeding is not controlled, notify prescriber. The patient may have developed antibodies to the drug. Be prepared to obtain specimen for antibody analysis.
- Reconstitute with sterile water (NovoSeven) or histidine diluent (NovoSeven RT) according to manufacturer guidelines. Clean rubber stopper with alcohol and insert the syringe needle into the center of the stopper, aiming the needle against the side of the vial so the stream of sterile water runs down the vial wall. Do not inject the diluent directly onto the powder. Gently swirl vial until powder is dissolved. Do not shake reconstituted solution. If solution is foamy, let solution settle before giving it. Once reconstituted, use within 3 hours.
- Monitor patient's clotting status closely. If intravascular coagulation is confirmed by test results or signs and symptoms occur, notify prescriber and expect to reduce dosage or stop drug.

PATIENT TEACHING

- Tell patient to immediately report evidence of an allergic reaction, such as hives, rash, chest tightness, or difficulty breathing.
- Inform patient that he will need regular laboratory tests to determine effectiveness of drug.

codeine phosphate

Class, Category, and Schedule

Chemical: Phenanthrene derivative
Therapeutic: Opioid analgesic
Pregnancy category: C
Controlled substance schedule: II

Indications and Dosages
▶ *To treat mild to moderate pain*
I.V. INJECTION
Adults. 15 to 60 mg every 4 hr. *Usual:* 30 mg/dose.

Mechanism of Action
May produce analgesia through partial metabolism to morphine. Codeine binds with mu, delta, and kappa receptors in the spinal cord and with mu_1 and $kappa_3$ receptors at higher levels in the CNS, altering the perception of—and emotional response to—pain. By binding with these receptors, the drug decreases levels of intracellular cAMP, which inhibits adenylate cyclase activity. This action prevents the release of pain neurotransmitters, such as substance P and dopamine.

Contraindications
Hypersensitivity to codeine, other opioids, or their components; significant respiratory depression

Interactions
DRUGS
anticholinergics, paregoric: Increased risk of severe constipation
antihypertensives, diuretics: Potentiated hypotensive effects
buprenorphine: Decreased effectiveness of codeine
CNS depressants: Additive CNS effects
hydroxyzine: Increased codeine analgesic effect, increased CNS depressant and hypotensive effects
MAO inhibitors: Increased risk of unpredictable, severe, and sometimes fatal reactions
metoclopramide: Antagonized effect of metoclopramide on GI motility
naloxone: Antagonized codeine analgesic effect
naltrexone: Precipitated withdrawal symptoms in codeine-dependent patients
neuromuscular blockers: Additive respiratory depressant effects
other opioid analgesics: Additive CNS and respiratory depressant effects and hypotensive effects
ACTIVITIES
alcohol use: Additive CNS effects

Adverse Reactions
CNS: Coma, delirium, depression, disorientation, dizziness, drowsiness, euphoria, hallucinations, headache, lack of coordina-

tion, lethargy, light-headedness, mental and physical impairment, mood changes, restlessness, sedation, seizures, tremor

CV: Bradycardia, heart block, orthostatic hypotension, palpitations, tachycardia

EENT: Altered taste, blurred vision, diplopia, dry mouth, laryngeal edema, laryngospasm, miosis

GI: Abdominal cramps and pain, anorexia, constipation, flatulence, ileus, nausea, vomiting

GU: Decreased libido, difficult ejaculation, dysuria, impotence, oliguria, ureteral spasm, urinary incontinence, urine retention

MS: Muscle rigidity

RESP: Apnea, bronchoconstriction, bronchospasm, depressed cough reflex, respiratory depression

SKIN: Diaphoresis, flushing, pallor, pruritus, rash, urticaria

Other: Anaphylaxis, facial edema, physical and psychological dependence

Nursing Considerations

- Instruct patient to lie down during codeine administration and for a period afterward to lessen dizziness, light-headedness, nausea, and vomiting.
- **WARNING** Give diluted codeine solution slowly over several minutes. Rapid delivery may cause serious adverse reactions, including anaphylaxis, severe respiratory depression, hypotension, peripheral circulatory collapse, and cardiac arrest. Make sure emergency equipment and drugs are available.
- Evaluate for therapeutic response, including decreased pain and facial grimacing.
- Monitor respiratory depth, effort, and rate. Notify prescriber immediately if respiratory rate drops below 10 breaths/minute; patients having an acute asthma attack and those with chronic respiratory disease are at increased risk. Pediatric, elderly, debilitated, or extremely ill patients are at increased risk for drug's respiratory depressant effects.
- Monitor patient for evidence of drug-induced CNS depression or increased CSF pressure, such as altered LOC, restlessness, and irritability, in patients with a head injury, intracranial lesions, or other conditions that could cause these effects. Patients who are taking or have recently taken drugs that cause CNS depression are also more susceptible to these effects. Take appropriate safety precautions.
- Be aware that codeine may induce or exacerbate arrhythmias or seizures in patients with a history of these conditions and

may mask symptoms of acute abdominal conditions.

- **WARNING** Assess patient for signs of physical and psychological dependence.
- Be aware that patients with a history of drug abuse (including acute alcoholism), emotional instability, or suicidal ideation or attempts are at increased risk for opioid abuse; however, the risk of drug dependence is lower with codeine than with some other opioid analgesics.
- Assess urine output; a decrease may signal urine retention.
- Store drug at 15° to 30° C (59° to 86° F). Protect from freezing and light.

PATIENT TEACHING

- Advise patient to avoid alcohol and other CNS depressants, including OTC preparations, during codeine therapy because of possible additive CNS effects.
- Advise patient to avoid potentially hazardous activities until drug's CNS effects are known.
- Caution patient to get up slowly from a sitting or lying position.
- To prevent constipation, urge patient to consume plenty of fluids and high-fiber foods, unless contraindicated.
- Advise patient to notify prescriber if he becomes short of breath or has difficulty breathing.

colchicine

Class and Category
Chemical: Colchicum alkaloid derivative
Therapeutic: Antigout agent, anti-inflammatory
Pregnancy category: D

Indications and Dosages
▶ *To prevent gouty arthritis attacks*
I.V. INFUSION, I.V. INJECTION
Adults. 0.5 to 1 mg once or twice daily. *Maximum:* 4 mg daily.
▶ *To treat acute gouty arthritis*
I.V. INFUSION, I.V. INJECTION
Adults. 2 mg over 2 to 5 min; then 0.5 mg every 6 hr or 1 mg every 6 to 12 hr until pain decreases. *Maximum:* 4 mg daily.
DOSAGE ADJUSTMENT For elderly patients, maximum dosage reduced to 2 mg/24 hr. After initial course of therapy, patient should receive no further colchicine in any form for 21 days.

Route	Onset	Peak	Duration
I.V.	In 6 to 12 hr	Unknown	Unknown

Mechanism of Action

In gouty arthritis, leukocytes release chemotactic factors, degradation enzymes, and other inflammatory substances through phagocytosis of urate crystals in affected joints. Colchicine probably disrupts microtubules in leukocytes, helping stop this process.

Normally, microtubules contribute to cell structure and movement. When colchicine binds to tubulin (the protein from which microtubules are made), the microtubule falls apart, as shown. This process disrupts cell function and keeps leukocytes from invading joints and causing inflammation.

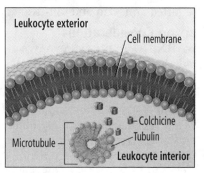

Contraindications

Blood dyscrasias; hypersensitivity to colchicine or its components; serious cardiac, GI, hepatic, or renal disorders

Incompatibilities

Don't combine colchicine with bacteriostatic agents, any solution or injection that contains D_5W, or any other solution that may change colchicine's pH because precipitation may occur.

Interactions

DRUGS

anticoagulants (such as heparin), platelet aggregation inhibitors (such as aspirin), thrombolytics (such as alteplase): Possibly significantly increased risk of GI ulceration or hemorrhage

antineoplastics: Possibly increased serum uric acid level and decreased therapeutic effectiveness of colchicine

cyclosporine: Increased blood cyclosporine level

NSAIDs (such as phenylbutazone): Possibly increased risk of bone marrow depression, GI bleeding, leukopenia, or thrombocytopenia

vitamin B_{12}: Possibly impaired absorption of and increased dosage requirements for vitamin B_{12}

ACTIVITIES

alcohol use: Increased risk of adverse GI effects

Adverse Reactions

CNS: Peripheral neuropathy
CV: Arrhythmias
GI: Abdominal pain, diarrhea, nausea, vomiting
HEME: Agranulocytosis, aplastic anemia, thrombocytopenia
MS: Myopathy
SKIN: Alopecia, rash
Other: Injection site pain and tenderness, median nerve neuritis in affected arm, skin and soft-tissue necrosis (in extravasation)

Nursing Considerations

- **WARNING** To prevent extravasation, ensure that the I.V. catheter is patent and correctly positioned before administering colchicine. Throughout therapy, check I.V. injection site frequently for pain, tenderness, and skin peeling. Consult prescriber about switching to oral form as soon as possible. Avoid subcutaneous or I.M. administration of colchicine because these routes may cause tissue necrosis and sloughing.
- **WARNING** Don't give colchicine by any route within 7 days after a full I.V. course (4 mg) because of the risk of toxicity. Be aware that elderly or debilitated patients and those with a history of cardiac disease or impaired renal or hepatic function are at increased risk for cumulative toxicity.
- Expect to monitor CBC and platelet and reticulocyte counts at baseline and every 3 months after therapy starts.
- Dilute drug with 10 to 20 ml of normal saline solution. Don't use a diluent that contains a bacteriostatic agent. Alternatively, administer colchicine through a free-flowing I.V. line with normal saline solution into a large vein. Don't use colchicine if solution is cloudy or contains sediment.
- Administer I.V. form over 2 to 5 minutes.
- Notify prescriber immediately and expect to stop therapy if patient develops signs or symptoms of colchicine toxicity, such as abdominal pain, diarrhea, nausea, or vomiting.
- Store drug at 15° to 30° C (59° to 86° F); protect from freezing and light.

PATIENT TEACHING

- Instruct patient to return for blood tests every 3 months, as ordered, during colchicine therapy.
- Explain that gouty arthritis pain and swelling typically subside in 24 to 48 hours after therapy begins.
- Advise patient to immediately report abdominal pain, diarrhea, nausea, or vomiting.

colistimethate sodium
Coly-Mycin M

Class and Category
Chemical: Polypeptide
Therapeutic: Antibiotic
Pregnancy category: C

Indications and Dosages
▶ *To treat acute or chronic gram-negative infections caused by*
Enterobacter aerogenes, Escherichia coli, Klebsiella pneumoniae,
or Pseudomonas aeruginosa
I.V. INFUSION, I.V. INJECTION
Adults. 2.5 to 5 mg/kg daily in 2 to 4 divided doses. *Maximum:*
5 mg/kg/day.
DOSAGE ADJUSTMENT Dosage should be based on ideal
body weight for obese patients. Dosage reduced to 1.5 mg/kg
daily and dosing frequency reduced to every 36 hours in patients with severe renal impairment. For patients with mild renal impairment, dosage frequency shouldn't exceed twice daily;
for patients with moderate renal impairment, frequency
shouldn't exceed twice daily but may need to be decreased to
once daily.

Mechanism of Action
A surface active agent, penetrates into and disrupts the bacterial cell membrane, resulting in cell death.

Contraindications
Hypersensitivity to colistimethate or its components

Interactions
DRUGS
aminoglycosides, polymyxin: Interference with nerve transmission
curaniform muscle relaxants such as tubocurarine, decamethonium, ether,
gallamine, succinylcholine: Potentiated neuromuscular blocking effect of these drugs
sodium cephalothin: Possibly enhanced nephrotoxicity

Adverse Reactions
CNS: Dizziness, fever, paresthesia, slurred speech, tingling limbs,
vertigo
GI: Nausea, vomiting

GU: Decreased creatinine clearance and urine output, increased BUN and serum creatinine levels, nephrotoxicity

MS: Muscle weakness

RESP: Apnea, respiratory distress

SKIN: Pruritus, rash, urticaria

Nursing Considerations

- Use colistimethate cautiously in patients with impaired renal function.
- Reconstitute each 150-mg colistimethate vial with 2 ml sterile water for injection to yield a concentration equivalent to 75 mg/ml of drug. During reconstitution, swirl drug gently to avoid frothing.
- When administering drug as an I.V. injection, slowly inject half the total daily dose over 3 to 5 minutes and repeat dose 12 hours later, as ordered.
- When administering drug as an I.V. infusion, slowly inject half the total daily dose over 3 to 5 minutes, and then add remaining half of total daily dose to an appropriate solution, such as normal saline solution or D₅W. The type and amount of solution used for I.V. infusion is dictated by patient's fluid and electrolyte needs. Infuse remaining drug slowly over 22 to 23 hours starting 1 to 2 hours after the initial dose. Use a decreased infusion rate if patient has renal impairment. Once the infusion is prepared, use it within 24 hours.
- Notify prescriber if patient develops neurological disturbances such as paresthesia, tingling limbs, generalized pruritus, vertigo, dizziness, and slurring of speech, because dosage may need to be reduced.
- **WARNING** Monitor patient's BUN and serum creatinine levels, as ordered. If elevated, notify prescriber because colistimethate may cause nephrotoxicity, possible renal shutdown, and toxic drug levels that interfere with nerve transmission at neuromuscular junctions, resulting in apnea and muscle weakness. If drug is discontinued, nephrotoxicity usually is reversible.
- Monitor patient's bowel elimination. If diarrhea develops, obtain stool culture to check for pseudomembranous colitis. If confirmed, expect to stop drug and give fluids, electrolytes, and antibiotics effective against *Clostridium difficile.*

PATIENT TEACHING

- Caution patient to avoid performing hazardous activities, such as driving, during colistimethate therapy.

• Tell patient to report tingling limbs, vertigo, dizziness, generalized pruritus, and slurred speech immediately because dosage may need to be decreased.
• Inform patient that she'll need frequent blood tests throughout therapy to monitor kidney function.
• Instruct patient to immediately report severe diarrhea.

conivaptan hydrochloride
Vaprisol

Class and Category
Chemical: Arginine vasopressin antagonist (antidiuretic hormone)
Therapeutic: Aquaretic (sodium/water stabilizer)
Pregnancy category: C

Indications and Dosages
▶ *To treat euvolemic and hypervolemic hyponatremia in hospitalized patients, such as those with syndrome of inappropriate antidiuretic hormone secretion, hypothyroidism, adrenal insufficiency, or pulmonary disorders*

I.V. INFUSION
Adults. *Loading dose:* 20 mg over 30 min, followed by 20 mg as a continuous infusion over 24 hr. An additional 20 mg daily may be given by continuous infusion for 1 to 3 days, as needed. *Maximum:* 40 mg daily with total duration of therapy, including loading dose, not to exceed 4 days.

Route	Onset	Peak	Duration
I.V.	Unknown	24 hr	Unknown

Mechanism of Action
Binds with arginine vasopressin V2 receptor sites in the collecting ducts of the kidneys. By doing so, conivaptan blocks the action of arginine vasopressin on V2 receptors, decreasing water resorption in the collecting ducts. This increases excretion of free water (urine output) and increases serum sodium concentration, thereby correcting the water and sodium imbalance.

Incompatibilities
Don't mix conivaptan with lactated Ringer's solution, normal saline solution, or other drugs.

Contraindications
Hypersensitivity to conivaptan or its components; patients with hypovolemic hyponatremia; use with potent CYP3A4 inhibitors, such as clarithromycin, indinavir, itraconazole, ketoconazole, and ritonavir

Interactions
DRUGS
amphotericin B, cisplatin, corticosteroids: Possibly additive hypokalemic effects
clarithromycin, indinavir, itraconazole, ketoconazole, ritonavir, and other strong CYP3A4 inhibitors: Increased blood conivaptan level
digoxin: Possibly increased digoxin level and risk of digioxin toxicity
drugs metabolized by CYP3A4, such as HMG-CoA reductase inhibitors: Possibly increased risk of rhabdomyolysis

Adverse Reactions
CNS: Confusion, fever, headache, insomnia
CV: Atrial fibrillation, hypertension, hypotension, orthostatic hypotension, peripheral edema
EENT: Dry mouth, oral candidiasis
ENDO: Hyperglycemia, hypoglycemia
GI: Constipation, diarrhea, nausea, thirst, vomiting
GU: Hematuria, pollakiuria, polyuria, UTI
HEME: Anemia
RESP: Pneumonia
SKIN: Erythema
Other: Dehydration, hypokalemia, hypomagnesemia, hyponatremia, infusion site reactions (erythema, pain, phlebitis, swelling)

Nursing Considerations
- Be aware that conivaptan shouldn't be used to treat patients with heart failure.
- Use conivaptan cautiously in patients with hepatic or renal dysfunction because conivaptan levels remain elevated longer in these patients, increasing exposure to the drug.
- Administer conivaptan only through large veins, and change the infusion site every 24 hours. This drug may cause serious infusion site reactions even when diluted and infused correctly. Inspect the site regularly; change it immediately if reactions occur, such as erythema, pain, phlebitis, or swelling.
- Dilute 20-mg (4-ml) loading dose with 100 ml of 5% dextrose injection before administration. Gently invert the bag several

times to mix thoroughly. Use mixture within 24 hours, infusing over 30 minutes.

- Dilute 20-mg (4-ml) or 40-mg (8-ml) continuous infusion dose with 250 ml of D_5W before administration. Gently invert the bag several times to mix thoroughly. Infuse immediately over 24 hours. If infusion is interrupted for any reason, discard any remaining solution 24 hours after mixing.

- Monitor patient's neurologic status and serum sodium level closely during conivaptan therapy because a rapid increase in serum sodium level (more than 12 mEq/L/24 hr) may cause serious neurologic impairment. If serum sodium level rises faster than expected, stop infusion temporarily and notify prescriber. If it continues to rise, expect to stop conivaptan. If hyponatremia persists or recurs and the patient has no neurologic abnormalities, conivaptan may be resumed at a reduced rate.

- Monitor patient's vital signs, and assess patient regularly for evidence of hypovolemia. If patient develops hypovolemia or hypotension while receiving conivaptan, stop infusion, notify prescriber, and provide supportive care, as prescribed. After hypovolemia and hypotension have been corrected, drug may be resumed at a reduced rate.

- Store ampules in cardboard container, protected from light, until ready for use.

PATIENT TEACHING

- Instruct patient to report infusion site discomfort immediately.
- Tell patient that frequent laboratory tests will be needed to monitor his serum sodium level and volume status.

co-trimoxazole
(sulfamethoxazole and trimethoprim)

Bactrim, Septra

Class and Category

Chemical: Sulfonamide derivative (sulfamethoxazole), dihydrofolic acid analogue (trimethoprim)
Therapeutic: Antibiotic
Pregnancy category: C

Indications and Dosages

▶ *To treat acute otitis media, shigellosis, UTI, and other infections caused by gram-negative organisms (including* Enterobacter *species,* Escherichia coli, Haemophilus ducreyi, Haemophilus influenzae,

indole-positive Proteus *species,* Klebsiella pneumoniae, Neisseria gonorrhoeae, Proteus mirabilis, Providencia *species,* Salmonella *species,* Serratia *species, and* Shigella *species) and gram-positive organisms (including group A beta-hemolytic streptococci,* Nocardia *species,* Staphylococcus aureus, *and* Streptococcus pneumoniae)
I.V. INFUSION
Adults and children over age 2 months. 40 to 50 mg/kg of sulfamethoxazole (SMZ) and 8 to 10 mg/kg of trimethoprim (TMP) daily in divided doses every 6, 8, or 12 hr for up to 5 days for shigellosis, 14 days for UTI.

▶ *To treat* Pneumocystis jiroveci (carinii) *pneumonia*
I.V. INFUSION
Adults and children over age 2 months. 75 to 100 mg/kg of SMZ and 15 to 20 mg/kg of TMP daily in three or four divided doses every 6 to 8 hr for up to 14 days.

Mechanism of Action
Blocks two consecutive steps in the formation of essential nucleic acids and proteins in susceptible organisms. Sulfamethoxazole inhibits synthesis of dehydrofolic acid (a nucleic acid) by competing with para-aminobenzoic acid. Trimethoprim inhibits the action of the enzyme dihydrofolate reductase, thus blocking production of tetrahydrofolic acid.

Incompatibilities
Don't mix co-trimoxazole with other drugs or solutions.

Contraindications
Age younger than 2 months; hypersensitivity to sulfamethoxazole, sulfonamides, trimethoprim, or their components; megaloblastic anemia caused by folate deficiency

Interactions
DRUGS
ACE inhibitors: Increased risk of hyperkalemia (elderly patients)
cyclosporine: Decreased blood level and therapeutic effectiveness of cyclosporine, increased risk of nephrotoxicity
digoxin: Possibly increased blood digoxin level resulting in increased risk of digoxin toxicity
diuretics: Increased risk of thrombocytopenic purpura (elderly patients)
indomethacin: Possibly increased blood co-trimoxazole level
methotrexate: Increased blood methotrexate level and risk of methotrexate toxicity

phenytoin: Possibly decreased hepatic clearance and prolonged half-life of phenytoin

pyrimethamine (dosage greater than 25 mg/wk): Increased risk of megaloblastic anemia

sulfonylureas: Possibly increased hypoglycemic effects of sulfonylureas

tricyclic antidepressants: Decreased effectiveness of tricyclic antidepressant

warfarin: Increased anticoagulant effects

Adverse Reactions

CNS: Anxiety, aseptic meningitis, ataxia, chills, depression, fatigue, hallucinations, headache, insomnia, seizures, vertigo

EENT: Glossitis, stomatitis

GI: Abdominal pain, anorexia, diarrhea, hepatitis, nausea, pancreatitis, pseudomembranous enterocolitis, vomiting

GU: Crystalluria, renal failure, toxic nephrosis

HEME: Agranulocytosis, eosinophilia, hemolytic anemia, leukopenia, methemoglobinemia, neutropenia, thrombocytopenia

RESP: Cough, dyspnea

SKIN: Dermatitis, erythema, photosensitivity, rash, Stevens-Johnson syndrome, toxic epidermal necrolysis, urticaria

Other: Anaphylaxis, hyperkalemia, injection site inflammation and pain

Nursing Considerations

- Use cautiously in patients with impaired hepatic or renal function, severe allergy or bronchial asthma, or possible folate deficiency (patient who are elderly, long-term alcoholic, taking anticonvulsants, or malnourished or have malabsorption).
- Expect to obtain culture and sensitivity test results before beginning co-trimoxazole therapy.
- For I.V. infusion, dilute each 5 ml of cotrimoxazole with 75 to 125 ml of D_5W before administration.
- When giving drug to neonates, don't mix with solutions that contain benzyl alcohol because this preservative has been linked to a fatal toxic syndrome involving circulatory, CNS, renal, and respiratory impairment and metabolic acidosis.
- Infuse slowly over 60 to 90 minutes.
- Watch for blood dyscrasia (bleeding, ecchymosis, joint pain), especially in elderly patients who take a thiazide diuretic.
- Monitor older patients closely because of increased risk of bone marrow suppression, hyperkalemia, and severe skin reactions.
- Monitor patient's bowel elimination; if needed, obtain a stool culture to test for pseudomembranous colitis. If it occurs, expect

to stop co-trimoxazole and give fluids, electrolytes, and antibiotics effective against *Clostridium difficile*.

PATIENT TEACHING

• Instruct patient to notify prescriber immediately if rash, severe diarrhea, or other serious adverse reactions occur.

• Urge patient to report watery, bloody stools to prescriber immediately, even up to 2 months after drug therapy has ended.

cyclophosphamide
Cytoxan, Neosar, Procytox (CAN)

Class and Category
Chemical: Nitrogen mustard derivative
Therapeutic: Alkylating antineoplastic
Pregnancy category: D

Indications and Dosages
▶ *To treat acute lymphocytic or nonlymphocytic leukemia, chronic myelocytic or lymphocytic leukemia, neuroblastoma, retinoblastoma, and Hodgkin's disease or non-Hodgkin's lymphoma*

I.V. INFUSION, I.V. INJECTION

Adults. *Initial:* 40 to 50 mg/kg in divided doses over 2 to 5 days, or 10 to 15 mg/kg every 7 to 10 days, or 3 to 5 mg/kg twice weekly. *Maintenance:* Varies with diagnosis and patient's clinical and hematologic response to, and tolerance of, therapy.

Children. *Initial:* 2 to 8 mg/kg or 60 to 250 mg/m^2 every wk or in divided doses for 6 or more days. *Maintenance:* 10 to 15 mg/kg every 7 to 10 days, or 30 mg/kg every 3 to 4 wk or when bone marrow recovers.

▶ *To treat breast, epithelial, or ovarian cancer; multiple myeloma; and mycosis fungoides*

I.V. INFUSION, I.V. INJECTION

Adults. *Initial:* 40 to 50 mg/kg in divided doses over 2 to 5 days, or 10 to 15 mg/kg every 7 to 10 days, or 3 to 5 mg/kg twice weekly. *Maintenance:* Varies with diagnosis and patient's clinical and hematologic response and tolerance to therapy.

DOSAGE ADJUSTMENT Dosage varies, depending on regimen used. Dosage may be reduced when cyclophosphamide is used with other cytotoxic drugs.

Contraindications
Hypersensitivity to cyclophosphamide, severely depressed bone marrow

Mechanism of Action

After biotransformation in the liver, crosslinks with strands of DNA and RNA to interfere with the growth of susceptible, rapidly proliferating malignant cells. Cyclophosphamide inhibits protein synthesis inside the cell and also has immunosuppressive qualities. Drug is cell-cycle-phase–nonspecific.

Interactions

DRUGS

allopurinol: Increased toxic effects of cyclophosphamide on bone marrow

blood-dyscrasia–causing drugs (cephalosporins, cisplatin): Increased leukopenic and thrombocytopenic effects of cyclophosphamide

bone marrow depressants (such as colchicine and methotrexate): Increased bone marrow depression

busulfan: Decreased cyclophosphamide clearance, possibly leading to cyclophosphamide toxicity

chloramphenicol: Decreased cyclophosphamide effectiveness

cocaine: Increased risk of prolonged cocaine effects and toxicity

cytarabine: Cardiomyopathy and risk of death

daunorubicin, doxorubicin: Risk of increased cardiotoxicity

hepatic enzyme inducers (such as allopurinol and erythromycin): Decreased half-life and increased activity of cyclophosphamide

immunosuppressants (such as azathioprine, chlorambucil, corticosteroids, and cyclosporine): Increased risk of infection and development of neoplasms

lovastatin: Increased risk of rhabdomyolysis and acute renal failure in heart transplant patients

oral anticoagulants: Decreased or increased anticoagulant activity

pentostatin, trastuzumab: Increased risk of cardiotoxicity

phenobarbital: Increased metabolism and leukopenic activity of cyclophosphamide

succinylcholine: Enhanced neuromuscular blockade effects of succinylcholine

tamoxifen: Increased risk of thromboembolism

thiazide diuretics: Increased risk of granulocytopenia

vaccines, killed virus: Possibly decreased antibody response to vaccine

vaccines, live virus: Possibly increased adverse effects of vaccine, severe infection, and decreased antibody response to vaccine

Adverse Reactions

CNS: Dizziness, headache

CV: Cardiotoxicity (including acute myopericarditis and cardiomyopathy)

EENT: Stomatitis

ENDO: Condition resembling syndrome of inappropriate ADH secretion (SIADH), hyperglycemia

GI: Anorexia, diarrhea, epigastric pain, hemorrhagic colitis, hepatitis, nausea, vomiting

GU: Amenorrhea, azoospermia, hemorrhagic and nonhemorrhagic cystitis, infertility, nephrotoxicity, oligospermia, uric acid nephropathy

HEME: Anemia, leukopenia, thrombocytopenia

RESP: Interstitial pulmonary fibrosis, pneumonitis

SKIN: Alopecia, darkened nails, diaphoresis, flushing or erythema of face, hyperpigmentation, pruritus, rash, urticaria

Other: Anaphylaxis, hyperkalemia, hyperuricemia, hyponatremia, impaired wound healing, infection, injection site edema, pain, or redness

Nursing Considerations

• Follow facility protocol for preparation and handling of antineoplastic drugs and for appropriate disposal of used equipment.

• Anticipate dosage reduction if patient is also receiving radiation therapy or a drug that depresses bone marrow.

• Monitor liver and renal function test results before and periodically during therapy because drug is metabolized in the liver and excreted by the kidneys.

• Monitor CBC, including hematocrit, platelet count, and WBC count with differential, before and periodically during therapy.

• Be prepared to hydrate patient before and after therapy to minimize the risk of hemorrhagic cystitis and to help eliminate drug-induced uric acid accumulation.

• Prepare a solution with a concentration of 20 mg/ml by adding appropriate amount of sterile water for injection or bacteriostatic water for injection (paraben-preserved only) if specified by manufacturer. Shake until dissolved. Be aware that nonlyophilized form of cyclophosphamide for injection may take up to 6 minutes to dissolve; lyophilized form takes about 45 seconds.

• **WARNING** When preparing drug for administration to neonates or premature infants, don't use diluents that contain benzyl alcohol because they have been linked to a fatal toxic syndrome characterized by CNS, respiratory, circulatory, and renal impairment and metabolic acidosis.

• Solution may be diluted further for I.V. infusion with D_5W,

D_5/normal saline solution, D_5/lactated Ringer's solution, lactated Ringer's solution, 0.45 normal saline solution, or sodium lactate injection. Use within 24 hours if stored at room temperature or within 6 days if refrigerated.

- Be aware that adverse reactions can vary when cyclophosphamide is used in combination therapy. Review all drugs given in the regimen, including drug interactions and adverse effects.
- Watch for signs of hemorrhagic cystitis, including hematuria and dysuria; expect to stop cyclophosphamide if they occur.
- Monitor serum uric acid level, especially in patients with a history of gout or urate calculi. Expect a dosage adjustment of antigout drugs if blood uric acid level is elevated from cyclophosphamide therapy. Be aware that uricosuric antigout drugs may increase the risk of uric acid nephropathy.
- Observe patient for signs of leukopenia or infection, including fever, chills, pharyngitis, tiredness or weakness, and unusual bleeding or ecchymosis.
- Monitor patients who have undergone an adrenalectomy for increased toxic effects of cyclophosphamide. Expect dosages of replacement steroids and cyclophosphamide to be adjusted.
- Be aware that effects of radiation therapy or bone marrow depressants may increased when used with cyclophosphamide. Patients with a history of bone marrow depression, chickenpox (including recent exposure), or herpes zoster are at increased risk for severe generalized disease.
- Assess urine output and urinary specific gravity to assess for a syndrome resembling SIADH. Obtain urine specimen, as ordered, for microscopic examination for hematuria periodically during therapy and for several hours after a large dose.
- Monitor patient for dizziness, confusion, agitation, tiredness, and weakness, which could indicate a syndrome like SIADH.
- Be aware that some patients receiving cyclophosphamide have developed a second malignancy, such as leukemia or bladder or renal cancer; a causal relationship hasn't been established.
- Store unopened cyclophosphamide below 25° C (77° F).

PATIENT TEACHING
- Tell patient receiving cyclophosphamide to immediately report unusual bruising or bleeding; black, tarry stools; blood in urine or stools; or pinpoint red spots on the skin.
- Review with patient the need for adequate fluid intake and frequent urination (including at least once at night) to help prevent hemorrhagic cystitis and to aid in elimination of excess uric acid, which may result from cyclophosphamide treatment.

- Instruct patient to consult prescriber if he requires dental surgery or emergency treatment with general anesthesia within 10 days of cyclophosphamide treatment.
- Advise patient not to receive live or killed virus vaccines during therapy and for 3 months to 1 year afterward, unless approved by prescriber. Urge patient to avoid people who have received such vaccines or to wear a protective mask around them.
- Caution patient to avoid sports and other activities that increase the risk of accidental injury. Also advise measures to avoid infection, such as maintaining oral hygiene (as by using a soft-bristled toothbrush) and washing hands often.
- Advise patient with thrombocytopenia to avoid alcohol and aspirin to reduce the risk of GI bleeding.
- Suggest that patient with stomatitis eat soft, bland foods served cold or at room temperature to decrease irritation.
- Inform patient that his hair should grow back following treatment but that color and texture may be different.
- Inform patient that although cyclophosphamide may reduce sperm count and function and ovarian function, he should use a barrier method of birth control during therapy.

cyclosporine
(cyclosporin A)
Neoral, Sandimmune, SangCya

Class and Category
Chemical: Tolypocladium inflatum Gams- or *Cylindrocarpon lucidum* Booth—derived polypeptide
Therapeutic: Antipsoriatic, antirheumatic, immunosuppressant
Pregnancy category: C

Indications and Dosages
▶ *To prevent or treat organ rejection in kidney, liver, and heart allogenic transplantation*
I.V. INFUSION
Adults. 2 to 6 mg/kg daily starting 4 to 12 hr before surgery and continuing postoperatively until patient can tolerate oral form.

Contraindications
Abnormal renal function, neoplastic diseases, and uncontrolled hypertension in patients with psoriasis or rheumatoid arthritis (modified capsules, oral solution); hypersensitivity to cyclosporine, its components, or polyoxyethylated castor oil (I.V. infusion)

Mechanism of Action

Causes immunosuppression by inhibiting the proliferation of T lymphocytes, the production and release of lymphokines, and the release of interleukin-2.

Interactions

DRUGS

ACE inhibitors, angiotensin II receptor antagonists, potassium-sparing diuretics, potassium supplements: Increased risk of hyperkalemia

amiodarone, azithromycin, bromocriptine, clarithromycin, colchicine, danazol, diltiazem, erythromycin, fluconazole, hormonal contraceptives, imatinib, itraconazole, ketoconazole, methylprednisolone, metoclopromide, nicardipine, quinupristin and dalfopristin, verapamil: Increased blood cyclosporine level

amphotericin B, azapropazon, cimetidine, ciprofloxacin, colchicine, cotrimoxazole, fibric acid derivatives (such as bezafibrate and fenofibrate), gentamicin, ketoconazole, melphalan, NSAIDs, ranitidine, tacrolimus, tobramycin, vancomycin: Increased risk of nephrotoxicity

atorvastatin, fluvastatin, lovastatin, pravastatin, simvastatin: Increased risk of myotoxicity

carbamazepine, nafcillin, octreotide, orlistat, phenobarbital, phenytoin, rifampin, St. John's wort, sulfinpyrazone, terbinafine, ticlopidine: Decreased blood cyclosporine level and therapeutic response

digoxin: Increased blood digoxin level and risk of digitalis toxicity

indinavir, nelfinavir, ritonavir, saquinavir: Possibly increased blood cyclosporine level

methotrexate: Increased blood methotrexate level

methylprednisolone (high dose): Increased risk of seizures

other immunosuppressants: Possibly excessive immunosuppression

prednisolone: Increased blood prednisolone level

sirolimus: Increased blood sirolimus level

vaccines (killed or live virus): Possibly suppressed immune response and increased adverse effects of vaccine

FOODS

Grapefruit, grapefruit juice: Increased risk of nephrotoxicity

Potassium-rich foods: Increased risk of hyperkalemia

Adverse Reactions

CNS: Altered level of consciousness, confusion, headache, intracranial hypertension, loss of motor function, paresthesia, psychiatric disturbances, seizures, tremor

CV: Chest pain, hypertension

EENT: Gingival hyperplasia, optic disc edema, oral candidiasis, visual impairment

ENDO: Gynecomastia

GI: Diarrhea, nausea, pancreatitis, vomiting

GU: Albuminuria, hematuria, proteinuria, renal failure

HEME: Anemia, leukopenia, thrombocytopenia

SKIN: Acne, flushing, hirsutism, rash

Other: Anaphylaxis, hyperkalemia, hypomagnesemia, life-threatening infection, lymphoma

Nursing Considerations

• Prepare I.V. infusion by diluting each milliliter of concentrate in 20 to 100 ml of normal saline solution or D$_5$W. Use glass containers because of possible leaching of diethylhexyphthalate from polyvinyl chloride bags into cyclosporine solution.

• Give infusion over 2 to 6 hours or, if needed, over 24 hours.

• **WARNING** Watch closely for anaphylaxis for first 30 minutes of I.V. use. Keep emergency equipment and drugs nearby.

• **WARNING** Be aware that rapid I.V. infusion may cause acute nephrotoxicity.

• Don't draw blood to measure cyclosporine level through same I.V. tubing used to administer drug, even if line was flushed after administration. Blood level may be falsely elevated.

• Discard diluted solution after 24 hours.

• Monitor blood pressure, especially in patients with a history of hypertension, because drug can worsen this condition. Expect to decrease cyclosporine dosage if hypertension develops.

• Monitor results of liver and renal function tests, as ordered, to detect signs of decreased function.

• Although uncommon, cyclosporine may cause neurotoxicity, especially after liver transplantation. Watch for evidence of encephalopathy: impaired consciousness, loss of motor function, psychiatric disturbance, seizures, and visual disturbance.

• Be aware that cyclosporine may increase serum cholesterol level and St. John's wort may decrease blood cyclosporine level.

PATIENT TEACHING

• Instruct patient not to receive virus vaccines during therapy. Urge him to avoid people who have received such vaccines or to wear a protective mask when he's around them.

• Caution patient to avoid exposure to infection during therapy because cyclosporine causes immunosuppression.

• Urge patient to maintain dental hygiene because of risk of gingival hyperplasia.

daclizumab
(dacliximab)
Zenapax

Class and Category
Chemical: Monoclonal antibody
Therapeutic: Immunosuppressant
Pregnancy category: C

Indications and Dosages
▶ *To prevent acute organ rejection after kidney transplantation*
I.V. INFUSION
Adults and children. 1 mg/kg given in five doses: dose 1 given no more than 24 hr before transplantation; doses 2 through 5 at 14-day intervals.

Mechanism of Action
Inhibits interleukin-2–mediated activation of lymphocytes, which prevents WBCs from attacking the transplanted kidney. Daclizumab also reduces the body's infection-fighting ability.

Contraindications
Hypersensitivity to daclizumab or its components

Interactions
None known.

Adverse Reactions
CNS: Anxiety, chills, depression, dizziness, fatigue, fever, headache, insomnia, paresthesia, tremor, weakness
CV: Chest pain, edema, hypertension, hypotension, tachycardia, thrombosis
EENT: Blurred vision, pharyngitis, rhinitis
ENDO: Hyperglycemia
GI: Abdominal distention and pain, constipation, diarrhea, flatulence, gastritis, heartburn, hemorrhoids, indigestion, nausea, vomiting

GU: Dysuria, hematuria, hydronephrosis, oliguria, renal insufficiency, renal tubular necrosis, urine retention

HEME: Bleeding

MS: Arthralgia, back pain, leg cramps, myalgia

RESP: Atelectasis, cough, crackles, dyspnea, hypoxia, lung congestion, pleural effusion, pulmonary edema

SKIN: Acne, diaphoresis, hirsutism, impaired wound healing, night sweats, pruritus, rash

Other: Dehydration, fluid overload, injection site pain and redness, lymphocele

Nursing Considerations

- Avoid shaking daclizumab vial before use. Dilute calculated dose of daclizumab in 50 ml of normal saline solution. Gently invert bag to mix; to prevent foaming, don't shake it.
- Don't use solution if it contains particles or is discolored.
- Use room temperature solution within 4 hours or refrigerated solution within 24 hours; discard unused solution.
- Because daclizumab's compatibility with other drugs isn't known, don't add or simultaneously infuse other drugs through same I.V. line.
- Administer drug through a peripheral or central vein over 15 minutes.
- Monitor blood glucose level for increases during therapy.
- **WARNING** Although daclizumab seldom causes severe hypersensitivity reactions, keep drugs that treat such reactions readily available.
- Before using drug, store it at 2° to 8° C (36° to 46° F). Don't freeze or shake; protect from direct light.

PATIENT TEACHING

- Urge patient to complete full course of daclizumab therapy and to return for scheduled follow-up visits.

dantrolene sodium

Dantrium, Dantrium Intravenous

Class and Category

Chemical: Hydantoin derivative, imidazolidinedione sodium salt

Therapeutic: Malignant hyperthermia therapy adjunct

Pregnancy category: C (parenteral), not rated (oral)

Indications and Dosages

▶ *To prevent malignant hyperthermia before surgery*

I.V. INFUSION
Adults and children. *Initial:* 2.5 mg/kg infused over 1 hr 60 to 75 min before anesthesia. Additional individualized doses given as needed during surgery.

CAPSULES
Adults and children. 4 to 8 mg/kg daily in divided doses t.i.d. or q.i.d. 1 or 2 days before surgery, with last dose given 3 to 4 hr before surgery.

▶ *To treat malignant hyperthermia*
I.V. INJECTION
Adults and adolescents. *Initial:* 1 mg/kg by rapid bolus, repeated as needed until symptoms subside or cumulative dose of 10 mg/kg has been reached. If symptoms reappear, dose repeated.

▶ *To treat postmalignant hyperthermic crisis*
I.V. INJECTION
Adults and children. *Initial:* Individualized dosage beginning with 1 mg/kg or more as needed if oral therapy can't be used. *Maximum:* 10 mg/kg total dose.

CAPSULES
Adults and children. 4 to 8 mg/kg daily in divided doses q.i.d. for 1 to 3 days.

Mechanism of Action

Prevents calcium release from the sarcoplasmic reticulum of skeletal muscle cells. Blocked calcium release inhibits the activation of acute catabolism associated with malignant hyperthermia.

Incompatibilities

Don't administer dantrolene with acidic solutions, including D_5W and normal saline solution.

Contraindications

For oral drug only: Active hepatic disease (such as cirrhosis and hepatitis), conditions in which spasticity helps maintain upright posture and improve balance or function, skeletal muscle spasms caused by rheumatic disorders

Interactions

DRUGS
calcium channel blockers (especially verapamil): Possibly hyperkalemia, life-threatening arrhythmias, and shock
sedatives: Possibly profound sedation

ACTIVITIES

alcohol use: Possibly increased CNS depression

Adverse Reactions

CNS: Dizziness, drowsiness, fatigue, light-headedness, malaise, slurred speech or other speech problems, weakness

CV: Heart failure, pericarditis

GI: Abdominal cramps, diarrhea, dysphagia, hepatitis, hepatotoxicity, nausea, vomiting

GU: Enuresis

MS: Decreased grip strength, myalgia

RESP: Dyspnea, feeling of suffocation, pleural effusion

SKIN: Erythema, extravasation with tissue damage, urticaria

Other: Thrombophlebitis

Nursing Considerations

- Reconstitute each vial of dantrolene with 60 ml of sterile water for injection (without a bacteriostatic agent). Shake vial until clear. Store reconstituted solution at room temperature, protected from direct sunlight. Discard after 6 hours.
- To prevent precipitation of reconstituted drug, transfer it to a plastic I.V. bag, rather than a glass bottle, for infusion. Don't use solution if it contains precipitate or is cloudy.
- Because drug has a high pH, infuse into a central vein, if possible, to avoid tissue damage from extravasation.
- Monitor blood pressure and heart rate often during drug administration to detect tachycardia and blood pressure changes.
- Monitor results of liver function tests—especially ALT, AST, alkaline phosphatase, and total bilirubin levels—for hepatotoxicity.
- Be aware that oral form of dantrolene is also used to treat chronic spastic conditions. Consult manufacturer's insert for additional dosage guidelines, nursing considerations, and adverse reactions associated with long-term oral use.
- Before reconstituting dantrolene, store it at 15° to 30° C (59° to 86° F), and avoid prolonged exposure to light.

PATIENT TEACHING

- Inform patient that dantrolene may weaken her grip strength as well as muscles used for walking and climbing stairs. Advise her to be careful when eating to avoid problems due to difficulty swallowing.
- Caution patient about drug's sedating effects. Instruct her to avoid sedatives, unless prescribed, and other sedating substances, such as alcohol.
- Advise patient to report yellow skin or sclerae, itching, or fatigue.

daptomycin

Cubicin

Class and Category

Chemical: Cyclic lipopetide
Therapeutic: Antibacterial
Pregnancy category: B

Indications and Dosages

▶ *To treat complicated skin and skin-structure infections caused by*
Staphylococcus aureus *(including methicillin-resistant
microorganisms);* Staphylococcus pyogenes, Streptococcus
agalactiae, Streptococcus dysgalactiae *subspecies* equisimilis, *and*
Enterococcus faecalis *(vancomycin-susceptible isolates only)*

I.V. INFUSION

Adults. 4 mg/kg over 30 min once daily every 24 hr for 7 to
14 days.

▶ *To treat* S. aureus *bacteremia including those with right-sided
infective endocarditis, caused by methicillin-susceptible and methicillin-
resistant isolates*

I.V. INFUSION

Adults. 6 mg/kg over 30 min once daily for 2 to 6 weeks

DOSAGE ADJUSTMENT For patients with a creatinine clearance less than 30 ml/min, dosage interval increased to once
every 48 hours

Route	Onset	Peak	Duration
I.V.	Unknown	72 hr	Unknown

Mechanism of Action

Binds to bacterial membranes, allowing efflux of potassium to cause depolarization of the membrane potential. With the loss of the membrane potential,
inhibition of protein, DNA, and RNA synthesis occur, which causes bacterial
cell death.

Incompatibilities

Daptomycin is incompatible with dextrose-containing diluents
and should not be given with other I.V. substances, additives, or
other medications

Contraindications

Hypersensitivity to daptomycin or its components

Interactions

DRUGS

HMG-CoA reductase inhibitors: Increased risk of myopathy

Adverse Reactions

CNS: Anxiety, asthenia, confusion, dizziness, fever, headache, insomnia, neuropathy

CV: Chest pain, edema, heart failure, hypertension, hypotension

EENT: Throat pain

ENDO: Hyperglycemia, hypoglycemia

GI: Abdominal pain, abnormal liver function tests, constipation, decreased appetite, diarrhea, dyspepsia, elevated CK level, GI hemorrhage, nausea, pseudomembranous colitis, vomiting

GU: Renal failure, UTI

HEME: Anemia

MS: Arthralgia, back pain, limb pain, muscle pain or weakness, myopathy, osteomyelitis, rhabdomyolysis

RESP: Cough, dyspnea, pleural effusion, pneumonia

SKIN: Cellulitis, diaphoresis, erythema, rash, pruritis, truncal erythema, urticaria

Other: Anaphylaxis, bacteremia, *Candida* infection, fungal infection, hyperkalemia, hypokalemia, injection site reactions, sepsis

Nursing Considerations

- Expect to obtain samples for culture and sensitivity tests before daptomycin treatment begins.
- Reconstitute daptomycin powder with 10 ml normal saline solution and then further dilute with normal saline solution. If kept at room temperature, use within 12 hours; if refrigerated, use within 48 hours.
- Administer as an I.V. infusion over 30 minutes.
- Be aware that daptomycin is compatible with normal saline and lactated Ringer's solutions. It is not compatible with dextrose-containing solutions.
- Monitor patient's bowel elimination. If diarrhea develops, obtain stool culture to check for pseudomembranous colitis. If confirmed, expect to stop drug and give fluids, electrolytes, and antibiotics effective against *Clostridium difficile.*
- Obtain repeated blood cultures, as ordered, if patient has persistent or relapsing *S. aureus* infection or has a poor response to daptomycin therapy. Surgical intervention at the site of the infection (such as debridement, removal of prosthetic device, or valve replacement) may be needed.
- Assess patient regularly for muscle pain or weakness, particu-

larly affecting the arms or legs. If present, notify prescriber.
- Check CK level weekly or more often if patient is receiving or has recently received an HMG-CoA reductase inhibitor or has renal insufficiency. If CK level is elevated, increase monitoring frequency. Expect to discontinue drug if patient develops unexplained signs and symptoms of myopathy with CK level of 1,000 to 2,000 units/L. If CK level exceeds 2,000 units/L, expect to stop giving drug if patient is symptom-free.
- Monitor patient closely for signs and symptoms of neuropathy. If present, notify prescriber.

PATIENT TEACHING
- Tell patient to report unexplained muscle or limb pain or weakness to prescriber.
- Instruct patient to alert prescriber if signs and symptoms of an allergic reaction occur, such as a rash, itching, hives, or difficulty breathing.
- Urge patient to report watery, bloody stools to prescriber immediately, even up to 2 months after daptomycin therapy has ended.
- Inform patient that regular blood tests will be needed throughout daptomycin therapy.
- Tell patient with bacteremia that daptomycin therapy may be needed for up to 6 weeks.

darbepoetin alfa

Aranesp

Class and Category

Chemical: 165-amino acid glycoprotein identical to human erythropoietin
Therapeutic: Antianemic
Pregnancy category: C

Indications and Dosages

▶ *To treat anemia from chronic renal failure*
I.V. INJECTION
Adults. *Initial:* 0.45 mcg/kg as a single dose every wk. *Maintenance:* Dosage individualized and increased once a month to maintain a hemoglobin level of 12 g/dl or less.
DOSAGE ADJUSTMENT Dosage reduced by about 25% if hemoglobin level increases and approaches 12 g/dl. If hemoglobin level continues to increase, doses temporarily withheld until hemoglobin level begins to decrease; then therapy is

restarted at a dose about 25% below previous dose. Dosage reduced by about 25% if hemoglobin level increases by more than 1.0 g/dl in a 2-week period. Dosage increased by about 25% of previous dose if hemoglobin level increases less than 1 g/dl over 4 weeks but only if serum ferritin level is 100 mcg/L or greater and serum transferrin saturation is 20% or greater. Further increases made at 4-week intervals until specified hemoglobin level is obtained.

DOSAGE ADJUSTMENT For conversion from epoetin alfa to darbepoetin alfa, drug given every wk for patient who previously received epoetin alfa two to three times/wk and once every 2 wk for patient who previously received epoetin alfa once/wk. For patients being converted from epoetin alfa, 6.25 mcg/wk darbepoetin alfa given every wk for patients who received less than 2,500 units/wk of epoetin alfa; 12.5 mcg/wk darbepoetin alfa given every wk for patients who received 2,500 to 4,999 units/wk of epoetin alfa; 25 mcg/wk darbepoetin alfa given every wk for patients who received 5,000 to 10,999 units/wk of epoetin alfa; 40 mcg/wk darbepoetin alfa given every wk for patients who received 11,000 to 17,999 units/wk of epoetin alfa; 60 mcg/wk darbepoetin alfa given every wk for patients who received 18,000 to 33,999 units/wk of epoetin alfa; 100 mcg/wk darbepoetin alfa given every wk for patients who received 34,000 to 89,999 units/wk of epoetin alfa; 200 mcg/wk darbepoetin alfa given every wk for patients who received 90,000 or more units/wk of epoetin alfa.

Route	Onset	Peak	Duration
I.V.	2 to 6 wk	Unknown	Unknown

Mechanism of Action

Stimulates the release of reticulocytes from the bone marrow into the bloodstream, where they develop into mature RBCs.

Incompatibilities

Don't mix darbepoetin alfa with any other drug.

Contraindications

Hypersensitivity to human albumin or products made from mammal cells; uncontrolled hypertension

Interactions
DRUGS
None known.

Adverse Reactions
CNS: Asthenia, dizziness, fatigue, fever, headache, seizures
CV: Arrhythmias, cardiac arrest, chest pain, congestive heart failure, hypertension, hypotension, peripheral edema, vascular access hemorrhage, vascular access thrombosis
GI: Abdominal pain, constipation, diarrhea, nausea, vomiting
MS: Arthralgia, back pain, limb pain, myalgia
RESP: Bronchitis, cough, dyspnea, pneumonia, pulmonary embolism, upper respiratory tract infection
SKIN: Rash, urticaria
Other: Antibody formation against darbepoetin alfa, dehydration, fluid overload, flulike symptoms, increased risk of death (with increased or rapid response and in cancer patients), infection, injection site pain, sepsis, tumor progression (cancer patients)

Nursing Considerations
- **WARNING** If patient has cancer, make sure she understands before therapy begins that darbepoetin alfa may increase tumor progression and the risk of death.
- Before starting therapy, expect to correct folic acid or vitamin B_{12} deficiencies because these conditions may interfere with drug's effectiveness.
- To ensure effective drug response, expect to obtain serum ferritin level and serum transferrin saturation before beginning and during therapy, as ordered. If serum ferritin level is less than 100 mcg/l or serum transferrin saturation is less than 20%, expect to begin supplemental iron therapy.
- Don't shake vial during preparation to avoid denaturing drug and rendering it biologically inactive.
- Discard drug if you see particulate matter or discoloration.
- Don't dilute drug before giving it.
- Discard unused portion of drug because it contains no preservatives.
- Monitor blood pressure frequently during therapy for hypertension. Expect to reduce dosage or withhold drug if blood pressure is poorly controlled with antihypertensive and dietary measures.
- Monitor hemoglobin level weekly, as ordered, until hemoglobin stabilizes and maintenance dosage has been achieved. There-

after, monitor hemoglobin level regularly, as ordered. After each dosage adjustment, expect to monitor hemoglobin level weekly for 4 weeks until hemoglobin level stabilizes in response to dosage change.

- **WARNING** Assess patient for a sudden but rare change in condition that may reflect a severe anemia as a result of loss of response to darbepoetin alfa. If this occurs, be prepared for patient to undergo tests as ordered to rule out infections, inflammatory or malignant processes, osteofibrosis cystica, occult blood loss, hemolysis, severe aluminum toxicity, or bone marrow fibrosis, any of which may compromise an erythropoietic response.

- **WARNING** Be aware that a hemoglobin level that exceeds 12 g/dl or that increases more than about 1 g/dl during any 2-week period increases the risk of cardiac arrest, seizures, CVA, worsening hypertension, congestive heart failure, vascular thrombosis, vascular ischemia, vascular infarction, acute MI, fluid overload with peripheral edema, and death. Expect to decrease darbepoetin dosage in response to such changes in hemoglobin level.

- **WARNING** Be aware that patients with chronic renal failure whose hemoglobin level responds insufficiently to darbepoetin alfa therapy face an even greater risk of serious cardiovascular or thromboembolic events or death. Monitor them closely.

- Institute seizure precautions according to facility policy.

- For patients with chronic renal failure who aren't receiving dialysis, expect to administer doses lower than those given to patients receiving dialysis. Also, monitor renal function test results and fluid and electrolyte balance in these patients for signs of deteriorating renal function.

- Store drug at 2° to 8° C (36° to 46° F). Don't freeze, and protect from light.

PATIENT TEACHING

- Advise patient that the risk of seizures is highest during the first 90 days of drug therapy. Discourage her from engaging in hazardous activities during this time.

- Stress the importance of complying with the dosage regimen and keeping follow-up medical and laboratory appointments.

- Advise patient to follow up with her prescriber for blood pressure monitoring.

- Encourage patient to eat adequate quantities of iron-rich foods.

- **WARNING** Review possible adverse reactions, and urge patient to notify prescriber if she has chest pain, headache, rash, seizures, shortness of breath, or swelling.

decitabine
Dacogen

Class and Category
Chemical: Analogue of natural nucleoside 2'-deoxycytidine
Therapeutic: Antineoplastic
Pregnancy category: D

Indications and Dosages
▶ *To treat myelodysplastic syndromes (MDS), including secondary MDS of all French-American-British subtypes and intermediate 1 and 2 and high-risk International Prognostic Scoring System groups*

I.V. INFUSION
Adults. 15 mg/m^2 over 3 hr; then repeated every 8 hr for 3 days, with cycle repeated every 6 wk for at least four cycles.
DOSAGE ADJUSTMENT For hematologic recovery that requires more than 6 wk but less than 8 wk, treatment delayed for up to 2 wk and dose temporarily reduced to 11 mg/m^2 every 8 hr. For hematologic recovery that requires more than 8 wk but less than 10 wk, treatment delayed up to 2 more wk and dose reduced to 11 mg/m^2 every 8 hr with dosage maintained or increased in subsequent cycles as clinically indicated.

Mechanism of Action
After phosphorylation and incorporation into DNA, inhibits DNA methyltransferase, resulting in hypomethylation of DNA and cellular differentiation. In neoplastic cells, hypomethylation may restore normal function to genes essential for control of cellular differentiation and proliferation. Decitabine also may kill rapidly dividing cells by forming covalent adducts between DNA methyltransferase and decitabine-saturated DNA.

Contraindications
Hypersensitivity to decitabine or its components

Interactions
DRUGS
live-virus vaccines: increased risk of infection resulting from vaccine

Adverse Reactions

CNS: Anxiety, cerebral edema, confusion, dizziness, fatigue, fever, headache, hypoesthesia, insomnia, intracranial hemorrhage, lethargy, malaise, rigors

CV: Atrial fibrillation, cardiac arrest, chest discomfort or pain, heart failure, hypotension, MI, peripheral edema

EENT: Bleeding gums, blurred vision, lip or tongue ulceration, oral mucous petechiae, oral candidasis, pharyngitis, postnasal drip, sinusitis, stomatitis

ENDO: Hyperglycemia

GI: Abdominal distention or pain, anorexia, ascities, abdominal pain, constipation, decreased appetite, diarrhea, dysphagia, dyspepsia, gastroesophageal reflux disease, hyperbilirubinemia, nausea, vomiting

GU: Dysuria, urinary frequency, UTI

HEME: Anemia, leukopenia, neutropenia, thrombocytopenia, thrombocythemia

MS: Arthralgia, back or limb pain, myalgia

RESP: Decreased breath sounds, cough, crackles, hypoxia, pneumonia, pulmonary edema

SKIN: Alopecia, cellulites, ecchymosis, erythema, hematoma, pallor, petechiae, pruritis, rash, urticaria

Other: Bacteremia, candidal infection, dehydration, facial edema, hyperkalemia, hypoalbuminemia, hypokalemia, hypomagnesemia, hyponatremia, injection site swelling, pain and redness; lymphodenpathy

Nursing Considerations

• Use cautiously in patients with liver or renal impairment.
• Follow facility protocols for preparing and handlingantineoplastic drugs and for appropriate disposal of used equipment.
• Reconstitute with 10 ml sterile water using aseptic technique. Upon reconstitution know that each ml contains approximately 5 mg of decitabine. Immediately after reconstitution, further dilute with normal saline solution, dextrose 5%, or lactated Ringer's solution to a final drug concentration of 0.1 to 1 mg/ml. Use within 15 minutes or if delay is anticipated, reconstitute drug using cold dilution solution and store in refrigerator for up to 7 hr.
• Monitor CBC, including hematocrit, platelet count, and WBC with differential as well as electrolytes, liver enzymes and serum creatinine before and intermittently during decitabine therapy, as ordered.

- If patient develops leukopenia, watch for signs of infection, such as fever. Obtain specimens for culture and sensitivity tests.
- **WARNING** Monitor patient closely for non-hematological toxicities such as active or uncontrolled infections, a serum creatinine level greater than 2 mg/dl, or serum glutamic pyruvic transaminase or total bilirubin levels 2 times or more the upper normal limits. If present, notify prescriber and expect decitabine therapy to be withheld until resolved.

PATIENT TEACHING
- Advise male patients not to father a child during decitabine therapy and for 2 months after. Also urge female patients to use contraception to avoid pregnancy during therapy and to notify prescriber immediately if pregnancy occurs.
- Advise patient to have dental work completed before beginning decitabine therapy, if possible, or to defer such work until blood counts return to normal because drug can delay healing and cause gingival bleeding. Teach patient proper oral hygiene, and advise him to use a soft-bristled toothbrush.
- If patient develops bone marrow depression, tell him to avoid people with infections and to report fever, cough, or lower back or side pain. These signs and symptoms may indicate infection.
- Stress the importance of avoiding accidental cuts from sharp objects, such as razor blades or fingernail clippers, because excessive bleeding or infection may occur.
- Advise patient with stomatitis to eat bland, soft foods served cold or at room temperature to decrease irritation.
- Stress the importance of complying with the dosage regimen and of keeping follow-up medical appointments and appointments for laboratory tests.

desmopressin acetate
DDAVP Injection, Octostim (CAN)

Class and Category
Chemical: Synthetic ADH analogue
Therapeutic: Antidiuretic, antihemorrhagic
Pregnancy category: B

Indications and Dosages
▶ *To control symptoms of central diabetes insipidus*
I.V. INFUSION
Adults. 2 to 4 mcg daily in divided doses b.i.d. Dosage adjusted as needed.

▶ *To prevent or manage bleeding episodes in hemophilia A or mild to moderate type I von Willebrand's disease*
I.V. INFUSION
Adults and children weighing more than 10 kg (22 lb).
0.3 mcg/kg diluted in 50 ml of normal saline solution and infused over 15 to 30 min. If used preoperatively, give 30 min before procedure.
Children weighing 10 kg or less. 0.3 mcg/kg diluted in 10 ml of normal saline solution and infused over 15 to 30 min. If used preoperatively, dose is given 30 min before procedure.

Route	Onset	Peak	Duration
I.V.	15 to 30 min*	30 to 60 min*	3 hr†

Mechanism of Action
Exerts an antidiuretic effect similar to that of vasopressin by increasing cellular permeability of renal collecting ducts and distal tubules, thus enhancing water reabsorption, reducing urine flow, and increasing osmolality. As an antihemorrhagic, drug increases blood level of clotting factor VIII (antihemophilic factor) and activity of von Willebrand's factor (factor VIII$_{VWF}$). It also may increase platelet aggregation and adhesion at injury sites by directly affecting blood vessel walls.

Contraindications
History or presence of hyponatremia, hypersensitivity to desmopressin or its components

Interactions
DRUGS
carbamazepine, chlorpromazine, lamotrigine, NSAIDs, selective serotonin reuptake inhibitors, tricyclcic antidepressants: Possibly increased risk of water intoxication with desmopressin-induced hyponatremia
carbamazepine, chlorpropamide, clofibrate: Possibly potentiated antidiuretic effect of desmopressin
demeclocycline, lithium: Possibly decreased antidiuretic effect
imipramine, oxybutynin: Increased risk of hyponatremic seizures
vasopressor drugs: Possibly potentiated vasopressor effect

Adverse Reactions
CNS: Asthenia, chills, CVA, dizziness, headache

---

* For antihemorrhagic effect.
† For von Willebrand's disease; 4 to 20 hr for mild hemophilia A.

CV: Acute MI, hypertension (with high doses), transient hypotension
EENT: Conjunctivitis, epistaxis, lacrimation, nasal congestion (nasal form), ocular edema, pharyngitis, rhinitis
GI: Nausea
GU: Vulvar pain (parenteral form)
SKIN: Flushing
Other: Anaphylaxis, hyponatremia, injection site pain and redness, water intoxication

Nursing Considerations

- Use desmopressin cautiously in patients with conditions associated with fluid and electrolyte imbalance, such as cystic fibrosis. Also use cautiously in patients with habitual or psychogenic polydipsia. Such patients are prone to hyponatremia.
- **WARNING** Monitor patient closely for evidence of hyponatremia, such as an abnormal mental status (hallucinations, decreased consciousness, confusion), headache, nausea and vomiting, weight gain, restlessness, fatigue, lethargy, depressed reflexes, loss of appetite, irritability, or muscle weakness, spasms, or cramps. Severe effects may include seizures, coma, and respiratory arrest. Restrict fluids, and monitor intake and output and serum sodium level closely, as ordered. Notify prescriber immediately about evidence of possible hyponatremia.
- Monitor patient's blood pressure often during therapy.

PATIENT TEACHING

- To prevent hyponatremia and water intoxication, especially in a child or an elderly patient, instruct family to restrict fluids as prescribed.
- Urge patient to notify prescriber if adverse reactions occur.
- Advise patient's caregiver or family members to immediately report signs and symptoms of possible hyponatremia.

dexamethasone sodium phosphate

Cortastat, Dalalone, Decadrol, Decaject, Dexacorten, Dexasone, Dexone, Hexadrol Phosphate, Primethasone, Solurex

Class and Category

Chemical: Synthetic adrenocortical steroid
Therapeutic: Anti-inflammatory, diagnostic aid, immunosuppressant
Pregnancy category: C

Indications and Dosages

▶ *To treat endocrine disorders, such as congenital adrenal hyperplasia, hypercalcemia with cancer, and nonsuppurative thyroiditis; acute episodes or exacerbations of rheumatic disorders; collagen diseases, such as systemic lupus erythematosus and acute rheumatic carditis; severe dermatologic diseases; severe allergic conditions, such as seasonal or perennial allergic rhinitis, bronchial asthma, serum sickness, and drug hypersensitivity reactions; respiratory diseases, such as symptomatic sarcoidosis, Löffler's syndrome, berylliosis, fulminating or disseminated pulmonary tuberculosis, and aspiration pneumonitis; hematologic disorders, such as idiopathic thrombocytopenic purpura and secondary thrombocytopenia in adults, autoimmune hemolytic anemia, aplastic crisis, and congenital hypoplastic anemia; tuberculous meningitis and trichinosis with neurologic or myocardial involvement*

▶ *To manage leukemias and lymphomas in adults and acute leukemia in children; to induce diuresis or remission of proteinuria in idiopathic nephrotic syndrome without uremia or nephrotic syndrome caused by systemic lupus erythematosus*

▶ *To provide palliative therapy during acute exacerbations of GI diseases, such as ulcerative colitis and regional enteritis*

I.V. INJECTION

Adults. Highly individualized dosage based on severity of disorder. *Usual:* 0.75 to 9 mg daily as a single dose or in divided doses.

▶ *To manage adrenocortical insufficiency*

I.V. INJECTION

Adults. 0.5 to 9 mg daily as a single dose or in divided doses.

▶ *To decrease cerebral edema*

I.V. INJECTION

Adults. 10 mg I.V. followed by 4 mg I.M. every 6 hr. Decreased after 2 to 4 days, if needed, gradually tapering off over 5 to 7 days unless inoperable or recurring brain tumor is present. If such a tumor is present, dosage gradually decreased after 2 to 4 days to maintenance dosage of 2 mg I.M. every 8 to 12 hr and switched to P.O. regimen as soon as possible.

▶ *To treat unresponsive shock*

I.V. INFUSION, I.V. INJECTION

Adults. 20 mg as a single dose followed by 3 mg/kg over 24 hr as a continuous infusion; 40 mg as a single dose followed by 40 mg every 2 to 6 hr, as needed; or 1 mg/kg as a single dose. All regimens used for no more than 3 days.

Contraindications

Administration of live virus vaccine to patient or family member, hypersensitivity to dexamethasone or its components (including sulfites), idiopathic thrombocytopenic purpura (I.M. use), systemic fungal infections

---

Mechanism of Action

Binds to intracellular glucocorticoid receptors and suppresses inflammatory and immune responses by:
- inhibiting neutrophil and monocyte accumulation at inflammation site and suppressing their phagocytic and bactericidal activity
- stabilizing lysosomal membranes
- suppressing antigen response of macrophages and helper T cells
- inhibiting synthesis of inflammatory response mediators, such as cytokines, interleukins, and prostaglandins.

Interactions

DRUGS

aminoglutethimide, antacids, barbiturates, carbamazepine, hydantoins, mitotane, rifampin: Decreased dexamethasone effectiveness

amphotericin B (parenteral), carbonic anhydrase inhibitors: Risk of hypokalemia

anticholinesterases: Decreased anticholinesterase effectiveness in myasthenia gravis

aspirin, NSAIDs: Increased risk of adverse GI effects

cholestyramine: Increased dexamethasone clearance

cyclosporine: Increased activity of both drugs, possibly resulting in seizures

digoxin: Increased risk of digitalis toxicity related to hypokalemia

ephedrine: Decreased half-life and increased clearance of dexamethasone

erythromycin, indinavir: Increased clearance and decreased plasma concentrations of these drugs

estrogens, ketoconazole, macrolide antibiotics: Decreased dexamethasone clearance

isoniazid: Decreased blood isoniazid level

neuromuscular blockers: Possibly potentiated or counteracted neuromuscular blockade

oral anticoagulants: Altered coagulation times, requiring reduced anticoagulant dosage

oral contraceptives: Increased half-life and concentration of dexamethasone

phenytoin: Increased risk of seizures

potassium-wasting diuretics: Increased potassium loss and risk of hypokalemia

salicylates: Decreased blood level and effectiveness of salicylates

somatrem: Possibly inhibition of somatrem's growth-promoting effect

thalidomide: Increased risk of toxic epidermal necrolysis

theophyllines: Altered effects of either drug

toxoids, vaccines: Decreased antibody response

ACTIVITIES

alcohol use: Increased risk of GI bleeding

Adverse Reactions

CNS: Depression, emotional lability, euphoria, fever, headache, increased ICP with papilledema, insomnia, light-headedness, malaise, neuritis, neuropathy, paresthesia, psychosis, seizures, syncope, tiredness, vertigo, weakness

CV: Arrhythmias, bradycardia, edema, fat embolism, heart failure, hypercholesterolemia, hyperlipidemia, hypertension, myocardial rupture, tachycardia, thromboembolism, thrombophlebitis, vasculitis

EENT: Cataracts, glaucoma, vision changes (all forms); epistaxis, loss of smell and taste, nasal burning and dryness, oral candidiasis, perforated nasal septum, pharyngitis, rebound nasal congestion, rhinorrhea, sneezing (nasal aerosol)

ENDO: Cushingoid symptoms, decreased iodine uptake, growth suppression in children, hyperglycemia, menstrual irregularities, secondary adrenocortical and pituitary unresponsiveness

GI: Abdominal distention, bloody stools, elevated liver function test results, heartburn, hepatomegaly, increased appetite, indigestion, intestinal perforation, melena, nausea, pancreatitis, peptic ulcer with possible perforation, ulcerative esophagitis, vomiting

GU: Glycosuria, increased or decreased number and motility of spermatozoa, perineal irritation, urinary frequency

HEME: Leukocytosis, leukopenia

MS: Aseptic necrosis of femoral and humeral heads; muscle atrophy, spasms, or weakness; myalgia; osteoporosis; pathologic fracture of long bones; tendon rupture (intra-articular injection); vertebral compression fracture

RESP: Bronchospasm

SKIN: Acne, allergic dermatitis, diaphoresis, ecchymosis, erythema, hirsutism, necrotizing vasculitis, petechiae, subcutaneous fat atrophy, striae, thin and fragile skin, urticaria

Other: Aggravated or masked signs of infection, anaphylaxis, angioedema, hypernatremia, hypocalcemia, hypokalemia, hypokalemic alkalosis, impaired wound healing, metabolic acidosis, sodium and fluid retention, suppressed skin test reaction, weight gain

Nursing Considerations

- Use dexamethasone cautiously in patients with congestive heart failure, hypertension, or renal insufficiency because drug can cause sodium retention, which may lead to edema and hypokalemia.
- Also use cautiously in patients who have had intestinal sugery and in those with peptic ulcer, diverticulitis, or ulcerative colitis because of the risk of perforation.
- Give once-daily dose of dexamethasone in the morning to coincide with the body's natural cortisol secretion.
- Be aware that dosage forms with a concentration of 24 mg/ml are for I.V. use only.
- **WARNING** Avoid subcutaneous injection; it may cause atrophy and sterile abscess.
- Inject undiluted I.V. dose directly into I.V. tubing of infusing compatible solution over 30 seconds or less, as prescribed.
- **WARNING** Don't give acetate form by I.V. injection.
- Expect to taper drug rather than stopping it abruptly; prolonged use can cause adrenal suppression.
- Monitor fluid intake and output and daily weight, and assess patient for crackles, dyspnea, peripheral edema, and steady weight gain.
- Periodically evaluate growth if patient is a child.
- Test stool for occult blood.
- Monitor results of hematology studies and blood glucose, serum electrolyte, cholesterol, and lipid levels. Dexamethasone may cause hyperglycemia, hypernatremia, hypocalcemia, hypokalemia, or leukopenia. It also may increase serum cholesterol and lipid levels, and it may decrease iodine uptake by the thyroid.
- Assess patient for evidence of osteoporosis, Cushing's syndrome, and other systemic effects during long-term use.
- Monitor neonate for signs of hypoadrenocorticism if mother received dexamethasone during pregnancy. Be aware that some preparations also contain benzyl alcohol, which may cause a fatal toxic syndrome in neonates and immature infants.
- Watch for hypersensitivity reactions after giving acetate or sodium phosphate form; both may contain bisulfites or parabens, inactive ingredients to which some people are allergic.

PATIENT TEACHING

- Caution patient to avoid alcoholic beverages during therapy because they increase the risk of GI bleeding.
- Advise patient to follow a low-sodium, high-potassium, high-protein diet, if prescribed, to help minimize weight gain (common with this drug). Instruct her to inform prescriber if she's on a special diet.
- Instruct patient not to stop using drug abruptly.
- Advise patient to notify prescriber if condition recurs or worsens after dosage is reduced or therapy stops.
- Urge patient to have regular eye examinations during long-term use.
- Advise patient receiving long-term therapy to carry medical identification and to notify all health care providers that she takes dexamethasone.
- Instruct patient (especially a child) to avoid close contact with anyone who has chickenpox or measles and to notify prescriber immediately if exposure occurs.
- Advise patient and family members to avoid live virus vaccinations, such as oral polio vaccine, during therapy unless prescriber approves.
- Inform diabetic patient that drug may affect her blood glucose level.
- Advise patient to notify prescriber about anorexia, depression, light-headedness, malaise, muscle pain, nausea, vomiting, and signs of early hyperadrenocorticism (abdominal distention, amenorrhea, easy bruising, extreme weakness, facial hair, increased appetite, moon face, weight gain). Inform patient and family about possible changes in appearance.
- Encourage patient to notify prescriber about illness, surgery, or changes in stress level.

dexrazoxane

Zinecard

Class and Category

Chemical: Piperazinedione
Therapeutic: Cardioprotective agent, chelating agent
Pregnancy category: C

Indications and Dosages

▶ *To prevent or reduce severity of cardiomyopathy associated with doxorubicin therapy in women with metastatic breast cancer*

I.V. INJECTION

Adults. *Initial:* 500 mg/m^2 for every 50 mg/m^2 of doxorubicin every 3 wk.

DOSAGE ADJUSTMENT In patients with hyperbilirubinemia, dosage proportionately reduced (depending on severity) to maintain a dexrazoxane-to-doxorubicin ratio of 10:1. In patients with creatinine clearance of less than 40 ml/min, dosage decreased 50%.

Mechanism of Action

Rapidly enters cardiac cells and acts as an intracellular heavy metal chelator. In cardiac tissues, anthracyclines, such as doxorubicin, form complexes with iron or copper, resulting in damage to cardiac cell membranes and mitochondria. Dexrazoxane combines with intracellular iron and protects against anthracycline-induced free radical damage to the myocardium. It also prevents the conversion of ferrous ions back to ferric ions for use by free radicals.

Incompatibilities

Don't mix dexrazoxane in same I.V. line with other drugs.

Contraindications

Hypersensitivity to dexrazoxane or its components; use with chemotherapy regimens that don't include an anthracycline, such as daunorubicin, doxorubicin, epirubicin, idarubicin, or mitoxantrone

Interactions

bone marrow depressants: Possibly enhanced bone marrow depression

Adverse Reactions

HEME: Myelosuppression including granulocytopenia, leukopenia, or thrombocytopenia
Other: Injection site pain

Nursing Considerations

- **WARNING** Use gloves when preparing reconstituted solution. If dexrazoxane powder or solution comes in contact with your skin or mucosa, immediately and thoroughly wash with soap and water.
- Reconstitute drug by mixing with 25 or 50 ml of 0.167 molar sodium lactate, supplied by the manufacturer, to produce a final concentration of 10 mg/ml. Administer reconstituted solution by slow I.V. push, or further dilute with either normal saline

solution or D_5W to a concentration of 1.3 to 5 mg/ml, as prescribed, for rapid I.V. infusion.

- Be aware that dexrazoxane may interfere with tumor response to doxorubicin, especially in patients receiving drug at start of fluorouracil-doxorubicin-cyclophosphamide therapy.
- Monitor patient with immunosuppression or decreased bone marrow reserves resulting from prior chemotherapy or radiation therapy to prevent worsening of her condition. Notify prescriber if condition deteriorates.

PATIENT TEACHING
- Inform patient that dexrazoxane is used to protect the heart from damage caused by myelosuppression and that she'll be given the drug by a health care professional in the hospital or clinic before receiving chemotherapy.
- Inform patient that dexrazoxane and chemotherapy may make her feel generally unwell, but urge her to continue treatment unless prescriber tells her to stop.
- Instruct patient to report chills, fever, mouth sores, pain at injection site, sore throat, unusual bleeding or bruising, unusual tiredness or weakness, and vomiting. Dosage may need to be changed or therapy stopped.
- Inform patient that drug may exacerbate symptoms of bone marrow suppression caused by anthracycline chemotherapy, including increased risk of infection.
- Teach patient importance of avoiding injury and infection during dexrazoxane therapy. For example, advise her to use a soft-bristled toothbrush to prevent damage to teeth and gums; to avoid people with colds, the flu, or bronchitis; and to avoid anyone who has recently had oral polio vaccine because of the increased risk of infection from live virus.

dextrose
(D–glucose)
2.5% Dextrose Injection, 5% Dextrose Injection, 10% Dextrose Injection, 20% Dextrose Injection, 25% Dextrose Injection, 50% Dextrose Injection, 60% Dextrose Injection, 70% Dextrose Injection

Class and Category
Chemical: Monosaccharide
Therapeutic: Antidiabetic, nutritional supplement
Pregnancy category: C

Indications and Dosages

▶ *To treat insulin-induced hypoglycemia*
I.V. INFUSION, I.V. INJECTION

Adults and children. *Initial:* 20 to 50 ml of 50% solution given at 3 ml/min. *Maintenance:* 10% to 15% solution by continuous infusion until blood glucose level reaches therapeutic range.

Infants and neonates. 2 ml/kg of 10% to 25% solution until blood glucose level reaches therapeutic range.

▶ *To replace calories*
I.V. INFUSION

Adults and children. Individualized dosage of 2.5%, 5%, or 10% solution, based on need for fluids or calories and given through peripheral I.V. line. Or a 10% to 70% solution given through a large central vein, if needed, typically mixed with amino acids or other solutions.

Route	Onset	Peak	Duration
I.V.	2 to 3 min	Unknown	Unknown

Mechanism of Action

Prevents protein and nitrogen loss, promotes glycogen deposition, prevents or decreases ketosis, and, in large amounts, acts as an osmotic diuretic. Dextrose is readily metabolized and undergoes oxidation to carbon dioxide and water. The oral form—glucose—is absorbed directly into the bloodstream from the intestines and is distributed, used, or stored in the liver.

Incompatibilities

Don't give dextrose through same infusion set as blood or blood products because pseudoagglutination of RBCs may occur.

Contraindications

For all solutions: Diabetic coma with excessively elevated blood glucose level

For concentrated solutions: Anuria, alcohol withdrawal syndrome in dehydrated patient, glucose-galactose malabsorption syndrome, hepatic coma, intracranial or intraspinal hemorrhage, overhydration

Interactions

DRUGS

corticosteroids, corticotropin: Increased risk of fluid and electrolyte imbalance if dextrose solution contains sodium ions

Adverse Reactions

CNS: Confusion, fever
GU: Glycosuria
Other: Dehydration; hyperosmolar coma; hypervolemia; hypovolemia; injection site extravasation with tissue necrosis, infection, phlebitis, and venous thrombosis

Nursing Considerations

- Use cautiously in patients with renal impairment because dextrose solutions contain aluminum, which may reach toxic levels when these patients receive prolonged parenteral therapy.
- Give highly concentrated dextrose solution by central venous catheter—not by subcutaneous or I.M. route.
- **WARNING** Avoid rapid or excessive administration of dextrose solution in a very low–birth-weight infant because it can increase serum osmolality and possibly cause intracerebral hemorrhage.
- Assess infusion site regularly for signs of infiltration, such as pain or swelling.
- Assess for glucosuria by using a urine reagent strip or collecting a urine sample and reviewing urinalysis results.
- When discontinuing a concentrated solution, expect to give a 5% to 10% dextrose infusion to avoid rebound hypoglycemia.
- Monitor patient for signs of hypervolemia, such as jugular vein distention and crackles.

PATIENT TEACHING
- Instruct patient to monitor her blood glucose level as directed.
- Stress the importance of reporting discomfort, pain, or signs of infection at I.V. site.

dezocine

Dalgan

Class and Category

Chemical: Aminotetralin, synthetic opioid
Therapeutic: Opioid analgesic
Pregnancy category: C

Indications and Dosages

▶ *To relieve pain*
I.V. INJECTION
Adult. *Initial:* 5 mg, followed by 2.5 to 10 mg every 2 to 4 hr, p.r.n. *Maximum:* 120 mg daily.

Route	Onset	Peak	Duration
I.V.	15 min	30 min	2 to 4 hr

Mechanism of Action

Binds with opiate receptors at many CNS sites, which alters the perception of and emotional response to pain.

Contraindications

Hypersensitivity to dezocine or its components

Interactions

DRUGS

CNS depressants, general anesthetics, hypnotics, sedatives, tranquilizers: Increased CNS depression

other opioid analgesics: Possibly decreased therapeutic effects of other opioid and withdrawal symptoms in patient receiving long-term opioid therapy

ACTIVITIES

alcohol use: Increased CNS depression

Adverse Reactions

CNS: CNS toxicity (delirium, delusions, mental depression), dizziness, sedation, vertigo

CV: Chest pain, hypertension, hypotension, irregular heartbeat

GI: Nausea, vomiting

GU: Decreased urine output, dysuria, urinary frequency

RESP: Atelectasis, cough, dyspnea, respiratory depression

Other: Injection site redness and swelling

Nursing Considerations

- Have patient lie down during dezocine administration and for a period afterward to lessen hypotensive effects (dizziness, lightheadedness) and other adverse effects (nausea, vomiting).
- **WARNING** Administer dezocine slowly. Rapid delivery of other opioid analgesics has caused anaphylaxis, severe respiratory depression, hypotension, peripheral circulatory collapse, and cardiac arrest. Keep emergency equipment and drugs nearby.
- Be aware that dosage reduction may be required for patients with respiratory disease (to avoid decreased respiratory drive and increased airway resistance); impaired hepatic function, including cirrhosis (because elimination half-life may be pro-

longed); or impaired renal function as well as for elderly, debilitated, or severely ill patients (who may be more sensitive to drug's effects).

- Discard solution if it contains precipitate.
- Frequently monitor blood pressure and pulse and respiratory rates after giving first dose.
- **WARNING** Avoid administering dezocine to a patient who is opioid-dependent. Doing so may precipitate withdrawal symptoms because drug can antagonize opioid effects. Patients with a history of drug abuse (including acute alcoholism), emotional instability, or suicidal ideation or attempts are at increased risk for abuse.
- Assess patient for pain relief; document your findings often.
- Assess respiratory status in patients with acute respiratory depression because dezocine can worsen this condition. Patients having an acute asthma attack and those with chronic disease are at increased risk for respiratory depression.
- Monitor patients with a history of common bile duct disorders for signs of increased biliary pressure, such as pain in upper midline area that may radiate to back and right shoulder.
- Monitor for worsening condition in patients with diarrhea caused by poisoning or pseudomembranous colitis.
- Assess patient's urine output; decreasing output may signal urine retention.
- Watch for evidence of drug-induced CNS depression or increased CSF pressure—such as altered LOC, restlessness, and irritability—in patients with a head injury, intracranial lesions, or other conditions that could cause these effects. Patients who are taking or have recently taken drugs that cause CNS depression are also more susceptible to these effects. Take appropriate safety precautions.
- Be aware that patients with hypothyroidism are at increased risk for respiratory depression and prolonged CNS depression.
- Be aware that dezocine may affect GI motility or mask symptoms of acute abdominal conditions.

PATIENT TEACHING

- Instruct patient to report if dezocine doesn't relieve pain within 1 hour.
- Advise patient to avoid potentially hazardous activities until drug's CNS effects are known.
- Advise patient to change position slowly to minimize dizziness and light-headedness.

• Urge patient to avoid alcohol and other drugs that cause CNS depression during dezocine therapy.

diazepam
Diazemuls, Dizac, Valium

Class, Category, and Schedule
Chemical: Benzodiazepine
Therapeutic: Anticonvulsant, anxiolytic, sedative-hypnotic, skeletal muscle relaxant
Pregnancy category: D
Controlled substance schedule: IV

Indications and Dosages
▶ *To relieve anxiety*
I.V. INJECTION
Adults. 2 to 5 mg every 3 to 4 hr, p.r.n., for moderate anxiety; 5 to 10 mg every 3 to 4 hr, p.r.n., for severe anxiety.
Children. Individualized dosage. *Maximum:* 0.25 mg/kg given over 3 min and repeated after 15 to 30 min if needed and after another 15 to 30 min if needed.
▶ *To treat symptoms of acute alcohol withdrawal*
I.V. INJECTION
Adults. 10 mg and then 5 to 10 mg in 3 to 4 hr, if needed.
▶ *To provide muscle relaxation, sedation*
I.V. INJECTION
Adults. 5 to 10 mg and then 5 to 10 mg in 3 to 4 hr, if needed.
DOSAGE ADJUSTMENT Dosage reduced to 2 to 5 mg/dose and increased as needed and tolerated for patients who are debilitated.
▶ *To treat status epilepticus and severe recurrent seizures*
I.V. INJECTION
Adults. 5 to 10 mg repeated every 10 to 15 min, as needed, up to a cumulative dose of 30 mg. Regimen repeated, if needed, in 2 to 4 hr. (Use I.M. route if I.V. access is impossible.)
Children age 5 and over. 1 mg repeated every 2 to 5 min, as needed, up to a cumulative dose of 10 mg. Regimen repeated, if needed, in 2 to 4 hr.
Children ages 1 month to 5 years. 0.2 to 0.5 mg repeated every 2 to 5 min, as needed, up to a cumulative dose of 5 mg. Regimen repeated, if needed, in 2 to 4 hr.
▶ *To provide preoperative sedation*

I.V. INJECTION

Adults. 5 to 10 mg 30 min before surgery.

▶ *To reduce anxiety before cardioversion*

I.V. INJECTION

Adults. 5 to 15 mg 5 to 10 min before procedure.

▶ *To reduce anxiety before endoscopic procedures*

I.V. INJECTION

Adults. Up to 20 mg titrated to desired sedation and administered immediately before procedure.

▶ *To treat tetanus*

I.V. INJECTION

Adults and children age 5 and over. *Initial:* 5 to 10 mg repeated every 3 to 4 hr, if needed. Sometimes larger doses are needed for adults.

DOSAGE ADJUSTMENT For debilitated patients, initial dose reduced to 2 to 5 mg and increased gradually as needed and tolerated.

Children ages 1 month to 5 years. 1 to 2 mg repeated every 3 to 4 hr, as needed.

Mechanism of Action

May potentiate the effects of gamma-aminobutyric acid (GABA) and other inhibitory neurotransmitters by binding to specific benzodiazepine receptors in the limbic and cortical areas of the CNS. GABA inhibits excitatory stimulation, which helps control emotional behavior. The limbic system contains a highly dense area of benzodiazepine receptors, which may explain the drug's antianxiety effects. Diazepam also suppresses the spread of seizure activity caused by seizure-producing foci in the cortex, thalamus, and limbic structures.

Incompatibilities

Don't mix diazepam injection with aqueous solutions. Don't mix diazepam emulsion with morphine or glycopyrrolate or administer it through an infusion set that contains polyvinyl chloride.

Contraindications

Acute angle-closure glaucoma, hypersensitivity to diazepam or its components, untreated open-angle glaucoma

Interactions

DRUGS

cimetidine, disulfiram, fluoxetine, isoniazid, itraconazole, ketoconazole, metoprolol, oral contraceptives, propoxyphene, propranolol, valproic acid:

Decreased diazepam metabolism, increased blood level and risk of adverse effects of diazepam

CNS depressants: Increased CNS depression

digoxin: Increased serum digoxin level and risk of digitalis toxicity

levodopa: Decreased antidyskinetic effect of levodopa

probenecid: Faster onset or more prolonged effects of diazepam

ranitidine: Delayed elimination and increased blood level of diazepam

rifampin: Decreased blood diazepam level

theophyllines: Antagonized sedative effect of diazepam

ACTIVITIES

alcohol use: Increased CNS depression

Adverse Reactions

CNS: Anterograde amnesia, anxiety, ataxia, confusion, depression, dizziness, drowsiness, fatigue, headache, insomnia, lethargy, light-headedness, sedation, sleepiness, slurred speech, tremor, vertigo

CV: Hypotension, palpitations, phlebitis, tachycardia, thrombophlebitis

EENT: Blurred vision, diplopia, increased salivation

GI: Anorexia, constipation, diarrhea, nausea, vomiting

GU: Libido changes, urinary incontinence, urine retention

RESP: Respiratory depression

SKIN: Dermatitis

Other: Physical and psychological dependence

Nursing Considerations

- Protect diazepam injection from light. Don't use solution if it is more than slightly yellow or contains precipitate.
- Don't mix emulsion form with anything other than its emulsion base. Otherwise, it may become unstable and increase the risk of serious adverse reactions.
- Before administering emulsion form, ask if patient is allergic to soybeans because this form contains soybean oil.
- Administer diazepam directly into an I.V. line inserted in a large vein or through I.V. tubing as close to insertion site as possible at a rate of at least 5 mg/minute. For an infant or a child, administer I.V. injection slowly over 3 minutes.
- Giive emulsion form within 6 hours of opening ampule because it contains no preservatives. Use polyethylene-lined or glass infusion sets and polyethylene or polypropylene plastic syringes. Don't use a filter with a pore size smaller than 5 microns because it may break down the emulsion.
- **WARNING** Be aware that patients with a history of seizure disorders may have seizures when diazepam is started or sud-

denly withdrawn. Monitor patients with Lennox-Gastaut syndrome or absence seizures for tonic status epilepticus.
- Monitor for increased sedation, especially in patients with hypoalbuminemia.
- Monitor hepatic and renal function blood test results in patients with impaired renal or hepatic function because diazepam is metabolized in the liver and excreted by the kidneys.
- **WARNING** Observe for signs of physical and psychological dependence: a strong desire or need to continue taking diazepam, a need to increase dosage to maintain drug effects, and posttherapy withdrawal symptoms, such as abdominal cramps, insomnia, irritability, nervousness, and tremor.
- Observe for signs of phlebitis or thrombophlebitis after administration.
- Store diazepam injection at 15° to 30° C (59° to 86° F). Store diazepam emulsion below 25° C (77° F). Protect from freezing and light.

PATIENT TEACHING
- Inform patient that diazepam may cause drowsiness, and advise her to avoid activities requiring alertness until drug's CNS effects are known.
- Urge patient to avoid CNS depressants and alcohol during therapy.
- Instruct patient not to take drug more often, in greater quantities, or for a longer time than prescribed. Inform her that physical and psychological dependence can occur, and teach her to recognize signs of dependence.
- Instruct patient not to abruptly stop taking drug without prescriber supervision. Caution patient with a history of seizures that abrupt drug withdrawal may trigger them.

diazoxide
Hyperstat

Class and Category
Chemical: Benzothiadiazine derivative
Therapeutic: Antihypertensive, antihypoglycemic
Pregnancy category: C

Indications and Dosages
▶ *To treat severe hypertension in hospitalized patients*
I.V. INJECTION
Adults and children. *Initial:* 1 to 3 mg/kg by rapid bolus, repeated every 5 to 15 min until diastolic pressure falls below 100 mm Hg.

Repeated in 4 hr and again in 24 hr, if needed, until oral antihypertensive therapy begins. *Maximum:* 150 mg/dose, 1.2 g daily.

Route	Onset	Peak	Duration
I.V.	1 min	2 to 5 min	2 to 12 hr

Mechanism of Action

Directly affects smooth muscle cells of peripheral arteries and arterioles, causing them to dilate. This action decreases peripheral resistance, which helps reduce blood pressure. Diazoxide also inhibits insulin release from the pancreas, stimulates catecholamine release, and increases hepatic glucose release.

Contraindications

Acute aortic dissection; hypersensitivity to diazoxide, thiazides, other sulfonamide derivatives, or their components; treatment of compensatory hypertension (as occurs with aortic coarctation)

Interactions

DRUGS

allopurinol, colchicine, probenecid, sulfinpyrazone: Increased serum uric acid level

antihypertensives: Additive hypotensive effects

beta blockers: Increased hypotensive effects of diazoxide

diuretics (especially thiazides): Potentiated hyperglycemic, hyperuricemic, and antihypertensive effects of diazoxide

estrogens, NSAIDs, sympathomimetics: Antagonized hypotensive effects of diazoxide

insulin, oral antidiabetic drugs: Possibly decreased effectiveness of these drugs

oral anticoagulants: Increased anticoagulant effects

peripheral vasodilators, ritodrine: Additive, possibly severe, hypotensive effects

Adverse Reactions

CNS: Anxiety, apprehension, cerebral ischemia, confusion, dizziness, euphoria, headache, insomnia, light-headedness, malaise, somnolence, weakness

CV: Bradycardia, chest pain, hypotension, orthostatic hypotension, palpitations, peripheral edema, tachycardia, transient hypertension

EENT: Blurred vision, dry mouth, increased salivation, taste perversion, tinnitus, transient hearing loss

ENDO: Transient hyperglycemia
GI: Abdominal pain, anorexia, constipation, diarrhea, ileus, nausea, vomiting
HEME: Thrombocytopenia
MS: Gout
SKIN: Diaphoresis, flushing, pruritus, rash, sensation of warmth
Other: Allergic reaction, extravasation with injection site cellulitis and pain; fluid and sodium retention

Nursing Considerations

- Administer diazoxide undiluted over 10 to 30 seconds. Don't give drug by I.M. or subcutaneous route.
- Keep patient supine during I.V. injection and for 1 hour afterward.
- Monitor blood pressure throughout treatment to check for hypertension. Before ending surveillance, measure patient's standing blood pressure if she's ambulatory.
- Monitor patients with uncompensated heart failure for signs of fluid retention and worsening heart failure due to diazoxide's effects.
- Monitor patients with impaired cardiac or cerebral circulation for exacerbations caused by drug-related abrupt blood pressure reduction, mild tachycardia, and decreased blood perfusion.
- Frequently assess I.V. site for extravasation because the alkaline drug can irritate tissue.
- If diabetic patient receives diazoxide to treat hypertension, monitor for signs and symptoms of hyperglycemia because parenteral form commonly causes transient hyperglycemia.
- Be aware that patients with impaired renal function may require reduced dosage because drug effects may be prolonged.
- Monitor patients with a history of gout for signs of exacerbation, such as joint redness or swelling and hyperuricemia.
- Monitor blood glucose level of all patients who receive diazoxide to determine if drug has raised blood glucose level to normal.
- Store drug at 15° to 30° C (59° to 86° F); protect from freezing and light.

PATIENT TEACHING

- Inform patient that she'll be on bed rest until oral diazoxide therapy starts.
- Caution patient not to take antidiabetic drugs unless prescribed.
- Advise patient to report signs of hyperglycemia, such as increased urinary frequency, increased thirst, and fruity breath.

digoxin

Lanoxin Injection, Lanoxin Injection Pediatric

Class and Category

Chemical: Digitalis glycoside
Therapeutic: Antiarrhythmic, cardiotonic
Pregnancy category: C

Indications and Dosages

▶ *To treat heart failure, atrial flutter, atrial fibrillation, and paroxysmal atrial tachycardia with rapid digitalization*

I.V. INJECTION

Adults. *Loading:* 10 to 15 mcg/kg in 3 divided doses every 6 to 8 hr, with first dose equal to 50% of total dose. *Maintenance:* 125 to 350 mcg daily, given once or twice daily.

Children over age 10. *Loading:* 8 to 12 mcg/kg in 3 or more divided doses, with first dose equal to 50% of total dose. Subsequent doses given every 6 to 8 hr. *Maintenance:* 2 to 3 mcg/kg once daily.

Children ages 6 to 10. *Loading:* 15 to 30 mcg/kg in 3 or more divided doses, with first dose equal to 50% of total dose. Subsequent doses given every 6 to 8 hr. *Maintenance:* 4 to 8 mcg/kg daily in two divided doses.

Children ages 2 to 5. *Loading:* 25 to 35 mcg/kg in 3 or more divided doses, with first dose equal to 50% of total dose. Subsequent doses given every 6 to 8 hr. *Maintenance:* 6 to 9 mcg/kg daily in two divided doses.

Infants ages 1 to 24 months. *Loading:* 30 to 50 mcg/kg in 3 or more divided doses, with first dose equal to 50% of total dose. Subsequent doses given every 6 to 8 hr. *Maintenance:* 7.5 to 12 mcg/kg daily in two divided doses.

Full-term neonates. *Loading:* 20 to 30 mcg/kg in 3 or more divided doses, with first dose equal to 50% of total dose. Subsequent doses given every 6 to 8 hr. *Maintenance:* 5 to 8 mcg/kg daily in two divided doses.

Premature neonates. *Loading:* 15 to 25 mcg/kg in 3 or more divided doses, with first dose equal to 50% of total dose. Subsequent doses given every 6 to 8 hr. *Maintenance:* 4 to 6 mcg/kg/daily in two divided doses.

DOSAGE ADJUSTMENT Dosage carefully adjusted for elderly or debilitated patients and those who have implanted pacemakers because they may develop toxicity at doses tolerated by most patients.

Route	Onset	Peak	Duration
I.V.	5 to 30 min	1 to 5 hr	3 to 4 days

Mechanism of Action

Increases the force and velocity of myocardial contraction, resulting in positive inotropic effects. Digoxin produces antiarrhythmic effects by decreasing the conduction rate and increasing the effective refractory period of the AV node.

Incompatibilities

Don't mix digoxin in the same container or I.V. line as other other drugs.

Contraindications

Hypersensitive carotid sinus syndrome, hypersensitivity to digoxin, presence or history of digitalis toxicity or idiosyncratic reaction to digoxin, ventricular fibrillation, ventricular tachycardia unless heart failure unrelated to digoxin therapy occurs

Interactions

DRUGS

amiodarone, propafenone: Elevated blood digoxin level, possibly to toxic level

antacids: Inhibited digoxin absorption

antiarrhythmics, pancuronium, parenteral calcium salts, rauwolfia alkaloids, sympathomimetics: Possibly increased risk of arrhythmias

diltiazem, verapamil: Increased blood digoxin level, possibly excessive bradycardia

edrophonium: Excessive slowing of heart rate

erythromycin, neomycin, tetracycline: Possibly increased blood digoxin level

hypokalemia-causing drugs, potassium-wasting diuretics: Increased risk of digitalis toxicity from hypokalemia

indomethacin: Decreased renal clearance and increased blood level of digoxin

magnesium sulfate (parenteral): Possibly cardiac conduction changes and heart block

quinidine, quinine: Increased blood digoxin level

spironolactone: Increased digoxin half-life and risk of adverse effects

succinylcholine: Increased risk of digoxin-induced arrhythmias

sucralfate: Decreased digoxin absorption

Adverse Reactions

CNS: Anxiety, confusion, depression, drowsiness, extreme weakness, hallucinations, headache, syncope
CV: Arrhythmias, heart block
EENT: Blurred vision, colored halos around objects
GI: Abdominal discomfort or pain, anorexia, diarrhea, nausea, vomiting
SKIN: Rash
Other: Electrolyte imbalances

Nursing Considerations

- Before giving each dose of digoxin, take patient's apical pulse and notify prescriber if pulse is below 60 beats/minute (or other specified level).
- Administer drug undiluted, or dilute with a fourfold or greater volume of sterile water for injection, normal saline solution, or D$_5$W for I.V. administration. Once diluted, administer immediately over at least 5 minutes. Discard if solution is markedly discolored or contains precipitate.
- Monitor closely for signs of digitalis toxicity: altered mental status, arrhythmias, heart block, nausea, vision disturbances, and vomiting. If they appear, notify prescriber, check serum digoxin level as ordered, and expect to withhold drug until level is known. Monitor ECG tracing continuously.
- If patient has acute or unstable chronic atrial fibrillation, assess drug effects. Ventricular rate may not normalize even when serum drug level is in therapeutic range; raising the dosage probably won't be therapeutic and may lead to toxicity.
- Frequently obtain ECG tracings as ordered in elderly patients because of their smaller body mass and reduced renal clearance. Elderly patients, especially those with coronary insufficiency, are more susceptible to arrhythmias—particularly ventricular fibrillation—if digitalis toxicity occurs.
- Monitor serum electrolyte—especially potassium—levels regularly because hypokalemia predisposes patient to digitalis toxicity and serious arrhythmias. Also monitor potassium levels frequently if patient is receiving potassium salts in addition to digoxin because hyperkalemia in such a patient can be fatal.
- Store drug at 15° to 25° C (59° to 77° F); protect from freezing and light.

PATIENT TEACHING

- Urge patient to report adverse reactions, such as GI distress, palpitations, or pulse changes.

digoxin immune Fab (ovine)
Digibind

Class and Category
Chemical: Digoxin-specific antigen-binding fragments
Therapeutic: Digitalis glycoside antidote
Pregnancy category: C

Indications and Dosages
▶ *To treat acute toxicity from known amount of digoxin elixir or tablets*
I.V. INJECTION
Adults and children. Individualized dosage based on amount ingested. Dose (mg) = dose ingested (mg) multiplied by 0.8 and then divided by 0.5, multiplied by 38, and rounded up to next whole vial.

▶ *To treat acute toxicity from known quantity of digoxin capsules, digitoxin tablets, or I.V. injection of digoxin or digitoxin*
I.V. INJECTION
Adults and children. Individualized dosage based on amount ingested. Dose (mg) = dose ingested (mg) divided by 0.5, then multiplied by 38 and rounded up to next whole vial.

▶ *To treat acute toxicity from unknown amount of digoxin or digitoxin during long-term therapy*
I.V. INJECTION
Adults and children. Individualized dosage for digoxin toxicity: Dose (mg) = serum digoxin level (ng/ml) multiplied by body weight (kg), then divided by 100, and then multiplied by 38. Individualized dosage for digitoxin toxicity: Dose (mg) = serum digitoxin level (ng/ml) multiplied by body weight (kg) and then divided by 1,000, multiplied by 38, and rounded up to next whole vial.

DOSAGE ADJUSTMENT Higher dose administered, as prescribed, if the dose based on ingested amount differs substantially from the dose based on serum digoxin or digitoxin level. Dose repeated after several hours, if needed.

Route	Onset	Peak	Duration
I.V.	15 to 30 min	Unknown	8 to 12 hr

Contraindications
Hypersensitivity to digoxin immune Fab

Interactions
None known.

Mechanism of Action

Binds with digoxin or digitoxin molecules. The resulting complex is excreted through the kidneys. As the free serum digoxin level declines, tissue-bound digoxin enters the serum and also is bound and excreted.

Adverse Reactions

CV: Increased ventricular rate (in atrial fibrillation), worsening of heart failure or low cardiac output

Other: Allergic reaction (difficulty breathing, urticaria), febrile reaction, hypokalemia

Nursing Considerations

- Expect each 38-mg vial of purified digoxin immune Fab to bind with about 0.5 mg of digoxin or digitoxin.
- Reconstitute by dissolving 38 mg of drug in 4 ml of sterile water for injection to yield 9.5 mg/ml. Mix gently. Further dilute with normal saline solution to a convenient volume for I.V. infusion. For very small doses, reconstituted 38-mg vial may be diluted with 34 ml of normal saline solution to yield 1 mg/ml. Use reconstituted solution promptly or, if necessary, store it for up to 4 hours at 2° to 8° C (36° to 46° F).
- **WARNING** Before giving digoxin immune Fab to high-risk patient, test for allergic reaction, as prescribed, by diluting 0.1 ml of reconstituted drug in 9.9 ml of sodium chloride for injection and injecting 0.1 ml (9.5 mcg/0.1 ml) intradermally. After 20 minutes, look for an urticarial wheal surrounded by erythema. Or, perform a scratch test by placing 1 drop of 9.5-mcg/0.1 ml dilution on patient's skin and making a ¼" scratch through drop with a sterile needle. Inspect site in 20 minutes. Test is considered positive if it produces a wheal surrounded by erythema. If it causes a systemic reaction, apply tourniquet above test site, notify prescriber, and prepare to respond to anaphylaxis. Be aware that if a skin or systemic reaction occurs, additional drug shouldn't be given unless essential; if more of the drug must be given, expect prescriber to pretreat patient with corticosteroids and diphenhydramine. Prescriber should be on standby to treat anaphylaxis.
- When preparing digoxin immune Fab for an infant, reconstitute drug as ordered and administer with a tuberculin syringe.
- When administering drug to a child, monitor for fluid volume overload.

- When giving a large dose, expect a faster onset but watch closely for febrile reaction. Monitor body temperature and ECG tracing during treatment. Make sure emergency equipment and drugs are readily available.
- Administer I.V. infusion through a 0.22-micron membrane filter over 30 minutes. Keep in mind that drug may be given by rapid I.V. injection if cardiac arrest is imminent.
- Monitor serum potassium level frequently, especially during first few hours of therapy, because potassium level may drop rapidly.
- Be aware that patient may not be redigitalized for several days or even longer, until fragments of digoxin immune Fab have been eliminated from body. This process may be delayed in patients with impaired renal function because drug is eliminated by kidneys.

PATIENT TEACHING

- Teach patient the purpose of digoxin immune Fab and how it will be administered.
- Advise patient to notify you immediately if she experiences adverse reactions, especially difficulty breathing and urticaria.

dihydroergotamine mesylate
D.H.E. 45, Dihydroergotamine-Sandoz (CAN), Migranal

Class and Category
Chemical: Semisynthetic ergot alkaloid
Therapeutic: Antimigraine
Pregnancy category: X

Indications and Dosages
▶ *To treat acute migraine with or without aura*
I.V. INJECTION
Adults. 1 mg, repeated in 1 hr, if needed. *Maximum:* 6 mg/wk.

Route	Onset	Peak	Duration
I.V.	5 min	15 min to 2 hr	About 8 hr

Contraindications
Coronary artery disease, including vasospasm; hemiplegic or basilar migraine; hypersensitivity to dihydroergotamine or other ergot alkaloids; malnutrition; peripheral vascular disease or after vascular surgery; pregnancy; sepsis; severe hepatic or renal impairment; severe pruritus; uncontrolled hypertension; use of macrolide

antibiotics or protease inhibitors; use within 24 hours of 5-hydroxytryptamine$_1$ (5-HT$_1$) agonist, ergotamine-containing or ergot-type drug, or methysergide

---

Mechanism of Action

Produces intracranial and peripheral vasoconstriction by binding to all known 5-hydroxytryptamine$_1$ (5-HT$_1$) receptors, alpha$_1$- and alpha$_2$-adrenergic receptors, and dopaminergic receptors. Activation of 5-HT$_1$ receptors on intracranial blood vessels probably constricts large intracranial arteries and closes arteriovenous anastomoses to relieve migraine headache. Activation of 5-HT$_1$ receptors on sensory nerves in the trigeminal system also may inhibit the release of pro-inflammatory neuropeptides.

Peripherally, dihydroergotamine causes vasoconstriction by stimulating alpha-adrenergic receptors. At therapeutic doses, it inhibits norepinephrine reuptake, increasing vasoconstriction. The drug constricts veins more than arteries, increasing venous return while decreasing venous stasis and pooling.

Interactions
DRUGS
beta blockers: Possibly peripheral vasoconstriction and peripheral ischemia, increased risk of gangrene
macrolides, protease inhibitors: Possibly increased risk of vasospasm, acute ergotism with peripheral ischemia
nitrates: Decreased antianginal effects of nitrates
other ergot drugs, including ergoloid mesylates, ergonovine, methylergonovine, methysergide, and sumatriptan: Increased risk of serious adverse effects from nasal dihydroergotamine
systemic vasoconstrictors: Risk of severe hypertension
ACTIVITIES
smoking: Possibly increased ischemic response to ergot therapy

Adverse Reactions
CNS: Anxiety, confusion, dizziness, fatigue, headache, paresthesia, somnolence, weakness
CV: Bradycardia, chest pain, peripheral vasospasm (calf or heel pain with exertion, cool and cyanotic hands and feet, leg weakness, weak or absent pulses), tachycardia
EENT: Abnormal vision; dry mouth; epistaxis, nasal congestion or rhinitis, and sore nose (nasal spray); miosis; pharyngitis; sinusitis; taste perversion
GI: Diarrhea, nausea, vomiting

MS: Muscle stiffness
SKIN: Localized edema of face, feet, fingers, and lower legs; sensation of heat or warmth; sudden diaphoresis

Nursing Considerations

- **WARNING** Monitor patient for signs of dihydroergotamine overdose, such as abdominal pain, confusion, delirium, dizziness, dyspnea, headache, nausea, pain in legs or arms, paresthesia, seizures, and vomiting.
- Assess peripheral pulses, skin sensation, warmth, and capillary refill. After giving nasal dihydroergotamine, monitor for signs of widespread blood vessel constriction and adverse reactions caused by decreased circulation to many body areas.

PATIENT TEACHING

- If patient experiences a headache different from her usual migraines, caution her not to use dihydroergotamine and to notify prescriber.
- Urge patient to avoid alcohol, which can cause or worsen headaches, and smoking, which may cause an ischemic response.
- Warn patient about possible dizziness during or after a migraine for which she took dihydroergotamine.

diltiazem hydrochloride

Cardizem

Class and Category

Chemical: Benzothiazepine derivative
Therapeutic: Antianginal, antiarrhythmic, antihypertensive
Pregnancy category: C

Indications and Dosages

▶ *To treat atrial fibrillation, atrial flutter, and paroxysmal supraventricular tachycardia*
I.V. INFUSION, I.V. INJECTION
Adults and adolescents. 0.25 mg/kg given by bolus over 2 min. If response is inadequate after 15 min, 0.35 mg/kg given by bolus over 2 min. Then 10 mg/hr for continued reduction of heart rate after bolus, increased by 5 mg/hr, as needed. *Maximum:* 15 mg/hr for up to 24 hr.

Route	Onset	Peak	Duration
I.V.	3 min	2 to 7 min	30 min to 10 hr*

* For infusion; 1 to 3 hr for injection.

Mechanism of Action

Diltiazem inhibits calcium movement into coronary and vascular smooth-muscle cells by blocking slow calcium channels in cell membranes, as shown. This action decreases intracellular calcium, which:

• inhibits smooth-muscle cell contractions
• decreases myocardial oxygen demand by relaxing coronary and vascular smooth muscle, reducing peripheral vascular resistance and systolic and diastolic blood pressures
• slows AV conduction time and prolongs AV nodal refractoriness
• interrupts the reentry circuit in AV nodal reentrant tachycardias.

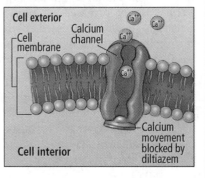

Incompatibilities

Don't give diltiazem through same I.V. line as acetazolamide, acyclovir, aminophylline, ampicillin sodium/sulbactam sodium, cefamandole, cefoperazone, diazepam, furosemide, heparin, hydrocortisone sodium succinate, methylprednisolone sodium succinate, mezlocillin, nafcillin, phenytoin, rifampin, or sodium bicarbonate.

Contraindications

Acute MI; cardiogenic shock; Lown-Ganong-Levine or Wolff-Parkinson-White syndrome, second- or third-degree AV block, and sick sinus syndrome, unless artificial pacemaker is in place; pulmonary edema; systolic blood pressure below 90 mm Hg; ventricular tachycardia (wide complex)

Interactions

DRUGS

anesthetics: Additive hypotension; possibly decreased cardiac contractility, conductivity, and automaticity

benzodiazepines: Increased risk of prolonged sedation

beta blockers: Possibly increased risk of adverse cardiovascular effects

buspirone: Increased effects and risk of buspirone toxicity

carbamazepine, cyclosporine, lovastatin, quinidine, theophyllines: Decreased hepatic clearance and increased serum levels of these drugs, leading to toxicity

cimetidine: Decreased diltiazem metabolism, increased blood diltiazem level

digoxin: Increased blood digoxin level

lithium: Possibly neurotoxicity

NSAIDs: Possibly antagonized antihypertensive effect of diltiazem

prazocin: Possibly increased risk of hypotension

procainamide: Possibly increased risk of prolonged QT interval

quinidine: Increased risk of adverse quinidine effects

rifampin: Decreased blood diltiazem level to undetectable amounts

Adverse Reactions

CNS: Abnormal gait, amnesia, asthenia, depression, dizziness, dream disturbances, extrapyramidal reactions, fatigue, hallucinations, headache, insomnia, nervousness, paresthesia, personality change, somnolence, syncope, tremor, weakness

CV: Angina, atrial flutter, AV block (first-, second-, and third-degree), bradycardia, bundle-branch block, heart failure, hypotension, palpitations, peripheral edema, PVCs, sinus arrest, sinus tachycardia, 12-lead ECG abnormalities, ventricular fibrillation, ventricular tachycardia

EENT: Amblyopia, dry mouth, epistaxis, eye irritation, gingival bleeding and hyperplasia, gingivitis, nasal congestion, retinopathy, taste perversion, tinnitus

ENDO: Hyperglycemia

GI: Anorexia, constipation, diarrhea, elevated liver function test results, indigestion, nausea, thirst, vomiting

GU: Acute renal failure, impotence, nocturia, polyuria, sexual dysfunction

HEME: Hemolytic anemia, leukopenia, prolonged bleeding time, thrombocytopenia

MS: Arthralgia, muscle spasms, myalgia

RESP: Cough, dyspnea

SKIN: Alopecia, diaphoresis, erythema multiforme, exfoliative dermatitis, flushing, leukocytoclastic vasculitis, petechiae, photosensitivity, pruritus, purpura, rash, Stevens-Johnson syndrome, toxic epidermal necrolysis, urticaria

Other: Angioedema, hyperuricemia, weight gain

Nursing Considerations

• Use diltiazem cautiously in patients with impaired hepatic or renal function, and monitor liver and renal function test results, as appropriate; diltiazem is metabolized mainly in the liver and excreted by the kidneys.

- **WARNING** Monitor blood pressure, pulse rate, and heart rate and rhythm by continuous ECG as appropriate during therapy. Keep emergency equipment and drugs available.
- Assess patient for signs of heart failure.
- If patient takes digoxin, watch for signs of digitalis toxicity, such as nausea, vomiting, halo vision, and elevated serum digoxin level.
- Administer sublingual nitroglycerin, as prescribed, during diltiazem therapy.
- Expect to discontinue drug if adverse skin reactions, usually transient, persist.

PATIENT TEACHING

- Urge patient to report chest pain, difficulty breathing, dizziness, fainting, irregular heartbeat, rash, or swollen ankles.

dimenhydrinate

Dinate, Dramanate, Gravol (CAN), Hydrate

Class and Category

Chemical: Ethanolamine derivative
Therapeutic: Antiemetic, antihistamine, antivertigo agent
Pregnancy category: B

Indications and Dosages

▶ *To treat nausea, vomiting, dizziness, or vertigo with motion sickness*
I.V. INFUSION, I.V. INJECTION
Adults and adolescents. 50 mg in 10 ml of normal saline solution given slowly, over at least 2 min, every 4 hr p.r.n.
Children. 1.25 mg/kg or 37.5 mg/m^2 in 10 ml of normal saline solution given slowly, over at least 2 min, every 6 hr p.r.n. *Maximum:* 300 mg daily.

Route	Onset	Peak	Duration
I.V.	Immediate	Unknown	3 to 6 hr

Mechanism of Action

May inhibit vestibular stimulation and labyrinthine stimulation and function by acting on the otolith system and, with larger doses, on the semicircular canals.

Contraindications

Hypersensitivity to dimenhydrinate or its components, premature and full-term neonates

Interactions

DRUGS

aminoglycosides and other ototoxic drugs: Masked symptoms of ototoxicity

anticholinergics and drugs with anticholinergic activity: Potentiated anticholinergic effects of dimenhydrinate

apomorphine: Possibly decreased emetic response to apomorphine in treatment of poisoning

barbiturates and other CNS depressants: Possibly increased CNS depression

MAO inhibitors: Increased anticholinergic and CNS depressant effects of dimenhydrinate

ACTIVITIES

alcohol use: Possibly increased CNS depression

Adverse Reactions

CNS: Confusion, drowsiness, hallucinations, nervousness, paradoxical stimulation

CV: Hypotension, palpitations, tachycardia

EENT: Blurred vision, diplopia, dry eyes, dry mouth, nasal congestion

GI: Anorexia, constipation, diarrhea, epigastric discomfort, nausea, vomiting

GU: Dysuria

HEME: Hemolytic anemia

RESP: Thickening of bronchial secretions, wheezing

SKIN: Photosensitivity, rash, urticaria

Other: Anaphylaxis

Nursing Considerations

- **WARNING** Don't give dimenhydrinate to premature or full-term neonates. Some I.V. forms may contain benzyl alcohol, which can cause a fatal toxic syndrome with CNS, respiratory, circulatory, and renal impairment and metabolic acidosis.
- **WARNING** Be aware that 50-mg/ml dimenhydrinate is intended for I.M. use. For I.V. use, the solution *must* be diluted further with at least 10 ml of diluent, such as D_5W or normal saline solution, for each milliliter of dimenhydrinate.
- Monitor patients with prostatic hypertrophy, stenosing peptic ulcer, pyloroduodenal obstruction, bladder neck obstruction,

narrow angle glaucoma, bronchial asthma, or cardiac arrhythmias for signs and symptoms of exacerbation of these conditions resulting from drug's anticholinergic effects.

- Monitor elderly patients for evidence of increased sensitivity to dimenhydrinate, such as excessive drowsiness, confusion, and restlessness.
- Assess for signs of paradoxical stimulation, such as nightmares, unusual excitement, nervousness, restlessness, or irritability, especially in children and elderly patients.
- Store drug at 15° to 30° C (59° to 86° F); don't freeze.

PATIENT TEACHING

- Because drug may cause drowsiness, instruct patient to avoid hazardous activities until its CNS effects are known.
- Advise patient to inform health care providers of dimenhydrinate therapy, especially if she's being evaluated for medical conditions that are affected by this drug, such as appendicitis.
- Instruct patient to avoid alcohol, sedatives, and tranquilizers while receiving this drug.
- Encourage patient to use sunscreen to prevent photosensitivity reactions.

diphenhydramine hydrochloride
Benadryl, Hyrexin

Class and Category
Chemical: Ethanolamine derivative
Therapeutic: Antianaphylactic adjunct, antidyskinetic, antiemetic, antihistamine, antivertigo agent
Pregnancy category: B

Indications and Dosages
▶ *To treat hypersensitivity reactions, such as perennial and seasonal allergic rhinitis, vasomotor rhinitis, allergic conjunctivitis, uncomplicated allergic skin eruptions, and transfusion reactions*
I.V. INJECTION
Adults and adolescents. 10 to 50 mg every 4 to 6 hr up to 100 mg/dose, if needed. *Maximum:* 400 mg daily.
Children. 1.25 mg/kg every 4 to 6 hr. *Maximum:* 300 mg daily.
▶ *To prevent motion sickness or treat vertigo*
I.V. INJECTION
Adults and adolescents. *Initial:* 10 mg; increased to 20 to 50 mg every 2 to 3 hr, if needed. *Maximum:* 100 mg/dose, 400 mg daily.

Children. 1 to 1.5 mg/kg I.M. every 4 to 6 hr, p.r.n. *Maximum:* 300 mg daily.

▶ *To treat symptoms of Parkinson's disease and drug-induced extrapyramidal reactions in elderly patients who can't tolerate more potent antidyskinetic drugs*

I.V. INJECTION

Adults and adolescents. 10 to 50 mg q.i.d., as needed. *Maximum:* 100 mg/dose, 400 mg daily.

Route	Onset	Peak	Duration
I.V.	Immediate	1 to 3 hr	6 to 8 hr

Mechanism of Action

Binds to central and peripheral H_1 receptors, competing with histamine for these sites and preventing it from reaching its site of action. By blocking histamine, diphenhydramine produces antihistamine effects: inhibiting respiratory, vascular, and GI smooth-muscle contraction; decreasing capillary permeability, which reduces wheals, flares, and itching; and decreasing salivary and lacrimal gland secretions.

Diphenhydramine also produces antidyskinetic effects, possibly by inhibiting acetylcholine in the CNS. The drug's antiemetic and antivertigo effects may be related to its ability to bind to CNS muscarinic receptors and depress vestibular stimulation and labyrinthine function.

Contraindications

Bladder neck obstruction, hypersensitivity to diphenhydramine or its components, lower respiratory tract symptoms (including asthma), narrow-angle glaucoma, pyloroduodenal obstruction, stenosing peptic ulcer, symptomatic benign prostatic hyperplasia, use within 14 days of MAO inhibitor therapy

Interactions

DRUGS

anticholinergics and drugs with anticholinergic activity: Potentiated anticholinergic effects of diphenhydramine

apomorphine: Possibly decreased emetic response to apomorphine in treatment of poisoning

barbiturates, other CNS depressants: Possibly increased CNS depression

MAO inhibitors: Increased anticholinergic and CNS depressant effects of diphenhydramine

ACTIVITIES

alcohol use: Possibly increased CNS depression

Adverse Reactions
CNS: Confusion, dizziness, drowsiness
CV: Arrhythmias, palpitations, tachycardia
EENT: Blurred vision, diplopia
GI: Epigastric distress, nausea
HEME: Agranulocytosis, hemolytic anemia, thrombocytopenia
RESP: Thickened bronchial secretions
SKIN: Photosensitivity

Nursing Considerations
- Expect to give parenteral form of diphenhydramine only when oral ingestion isn't possible.
- Don't exceed 25 mg/minute when giving diphenhydramine.
- Expect to discontinue drug at least 72 hours before skin tests for allergies because drug may inhibit cutaneous histamine response, thus producing false-negative results.
- Store drug at 15° to 30° C (59° to 86° F); protect from freezing and light.

PATIENT TEACHING
- Because diphenhydramine may cause drowsiness, advise patient to avoid hazardous activities until its CNS effects are known.
- Urge patient to avoid alcohol and other CNS depressants, such as sedatives and tranquilizers, while receiving diphenhydramine.
- Advise use of sunscreen to prevent photosensitivity reactions.

dipyridamole
Persantine

Class and Category
Chemical: Pyrimidine
Therapeutic: Coronary vasodilator, diagnostic aid, platelet aggregation inhibitor
Pregnancy category: B

Indications and Dosages
▶ *To aid diagnosis during thallium perfusion imaging of myocardium*
I.V. INFUSION
Adults. 0.57 mg/kg in 50 ml of D_5W infused over 4 min. *Maximum:* 60 mg.

Route	Onset	Peak	Duration
I.V.	Unknown	3.8 to 8.7 min*	Unknown

* After start of infusion, for increased velocity of coronary artery blood flow.

Mechanism of Action

May increase the intraplatelet level of adenosine, which causes coronary vasodilation and inhibits platelet aggregation. Dipyridamole also may increase the intraplatelet level of cAMP and may inhibit formation of the potent platelet activator stimulant thromboxane A2, which decreases platelet activation. Vasodilation and increased blood flow occur preferentially in nondiseased coronary vessels, which results in redistribution of blood away from significantly diseased vessels. These changes in perfusion are observed during thallium imaging studies.

Contraindications

Asthma, hypersensitivity to dipyridamole or its components, hypotension, unstable angina pectoris

Interactions

DRUGS

adenosine: Potentiated effects of adenosine

cefamandole, cefoperazone, cefotetan, plicamycin, valproic acid: Possibly hypoprothrombinemia and increased risk of bleeding

heparin, NSAIDs, thrombolytics: Possibly increased risk of bleeding

theophylline: Reversal of coronary vasodilation caused by dipyridamole, possibly false-negative thallium imaging result

warfarin: Increased risk of dizziness, abdominal distress, headache and rash

Adverse Reactions

CNS: Dizziness, headache

CV: Angina, arrhythmias, ECG changes (specifically ST-segment and T-wave changes)

GI: Abdominal pain, diarrhea, nausea, vomiting

RESP: Dyspnea

SKIN: Flushing, pruritus, rash

Nursing Considerations

- Protect I.V. form of dipyridamole from direct light and from freezing.
- Monitor blood pressure, pulse rate and rhythm, and breath sounds every 10 to 15 minutes during I.V. infusion.
- Keep parenteral aminophylline available to relieve adverse reactions to dipyridamole infusion.
- At therapeutic doses, expect adverse reactions to be minimal and transient. They typically resolve with long-term use.

PATIENT TEACHING
- Tell patient that dipyridamole usually is given with other anti-coagulants.
- Urge her to keep appointments for coagulation tests.
- Instruct patient to seek immediate emergency treatment if chest pain occurs.
- Caution patient to consult prescriber before taking aspirin and other OTC NSAIDs because of increased risk of bleeding.

dobutamine hydrochloride
Dobutrex

Class and Category
Chemical: Synthetic catecholamine
Therapeutic: Cardiac stimulant
Pregnancy category: Not rated

Indications and Dosages
▶ *To treat low cardiac output and heart failure*
I.V. INFUSION
Adults. 2.5 to 10 mcg/kg/min as continuous infusion, adjusted according to hemodynamic response.
Children. 5 to 20 mcg/kg/min as continuous infusion, adjusted according to hemodynamic response.

Route	Onset	Peak	Duration
I.V.	1 to 2 min	Unknown	Less than 5 min

Mechanism of Action
Primarily stimulates beta$_1$-adrenergic receptors and mildly stimulates beta$_2$- and alpha$_1$-adrenergic receptors. Beta$_1$-receptor stimulation produces a positive inotropic effect on the myocardium. This increases cardiac output by boosting myocardial contractility and stroke volume. Increased myocardial contractility raises coronary blood flow and myocardial oxygen consumption. Systolic blood pressure typically rises as a result of increased stroke volume. Other hemodynamic effects include decreased systemic vascular resistance, which reduces afterload, and decreased ventricular filling pressure, which reduces preload.

Incompatibilities
Don't combine dobutamine with cefamandole, cefazolin, cepha-

lothin, ethacrynate sodium, heparin sodium, hydrocortisone sodium succinate, or penicillin because these drugs are incompatible. Don't mix dobutamine with alkaline solutions, such as sodium bicarbonate, because of possible incompatibility. Don't use diluents that contain sodium bisulfite or ethanol. Don't mix dobutamine in same solution with other drugs.

Contraindications
Hypersensitivity to dobutamine or its components, idiopathic hypertrophic subaortic stenosis

Interactions
DRUGS
beta blockers: Possibly increased alpha-adrenergic activity and peripheral resistance
bretylium: Potentiated vasopressor activity, possibly arrhythmias
cyclopropane, halothane: Possibly serious arrhythmias
guanethidine: Decreased hypotensive effect of guanethidine, possibly resulting in severe hypertension
thyroid hormones: Increased cardiovascular effects of thyroid hormones or dobutamine
tricyclic antidepressants: Possibly potentiated cardiovascular and vasopressor effects of dobutamine, resulting in arrhythmias, hyperpyrexia, or severe hypertension

Adverse Reactions
CNS: Fever, headache, nervousness, restlessness
CV: Angina, bradycardia, hypertension, hypotension, palpitations, PVCs, tachycardia
GI: Nausea, vomiting
RESP: Dyspnea
SKIN: Extravasation with tissue necrosis and sloughing, rash
Other: Allergic reaction, hypokalemia

Nursing Considerations
- Avoid giving dobutamine to patients with uncorrected hypovolemia; expect prescriber to order whole blood or plasma volume expanders to correct it. Also avoid giving drug to patients with acute MI; it can intensify or extend myocardial ischemia.
- Dilute concentrate with at least 50 ml of compatible I.V. solution. A common dilution is 500 mg (40 ml from 250-ml bag) in 210 ml D_5W or normal saline solution to yield 2,000 mcg/ml. Or dilute 1,000 mg (80 ml from 250-ml bag) in 170 ml D_5W or normal saline solution to yield 4,000 mcg/ml. Adjust maximum concentration to patient's fluid requirements, as prescribed.

Don't exceed 5,000 mcg/ml. Discard solution after 24 hours.
- Inspect parenteral solution for particles and discoloration before administering it.
- Administer drug using an infusion pump.
- Monitor patients who are allergic to sulfites because commercially available dobutamine injections contain sodium bisulfite and may cause anaphylaxis-like signs and symptoms.
- Keep in mind that patients with atrial fibrillation should be adequately digitalized before giving dobutamine. Watch for signs of increased AV conduction, such as increased heart rate.
- Monitor blood pressure frequently during therapy, preferably by continuous intra-arterial monitoring; a systolic pressure increase of 10 to 20 mm Hg may indicate a dobutamine-induced increase in cardiac output.
- If hypotension develops, expect to reduce dosage or stop drug.
- Monitor heart rate and rhythm continuously for PVCs, which may result from drug's stimulatory effect on the heart's conduction system, and sinus tachycardia, which results from positive chronotropic effect of beta stimulation and may increase the heart rate by 5 to 15 beats/minute.
- Monitor hemodynamic parameters, such as central venous pressure, pulmonary artery wedge pressure, and cardiac output, as indicated, to assess drug's effectiveness.
- **WARNING** Monitor serum potassium level. Rarely, hypokalemia results from $beta_2$ stimulation and electrolyte imbalances.
- Monitor urine output hourly, as appropriate, to assess for improved renal blood flow.
- Be aware that dobutamine isn't indicated for long-term treatment of heart failure because it may not be effective and may increase the risk of hospitalization and death.
- Before diluting drug, store it at 15° to 30° C (59° to 86° F).

PATIENT TEACHING
- Explain the need for frequent hemodynamic monitoring during dobutamine therapy.

dolasetron mesylate
Anzemet

Class and Category
Chemical: Carboxylate monomethanesulfonate
Therapeutic: Antiemetic
Pregnancy category: B

Indications and Dosages

▶ *To prevent nausea and vomiting from chemotherapy*

I.V. INJECTION

Adults and children over age 16. 1.8 mg/kg or 100 mg as a single dose within 30 min before chemotherapy.

Children ages 2 to 16. 1.8 mg/kg as a single dose within 30 min before chemotherapy. *Maximum:* 100 mg.

ORAL SOLUTION

Adults and children over age 16. 100 mg within 1 hr before chemotherapy.

Children ages 2 to 16. 1.8 mg/kg within 1 hr before chemotherapy. *Maximum:* 100 mg.

▶ *To prevent postoperative nausea and vomiting*

I.V. INJECTION

Adults and children over age 16. 12.5 mg 15 min before end of anesthesia.

Children ages 2 to 16. 0.35 mg/kg 15 min before end of anesthesia. *Maximum:* 12.5 mg/dose.

ORAL SOLUTION

Adults and children over age 16. 100 mg within 2 hr before surgery.

Children ages 2 to 16. 1.2 mg/kg within 2 hr before surgery. *Maximum:* 100 mg.

▶ *To treat postoperative nausea and vomiting*

I.V. INJECTION

Adults and children over age 16. 12.5 mg as a single dose as soon as symptoms develop.

Children ages 2 to 16. 0.35 mg/kg as a single dose as soon as symptoms develop. *Maximum:* 12.5 mg/dose.

Mechanism of Action

Decreases vomiting reflex (with its active metabolite hydrodolasetron) by preventing activation of serotonin 5-hydroxytryptamine$_3$ (5-HT$_3$) receptors on vagal nerve terminals peripherally and chemoreceptor trigger zone centrally.

Contraindications

Hypersensitivity to dolasetron or its components

Interactions

DRUGS

atenolol: Possibly decreased clearance of dolasetron

cimetidine: Possibly increased blood dolasetron level
rifampin: Possibly decreased blood dolasetron level

Adverse Reactions
CNS: Headache
CV: Bradycardia, cardiac arrest, ECG changes, hypertension, hypotension, MI, tachycardia, ventricular fibrillation and tachycardia, wide-complex tachycardia
GI: Diarrhea
SKIN: Rash
Other: Anaphylaxis, injection site pain

Nursing Considerations
• Administer up to 100 mg of dolasetron I.V. in 30 seconds or dilute drug in normal saline solution, D5W, D5/0.45 normal saline solution, or lactated Ringer's solution and infuse for up to 15 minutes, as prescribed.
• Flush I.V. line with compatible solution before and after drug administration.
• Expect to prepare an oral solution of dolasetron for patients unable to swallow tablets by diluting injection solution with apple or apple-grape juice.
• **WARNING** Monitor patients receiving dolasetron for ECG changes, including prolonged PR, QTc, and JT intervals and widened QRS complex.
• Store drug at 20° to 25° C (68° to 77° F) and protect from light.
PATIENT TEACHING
• Advise parents of pediatric patients and patients who have difficulty swallowing that oral solution can be prepared by diluting injection form of dolasetron with apple or apple-grape juice.
• Inform patient that oral solution may be refrigerated for up to 48 hours but should be discarded after 2 hours at room temperature.

dopamine hydrochloride
Intropin, Revimine (CAN)

Class and Category
Chemical: Catecholamine
Therapeutic: Cardiac stimulant, vasopressor
Pregnancy category: C

Indications and Dosages
▶ *To correct hypotension that is unresponsive to adequate fluid volume*

replacement or occurs as part of shock syndrome caused by bacteremia, chronic cardiac decompensation, drug overdose, MI, open-heart surgery, renal failure, trauma, or other major systemic illnesses; to improve low cardiac output

I.V. INFUSION

Adults. 0.5 to 3 mcg/kg/min for vasodilation of renal arteries; 2 to 10 mcg/kg/min for positive inotropic effects and increased cardiac output; 10 mcg/kg/min, increased gradually according to patient's response, for increased systolic and diastolic blood pressures.

Children. 0.5 to 3 mcg/kg/min for vasodilation of renal arteries; 5 to 20 mcg/kg/min for increased cardiac output and systolic and diastolic blood pressures.

DOSAGE ADJUSTMENT Initial dosage reduced to 10% of usual amount if patient has received an MAO inhibitor in previous 2 to 3 wk.

Route	Onset	Peak	Duration
I.V.	In 5 min	Unknown	Up to 10 min

Mechanism of Action

Stimulates dopamine$_1$ (D$_1$) and dopamine$_2$ (D$_2$) postsynaptic receptors. D$_1$ receptors mediate vasodilation in renal, mesenteric, coronary, and cerebral blood vessels. D$_2$ receptors, when stimulated, inhibit norepinephrine release. In higher doses, dopamine also stimulates alpha$_1$ and alpha$_2$ receptors, causing vascular smooth-muscle contraction.

At doses of 0.5 to 3 mcg/kg/minute, this naturally occurring catecholamine mainly affects dopaminergic receptors in renal, mesenteric, coronary, and cerebral vessels, resulting in vasodilation, increased renal blood flow, improved GFR, and increased urine output. At doses of 2 to 10 mcg/kg/minute, dopamine stimulates beta$_1$-adrenergic receptors, increasing cardiac output while maintaining dopaminergic-induced vasodilation. At doses of 10 mcg/kg/minute or more, alpha-adrenergic agonism takes over, causing increased peripheral vascular resistance and renal vasoconstriction.

Incompatibilities

Don't add dopamine to 5% sodium bicarbonate, alkaline I.V. solutions, oxidizing agents, or iron salts.

Contraindications

Pheochromocytoma, uncorrected ventricular fibrillation, ventricular tachycardia and other tachyarrhythmias

Interactions

DRUGS

alpha blockers, haloperidol, loxapine, phenothiazines, thioxanthenes: Antagonized peripheral vasoconstriction with high doses of dopamine

anesthetics (such as chloroform, enflurane, halothane, isoflurane, and methoxyflurane): Increased risk of severe atrial and ventricular arrhythmias

antihypertensives, diuretics used as antihypertensives: Possibly decreased antihypertensive effects of these drugs

beta blockers: Antagonized beta receptor–mediated inotropic effects of dopamine

digitalis glycosides: Possibly increased risk of arrhythmias and additive inotropic effects

diuretics: Possibly increased diuretic effects of dopamine or diuretic

doxapram: Possibly increased vasopressor effects

ergot alkaloids: Enhanced peripheral vasoconstriction

guanadrel, guanethidine: Possibly decreased antihypertensive effects of these drugs and potentiated vasopressor response to dopamine, resulting in hypertension and arrhythmias

levodopa: Possibly increased risk of arrhythmias

MAO inhibitors: Prolonged and intensified cardiac stimulation and vasopressor effect of dopamine

maprotiline, tricyclic antidepressants: Possibly potentiated cardiovascular and vasopressor effects of dopamine, resulting in arrhythmias, hyperpyrexia, or severe hypertension

mecamylamine, methyldopa: Possibly decreased hypotensive effects of these drugs and enhanced vasopressor effect of dopamine

methylphenidate: Possibly potentiated vasopressor effect of dopamine

nitrates: Possibly decreased antianginal effect of nitrates; possibly decreased vasopressor effect of dopamine, resulting in hypotension

oxytoxic drugs: Possibly severe hypertension

phenoxybenzamine: Possibly antagonized peripheral vasoconstriction of dopamine, causing hypotension and tachycardia

phenytoin: Possibly sudden bradycardia and hypotension

rauwolfia alkaloids: Possibly decreased hypotensive effects of these drugs

sympathomimetics: Possibly increased adverse cardiovascular and other effects

thyroid hormones: Increased risk of coronary insufficiency

Adverse Reactions

CNS: Headache

CV: Angina, bradycardia, hypertension, hypotension, palpitations, peripheral vasoconstriction, sinus tachycardia, ventricular arrhythmias
GI: Nausea, vomiting
RESP: Dyspnea
SKIN: Extravasation with tissue necrosis
Other: Allergic reaction

Nursing Considerations

• If possible, avoid giving dopamine to patients with occlusive vascular disease, such as atherosclerosis, Buerger's disease, diabetic endarteritis, or Raynaud's disease, because of the risk of decreased peripheral circulation.

• Inspect parenteral solution for particles and discoloration before administration.

• Dilute dopamine concentrate with a compatible I.V. solution before administering. Typical dilution is 400 mg in 250 ml to yield 1.6 mg/ml. Don't exceed 3.2 mg/ml.

• Be aware that drug also comes premixed with D_5W in concentrations of 800 mcg, 1.6 mg, and 3.2 mg. Monitor for elevated glucose levels, as ordered, in patients with subclinical or overt diabetes mellitus because this finding may signal an exacerbation.

• If patient has hypovolemia, ensure adequate fluid resuscitation before giving drug.

• Give drug by I.V. infusion using an infusion pump.

• **WARNING** When infusion rate exceeds 20 mcg/kg/minute, monitor patient for excessive vasoconstriction and loss of renal vasodilating effects. Don't exceed 50 mcg/kg/minute.

• If you must infuse more than 20 mcg/kg/minute of dopamine to maintain blood pressure, expect to infuse norepinephrine as prescribed.

• Give infusion through a central catheter to avoid extravasation and tissue necrosis. If you must give drug through a peripheral line, inspect site often for signs of extravasation and necrosis. If you detect such signs, start a new I.V. line for dopamine infusion, discontinue previous I.V. line, and notify prescriber immediately.

• If drug extravasates, expect prescriber to order 5 to 10 mg of phentolamine diluted in 10 to 15 ml of normal saline solution. Phentolamine infiltrates directly into area to antagonize vasoconstriction and minimize sloughing and tissue necrosis.

• Titrate dopamine gradually to minimize hypotension, especially after a high infusion rate.

- Monitor blood pressure continuously with an intra-arterial line, as indicated.
- Place patient on continuous ECG monitoring, and assess heart rate and rhythm for arrhythmias.
- Assess patients with cardiac disease, particularly coronary artery disease, for signs of exacerbation or adverse cardiac reactions because dopamine increases myocardial oxygen demand.
- Monitor hemodynamic parameters, such as central venous pressure, pulmonary artery wedge pressure, and cardiac output, as indicated, to assess drug's effectiveness.
- Monitor urine output hourly as appropriate to assess for improved renal blood flow.
- Monitor patients who are allergic to sulfites for signs and symptoms of an allergic reaction because some forms of dopamine contain sulfites.
- Store dopamine at 15° to 30° C (59° to 86° F); don't freeze it.

PATIENT TEACHING
- Explain the need for frequent hemodynamic monitoring during dopamine therapy.

doripenem
Doribax

Class and Category
Chemical: Carbapenem
Therapeutic: Antibiotic
Pregnancy category: B

Indications and Dosages
▶ *To treat complicated intra-abdominal infections caused by* Escherichia coli, Klebsiella pneumoniae, Pseudomonas aeruginosa, Bacteroides caccae, B. fragilis, B. thetaiotaomicron, B. uniformis, B. vulgatus, Streptococcus intermedius, S. constellatus *or* Peptostreptococcus micros *and complicated UTI, including pyelonephritis, caused by* E. coli, K. pneumoniae, Proteus mirabilis, P. aeruginosa, *or* Acinetobacter baumannii

I. V. INFUSION
Adults. 500 mg infused over 1 hr every 8 hr.

DOSAGE ADJUSTMENT Dosage reduced to 250 mg infused over 1 hr every 8 hr if patient has impaired renal function and creatinine clearance of 30 to 50 ml/min/1.73 m^2. Dosage reduced to 250 mg infused over 1 hr every 12 hr if creatinine clearance is 10 to 30 ml/min/1.73 m^2.

Route	Onset	Peak	Duration
I.V.	Unknown	1 hr	8 hr

Mechanism of Action
Inhibits cell wall synthesis in susceptible bacteria. Doripenem inactivates multiple penicillin-binding proteins essential to cell wall synthesis, thus causing cell death.

Incompatibilities
Don't mix doripenem with other drugs or add to solutions containing other drugs because of possible incompatibility.

Contraindications
History of anaphylactic reactions to beta-lactam antibiotics; hypersensitivity to doripenem, its components, or other carbapenems

Interactions
DRUGS
probenecid: Increased plasma doripenem level
valproic acid: Decreased effectiveness of valproic acid and possible loss of seizure control

Adverse Reactions
CNS: Headache, seizure
CV: Phlebitis
EENT: Oral candidiasis
GI: Diarrhea, liver enzyme elevation, nausea
GU: Vaginitis
HEME: Neutropenia
SKIN: Dermatitis, erythema, erythema multiforme, macular or papular eruptions, pruritus, rash, Stevens-Johnson syndrome, toxic epidermal necrolysis, urticaria
Other: Anaphylaxis

Nursing Considerations
• Use cautiously in patients with a history of hypersensitivity to cephalosporins or penicillins because cross-sensitivity may occur.
• Reconstitute vial with 10 ml sterile water for injection or normal saline solution and shake gently to form a suspension. Withdraw suspension using a syringe with a 21G needle, and add to an infusion bag containing 100 ml normal saline solution or D_5W. Shake gently until clear. If administering a re-

duced dosage of 250 mg, remove 55 ml of prepared solution from the infusion bag and discard it before infusion.

- Be aware that suspension in vial must be diluted within 1 hour of reconstitution. Once drug is diluted in infusion solution, if stored at room temperature, it must be used within 8 hours if mixed in normal saline solution and 4 hours if mixed in D₅W. If infusion solution is refrigerated, it must be used within 24 hours or discarded.
- Watch closely for evidence of hypersensitivity, especially in patients with multiple allergies, because serious and occasionally fatal hypersensitivity reactions have occurred in patients receiving beta-lactam antibiotics. If an allergic reaction occurs, discontinue drug immediately, notify prescriber, and expect to administer emergency treatment as prescribed, such as epinephrine, oxygen, IV fluids, IV antihistamines, corticosteroids, and pressor amine. Provide airway management as needed.
- Assess patient's bowel pattern daily; severe diarrhea may indicate *Clostridium difficile*–related diarrhea. If suspected, stop drug and provide treatment, as prescribed.

PATIENT TEACHING
- Instruct patient to report any sign of allergic reaction, such as rash, hives, itching, or difficulty breathing.
- Advise patient to report diarrhea if severe or persistent.

doxapram hydrochloride
Dopram

Class and Category
Chemical: Pyrrolidinone derivative
Therapeutic: Respiratory stimulant
Pregnancy category: B

Indications and Dosages
▶ *To stimulate respiration in COPD-related acute respiratory insufficiency*
I.V. INFUSION
Adults and adolescents. 1 to 2 mg/min titrated according to respiratory response. *Maximum:* 3 mg/min for up to 2 hr.
▶ *To treat respiratory depression after anesthesia*
I.V. INFUSION
Adults and adolescents. 5 mg/min until desired response occurs and then reduced to 1 to 3 mg/min. *Maximum:* Cumulative dose of 4 mg/kg or 300 mg.

I.V. INJECTION

Adults and adolescents. 0.5 to 1 mg/kg, repeated every 5 min, if needed. *Maximum:* 1.5 mg/kg as a single dose or 2 mg/kg every 5 min.

Route	Onset	Peak	Duration
I.V.	20 to 40 sec	1 to 2 min	5 to 12 min

Mechanism of Action

Activates peripheral carotid, aortic, and other chemoreceptors to stimulate respiration, resulting in increased tidal volume and respiratory rate. Doxapram also may increase respiratory rate and tidal volume by directly stimulating the respiratory center in the medulla oblongata.

Incompatibilities

To avoid precipitation and gas formation, don't mix doxapram with alkaline solutions, such as aminophylline, sodium bicarbonate, or 2.5% thiopental.

Contraindications

Age less than 1 month; cerebral edema; CVA; head injury; hypersensitivity to doxapram or its components; mechanical disorders of ventilation, including acute bronchial asthma, flail chest, muscle paresis, obstruction, pneumothorax, and pulmonary fibrosis; pulmonary embolism; seizure disorder; severe cardiovascular disorder; severe hypertension; uncompensated heart failure

Interactions

DRUGS

chloroform, cyclopropane, enflurane, halothane, isoflurane, methoxyflurane, trichloroethylene: Possibly adverse myocardial effects if doxapram given within 10 minutes of these drugs
CNS stimulants: Possibly excessive CNS stimulation, resulting in arrhythmias, insomnia, irritability, nervousness, or seizures
MAO inhibitors, sympathomimetics: Additive vasopressor effects
skeletal muscle relaxants: Masked residual effects of muscle relaxants

Adverse Reactions

CNS: Disorientation, dizziness, headache
CV: Arrhythmias, including sinus tachycardia; hypertension
GI: Diarrhea, hiccups, nausea, vomiting
GU: Urine retention

RESP: Bronchospasm, cough, dyspnea
SKIN: Diaphoresis
Other: Injection site pain, redness, swelling, and thrombophlebitis

Nursing Considerations
• Avoid giving doxapram to patients receiving mechanical ventilation.
• Maintain a patent airway, and assess for optimal oxygenation before administering drug.
• Monitor I.V. insertion site for extravasation and signs of thrombophlebitis or local skin irritation.
• If hypertension or dyspnea develops suddenly, stop infusion as directed.
• Assess for early signs of overdose, including enhanced deep tendon reflexes, skeletal muscle hyperactivity, and tachycardia.
PATIENT TEACHING
• Explain the need for frequent pulse and blood pressure monitoring.

doxorubicin hydrochloride
Adriamycin PFS, Adriamycin RDF, Rubex

Class and Category
Chemical: Anthracycline glycoside
Therapeutic: Antibiotic antineoplastic
Pregnancy category: D

Indications and Dosages
▶ *To treat disseminated neoplastic conditions, such as acute lymphoblastic or acute myeloblastic leukemia; Wilms' tumor; neuroblastoma; soft-tissue and bone sarcomas; breast, bronchogenic, gastric, ovarian, transitional cell bladder, or thyroid cancer; Hodgkin's disease; or malignant lymphoma*
I.V. INFUSION, I.V. INJECTION
Adults. 60 to 75 mg/m² administered over at least 3 to 5 min every 21 days when given as a single agent, or 40 to 60 mg/m² administered over at least 3 to 5 min every 21 to 28 days when given in combination therapy.
Children. 30 mg/m² for 3 days every 4 wk.
DOSAGE ADJUSTMENT Dosage varies, depending on regimen used. Dosage may be reduced when doxorubicin is used in combination with other cytotoxic drugs. Dosage reduced by

50% when plasma bilirubin level is 1.2 to 3 mg/ml and by 75% when plasma bilirubin level is 3.1 to 5 mg/ml.

Mechanism of Action
Binds directly to DNA by inserting (intercalating) itself between two DNA bases, which inhibits the synthesis of DNA and RNA and produces single-strand breaks in DNA. In addition, doxorubicin undergoes an enzymatic reduction, resulting in the multi-step production of a hydroxyl radical, which may lead to cell death by reacting with DNA, RNA, cell membranes, and proteins. Doxorubicin is active in all phases of the cell cycle, though cell cycle phase S is most sensitive.

Incompatibilities
Don't mix doxorubicin with heparin or fluorouracil because a precipitate will form. Don't mix doxorubicin with other drugs or with bacteriostatic agents.

Contraindications
Patients who've received maximum acceptable doses of doxorubicin, daunorubicin, idarubicin, or other anthracyclines and anthracenes; marked myelosuppression from prior antitumor therapy or radiation therapy

Interactions
DRUGS

actinomycin D: Acute "recall" pneumonitis after local radiation therapy in children

blood-dyscrasia–causing drugs (such as cephalosporins and cisplatin): Increased leukopenic and thrombocytopenic effects of doxorubicin

bone marrow depressants (such as colchicine and methotrexate): Increased bone marrow depression

carbamazepine: Decreased blood carbamazepine level

cisplatin: Risk of leukemia

cyclophosphamide: Potentiated cyclophosphamide-induced hemorrhagic cystitis, increased risk of doxorubicin-induced cardiotoxicity

cyclosporine: Possibly decreased doxorubicin metabolism; increased risk of severe and prolonged hematologic toxicity, coma, and seizures

cytarabine: Possibly necrotizing colitis

dactinomycin, mitomycin, nifedipine, and other calcium channel blockers: Increased risk of doxorubicin-induced cardiotoxicity *digoxin:* Decreased absorption of digoxin

fosphenytoin, phenytoin: Possibly decreased blood phenytoin level

methotrexate and other hepatotoxic drugs: Possibly impaired hepatic function, increased risk of doxorubicin toxicity

paclitaxel: Decreased doxorubicin clearance

phenobarbital: Possibly increased doxorubicin excretion

progesterone: Possibly enhanced doxorubicin-induced neutropenia and thrombocytopenia

streptozocin: Possibly inhibited hepatic metabolism of doxorubicin

trastuzumab: Possibly increased incidence and severity of cardiac dysfunction

vaccines, killed virus: Possibly decreased antibody response to vaccine

vaccines, live virus: Possibly increased adverse effects of vaccine, severe infection, and decreased antibody response to vaccine

Adverse Reactions

CNS: Chills, fever

CV: Arrhythmias, cardiomyopathy, cardiotoxicity

EENT: Conjunctivitis, esophagitis, stomatitis

GI: Diarrhea, GI ulceration or necrosis, nausea, vomiting

GU: Uric acid nephropathy, reddish urine

HEME: Anemia, leukopenia, myelosuppression, thrombocytopenia

SKIN: Alopecia; cellulitis; extravasation; hyperpigmentation of soles, palms, or nails; erythematous streaking along vein used for insertion; infusion site pain; recall postirradiation erythema; urticaria

Other: Hyperuricemia

Nursing Considerations

- **WARNING** Be aware that doxorubicin hydrochloride liposome should not be substituted for doxorubicin hydrochloride. These drugs are not interchangeable; severe adverse reactions may result.
- Be aware that doxorubicin should be administered only under the supervision of a qualified physician and that initial treatment usually takes place in a hospital.
- Follow facility protocols for preparation and handling of antineoplastic drugs and appropriate disposal of used equipment.
- Monitor patient's liver and renal function tests and CBC, including hematocrit, platelet count, and WBC count with differential, before and periodically during therapy. Be aware that cardiac evaluation, including ECG, radionuclide angiography to

determine ejection fraction, and echocardiography, will be performed before, during, and sometimes after doxorubicin therapy.

- Be aware that doxorubicin is available in various concentrations. Reconstitute doxorubicin with 0.9% sodium chloride injection to a final concentration of 2 mg/ml. Withdraw appropriate amount of air from vial when preparing drug to prevent pressure build-up. Shake vial to allow contents to dissolve. Inspect solution for particles or discoloration before administration.

- Use most reconstituted solutions within 7 days if stored at room temperature and in normal room light, or within 15 days if refrigerated at 2° to 8° C (36° to 46° F) and protected from sunlight. However, consult manufacturer's recommendations because some preparations may be stable for a shorter period.

- Administer doxorubicin into a large vein by a free-flowing I.V. infusion of D_5W or normal saline solution over at least 3 minutes. Watch for red streaking along vein or facial flushing, which may indicate too-rapid administration.

- Wash your skin thoroughly with soap and water and irrigate your eyes if exposed to doxorubicin.

- Avoid contact with patient's urine or other body fluids—for example, by wearing latex gloves when caring for pediatric patients—for at least 5 days after each treatment.

- **WARNING** Monitor patient for signs of doxorubicin-induced cardiotoxicity, including cardiomyopathy and life-threatening heart failure, which may occur during therapy or months to years afterward. Patients with a history of prior mediastinal irradiation and young or elderly patients receiving concurrent cyclophosphamide therapy are at increased risk for developing cardiotoxicity at lower doses. Be prepared to administer digitalis preparations, diuretics, and afterload reducers such as ACE inhibitors if heart failure occurs.

- Monitor patient's serum uric acid level before and during therapy, especially in patients with a history of gout or urate calculi. Expect antigout drug dosage to be adjusted if blood uric acid level is elevated from doxorubicin therapy. Oral hydration and allopurinol may be administered to prevent uric acid nephropathy.

- Monitor patients with a history of bone marrow depression, chickenpox (including recent exposure), and herpes zoster because they're at increased risk for severe generalized disease.

Assess patients with leukopenia for signs of infection, including fever, chills, and cough.

- Be aware that adverse reactions can vary when doxorubicin is administered in combination therapy. Review information for all drugs administered as part of a specific regimen, including drug interactions and adverse effects.
- Assess I.V. insertion site for signs of extravasation, such as redness or pain. Tissue necrosis can occur because drug is a vesicant. (However, extravasation can be painless or can occur even with blood return in I.V. line.) If extravasation occurs, immediately stop injection or infusion and apply ice. Then restart injection or infusion in another vein.
- Before reconstituting doxorubicin, store it at 15° to 30° C (59° to 86° F) and protect from light.

PATIENT TEACHING
- Instruct patient receiving doxorubicin to immediately report adverse reactions, such as unusual bruising or bleeding; black, tarry stools; blood in urine or stools; or pinpoint red spots on skin.
- Inform patient that urine may be red-tinged for 1 or 2 days after treatment.
- Stress the importance of keeping scheduled follow-up appointments and undergoing prescribed diagnostic tests, such as cardiac evaluation, especially to parents of pediatric patients, who are at increased risk for delayed cardiotoxicity, delayed growth, and temporary gonadal impairment.
- Caution patient to avoid sports and other activities that increase the risk of accidental injury. Also advise her to take measures to avoid infection, such as maintaining good oral hygiene (for example, by using soft-bristled toothbrush) and washing hands before touching eyes or nose.
- Advise patient with thrombocytopenia to avoid alcohol and aspirin to reduce the risk of GI bleeding.
- Advise patient not receive live or killed virus vaccines during therapy and for 3 months to 1 year after therapy is completed, unless approved by prescriber. Urge her to avoid people who have received such vaccines or to wear a protective mask when she's around them.
- Suggest that patient with stomatitis eat soft, bland foods served cold or at room temperature to decrease irritation.
- Inform patient that her hair should grow back after therapy but that the color and texture may be different.

- Advise female patient not to breast-feed during therapy.
- Urge both male and female patients to use two methods of birth control during therapy.

doxorubicin hydrochloride liposome

Caelyx (CAN), Doxil

Class and Category

Chemical: Anthracycline
Therapeutic: Antibiotic antineoplastic
Pregnancy category: D

Indications and Dosages

▶ *To treat Kaposi's sarcoma associated with AIDS*
I.V. INFUSION
Adults. 20 mg/m^2 over 30 min every 3 wk.
▶ *To treat refractory ovarian cancer*
I.V. INFUSION
Adults. 40 to 50 mg/m^2 infused at 1 mg/min initially to minimize risk of infusion reaction; then drug infused over 1 to 2 hr. Repeated every 4 wk.
DOSAGE ADJUSTMENT Dosage reduced by 50% when serum bilirubin level is 1.2 to 3 mg/dl and by 75% when serum bilirubin level is 3 mg/dl.

Mechanism of Action

May induce fragmentation of tumor cell DNA by inhibiting topo-isomerase II, an enzyme that usually catalyzes the breakage and reformation of DNA linkages. Antitumor activity and toxicity may be related to formation of intracellular oxygen free radicals, which may lead to cell death after reaction with DNA, RNA, cell membranes, and proteins. Liposomal encapsulation may enhance doxorubicin accumulation in Kaposi's sarcoma (KS) lesions and allow passage through endothelial cell gaps in lesions similar to those of KS.

Incompatibilities

Don't mix liposomal doxorubicin with diluents other than D$_5$W or with other drugs or bacteriostatic agents.

Contraindications

Breast-feeding women, hypersensitivity to doxorubicin hydrochloride or to liposomal components

Interactions
DRUGS
actinomycin D: Acute "recall" pneumonitis after local radiation therapy in children
blood-dyscrasia–causing drugs (such as cephalosporins and cisplatin): Increased leukopenic and thrombocytopenic effects of doxorubicin
bone marrow depressants (such as colchicine and methotrexate): Increased bone marrow depression
carbamazepine: Decreased blood carbamazepine level
cisplatin: Risk of leukemia
cyclophosphamide: Potentiated cyclophosphamide-induced hemorrhagic cystitis, increased risk of doxorubicin-induced cardiotoxicity
cyclosporine: Possibly decreased doxorubicin metabolism; increased risk of severe and prolonged hematologic toxicity, coma, and seizures
cytarabine: Possibly necrotizing colitis
dactinomycin, mitomycin, nifedipine, and other calcium channel blockers: Increased risk of doxorubicin-induced cardiotoxicity
digoxin: Decreased blood digoxin level
fosphenytoin, phenytoin: Possibly decreased blood phenytoin level
methotrexate and other hepatoxic drugs: Possibly impaired hepatic function, increased risk of doxorubicin toxicity
paclitaxel: Decreased doxorubicin clearance
phenobarbital: Possibly increased doxorubicin excretion
progesterone: Possibly enhanced doxorubicin-induced neutropenia and thrombocytopenia
streptozocin: Possibly inhibited hepatic metabolism of doxorubicin
trastuzumab: Possibly increased incidence and severity of cardiac dysfunction
vaccines, killed virus: Possibly decreased antibody response to vaccine
vaccines, live virus: Possibly increased adverse effects of vaccine, severe infection, and decreased antibody response to vaccine

Adverse Reactions
CNS: Anxiety, asthenia, chills, dizziness, fever, headache, insomnia
CV: Cardiotoxicity (dose-related or cumulative effect), chest pain
EENT: Conjunctivitis, mucous membrane disorder (changes in mouth or nose lining), oral candidiasis, pharyngitis, stomatitis, taste perversion
GI: Abdominal pain, anorexia, constipation, diarrhea, dysphagia, ileus, nausea, vomiting

GU: Reddish urine
HEME: Anemia, leukopenia, neutropenia, thrombocytopenia
MS: Back pain
RESP: Dyspnea, pneumonia
SKIN: Alopecia, injection site pain, jaundice, palmar-plantar erythrodysesthesia, rash, recall postirradiation erythema, pruritus
Other: Allergic reaction, infection, infusion reaction

Nursing Considerations

- **WARNING** Be aware that doxorubicin hydrochloride should not be substituted for doxorubicin hydrochloride liposome. These drugs are not interchangeable; severe adverse reactions may result.
- Be aware that liposomal doxorubicin should be administered only under the supervision of a qualified physician.
- Follow facility protocols for preparation and handling of antineoplastic drugs and appropriate disposal of used equipment.
- Monitor hepatic and renal function tests and CBC, including hematocrit, platelet count, and WBC count with differential, before and periodically during therapy. Be aware that cardiac evaluation, including ECG, radionuclide angiography to determine ejection fraction, and echocardiography, will be performed before, during, and sometimes after doxorubicin hydrochloride liposome therapy.
- Wear gloves and other protective garments (according to facility protocol) when working with this drug. Wash skin thoroughly with soap and water to remove drug if exposed.
- Dilute up to 90 mg of liposomal doxorubicin in 250 ml of D_5W. Inspect solution for particles before administration and discard if particles are present. Be aware that liposomal doxorubicin is a red, translucent solution.
- Use diluted solution within 24 hours if stored at 2° to 8° C (36° to 46° F). Administer without an in-line filter.
- Monitor patient for signs of an infusion reaction, such as flushing, dyspnea, facial edema, headache, chills, back pain, chest or throat tightness, and hypotension. Such a reaction may resolve if infusion rate is decreased; however, in most patients, it will resolve within several hours or a day after infusion is terminated.
- **WARNING** Monitor patient for drug-induced cardiotoxicity, including cardiomyopathy and life-threatening heart failure, which may occur during therapy or months to years after-

ward. Patients with a history of prior mediastinal irradiation, those who are receiving concurrent cyclophosphamide therapy, and those who have previously received anthracyclines or anthracenediones are at increased risk for developing cardiotoxicity at lower doses. Be prepared to administer digitalis preparations, diuretics, and afterload reducers such as ACE inhibitors if heart failure occurs.

- Monitor patient for stomatitis and signs or symptoms of bone marrow depression or palmar-plantar erythrodysesthesia (swelling, pain, erythema, and skin peeling of hands and feet); these adverse reactions may require dosage reduction or drug discontinuation.
- Monitor patients with a history of bone marrow depression, chickenpox (including recent exposure), and herpes zoster because they're at increased risk for severe generalized disease. Assess patients with leukopenia for signs of infection, including fever, chills, and cough.
- Assess I.V. insertion site for signs of extravasation, such as redness or pain. (However, extravasation can be painless.) If extravasation occurs, immediately stop injection or infusion and apply ice. Follow facility protocol, if available, for management of extravasation. Then restart injection or infusion in another vein.
- Before diluting liposomal doxorubicin, store it at 2° to 8° C (36° to 46° F). Drug may be frozen for up to 1 month.

PATIENT TEACHING

- Instruct patient receiving liposomal doxorubicin to immediately report adverse reactions, such as swelling, blisters, or burning of hands or feet; unusual bruising or bleeding; black, tarry stools; blood in urine or stools; or red pinpoint spots on the skin.
- Inform patient that urine may be red-tinged for 1 or 2 days after treatment.
- Stress the importance of keeping scheduled follow-up appointments and undergoing prescribed diagnostic tests, such as cardiac evaluation.
- Caution patient to avoid sports and other activities that increase the risk of accidental injury. Also advise her to take measures to avoid infection, such as maintaining good oral hygiene (for example, by using soft-bristled toothbrush) and washing hands before touching eyes or nose.
- Advise patient with thrombocytopenia to avoid alcohol and aspirin to reduce the risk of GI bleeding.

- Advise patient not to receive live or killed virus vaccines during doxorubicin therapy and for a period afterward, unless approved by prescriber. Urge her to avoid people who have received such vaccines or to wear a protective mask when she's around them.
- Advise patient with stomatitis to try eating soft, bland foods served cold or at room temperature to decrease irritation.
- Inform patient that her hair should grow back after treatment but that the color and texture may be different.
- Advise female patient not to breast-feed during therapy.
- Urge both male and female patients to use two methods of birth control during therapy.

doxycycline hyclate

(contains 100 or 200 mg of base per injection vial)
Vibramycin

Class and Category

Chemical: Oxytetracycline derivative
Therapeutic: Antibiotic
Pregnancy category: D

Indications and Dosages

▶ *To treat cutaneous, GI, or inhalation anthrax*

I.V. INFUSION

Adults, adolescents, and children weighing more than 45 kg (99 lb). 100 mg (base) every 12 hr for 60 days.
Children weighing less than 45 kg. 2.2 mg/kg (base) every 12 hr for 60 days.

I.V. INFUSION

Adults and children over age 8 weighing more than 45 kg. 200 mg (base) daily or 100 mg (base) every 12 hr on day 1 and then 100 to 200 mg (base) daily or 50 to 100 mg (base) every 12 hr. *Maximum:* 300 mg (base) daily.
Children weighing 45 kg or less. 4.4 mg (base)/kg daily or 2.2 mg (base)/kg every 12 hr on day 1 and then 2.2 to 4.4 mg (base)/kg daily or 1.1 to 2.2 mg (base)/kg every 12 hr.

▶ *To treat epididymo-orchitis caused by* Chlamydia trachomatis *or* Neisseria gonorrhoeae *or nongonococcal urethritis caused by* C. trachomatis *or* Ureaplasma urealyticum

I.V. INFUSION

Adults and children over age 8 weighing more than 45 kg.

200 mg (base) daily or 100 mg (base) every 12 hr on day 1 and then 100 to 200 mg (base) daily or 50 to 100 mg (base) every 12 hr. *Maximum:* 300 mg (base) daily.

Children weighing 45 kg or less. 4.4 mg (base)/kg daily or 2.2 mg (base)/kg every 12 hr on day 1 and then 2.2 to 4.4 mg (base)/kg daily or 1.1 to 2.2 mg (base)/kg every 12 hr.

▶ *To treat early syphilis in penicillin-allergic patients*

I.V. INFUSION

Adults and children over age 8 weighing more than 45 kg. 150 mg (base) every 12 hr for at least 10 days. *Maximum:* 300 mg (base) daily.

Children weighing 45 kg or less. 4.4 mg (base)/kg daily or 2.2 mg (base)/kg every 12 hr on day 1 and then 2.2 to 4.4 mg (base)/kg daily or 1.1 to 2.2 mg (base)/kg every 12 hr.

▶ *To treat syphilis of more than 1 year's duration in patients allergic to penicillin*

I.V. INFUSION

Adults and children over age 8 weighing more than 45 kg. 150 mg (base) every 12 hr for at least 10 days. *Maximum:* 300 mg (base) daily.

Children weighing 45 kg or less. 4.4 mg (base)/kg daily or 2.2 mg (base)/kg every 12 hr on day 1 and then 2.2 to 4.4 mg (base)/kg daily or 1.1 to 2.2 mg (base)/kg every 12 hr.

▶ *To treat all other infections caused by susceptible organisms*

I.V. INFUSION

Adults and children over age 8 weighing more than 45 kg. 200 mg (base) daily or 100 mg (base) every 12 hr on day 1 and then 100 to 200 mg (base) daily or 50 to 100 mg (base) every 12 hr. *Maximum:* 300 mg (base) daily.

Children weighing 45 kg or less. 4.4 mg (base)/kg daily or 2.2 mg (base)/kg every 12 hr on day 1 and then 2.2 to 4.4 mg (base)/kg daily or 1.1 to 2.2 mg (base)/kg every 12 hr.

Mechanism of Action

Exerts a bacteriostatic effect against a wide variety of gram-positive and gram-negative organisms. Doxycycline is more lipophilic than other tetracycline antibiotics, which allows it to pass more easily through the bacterial lipid bilayer, where it binds reversibly to 30S ribosomal subunits. Bound doxycycline blocks the binding of aminoacyl transfer RNA to messenger RNA, thus inhibiting bacterial protein synthesis.

Contraindications

Hypersensitivity to any tetracycline

Interactions

DRUGS

antacids that contain aluminum, calcium, magnesium, or zinc; calcium supplements; choline and magnesium salicylates; iron salts; laxatives that contain magnesium: Decreased doxycycline absorption and therapeutic effects

barbiturates, carbamazepine, phenytoin: Increased clearance and decreased effects of doxycycline

cholestyramine, colestipol: Decreased doxycycline absorption

digoxin: Increased bioavailability of digoxin, possibly leading to digitalis toxicity

oral anticoagulants: Possibly increased hypoprothrombinemic effects of these drugs

oral contraceptives: Decreased effectiveness of estrogen-containing oral contraceptives, increased risk of breakthrough bleeding

penicillins: Inhibited bactericidal action

sodium bicarbonate: Altered doxycycline absorption from increased gastric pH

FOODS

dairy products, other foods high in calcium or iron: Decreased doxycycline absorption

Adverse Reactions

CNS: Paresthesia

CV: Phlebitis

EENT: Black "hairy" tongue, glossitis, hoarseness, oral candidiasis, pharyngitis, stomatitis, tooth discoloration

GI: Anorexia; bulky, loose stools; diarrhea; dysphagia; enterocolitis; epigastric distress; esophageal ulceration; hepatotoxicity; nausea; pseudomembranous colitis; rectal candidiasis; vomiting

GU: Anogenital lesions, dark yellow or brown urine, elevated BUN level, vaginal candidiasis

HEME: Eosinophilia, hemolytic anemia, neutropenia, thrombocytopenia, thrombocytopenic purpura

SKIN: Dermatitis, photosensitivity, rash, urticaria

Other: Anaphylaxis, injection site phlebitis

Nursing Considerations

• Avoid giving doxycycline to breast-feeding women because of the risk of enamel hypoplasia, inhibited linear skeletal growth, oral and vaginal candidiasis, photosensitivity reactions, and tooth discoloration in breast-feeding infant.

• Avoid giving drug to children younger than age 8; it may cause permanent discoloration and enamel hypoplasia of developing teeth.

• Expect to adjust dosage for patients who have hepatic disease to avoid drug accumulation.

• **WARNING** Don't give doxycycline by I.M. or subcutaneous route.

• Observe patient frequently for injection site phlebitis, a common adverse reaction to I.V. administration.

• Monitor liver function test results as appropriate to detect hepatotoxicity.

• Expect doxycycline to increase risk of oral, rectal, or vaginal candidiasis—especially in elderly or debilitated patients and those on prolonged therapy—by changing the normal balance of microbial flora.

• Monitor patient closely for diarrhea, which may indicate pseudomembranous colitis. If diarrhea occurs, obtain stool specimen to check for *Clostridium difficile,* notify prescriber, and expect to withhold doxycycline. Expect to treat pseudomembranous colitis with fluids, electrolytes, protein, and an antibiotic effective against *C. difficile.*

PATIENT TEACHING
• Encourage patient to drink plenty of fluids while taking doxycycline to reduce the risk of esophageal burning and ulceration.

• Advise patients who take an oral contraceptive to use an additional contraceptive method during therapy.

• If patient is being treated for a sexually transmitted disease, explain that her sexual partner or partners may need treatment as well.

• Instruct patient to notify prescriber immediately if she experiences anorexia, epigastric distress, nausea, and vomiting during therapy.

• Urge patient to report watery, bloody stools to prescriber immediately, even if it occurs up to 2 months after drug therapy has ended.

• Alert female patients that doxycycline may raise the risk of vaginal candidiasis. Tell them to report vaginal itching or discharge.

droperidol

Inapsine

Class and Category

Chemical: Butyrophenone derivative
Therapeutic: Anesthesia adjunct, antiemetic, sedative-hypnotic
Pregnancy category: C

Indications and Dosages

▶ *To provide anesthesia premedication*
I.V. INJECTION

Children. 0.075 to 0.15 mg/kg I.V. 30 to 60 min before surgery. (For adults and adolescents, drug is given by I.M. injection, 2.5 to 5 mg I.M. 30 to 60 min before surgery.)

▶ *To induce anesthesia*
I.V. INJECTION

Adults and adolescents. *Initial:* 1.25 to 2.5 mg/9 to 11 kg (20 to 25 lb) or 0.1 to 0.14 mg/kg given with general anesthesia. *Maintenance:* Additional 1.25 to 2.5 mg, as needed.
Children. 0.075 to 0.15 mg/kg, to be given with general anesthesia.

▶ *As adjunct to regional anesthesia*
I.V. INJECTION

Adults and adolescents. 2.5 to 5 mg.

▶ *To provide sedative-hypnotic effects for diagnostic procedures performed without anesthesia (conscious sedation)*
I.V. INJECTION

Adults and adolescents. 1.25 to 5 mg 30 to 60 min before diagnostic procedure, followed by another 1.25 to 2.5 mg I.V., if indicated.

▶ *To prevent postoperative nausea and vomiting*
I.V. INJECTION

Adults and adolescents. 7 to 20 mcg/kg after procedure.
Children. 0.02 to 0.075 mg/kg after procedure.

DOSAGE ADJUSTMENT Initial dosage reduced for elderly patients because of increased risk of hypotension and excessive sedation.

Route	Onset	Peak	Duration
I.V.	3 to 10 min	30 min	2 to 4 hr

Contraindications

Hypersensitivity to droperidol or its components

Mechanism of Action

Produces sedation by blocking postsynaptic dopamine receptors in the limbic system. Droperidol may reduce nausea by blocking dopamine receptors in the chemoreceptor trigger zone in the reticular formation of the medulla oblongata. It also may produce antiemetic effects by attaching to postsynaptic gamma-aminobutyric acid receptors in the chemoreceptor trigger zone.

Interactions

DRUGS

amoxapine, haloperidol, loxapine, metoclopramide, metyrosine, molindone, olanzapine, phenothiazines, pimozide, rauwolfia alkaloids, risperidone, tacrine, thioxanthenes: Possibly increased risk of severe extrapyramidal reactions
anesthetics: Possibly hypotension and peripheral vasodilation
antihypertensives: Possibly orthostatic hypotension
bromocriptine, levodopa: Possibly inhibited actions of these drugs
CNS depressants: Additive CNS depression
epinephrine: Possibly paradoxical reduction of blood pressure
propofol: Possibly decreased antiemetic effect of both drugs
ACTIVITIES
alcohol use: Additive CNS depression

Adverse Reactions

CNS: Anxiety, drowsiness, dystonia, restlessness
CV: Hypertension, hypotension, sinus tachycardia
EENT: Fixed upward position of eyeballs, laryngospasm
MS: Spasms of tongue, face, neck, and back muscles
RESP: Bronchospasm

Nursing Considerations

- Monitor blood pressure frequently in patients with cardiac disease, who may not be able to compensate for droperidol's hypotensive effect.
- Assess patients with parkinsonism for worsening of condition, which may be an adverse effect of droperidol use.
- Monitor heart rate and ECG in patients with hypokalemia, hypomagnesemia, or preexisitng QT interval prolongation and in those with acute alcoholism because they're at increased risk for arrhythmias and, rarely, sudden death.
- Assess patients with pheochromocytoma for hypertension and tachycardia.

- Monitor patients with epilepsy, severe depression, parkinsonism, or impaired cardiovascular function for signs of exacerbation.
- Expect altered LOC to last for up to 12 hours after drug is given.
- If drug causes extrapyramidal reactions, such as restlessness, dystonia, and oculogyric crisis, expect to administer an anticholinergic, such as benztropine or diphenhydramine. Be sure to maintain a patent airway and oxygenation.
- If severe hypotension develops, expect to administer phenylephrine. If hypotension is related to hypovolemia, expect to administer fluids.
- Store drug at 15° to 30° C (59° to 86° F) and protect from light.

PATIENT TEACHING

- Instruct patient to ask for help with ambulation on first postoperative day because LOC may be altered for up to 12 hours.
- Caution patient to avoid drinking alcohol, taking CNS depressants, driving, and operating machinery for 24 hours after receiving droperidol.

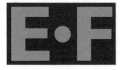

eflornithine hydrochloride
(alpha-difluoromethylornithine, DFMO)
Ornidyl

Class and Category
Chemical: Difluoromethylornithine
Therapeutic: Antiprotozoal
Pregnancy category: C

Indications and Dosages
▶ *To treat the meningoencephalitic stage of* Trypanosoma brucei gambiense *infection (sleeping sickness)*
I.V. INFUSION
Adults. 100 mg/kg given over at least 45 min every 6 hr for 14 days.

Route	Onset	Peak	Duration
I.V.	Unknown	4 to 6 hr	Unknown

Mechanism of Action
Inhibits the enzyme ornithine decarboxylase, which is needed for decarboxylation of ornithine. This process is the first step in polyamine synthesis, which is needed for protozoal cell division and differentiation.

Incompatibilities
Don't administer eflornithine with any other drug.

Contraindications
Hypersensitivity to eflornithine or its components

Interactions
DRUGS
other bone marrow depressants (such as chloramphenicol and doxorubicin): Possibly increased bone marrow depression
ototoxic drugs (such as aminoglycosides and NSAIDs): Increased risk of ototoxicity with long-term eflornithine therapy

Adverse Reactions

CNS: Asthenia, dizziness, headache, seizures
EENT: Hearing loss
GI: Abdominal pain, anorexia, diarrhea, vomiting
HEME: Anemia, eosinophilia, leukopenia, myelosuppression, thrombocytopenia
Other: Alopecia, facial edema

Nursing Considerations

- Monitor creatinine clearance of patients with impaired renal function, and plan to reduce eflornithine dosage, as prescribed, based on results.
- Before drug infusion, dilute eflornithine concentrate with sterile water for injection. Using strict aseptic technique, withdraw the contents of a 100-ml vial and inject 25 ml into each of four I.V. diluent bags that contain 100 ml of sterile water. The resulting solution contains 40 mg/ml of eflornithine (5,000 mg of eflornithine in 125 ml total volume).
- Store bags of diluted eflornithine at 4° C (39° F) to reduce the risk of contamination. Use diluted eflornithine solution within 24 hours.
- Expect to monitor CBC, including platelet count, before treatment, twice weekly during treatment, and weekly after therapy stops until hematologic values return to baseline.
- Don't give other I.V. drugs while infusing eflornithine.
- Take infection-control and bleeding precautions because drug may cause myelosuppression. Adjust dosage or stop therapy as prescribed, based on severity.
- Take seizure precautions during therapy.
- Consult prescriber about the need for serial audiography, if appropriate, to detect hearing loss.
- Store undiluted vials at room temperature, and protect from freezing and light.

PATIENT TEACHING
- Stress the importance of keeping follow-up medical appointments because relapse may occur for up to 24 months after eflornithine treatment ends.
- Teach patient how to follow infection-control and bleeding precautions if myelosuppression occurs.
- Instruct patient to report bothersome adverse reactions to prescriber.
- Caution patient about the risk of seizures; advise him not to perform potentially hazardous activities during therapy.

enalaprilat

Vasotec I.V.

Class and Category

Chemical: Dicarbocyl-containing angiotensin-converting enzyme (ACE) inhibitor
Therapeutic: Antihypertensive
Pregnancy category: C (first trimester), D (later trimesters)

Indications and Dosages

▶ *To control hypertension*

I.V. INJECTION

Adults. 1.25 mg every 6 hr.

DOSAGE ADJUSTMENT Initial dose 0.625 mg for patients who have sodium and water depletion from diuretic therapy, are taking diuretics, or have creatinine clearance below 30 ml/min/1.73 m^2. If response is inadequate after 1 hr, 0.625 mg is repeated and therapy continued at 1.25 mg every 6 hr.

Route	Onset	Peak	Duration
I.V.	15 min	1 to 4 hr	About 6 hr

Mechanism of Action

May reduce blood pressure by affecting the renin-angiotensin-aldosterone system. By inhibiting ACE, enalaprilat:

- prevents conversion of angiotensin I to angiotensin II, a potent vasoconstrictor that also stimulates the adrenal cortex to secrete aldosterone
- may inhibit renal and vascular production of angiotensin II
- decreases the serum angiotensin II level and increases serum renin activity, thereby decreasing aldosterone secretion and slightly increasing the serum potassium level and fluid loss
- decreases vascular tone and blood pressure
- inhibits aldosterone release, which reduces sodium and water reabsorption and increases their excretion, further reducing blood pressure.

Contraindications

History of angioedema from previous ACE inhibitor therapy; hypersensitivity to enalapril, enalaprilat, or their components

Interactions

DRUGS

allopurinol, bone marrow depressants (such as amphotericin B and methotrexate), procainamide, systemic corticosteroids: Possibly increased risk of fatal neutropenia or agranulocytosis

cyclosporine, potassium-sparing diuretics, potassium supplements: Increased risk of hyperkalemia

diuretics, other antihypertensives: Additive hypotensive effects

lithium: Increased blood lithium level and lithium toxicity

NSAIDs: Possibly reduced antihypertensive effects of enalapril and enalaprilat

sympathomimetics: Possibly reduced therapeutic effects of enalapril and enalaprilat

FOODS

potassium-containing salt substitutes: Increased risk of hyperkalemia

ACTIVITIES

alcohol use: Possibly additive hypotensive effect

Adverse Reactions

CNS: Ataxia, confusion, CVA, depression, dizziness, dream disturbances, fatigue, headache, insomnia, nervousness, peripheral neuropathy, somnolence, syncope, vertigo, weakness

CV: Angina, arrhythmias, cardiac arrest, hypotension, MI, orthostatic hypotension, palpitations, pulmonary embolism and infarction, Raynaud's phenomenon

EENT: Blurred vision, conjunctivitis, dry eyes and mouth, glossitis, hoarseness, lacrimation, loss of smell, pharyngitis, rhinorrhea, stomatitis, taste perversion, tinnitus

ENDO: Gynecomastia

GI: Abdominal pain, anorexia, constipation, diarrhea, hepatic failure, hepatitis, ileus, indigestion, melena, nausea, pancreatitis, vomiting

GU: Flank pain, impotence, oliguria, renal failure, UTI

MS: Muscle spasms

RESP: Asthma, bronchitis, bronchospasm, cough, dyspnea, pneumonia, pulmonary edema, pulmonary infiltrates, upper respiratory tract infection

SKIN: Alopecia, diaphoresis, erythema multiforme, exfoliative dermatitis, flushing, pemphigus, photosensitivity, pruritus, rash, Stevens-Johnson syndrome, toxic epidermal necrolysis, urticaria

Other: Anaphylaxis, angioedema, herpes zoster, hyperkalemia

Nursing Considerations

- Be aware that patients with impaired renal function may require a decreased dosage or less frequent doses of enalaprilat because of the risk of increased blood enalaprilat level and hyperkalemia. Monitor urinary protein level before and periodically during enalaprilat therapy.

- Administer enalaprilat undiluted, or dilute with up to 50 ml of D_5W, normal saline solution, dextrose 5% in normal saline solution, or dextrose 5% in lactated Ringer's solution. Use diluted enalaprilat within 24 hours if stored at room temperature. Administer each dose over at least 5 minutes.
- Measure blood pressure immediately after first dose and frequently for at least 2 hours thereafter. If hypotension requires a dosage reduction, monitor blood pressure frequently for 2 hours after reduced dose is administered and frequently for another hour after blood pressure has stabilized.
- Monitor blood pressure regularly during therapy. If patient develops hypotension, place him in supine position and expect to give I.V. normal saline solution or another volume expander, as prescribed.
- Monitor heart rate and rhythm. Expect to obtain repeated 12-lead ECG tracings.
- Monitor laboratory test results to check hepatic and renal function, leukocyte count, and serum potassium level.
- Monitor closely for angioedema of the face, lips, tongue, glottis, larynx, and limbs. If patient develops angioedema of the face and lips, stop drug and give an antihistamine, as prescribed, for symptoms. If tongue, glottis, or larynx is involved, assess for airway obstruction and prepare to give epinephrine 1:1,000 (0.3 to 0.5 ml) subcutaneously and maintain a patent airway.
- Closely assess for anaphylaxis in patients who receive dialysis with high-flux membranes, treatment with Hymenoptera venom, or LDL apheresis with dextran sulfate.
- Store drug between 15° and 30° C (59° and 86° F).

PATIENT TEACHING

- Tell women of childbearing age that ACE inhibitors taken during the first trimester of pregnancy have adverse effects on fetal development. Urge women to report suspected or confirmed pregnancy before starting enalaprilat therapy.
- Inform patient that he may experience light-headedness and fainting, especially during first few days of enalaprilat therapy. Advise him to change position slowly and to avoid potentially hazardous activities until drug's CNS effects are known.
- Inform patient that diarrhea, excessive sweating, vomiting, and other conditions may cause dehydration, which can lead to dizziness, fainting, and very low blood pressure during therapy.

Urge sufficient fluid intake to prevent dehydration and related adverse reactions. Instruct patient to report severe or prolonged diarrhea or vomiting.
- Urge patient to immediately report angioedema and other adverse reactions, including persistent dry cough.
- Advise patient to consult prescriber before using salt substitutes, potassium supplements, or other drugs (including OTC drugs) while receiving enalaprilat.

enoxaparin sodium

Lovenox

Class and Category

Chemical: Low–molecular-weight heparin
Therapeutic: Antithrombotic
Pregnancy category: B

Indications and Dosages

▶ *To prevent deep vein thrombosis (DVT) after hip or knee replacement and for continued prophylaxis after hospitalization for hip replacement*
SUBCUTANEOUS INJECTION
Adults. 30 mg every 12 hr starting 12 to 24 hr after surgery for up to 14 days. Or, 40 mg daily starting 9 to 15 hr after hip replacement surgery. *Prophylaxis:* 40 mg daily for 3 wk.

▶ *To prevent DVT after abdominal surgery for patients with thromboembolic risk factors (over age 40, obesity, general anesthesia lasting longer than 30 minutes, cancer, or a history of DVT or pulmonary embolism)*
SUBCUTANEOUS INJECTION
Adults. 40 mg daily starting 2 hr before surgery and lasting 7 to 10 days.

▶ *To prevent ischemic complications of unstable angina and non–Q-wave MI*
SUBCUTANEOUS INJECTION
Adults. 1 mg/kg every 12 hr with 100 to 325 mg of aspirin daily for 2 to 8 days or until condition is stable.

DOSAGE ADJUSTMENT Dosage reduced to 30 mg daily if creatinine clearance is less than 30 ml/min/1.73 m^2 and patient is receiving drug as prophylaxis in abdominal, hip, or knee replacement surgery or is acutely ill. Reduced to 1 mg/kg daily if creatinine clearance is less than 30 ml/min/1.73 m^2 and drug is given with aspirin to prevent ischemic complications of unstable angina and non–Q-wave MI, with warfarin as inpatient treatment for acute DVT with or without pulmonary embolism, or with warfarin as outpatient treatment of acute DVT without pulmonary embolism.

▶ *To treat acute ST-segment–elevation MI (STEMI)*

I.V. INJECTION, THEN SUBCUTANEOUS INJECTION

Adults. 30 mg I.V. as a single dose, followed by 1 mg/kg subcutaneously (maximum, 100 mg for first two doses). Then, 1 mg/kg subcutaneously every 12 hr.

DOSAGE ADJUSTMENT If patient also receives a thrombolytic, enoxaparin should be given 15 to 30 min before and 30 min after fibrinolytic therapy starts. If patient has percutaneous coronary intervention, give 0.3-mg/kg I.V. bolus if last enoxaparin dose was given more than 8 hr before balloon inflation.

Route	Onset	Peak	Duration
SubQ	Unknown	3 to 5 hr	Up to 24 hr

Mechanism of Action

Potentiates the action of antithrombin III, a coagulation inhibitor. By binding with antithrombin III, enoxaparin rapidly binds with and inactivates clotting factors (primarily thrombin and factor Xa). Without thrombin, fibrinogen can't convert to fibrin and clots can't form.

Incompatibilities

Don't mix enoxaparin with other I.V. fluids or drugs.

Contraindications

Active major bleeding; hypersensitivity to benzyl alcohol (if only the multidose vial is available), enoxaparin, heparin (including low–molecular-weight heparins), or pork products; thrombocytopenia and positive antiplatelet antibody test while taking low–molecular-weight heparins

Interactions

DRUGS

cefamandole, cefoperazone, cefotetan, plicamycin, valproic acid: Possibly increased risk of hemorrhage

NSAIDs; oral anticoagulants; platelet aggregation inhibitors, such as aspirin, dipyridamole, sulfinpyrazone, and ticlopidine; thrombolytics, such as alteplase, anistreplase, streptokinase, and urokinase: Possibly increased risk of bleeding

Adverse Reactions

CNS: Confusion, CVA, fever, paralysis
CV: Atrial fibrillation, congestive heart failure, peripheral edema, pulmonary embolism
EENT: Epistaxis
GI: Bloody stools, diarrhea, elevated liver function test results, hematemesis, melena, nausea, vomiting
GU: Hematuria, menstrual irregularities
HEME: Anemia, hemorrhage, thrombocytopenia
RESP: Dyspnea, pneumonia, pulmonary edema
SKIN: Cutaneous vasculitis, ecchymosis, persistent bleeding or oozing from mucous membranes or surgical wounds, pruritus, urticaria, vesiculobullous rash
Other: Anaphylaxis; injection site erythema, hematoma, irritation, and pain

Nursing Considerations

• Use enoxaparin with extreme caution in patients with a history of heparin-induced thrombocytopenia or an increased risk of hemorrhage. Use it cautiously in patients with bleeding diathesis, hepatic impairment, recent GI ulceration or hemorrhage, or uncontrolled hypertension. Expect possible delayed elimination in elderly patients and those with renal insufficiency.
• Enoxaparin is not recommended for patients with prosthetic heart valves, especially pregnant women, because of the risk of prosthetic valve thrombosis. If enoxaparin is needed, monitor patient's peak and trough anti-factor Xa levels often and adjust dosage as needed.
• Use multidose vials cautiously in pregnant women because benzyl alcohol may cross the placenta and cause fetal harm.
• Don't give drug by I.M. injection.
• Expect to give drug with aspirin to patient with unstable angina, STEMI, or non–Q-wave MI. To minimize risk of bleeding after vascular procedures, be careful to give enoxaparin at recommended intervals.
• After percutaneous revascularization procedure, it is important to achieve hemostasis at the puncture site. A closure device may be removed right away; however, if a manual compression method is used, the sheath should be removed 6 hours after last enoxaparin dose. If enoxaparin therapy will continue, give next dose no sooner than 6 to 8 hours after sheath removal.
• Watch closely for bleeding. Notify prescriber immediately if platelet count falls below 100,000/mm³. Expect to stop drug

and start treatment if patient has a thromboembolic event, such as a CVA.

- Test stool for occult blood, as ordered.
- Keep protamine sulfate nearby in case of accidental overdose.

PATIENT TEACHING

- Advise patient to notify prescriber about adverse reactions, especially bleeding.
- Instruct patient to seek immediate help for signs or symptoms of thromboembolism, such as neurologic changes and severe shortness of breath.
- Stress the need to comply with follow-up visits with prescriber.
- Teach patient or family member how to give enoxaparin at home, if needed. Show patient how to give by deep subcutaneous injection while lying down. Instruct him not to expel the air bubble from a prefilled syringe to avoid losing some of the drug. Tell him to insert the entire needle into a skin fold held between thumb and forefinger. Remind him to alternate injection sites between left and right anterolateral abdominal wall.
- To minimize bruising, caution patient not to rub the site after giving the injection.
- Review safe handling and disposal of syringes and needles.

epinephrine
(adrenaline)
Adrenalin, Ana-Guard
epinephrine hydrochloride
Adrenalin

Class and Category
Chemical: Catecholamine
Therapeutic: Antianaphylactic, bronchodilator, cardiac stimulant, vasopressor
Pregnancy category: C

Indications and Dosages
▶ *To treat anaphylaxis*
I.V. INFUSION
Adults and adolescents. 100 to 250 mcg given slowly.
▶ *To treat severe anaphylactic shock*
I.V. INFUSION
Adults. 1 mcg/min titrated to 2 to 10 mcg/min for desired hemodynamic response.

▶ *To treat cardiac arrest*
I.V. INJECTION
Adults. 0.5 to 1 mg every 3 to 5 min during resuscitation.
Children. 10 mcg/kg followed by 100 mcg/kg every 3 to 5 min, if needed. If two doses produce no response, subsequent doses are increased to 200 mcg/kg every 5 min.
Neonates. 10 to 30 mcg/kg every 3 to 5 min.

Route	Onset	Peak	Duration
I.V.	Rapid	Unknown	1 to 2 min

Mechanism of Action

Acts on alpha and beta receptors. This nonselective adrenergic agonist stimulates:

- alpha$_1$ receptors, which constricts arteries and may decrease bronchial secretions.
- presynaptic alpha$_2$ receptors, which inhibits norepinephrine release by way of negative feedback.
- postsynaptic alpha$_2$ receptors, which constricts arteries.
- beta$_1$ receptors, which induces positive chronotropic and inotropic responses.
- beta$_2$ receptors, which dilates arteries, relaxes bronchial smooth muscles, increases glycogenolysis, and prevents mast cells from secreting histamine and other substances, thus reversing bronchoconstriction and edema.

Incompatibilities

Don't mix epinephrine with alkalies or oxidizing agents, including bromine, chlorine, chromates, iodine, metal salts (as from iron), nitrites, oxygen, and permanganates, because these substances can destroy epinephrine.

Contraindications

Cerebral arteriosclerosis, coronary insufficiency, counteraction of phenothiazine-induced hypotension, dilated cardiomyopathy, general anesthesia with halogenated hydrocarbons or cyclopropane, hypersensitivity to epinephrine or its components, labor, angle-closure glaucoma, organic brain damage, shock (nonanaphylactic)

Interactions

DRUGS
alpha-adrenergic blockers, drugs with alpha-adrenergic action, rapid-acting vasodilators: Blockage of epinephrine's alpha-adrenergic ef-

fect, possibly causing severe hypotension and tachycardia

amyl nitrite, nitrates: Decreased antianginal effects

antihypertensives, diuretics used to treat hypertension: Decreased antihypertensive effects

beta blockers: Mutual inhibition of therapeutic effects, possibly severe hypertension and cerebral hemorrhage

digoxin, quinidine: Increased risk of arrhythmias

dihydroergotamine, ergoloid mesylates, ergonovine, ergotamine, methylergonovine, methysergide, oxytocin: Increased risk of vasoconstriction, causing gangrene, peripheral vascular ischemia, or severe hypertension

hydrocarbon inhalation anesthetics: Increased risk of severe atrial and ventricular arrhythmias

insulin, oral antidiabetic drugs: Decreased effects of these drugs

MAO inhibitors: Possibly increased vasopressor effect of epinephrine and hypertensive crisis

maprotiline, tricyclic antidepressants: Potentiated cardiovascular effects of epinephrine, possibly causing arrhythmias, hyperpyrexia, severe hypertension, or tachycardia

sympathomimetics: Additive CNS stimulation, increased cardiovascular effects of either drug

thyroid hormones: Increased effects of either drug

xanthines: Increased CNS stimulation, additive toxic effects

Adverse Reactions

CNS: Anxiety, chills, fever, dizziness, drowsiness, hallucinations, headache, insomnia, light-headedness, nervousness, restlessness, seizures, tremor, weakness

CV: Chest discomfort or pain; fast, irregular, or slow heartbeat; palpitations; severe hypertension

EENT: Blurred vision, dry mouth or throat, miosis

GI: Anorexia, heartburn, nausea, vomiting

GU: Dysuria

MS: Muscle twitching, severe muscle spasms

RESP: Dyspnea

SKIN: Cold skin, diaphoresis, ecchymosis, flushed or red face or skin, pallor, tissue necrosis

Other: Hyperkalemia, hypokalemia, injection site pain or stinging

Nursing Considerations

• Use epinephrine with extreme caution in patients with angina, arrhythmias, asthma, degenerative heart disease, or emphysema. Epinephrine's inotropic effect equals that of dopamine and dobutamine; its chronotropic effect exceeds that of both.

- Use drug cautiously in elderly patients and those with cardiovascular disease (other than listed above), diabetes mellitus, hypertension, hyperthyroidism, prostatic hypertrophy, and psychoneurologic disorders.
- Be aware that some preparations contain sulfites, which may cause allergic-type reactions. However, the presence of sulfites in epinephrine should not deter its use in a patient with anaphylaxis, even if patient is sensitive to sulfites. Monitor patient closely for adverse effects.
- Dilute the 1:1,000 (1-mg/ml) solution of parenteral epinephrine before I.V. administration.
- Shake suspension thoroughly before withdrawing dose; refrigerate it between uses.
- Inspect epinephrine solution or suspension before use. If it's pink or brown, air has entered a multidose vial. If it's discolored or contains particles, discard it. Also discard unused portions of parenteral epinephrine.
- When injecting drug, rotate sites because repeated injections in the same site may cause vasoconstriction and localized necrosis.
- Be aware that drug shouldn't be given by intra-arterial injection because marked vasoconstriction may cause gangrene.
- Monitor for potassium imbalances. Initially, hyperkalemia occurs when hepatocytes release potassium. Hypokalemia may quickly follow as skeletal muscles take up potassium.
- To minimize insomnia, give last dose a few hours before bedtime.
- **WARNING** To treat cardiac arrest, at least twice the peripheral I.V. dose of epinephrine may be given by endotracheal instillation. Two dilutions are needed for this regimen; use great caution to avoid medication errors.

PATIENT TEACHING
- Advise patient to notify prescriber if symptoms don't improve or if they improve but then worsen.
- Advise patient to notify prescriber immediately if he experiences blurred vision, chest pain, difficulty breathing, a fast or irregular heartbeat, or increased sweating.

epoetin alfa
(EPO, erythropoietin alfa, recombinant erythropoietin, r-HuEPO)

Epogen, Eprex (CAN), Procrit

Class and Category
Chemical: 165–amino acid glycoprotein identical to human erythropoietin
Therapeutic: Antianemic
Pregnancy category: C

Indications and Dosages
▶ *To treat anemia from renal failure*
I.V. INJECTION
Adults and adolescents. *Initial:* 50 to 100 units/kg 3 times/wk, increased by 25 units/kg after 8 wk if hematocrit hasn't risen by 5 or 6 points or is below desired range (30% to 36%). *Maintenance:* Dosage gradually decreased by 25 units/kg every 4 wk or more to lowest dose that keeps hematocrit at 30% to 36%. *Maximum:* 300 units/kg 3 times/wk.
Children on dialysis. 50 units/kg 3 times/wk; increased after 8 wk if hematocrit hasn't risen by 5 or 6 points and is still below desired range of 30% to 36%. *Maintenance:* Dosage gradually decreased to lowest dose that keeps hematocrit at 30% to 36%.
▶ *To treat anemia in HIV-infected patients who take zidovudine*
I.V. INJECTION
Adults with serum erythropoietin level of 500 mU/ml or less who receive 4,200 mg or less of zidovudine/wk. *Initial:* 100 units/kg 3 times/wk, increased by 50 to 100 units/kg every 4 to 8 wk after 8 wk of therapy. *Maintenance:* Dosage gradually titrated to maintain desired response, based on such factors as variations in zidovudine dosage and occurrence of infection or inflammation. *Maximum:* 300 units/kg 3 times/wk.

Route	Onset	Peak	Duration
I.V., SubQ	In 2 to 6 wk	In 2 mo	About 2 wk

Mechanism of Action
Stimulates the release of reticulocytes from the bone marrow into the bloodstream, where they develop into mature RBCs.

Incompatibilities
Don't mix epoetin alfa with any other drug.

Contraindications
Hypersensitivity to human albumin or products made from mammal cells, uncontrolled hypertension

Interactions
DRUGS
antihypertensives: Increased blood pressure (to hypertensive level), especially when hematocrit rises rapidly
heparin: Increased heparin requirement in hemodialysis patients
iron supplements: Increased iron requirement and need for increased dose

Adverse Reactions
CNS: Anxiety, asthenia, CVA, dizziness, fatigue, fever, headache, insomnia, paresthesia, seizures
CV: Cardiac arrest, chest pain, congestive heart failure, deep vein thrombosis, edema, hypertension, MI, peripheral edema, tachycardia, vascular access thrombosis
GI: Constipation, diarrhea, indigestion, nausea, vomiting
GU: UTI
HEME: Polycythemia
MS: Arthralgia, bone pain, muscle weakness
RESP: Cough, dyspnea, pulmonary congestion, upper respiratory tract infection
SKIN: Rash, pruritus, urticaria
Other: Flulike symptoms, hyperkalemia, increased risk of death (with decreased or rapid response and in patients with cancer), injection site reaction, trunk pain, tumor progression (in patients with cancer)

Nursing Considerations
- **WARNING** If patient has cancer, make sure he understands before he starts epoetin alfa therapy that epoetin alfa may increase tumor progression and the risk of death.
- Use epoetin alfa cautiously in patients who have conditions that could decrease or delay response to drug, such as aluminum intoxication, folic acid deficiency, hemolysis, infection, inflammation, iron deficiency, malignant neoplasm, osteitis (fibrosa cystica), or vitamin B_{12} deficiency.
- Also use drug cautiously in patients with cardiovascular disorders caused by hypertension, a history of seizures, vascular disease, or a hematologic disorder, such as hypercoagulation, myelodysplastic syndrome, or sickle cell disease.
- **WARNING** Be aware that multidose vial of epoetin contains benzyl alcohol, which can cause a fatal toxic syndrome in neonates and immature infants characterized by CNS, respiratory, circulatory, and renal impairment and metabolic acidosis.

- Don't shake vial during preparation to avoid denaturing glycoprotein and inactivating epoetin alfa.
- Discard unused portion of single-dose vial because it contains no preservatives. Discard unused portion of multidose vial after 21 days.
- Be aware that baseline hemoglobin level should be above 10 but below 12 g/dl if drug is given to patient scheduled for surgery.
- **WARNING** Be aware that the risk of cardiac arrest, seizures, CVA, worsening hypertension, congestive heart failure, vascular thrombosis, vascular ischemia, vascular infarction, acute MI, fluid overload with peripheral edema, and death increases if hemoglobin level increases by more than about 1 g/dl during any 2-week period or if it exceeds 12 g/dl. Expect to decrease epoetin alfa dosage if this occurs.
- **WARNING** Also be aware that patients with chronic renal failure and an insufficient hemoglobin response to epoetin alfa therapy are at an even higher risk of serious cardiovascular events, thromboembolic events, and death. Monitor them closely.
- Expect to increase heparin dose if patient receives hemodialysis because epoetin alfa can increase the RBC volume, which could cause clots to form in the dialyzer, hemodialysis vascular access, or both.
- Expect to give an iron supplement (I.V. iron dextran, if needed) because iron requirements rise when erythropoiesis consumes existing iron stores.
- Monitor drug effectiveness by checking hematocrit, typically twice weekly until it stabilizes at 30% to 36%. After that, monitoring can be less frequent.
- Take seizure precautions.

PATIENT TEACHING
- Advise patient that the risk of seizures is highest during the first 90 days of epoetin alfa therapy. Urge him not to engage in hazardous activities during this time.
- Stress the need to comply with dosage regimen and keep follow-up medical and laboratory appointments.
- Encourage patient to eat iron-rich foods.
- **WARNING** Review possible adverse reactions, and urge patient to notify prescriber if he experiences chest pain, headache, rash, seizures, rapid heartbeat, shortness of breath, or swelling.

epoprostenol sodium
(PGI$_2$, PGX, prostacyclin)
Flolan

Class and Category
Chemical: Natural prostaglandin
Therapeutic: Antihypertensive, vasodilator
Pregnancy category: B

Indications and Dosages
▶ *To provide long-term treatment of primary pulmonary hypertension and pulmonary hypertension secondary to scleroderma spectrum of diseases*

I.V. INFUSION

Adults. *Initial:* 2 nanograms/kg/min, increased by 2 nanograms/kg/min every 15 min or longer until dose-limiting adverse reactions (such as abdominal, chest, or musculoskeletal pain; anxiety; bradycardia; dizziness; dyspnea; flushing; headache; hypotension; nausea; tachycardia; and vomiting) occur. *Maintenance:* Dosage started at 4 nanograms/kg/min less than maximum rate tolerated during initial titration. If maximum rate tolerated was less than 5 nanograms/kg/min, long-term infusion rate is started at 50% of maximum rate.

DOSAGE ADJUSTMENT Continuous infusion rate adjusted based on persistence, recurrence, or worsening of primary pulmonary hypertension and dose-related adverse reactions.

Mechanism of Action
Acts as a natural prostaglandin to directly relax vascular smooth muscles, resulting in arterial dilation and inhibition of platelet aggregation. These actions decrease pulmonary vascular resistance, increase cardiac index and oxygen delivery, and limit thrombus formation.

Incompatibilities
Don't mix epoprostenol with other parenteral solutions or drugs.

Contraindications
Hypersensitivity to epoprostenol or its components; long-term use in patients with heart failure caused by severe left ventricular systolic dysfunction; pulmonary edema that developed while establishing epoprostenol dosage

Interactions
DRUGS

anticoagulants, antiplatelet drugs, NSAIDs: Increased risk of bleeding
antihypertensives, diuretics, vasodilators: Decreased blood pressure
digoxin: Possibly increased digoxin bioavailability

Adverse Reactions
CNS: Anxiety, chills, confusion, dizziness, fever, headache, nervousness, paresthesia, syncope, weakness
CV: Bradycardia, chest pain, hypotension, tachycardia
GI: Abdominal pain, diarrhea, nausea, vomiting
HEME: Thrombocytopenia
MS: Arthralgia, jaw pain, myalgia
RESP: Dyspnea, hypoxia
SKIN: Flushing
Other: Flulike symptoms, injection site infection and pain, sepsis, weight gain or loss

Nursing Considerations
- Reconstitute epoprostenol only with sterile diluent that comes in package. Don't dilute reconstituted epoprostenol.
- To make 100 ml of reconstituted solution at 3,000 nanograms/ml, dissolve contents of 0.5-mg vial with 5 ml of diluent; withdraw 3 ml and add enough diluent to make 100 ml. To make 100 ml of solution at 5,000 nanograms/ml, dissolve contents of 0.5-mg vial with 5 ml of diluent; withdraw contents and add enough diluent to make 100 ml. To make 100 ml of solution at 10,000 nanograms/ml, dissolve contents of two 0.5-mg vials each with 5 ml of diluent; withdraw contents and add enough diluent to make 100 ml. To make 100 ml of solution at 15,000 nanograms/ml, dissolve contents of 1.5-mg vial with 5 ml of diluent; withdraw contents and add enough diluent to make 100 ml.
- Give continuous infusion through a central venous catheter. Use peripheral I.V. route only until central access is established.
- Use an ambulatory infusion pump that is small, lightweight, and able to deliver 2 nanograms/kg/minute. It should have alarms for occlusion, end of infusion, and low battery. Use a polyvinyl chloride, polypropylene, or glass reservoir. Keep a backup pump and infusion set nearby to minimize disruptions in delivery.
- Administer a single container of reconstituted solution at room temperature over 8 hours. For extended use at temperatures above 25° C (77° F), use a cold pouch with frozen gel packs to

keep drug at 2° to 8°C (36° to 46° F) for 12 hours. Don't expose to direct sunlight.

- After a new infusion rate has been established, monitor closely for adverse reactions. Measure blood pressure each time with patient standing and supine. Also, monitor heart rate for several hours after dosage adjustment. Assess for signs of pulmonary edema, such as dyspnea, anxiety, and hemoptysis, which may be associated with veno-occlusive disease.
- During prolonged infusion, watch for dose-related adverse reactions. If they occur, expect to decrease infusion rate by 2 nanograms/kg/minute every 15 minutes, as prescribed, until adverse reactions resolve.
- **WARNING** Avoid abrupt withdrawal or a sudden large reduction in infusion rate, which could cause rebound pulmonary hypertension (asthenia, dizziness, dyspnea) or death.
- Expect lower dosage to be ordered for elderly patients, especially those with hepatic, renal, or cardiac impairment or other diseases and those who may receive other drugs that can interact with epoprostenol.
- Protect reconstituted drug from light, and refrigerate for no longer than 48 hours. Discard solution that has been frozen or that has been refrigerated for longer than 48 hours.
- Before reconstituting epoprostenol, store it and diluent at 15° to 25° C (59° to 77° F); protect from freezing and light.

PATIENT TEACHING
- Inform patient that epoprostenol is infused continuously through a permanent indwelling central venous catheter by a small infusion pump.
- Stress that patient must commit to long-term therapy, possibly for years.
- Teach patient or caregiver how to reconstitute drug, administer it, and care for the permanent central venous catheter.
- Urge patient to maintain prescribed infusion rate and to consult prescriber before altering it.
- Caution patient that even brief interruptions in drug delivery may cause rapid worsening of symptoms.
- Instruct patient to notify prescriber if adverse reactions occur. Stress the importance of keeping follow-up appointments to assess for adverse reactions and evaluate his response to therapy.
- Make sure patient or caregiver has ready access to emergency phone numbers. Advise patient to carry medical identification documenting his use of epoprostenol and its purpose.

• Caution patient to avoid saunas, hot baths, and sunbathing, which can increase the risk of hypertension.

eptifibatide
Integrilin

Class and Category
Chemical: Cyclic heptapeptide
Therapeutic: Platelet aggregation inhibitor
Pregnancy category: B

Indications and Dosages
▶ *To treat unstable angina and non–Q-wave MI*
I.V. INFUSION
Adults. *Initial:* 180 mcg/kg over 1 to 2 min as soon as possible after diagnosis. *Maintenance:* 2 mcg/kg/min by continuous infusion beginning immediately after initial dose and continuing until discharge or coronary artery bypass grafting, up to 72 hr.
DOSAGE ADJUSTMENT For patients with serum creatinine level of 2 to 4 mg/dl, initial dosage reduced to 135 mcg/kg over 1 to 2 min and maintenance dosage reduced to 0.5 mcg/kg/min by continuous infusion. Drug discontinued before coronary artery bypass graft surgery or if platelet count falls below 100,000/mm^3.

▶ *To prevent thrombosis related to percutaneous transluminal coronary angioplasty (PTCA)*
I.V. INFUSION
Adults. *Initial:* 135 mcg/kg over 1 to 2 min immediately before procedure. *Maintenance:* 0.5 mcg/kg/min by continuous infusion beginning immediately after initial dose and continuing for 20 to 24 hr. *Maximum:* 96 hr of therapy.

Route	Onset	Peak	Duration
I.V.	Immediate	In 15 min	4 to 8 hr

Mechanism of Action
Reversibly inhibits platelet aggregation by preventing the binding of fibrinogen, von Willebrand factor, and other adhesive ligands to the platelet receptor glycoprotein IIb/IIIa on activated platelets. Thus, eptifibatide disrupts the final cross-linking stage of platelet aggregation—and thrombus formation.

Incompatibilities

Don't administer eptifibatide through the same I.V. line as furosemide.

Contraindications

Active bleeding or CVA during previous 30 days, bleeding diathesis, dependence on dialysis, history of hemorrhagic CVA, hypersensitivity to eptifibatide, major surgery during previous 4 weeks, serum creatinine level of 2 mg/dl or higher for 180-mcg/kg dose or 2-mcg/kg/min infusion, serum creatinine level of 4 mg/dl or higher for 135-mcg/kg dose or 0.5-mcg/kg/min infusion, severe uncontrolled hypertension (systolic pressure above 200 mm Hg, diastolic pressure above 110 mm Hg), thrombocytopenia (platelet count below 100,000/mm^3)

Interactions

DRUGS

anticoagulants, clopidogrel, dipyridamole, NSAIDs, thrombolytics, ticlopidine: Additive pharmacologic effects, increased risk of bleeding
other platelet aggregation inhibitors (especially inhibitors of platelet receptor glycoprotein IIb/IIIa, such as abciximab): Increased risk of additive pharmacologic effects

Adverse Reactions

CNS: Intracranial hemorrhage
CV: Hypotension
GI: Hematemesis
GU: Hematuria
HEME: Bleeding, decreased hemoglobin level, thrombocytopenia
Other: Anaphylaxis

Nursing Considerations

- Expect to obtain hematocrit, platelet count, and hemoglobin and serum creatinine levels before starting eptifibatide therapy to detect abnormalities. Also expect to obtain baseline APTT and PT.
- Withdraw bolus dose of eptifibatide from a 10-ml (2-mg/ml) vial into a syringe.
- Using a vented I.V. infusion set, administer a continuous infusion directly from the 100-ml (0.75 mg/ml) vial. Be sure to center the spike in the circle on top of the vial stopper.
- Be aware that eptifibatide may be administered in same I.V. line as normal saline solution or dextrose 5% in normal saline solution containing potassium at a concentration of 60 mEq/L. It also may be administered in same I.V. line as alteplase, at-

ropine, dobutamine, heparin, lidocaine, meperidine, metoprolol, midazolam, morphine, nitroglycerin, or verapamil.

- Expect to keep APTT at 50 to 70 seconds or according to facility protocol during therapy unless patient undergoes PTCA.
- If patient undergoes PTCA, expect to maintain his activated clotting time between 300 and 350 seconds during the procedure.
- During therapy, avoid arterial and venous punctures, I.M. injections, urinary catheter use, nasotracheal or nasogastric intubation, and use of noncompressible I.V. sites, such as subclavian and jugular veins.
- Expect to discontinue eptifibatide and heparin and monitor patient closely if platelet count falls below 100,000/mm^3.
- Plan to discontinue drug, as prescribed, if patient undergoes coronary artery bypass surgery.

PATIENT TEACHING
- Instruct patient to immediately report bleeding during eptifibatide therapy.
- Reassure patient that he'll be monitored closely during therapy.
- Advise patient to avoid activities that may lead to bruising and bleeding.

ertapenem sodium

Invanz

Class and Category

Chemical: Synthetic 1-b methyl-carbapenem
Therapeutic: Antibiotic
Pregnancy category: B

Indications and Dosages

▶ *To treat moderate to severe infections, such as complicated intra-abdominal infections caused by* Escherichia coli, Clostridium clostridioforme, Eubacterium lentum, Peptostreptococcus *species,* Bacteroides fragilis, B. distasonis, B. ovatus, B. thetaiotaomicron, *or* B. uniformis; *complicated skin and skin-structure infections caused by* Staphylococcus aureus *(methicillin-susceptible strains only),* Streptococcus pyogenes, E. coli, *or* Peptostreptococcus *species; community-acquired pneumonia caused by* Streptococcus pneumoniae *(penicillin-susceptible strains only, including cases with concurrent bacteremia),* Haemophilus influenzae *(beta-lactamase–negative strains only), or* Moraxella catarrhalis; *complicated UTI (including pyelonephritis) caused by* E. coli *(including cases with concurrent bacteremia) or* Klebsiella pneumoniae; *and acute pelvic infections (including postpartum endomyometritis, septic abortion, and postsurgical gynecologic infections) caused by* Streptococcus agalactiae, E. coli, B. fragilis, Porphyromonas asaccharolytica, Peptostreptococcus *species, or* Prevotella bivia

I.V. INFUSION

Adults and adolescents. 1 g daily, infused over 30 min, for up to 14 days.

Children ages 3 months to 13 years. 15 mg/kg b.i.d., infused over 30 min, for up to 14 days. *Maximum:* 1 g daily.

DOSAGE ADJUSTMENT Dosage decreased to 500 mg daily for patients with advanced renal insufficiency (creatinine clearance 30 ml/min/1.73 m² or less) or end-stage renal insufficiency (creatinine clearance 10 ml/min/1.73 m² or less). For patients on hemodialysis who have received 500 mg of ertapenem within 6 hr of hemodialysis, supplemental dose of 150 mg given after hemodialysis.

Mechanism of Action

Inhibits bacterial cell wall synthesis by binding to specific penicillin-binding proteins inside the cell wall. Penicillin-binding proteins are responsible for various steps in bacterial cell wall synthesis. By binding to these proteins, ertapenem leads to bacterial cell wall lysis.

Incompatibilities

Don't mix ertapenem with other drugs. Don't dilute it with solutions containing dextrose.

Contraindications

Hypersensitivity to ertapenem, its components, or other drugs in the same class; hypersensitivity to local anesthetics (I.M. form only, because lidocaine hydrochloride 1% is used as a diluent); patients who have had anaphylactic reactions to beta-lactams

Interactions

DRUGS

probenecid: Increased ertapenem half-life; increased and prolonged blood ertapenem level

Adverse Reactions

CNS: Agitation, anxiety, asthenia, confusion, disorientation, dizziness, fatigue, fever, hallucinations, headache, hypothermia, insomnia, mental changes, seizures, somnolence, stupor

CV: Chest pain, edema, hypertension, hypotension, tachycardia, thrombophlebitis

EENT: Nasopharyngitis, oral candidiasis, viral pharyngitis

ENDO: Hyperglycemia

GI: Abdominal pain, acid regurgitation, *Clostridium difficile* colitis, constipation, diarrhea, elevated liver function test results, indigestion, nausea, small-intestine obstruction, vomiting

GU: Dysuria, elevated serum creatinine level, proteinuria, RBCs and WBCs in urine, UTI, vaginitis

HEME: Anemia, decreased hematocrit, decreased WBC count, eosinophilia, increased WBC count, neutropenia, prolonged PT, thrombocytopenia, thrombocytosis

MS: Leg pain

RESP: Atelectasis, cough, crackles, dyspnea, pneumonia, respiratory distress, upper respiratory tract infection, wheezing

SKIN: Cellulitis, dermatitis, erythema, extravasation, pruritus, rash

Other: Anaphylaxis; death; hyperkalemia; hypokalemia; infusion site induration, pain, phlebitis, redness, swelling, or warmth

Nursing Considerations

- Obtain sputum, urine, or other specimens for culture and sensitivity testing, as ordered, before giving ertapenem. Expect to begin therapy before results are available.
- When preparing drug for I.V. use, reconstitute 1 g with 10 ml of sterile water for injection, 0.9% sodium chloride injection, or bacteriostatic water for injection. Don't use solutions that contain dextrose. Shake well to dissolve. Immediately transfer reconstituted drug to 50 ml normal saline solution. Use within 6 hours if stored at room temperature, 24 hours if refrigerated at 5° C (41° F). Don't freeze. Give I.V. infusion over 30 minutes.
- Inspect drug for particles and discoloration after reconstitution.
- WARNING Don't give reconstituted I.M. solution by I.V. route because of risk of adverse reactions to the lidocaine hydrochloride injection used to reconstitute drug.
- Monitor patient closely for a life-threatening anaphylactic reaction. Patients with a history of hypersensitivity to penicillin, cephalosporins, other beta-lactams, or other allergens are at increased risk.
- WARNING If ertapenem triggers an anaphylactic reaction, stop drug, notify prescriber immediately, and provide appropriate therapy. Anaphylaxis requires immediate treatment

with epinephrine as well as airway management and administration of oxygen and I.V. corticosteroids, as needed.

- Be aware that patients with a history of seizures, other CNS disorders that predispose them to seizures (such as brain lesions), or compromised renal function may be at increased risk for seizures. Administer anticonvulsant, as ordered.
- Diarrhea that develops during or shortly after drug therapy may signal pseudomembranous colitis. Notify prescriber, and expect to obtain a stool specimen for testing, to withhold erythromycin, and to treat diarrhea with fluid, electrolytes, and antibiotics effective against *Clostridium difficile.*
- Be aware that because ertapenem appears in breast milk, its use by nursing mothers is carefully evaluated.

PATIENT TEACHING
- Instruct patient receiving ertapenem to immediately report signs of anaphylaxis, such as rash, itching, or shortness of breath; or signs of superinfection, such as severe diarrhea or white patches on tongue or in mouth.
- Urge patient to report watery, bloody stools to prescriber immediately, even up to 2 months after drug therapy has ended.

erythromycin gluceptate
(contains 500 or 1,000 mg of base per vial)
Ilotycin
erythromycin lactobionate
(contains 500 or 1,000 mg of base per vial)
Erythrocin

Class and Category
Chemical: Macrolide
Therapeutic: Antiacne agent, antibiotic
Pregnancy category: B

Indications and Dosages
▶ *To treat mild to moderate upper respiratory tract infections caused by* Haemophilus influenzae, Streptococcus pneumoniae, *or* Streptococcus pyogenes *(group A beta-hemolytic streptococcus)*
I.V. INFUSION
Adults. 250 to 500 mg (base) every 6 hr for 10 days.
Children. 250 to 500 mg (base) q.i.d. or 20 to 50 mg (base)/kg daily in divided doses for 10 days. For *H. influenzae* infections, erythromycin ethylsuccinate is administered with sulfisoxazole

150 mg/kg daily. *Maximum:* Adult dosage, or 6 g daily for erythromycin ethylsuccinate.

▶ *To treat lower respiratory tract infections caused by* S. pneumoniae *or* S. pyogenes *(group A beta-hemolytic streptococcus)*

I.V. INFUSION

Adults. 250 to 500 mg (base) every 6 hr for 10 days.

Children. 250 to 500 mg (base) q.i.d. or 20 to 50 mg (base)/kg daily in divided doses for 10 days. *Maximum:* Adult dosage.

▶ *To treat respiratory tract infections caused by* Mycoplasma pneumoniae

I.V. INFUSION

Adults. 500 mg (base) every 6 hr for 5 to 10 days or up to 3 wk for severe infections.

▶ *To treat mild to moderate skin and soft-tissue infections caused by* S. pyogenes *or* Staphylococcus aureus

I.V. INFUSION

Adults. 250 mg (base) every 6 hr or 500 mg (base) every 12 hr for 10 days. *Maximum:* 4 g (base) daily.

Children. 250 to 500 mg (base) q.i.d. or 20 to 50 mg (base)/kg daily in divided doses for 10 days. *Maximum:* Adult dosage.

▶ *To treat pertussis (whooping cough) caused by* Bordetella pertussis

I.V. INFUSION

Children. 500 mg (base) q.i.d. or 40 to 50 mg (base)/kg daily in divided doses for 5 to 14 days.

▶ *To treat diphtheria*

I.V. INFUSION

Adults and children. 500 mg (base) every 6 hr for 10 days.

▶ *To treat erythrasma*

I.V. INFUSION

Adults and children. 250 mg (base) t.i.d. for 21 days.

▶ *To treat intestinal amebiasis*

I.V. INFUSION

Adults. 250 mg (base) every 6 hr for 10 to 14 days.

Children. 30 to 50 mg (base)/kg daily in divided doses for 10 to 14 days

▶ *To treat pelvic inflammatory disease caused by* Neisseria gonorrhoeae

I.V. INFUSION

Adults. 500 mg (base) I.V. every 6 hr for 3 days and then 250 mg (base) P.O. or I.V. every 6 hr for 7 days.

▶ *To treat conjunctivitis in newborns*

I.V. INFUSION

Neonates. 50 mg (base)/kg daily in four divided doses for 14 days.

▶ *To treat pneumonia in neonates*

I.V. INFUSION

Neonates. 50 mg (base)/kg daily in divided doses for 21 days.

▶ *To treat Legionnaire's disease*

I.V. INFUSION

Adults. 1 to 4 g (base) daily in divided doses for 10 to 14 days.

▶ *To treat rheumatic fever*

I.V. INFUSION

Adults. 250 mg (base) every 12 hr.

▶ *To prevent bacterial endocarditis in patients with penicillin allergy who plan dental or upper respiratory tract surgery*

I.V. INFUSION

Adults. 1 g (base) given 1 to 2 hr before procedure and then 500 mg (base) 6 hr after initial dose.

Children. 20 mg (base)/kg given 2 hr before procedure and then 10 mg (base)/kg 6 hr after initial dose.

▶ *To treat listeriosis*

I.V. INFUSION

Adults. 250 mg (base) every 6 hr or 500 mg (base) every 12 hr. *Maximum:* 4 g (base) daily.

Mechanism of Action

Binds with the 50S ribosomal subunit of the 70S ribosome in many types of aerobic, anaerobic, gram-positive, and gram-negative bacteria. This action inhibits RNA-dependent protein synthesis in bacterial cells, causing them to die.

Contraindications

Astemizole, cisapride, pimozide, or terfenadine therapy; hypersensitivity to erythromycin, macrolide antibiotics, or their components

Interactions

DRUGS

alfentanil: Decreased alfentanil clearance and prolonged action
astemizole, cisapride, terfenadine: Increased risk of cardiotoxicity, torsades de pointes, ventricular tachycardia, and death
atorvastatin, lovastatin, pravastatin, simvastatin: Increased risk of rhabdomyolysis

carbamazepine, valproic acid: Possibly inhibited metabolism of these drugs, increasing their blood levels and risk of toxicity

chloramphenicol, lincomycins: Antagonized effects of these drugs

cyclosporine: Increased risk of nephrotoxicity

digoxin: Increased serum digoxin level and risk of digitalis toxicity

diltiazem, verapamil: Increased risk of life-threatening cardiac events

ergotamine: Decreased ergotamine metabolism, increased risk of vasospasm from ergotamine use

hepatotoxic drugs: Increased risk of hepatotoxicity

midazolam, triazolam: Increased pharmacologic effects of these drugs

oral contraceptives: Failed contraception, hepatotoxicity

ototoxic drugs: Increased risk of ototoxicity if patient with impaired renal function receives high doses of erythromycin

penicillins: Interference with bactericidal effects of penicillins

sildenafil: Increased effects of sildenafil

warfarin: Prolonged PT and risk of hemorrhage, especially in elderly patients

xanthines (except dyphylline): Increased serum theophylline level and risk of theophylline toxicity

ACTIVITIES

alcohol use: Increased alcohol level (by 40%) with I.V. erythromycin

Adverse Reactions

CNS: Fatigue, fever, malaise, weakness

CV: Prolonged QT interval, torsades de pointes, ventricular arrhythmias

EENT: Hearing loss, oral candidiasis

GI: Abdominal cramps and pain, diarrhea, hepatotoxicity, nausea, pseudomembranous colitis, vomiting

GU: Vaginal candidiasis

SKIN: Erythema, jaundice, pruritus, rash

Other: Fluid overload (from I.V. infusion), injection site inflammation and phlebitis

Nursing Considerations

- Use erythromycin cautiously in patients with impaired hepatic function because drug is metabolized by the liver.
- Use erythromycin cautiously in elderly patients, especially those with renal or hepatic dysfunction, because they have an increased risk of hearing loss and torsades de pointes. Those who take an oral anticoagulat have an increased risk of bleeding.

- Before administering the first erythromycin dose, expect to obtain body fluid or tissue sample for culture and sensitivity testing.
- Reconstitute parenteral form before administration. Add at least 10 ml of preservative-free sterile water for injection to each 500-mg vial or at least 20 ml of diluent to each 1-g vial.
- For prolonged infusion, expect to infuse a buffered solution up to 24 hours after dilution.
- For intermittent infusion, dilute the dose if needed in 100 to 250 ml of normal saline solution or D_5W and administer slowly over 20 to 60 minutes.
- When giving I.V. erythromycin gluceptate, dilute the solution if needed to 1 g/L in normal saline solution or D_5W injection for slow, continuous infusion. Diluted solution remains potent for 7 days if refrigerated.
- When giving I.V. erythromycin lactobionate, dilute the solution if needed to 1 to 5 mg/ml in normal saline, lactated Ringer's, or other electrolyte solution for slow, continuous infusion. Diluted solution remains potent for 14 days if refrigerated and for 24 hours at room temperature.
- Be aware that infusions prepared in piggyback infusion bottles remain potent for 30 days if frozen, 24 hours if refrigerated, or 8 hours at room temperature. Don't store infusions prepared in the ADD-vantage system.
- Don't use diluent with benzyl alcohol if parenteral erythromycin is for a neonate. It may cause a fatal toxic syndrome of CNS depression, hypotension, metabolic acidosis, renal failure, respiratory problems, and, possibly, seizures and intracranial hemorrhage.
- Periodically monitor liver function test results to detect hepatotoxicity, which is most common with erythromycin estolate. Signs typically appear within 2 weeks after continuous therapy starts and resolve when it stops.
- Assess hearing regularly, especially in elderly patients and those who receive 4 g or more daily or have hepatic or renal disease. Hearing impairment begins 36 hours to 8 days after treatment starts and usually begins to improve 1 to 14 days after treatment stops.
- During I.V. therapy, watch for signs of fluid overload, such as acute dyspnea and crackles.
- Monitor infants for vomiting or irritability with feeding because infantile hypertrophic pyloric stenosis has been reported.

- Monitor myasthenia gravis patients for weakness because drug may aggravate it.
- Monitor patient closely for signs and symptoms of superinfection. If they occur, notify prescriber and expect to stop drug and provide appropriate therapy.
- If patient receives an order for urine catecholamine analysis, notify prescriber; erythromycin interferes with fluorometric measurement of urine catecholamines.
- Diarrhea that develops during or shortly after drug therapy may signal pseudomembranous colitis. Notify prescriber, and expect to obtain a stool specimen for testing, to withhold erythromycin, and to treat diarrhea with fluid, electrolytes, and antibiotics effective against *Clostridium difficile.*

PATIENT TEACHING

- Instruct patient to promptly notify prescriber about allergic reactions, hearing changes, or signs of hepatic dysfunction.
- Urge patient to report watery, bloody stools to prescriber immediately, even up to 2 months after drug therapy has ended.

esmolol hydrochloride
Brevibloc

Class and Category
Chemical: Beta blocker
Therapeutic: Antiarrhythmic, antihypertensive
Pregnancy category: C

Indications and Dosages
▶ *To treat supraventricular tachycardia*
I.V. INFUSION
Adults. *Loading:* 500 mcg/kg over 1 min. *Maintenance:* If response to loading dose is adequate after 5 min, 50 mcg/kg/min infused for 4 min. If response is inadequate after 5 min, another 500 mcg/kg may be given over 1 min, followed by 100 mcg/kg/min for 4 min. Sequence repeated, as needed, until adequate response occurs, increasing maintenance dosage by 50 mcg/kg/min at each step. *Maximum:* 200 mcg/kg/min for 48 hr.
Children. 50 mcg/kg/min, titrated every 10 min up to 300 mcg/kg/min.
▶ *To treat intraoperative and postoperative tachycardia and hypertension*
I.V. INFUSION
Adults. *Initial:* 250 to 500 mcg/kg over 1 min. *Maintenance:*

50 mcg/kg/min infused over 4 min. If response is inadequate after 5 min, another 250 to 500 mcg/kg may be given over 1 min, followed by 100 mcg/kg/min for 4 min. Sequence repeated, as needed, up to 4 times, increasing by 50 mcg/kg/min each time. *Maximum:* 200 mcg/kg/min for 48 hr.

DOSAGE ADJUSTMENT Subsequent loading doses omitted, increments decreased to 25 mcg/kg/min, and titration intervals increased to 10 min as heart rate approaches desired level or if blood pressure decreases too much.

Route	Onset	Peak	Duration
I.V.	Immediate	Unknown	10 to 20 min

Mechanism of Action

Inhibits stimulation of $beta_1$ receptors primarily in the heart, which decreases cardiac excitability, cardiac output, and myocardial oxygen demand. Esmolol also decreases renin release from the kidneys, which helps reduce blood pressure.

Incompatibilities

Don't mix esmolol with 5% sodium bicarbonate injection.

Contraindications

Cardiogenic shock, hypersensitivity to beta-blocking drugs, overt heart failure, second- or third-degree heart block, sinus bradycardia

Interactions

DRUGS

antihypertensives: Possibly hypotension

digoxin: Increased blood digoxin level

insulin, oral antidiabetic drugs: Possibly masking of signs and symptoms of hypoglycemia caused by these drugs

MAO inhibitors: Possibly severe hypertension if esmolol is administered within 14 days of discontinuing MAO inhibitor therapy

neuromuscular blockers: Possibly potentiated and prolonged action of these drugs

phenytoin: Possibly increased cardiac depression

reserpine and other catecholamine-depleting drugs: Possibly bradycardia and hypotension

sympathomimetics, xanthine derivatives: Possibly inhibited therapeutic effects of both drugs, decreased theophylline clearance

Adverse Reactions
CNS: Anxiety, confusion, depression, dizziness, drowsiness, fatigue, fever, headache, syncope
CV: Bradycardia, chest pain, decreased peripheral circulation, heart block, hypotension
GI: Nausea, vomiting
RESP: Dyspnea, wheezing
SKIN: Diaphoresis, flushing, pallor
Other: Infusion site pain, redness, and swelling

Nursing Considerations
- Be aware that esmolol is not administered for intraoperative or postoperative hypertension that results mainly from vasoconstriction caused by hypothermia.
- Expect to give lowest possible dose to patients with allergies, asthma, bronchitis, or emphysema. If bronchospasm occurs, expect to discontinue infusion immediately and give a $beta_2$-stimulating drug, as ordered.
- **WARNING** Examine esmolol label closely to make sure you're using correct concentration; concentrations of 10 mg/ml (100 mg/10-ml vial) and 250 mg/ml (2,500 mg/10-ml vial) are available. The 250-mg/ml concentration is not for direct I.V. injection.
- Before administering esmolol, inspect it for particles or discoloration.
- Don't give 250-mg/ml (2,500-mg/10 ml) concentration by direct I.V. push. Dilute it to a 10-mg/ml infusion by first removing 20 ml from 500 ml of a compatible I.V. solution, such as D_5W or dextrose 5% in normal saline solution, and then adding 5 g of esmolol to the solution.
- Use diluted solution within 24 hours if stored at room temperature.
- Use a 100-mg vial (prediluted to 10 mg/ml) to give loading dose. For a 70-kg (154-lb) patient, loading dose for 500 mcg/kg/minute would be 3.5 ml.
- Monitor blood pressure and heart rate frequently during therapy. Keep in mind that hypotension can occur at any dose but usually is dose-related. Hypotension typically reverses within 30 minutes after dose is decreased or infusion is stopped.
- Monitor patient for signs of increased adverse reactions in patients with supraventricular arrhythmias, decreased cardiac output, hypotension, or other symptoms of hemodynamic compromise and in those who are taking drugs that decrease

peripheral resistance or myocardial filling, contractility, or impulse generation.

- Also monitor patient for evidence of increased adverse reactions in patients with impaired renal function, especially those with end-stage renal disease, because drug is excreted by the kidneys.
- Inspect infusion site regularly for evidence of thrombophlebitis (pain, redness, or swelling at site). Infusions of 20-mg/ml concentration are more likely to cause serious vein irritation than those of 10-mg/ml concentration. Extravasation of 20-mg/ml concentration may cause a serious local reaction and, possibly, skin necrosis. Don't infuse more than 10 mg/ml into a small vein or through a butterfly catheter.
- Before diluting drug, store it at 15° to 30° C (59° to 86° F). Avoid elevated temperatures.

PATIENT TEACHING
- Urge patient receiving esmolol to report adverse reactions immediately.
- Reassure patient that his blood pressure, heart rate, and response to therapy will be monitored throughout esmolol therapy.

esomeprazole magnesium
Nexium I.V.

Class and Category
Chemical: Substituted benzimidazole
Therapeutic: Antiulcer agent
Pregnancy category: B

Indications and Dosages
▶ *To treat gastroesophageal reflux disease in a patient with a history of erosive esophagitis who can't take the drug by mouth*
I.V. INFUSION, I.V. INJECTION
Adults. 20 or 40 mg daily infused for at least 3 min (I.V. injection) or 10 to 30 min (I.V. infusion).
DOSAGE ADJUSTMENT Maximum, 20 mg daily for patients with severe hepatic insufficiency.

Incompatibilities
Don't give esomeprazole with any other drug through the same I.V. site or tubing.

Contraindications
Hypersensitivity to esomeprazole or its components

Mechanism of Action

Interferes with gastric acid secretion by inhibiting the hydrogen-potassium-adenosine triphosphatase (H^+-K^+-ATPase) enzyme system, or proton pump, in gastric parietal cells. Normally, the proton pump uses energy from the hydrolysis of ATPase to drive H^+ and chloride (Cl^-) out of parietal cells and into the stomach lumen in exchange for potassium (K^+), which leaves the stomach lumen and enters parietal cells. After this exchange, H^+ and Cl^- combine in the stomach to form hydrochloric acid (HCl). Esomeprazole irreversibly inhibits the final step in gastric acid production by blocking the exchange of intracellular H^+ and extracellular K^+, thus preventing H^+ from entering the stomach and additional HCl from forming.

Interactions

DRUGS

antimicrobials: Increased blood esomeprazole levels
atazanavir: Possibly reduced blood atazanavir levels
diazepam: Possibly increased blood diazepam level
digoxin, iron salts, ketoconazole: Possibly decreased absorption of these drugs
warfarin: Possibly increased INR and PT, leading to abnormal bleeding

FOODS

all foods: Decreased bioavailability of esomeprazole

Adverse Reactions

CNS: Aggression, agitation, depression, dizziness, encephalopathy, hallucinations, headache
EENT: Blurred vision, dry mouth, sinusitis, taste disturbance
ENDO: Gynecomastia
GI: Abdominal pain, constipation, diarrhea, dyspepsia, flatulence, GI candidiasis, hepatic failure, hepatitis, jaundice, nausea, pancreatitis, stomatitis
GU: Interstitial nephritis
HEME: Agranulocytosis, pancytopenia
MS: Myalgia
RESP: Bronchospasm, respiratory tract infection
SKIN: Alopecia, erythema multiforme, excessive perspiration, Stevens-Johnson syndrome, toxic epidermal necrolysis
Other: Anaphylaxis, infusion site redness or pruritus

Nursing Considerations

• **WARNING** If patient takes drug with amoxicillin or clarithromycin for *Helicobacter pylori*–related ulcer, severe diarrhea may indicate pseudo-membranous colitis. Obtain stool cultures, as ordered.

• Always flush I.V. line with normal saline injection, lactated Ringer's injection, or 5% dextrose injection before and after giving esomeprazole intravenously.

• For I.V. injection, reconstitue powder with 5 ml of normal saline injection and give as a bolus dose over 3 or more minutes. Once reconstituted, drug may be stored at room temperature for up to 12 hours.

• For I.V. infusion, reconstitute powder with 5 ml of normal saline injection, lactated Ringer's injection, or dextrose 5% injection. Further dilute reconstituted solution to make a final volume of 50 ml, and infuse solution over 10 to 30 minutes. Reconstituted drug may be stored at room temperature up to 6 hours if mixed with 5% dextrose injection or up to 12 hours if mixed with normal saline injection or lactated Ringer's injection.

• Be aware that patient receiving I.V. esomeprazole should be switched to oral form as soon as possible.

PATIENT TEACHING

• Urge patient to tell prescriber if he experiences any adverse reactions.

estrogens (conjugated)

Premarin

Class and Category

Chemical: Estrogen derivative, steroid hormone
Therapeutic: Antiosteoporotic, ovarian hormone replacement
Pregnancy category: X

Indications and Dosages

▶ *To treat dysfunctional uterine bleeding*

I.V. INFUSION

Adults. 25 mg, repeated in 6 to 12 hr if needed.

Contraindications

Active deep vein thrombosis, pulmonary embolism, or history of these conditions; active or recent (within past year) arterial thromboembolic disease such as MI or stroke; hypersensitivity to estrogens or their components; known or suspected breast cancer or history of breast cancer; known or suspected estrogen-dependent cancer; liver dysfunction or disease; pregnancy; undiagnosed abnormal genital bleeding

---

Mechanism of Action

Increase the rate of DNA and RNA synthesis in the cells of female reproductive organs, hypothalamus, pituitary glands, and other target organs. In the hypothalamus, estrogens reduce the release of gonadotropin-releasing hormone, which decreases pituitary release of follicle-stimulating hormone and luteinizing hormone. In women, these hormones are required for normal genitourinary and other essential body functions. At the cellular level, estrogens increase cervical secretions, cause endometrial cell proliferation, and increase uterine tone. Estrogen replacement helps maintain genitourinary function and reduce vasomotor symptoms when estrogen production declines from menopause, surgical removal of ovaries, or other estrogen deficiency. It also may help prevent osteoporosis by keeping bone resorption from exceeding bone formation.

In men, estrogens inhibit pituitary secretion of luteinizing hormone and decrease testicular secretion of testosterone. These actions may decrease prostate tumor growth and lower the level of prostate-specific antigen.

Incompatibilities

Don't combine I.V. estrogens with acid solutions, ascorbic acid, and protein hydrolysate because they're incompatible.

Interactions

DRUGS

aminocaproic acid: Possibly increased level of hypercoagulability caused by amino-caproic acid

barbiturates, carbamazepine, hydantoins, rifabutin, rifampin: Possibly reduced activity of estrogen and medroxyprogesterone

bromocriptine: Possibly interference with bromocriptine's therapeutic effects

calcium: Possibly increased calcium absorption

corticosteroids: Increased therapeutic and toxic effects of corticosteroids

cyclosporine: Increased risk of hepatotoxicity and nephrotoxicity

didanosine, lamivudine, zalcitabine: Possibly pancreatitis

hepatotoxic drugs, such as isoniazid: Increased risk of hepatitis and hepatotoxicity

oral antidiabetic drugs: Decreased therapeutic effects of these drugs

somatrem, somatropin: Possibly accelerated epiphyseal maturation
tamoxifen: Possibly interference with tamoxifen's effects
warfarin: Decreased anticoagulant effect

ACTIVITIES

smoking: Increased risk of CVA, pulmonary embolism, thrombophlebitis, and transient ischemic attack

Adverse Reactions

CNS: CVA, dementia, depression, dizziness, headache, migraine headache

CV: Hypertriglyceridemia, MI, peripheral edema, pulmonary embolism, thromboembolism, thrombophlebitis

EENT: Intolerance of contact lenses, retinal vascular thrombosis

ENDO: Breast enlargement, pain, tenderness, or tumors; gynecomastia; hyperglycemia

GI: Abdominal cramps or pain, anorexia, constipation, diarrhea, gallbladder obstruction, hepatitis, increased appetite, nausea, pancreatitis, vomiting

GU: Amenorrhea, breakthrough bleeding, cervical erosion, clear vaginal discharge, decreased libido (males), dysmenorrhea, endometrial cancer, impotence, increased libido (females), ovarian cancer, prolonged or heavy menstrual bleeding, testicular atrophy, vaginal candidiasis

SKIN: Acne, alopecia, hirsutism, jaundice, melasma, oily skin, purpura, rash, seborrhea, urticaria

Other: Angioedema, folic acid deficiency, hypercalcemia (in metastatic bone disease), weight gain

Nursing Considerations

- Use conjugated estrogens cautiously in patients with severe hypocalcemia because a sudden increase in serum calcium levels may cause adverse effects.
- Reconstitute conjugated estrogens with normal saline solution, dextrose, or invert sugar solution and use within a few hours. Discard solution that contains precipitate.
- Monitor serum calcium level to detect severe hypercalcemia in patients with bone metastasis from breast cancer.
- Watch for elevated liver function test values because estrogen and progestins may worsen such conditions as acute intermittent or variegate hepatic porphyria.
- Assess hypertensive patients for increases in blood pressure because estrogens may cause fluid retention.
- Monitor patients who have asthma, diabetes mellitus, endometriosis, heart disease, renal disease, migraine headaches, seizure

disorder, or lupus erythematosus for worsening of these conditions.

- If patient takes warfarin, assess PT test results as prescribed for loss of anticoagulant effects because estrogens increase production of clotting factors and promote platelet aggregation.
- Expect to stop estrogen combination therapy if woman develops evidence of dementia, cancer, or cardiovascular disease, such as CVA, MI, pulmonary embolism, or venous thrombosis.

PATIENT TEACHING

- Explain the risks of estrogen therapy, including increased risk of cardiovascular disease; dementia; breast, endometrial, or ovarian cancer; and gallbladder disease.
- Urge patient to immediately report breakthrough bleeding.
- Instruct patient to perform a monthly breast self-examination and to comply with all prescribed follow-up examinations.
- Warn female patient that long-term use may increase risk of dementia, heart disease, CVA, gallbladder disease, and breast or endometrial cancer.

ethacrynate sodium

Edecrin

Class and Category

Chemical: Ketone derivative of anyloxyacetic acid
Therapeutic: Diuretic
Pregnancy category: B

Indications and Dosages

▶ *To promote diuresis in heart failure; hepatic cirrhosis; renal disease; ascites of short duration caused by cancer, idiopathic edema, or lymphedema; and edema in children (excluding infants with congenital heart disease or nephrotic syndrome)*

I.V. INFUSION

Adults. *Initial:* 50 mg or 0.5 to 1 mg/kg. Dose repeated in 2 to 4 hr, if needed, then every 4 to 6 hr based on patient response. In an emergency, dose repeated every 1 hr, if needed. *Maximum:* 100 mg as a single dose.

Route	Onset	Peak	Duration
I.V.	5 min	15 to 30 min	2 hr

Incompatibilities

Don't mix or infuse ethacrynate sodium with whole blood or its derivatives.

Mechanism of Action

May inhibit the sulfhydryl-catalyzed enzyme systems that cause sodium and chloride resorption in the proximal and distal tubules and the ascending limb of the loop of Henle. These inhibitory effects increase urinary excretion of sodium, chloride, and water, causing profound diuresis. The drug also increases the excretion of potassium, hydrogen, calcium, magnesium, bicarbonate, ammonium, and phosphate.

Contraindications

Anuria; hypersensitivity to ethacrynate sodium, ethacrynic acid, sulfonylureas, or their components; infancy; severe diarrhea

Interactions

DRUGS

ACE inhibitors, antihypertensives: Possibly hypotension
aminoglycosides: Increased risk of ototoxicity
amiodarone: Increased risk of arrhythmias
amphotericin B: Increased risk of electrolyte imbalances, nephrotoxicity, and ototoxicity
anticoagulants, thrombolytics: Possibly potentiated anticoagulation and risk of hemorrhage
corticosteroids: Increased risk of gastric hemorrhage
digoxin: Increased risk of digitalis toxicity
insulin, oral antidiabetic drugs: Possibly increased blood glucose level and decreased therapeutic effects of these drugs
lithium: Increased risk of lithium toxicity
neuromuscular blockers: Possibly increased neuromuscular blockade effects
NSAIDs: Possibly decreased effects of ethacrynate sodium
sympathomimetics: Possibly interference with hypotensive effects of ethacrynate sodium
ACTIVITIES
alcohol use: Possibly potentiated hypotensive and diuretic effects of ethacrynate sodium

Adverse Reactions

CNS: Confusion, fatigue, headache, malaise, nervousness
CV: Orthostatic hypotension
EENT: Blurred vision, hearing loss, ototoxicity (ringing or buzzing in ears), sensation of fullness in ears, yellow vision
ENDO: Hyperglycemia, hypoglycemia

GI: Abdominal pain, anorexia, diarrhea, dysphagia, GI bleeding, nausea, vomiting
GU: Hematuria, interstitial nephritis, polyuria
HEME: Agranulocytosis, severe neutropenia, thrombocytopenia
SKIN: Rash
Other: Hyperuricemia, hypochloremic alkalosis, hypokalemia, hypomagnesemia, hyponatremia, hypovolemia, infusion site irritation and pain

Nursing Considerations

- Dilute ethacrynate sodium with D_5W or normal saline solution for I.V. infusion. Discard unused portion after 24 hours. Don't use diluted solution that is cloudy or opalescent. Infuse slowly over 30 minutes.
- Weigh patient daily and assess for signs of electrolyte imbalance and dehydration. Monitor blood pressure and fluid intake and output, and check laboratory test results. Be aware that elderly patients may be more sensitive to drug's effects. Notify prescriber about significant changes, which may require dosage reduction or temporary drug discontinuation.
- If patient develops hypokalemia, administer replacement potassium, as ordered.
- **WARNING** Monitor hepatic function test results in patients with advanced hepatic cirrhosis, especially those with a history of electrolyte imbalance or hepatic encephalopathy, because drug may lead to life-threatening hepatic coma.
- Monitor blood glucose level frequently, especially if patient has diabetes mellitus, because drug may cause hyperglycemia or hypoglycemia.
- Notify prescriber if patient experiences hearing loss, vertigo, or ringing, buzzing, or sense of fullness in his ears. Drug may need to be discontinued.
- Store drug between 15° and 30° C (59° and 86° F).

PATIENT TEACHING
- Instruct patient to immediately report diarrhea; buzzing, fullness, or ringing in ears; hearing loss; severe nausea; vertigo; or vomiting because ethacrynate sodium therapy may need to be discontinued.
- Advise patient to change position slowly to minimize effects of orthostatic hypotension, especially if he takes an antihypertensive.
- Caution patient not to drink alcohol, stand for prolonged periods, or exercise during hot weather because these activities may

worsen orthostatic hypotension.
- Unless contraindicated, urge patient to eat more high-potassium foods and to take a potassium supplement, if prescribed, to prevent hypokalemia.
- Inform diabetic patient that his blood glucose level will be checked frequently to detect alterations.

etidronate disodium
Didronel

Class and Category
Chemical: Bisphosphonate
Therapeutic: Antihypercalcemic, bone resorption inhibitor
Pregnancy category: C

Indications and Dosages
▶ *To treat moderate to severe hypercalcemia caused by cancer*
I.V. INFUSION
Adults. *Initial:* 7.5 mg/kg daily infused over at least 2 hr for 3 to 7 successive days. Oral etidronate therapy may begin at 20 mg/kg daily for 30 days on the day after last infusion.
DOSAGE ADJUSTMENT Dosage reduced if patient has renal impairment. Drug not given if serum creatinine level exceeds 5 mg/dl.

Mechanism of Action
Inhibits normal and abnormal bone resorption by reducing bone turnover and slowing the remodeling of pagetic or heterotopic bone. Etidronate also decreases the elevated cardiac output that's seen in Paget's disease of bone and reduces local increases in skin temperature. It also inhibits the abnormal bone resorption that may occur with cancer and reduces the amount of calcium that enters the blood from resorbed bone.

Contraindications
Hypersensitivity to etidronate, bisphosphonates, or their components; severe renal impairment

Interactions
DRUGS
aluminum-, calcium-, or magnesium-containing antacids; aluminum-, calcium-, iron-, or magnesium-containing vitamin and mineral supplements: Decreased etidronate absorption

FOODS
high-calcium food, such as milk and other dairy products: Decreased etidronate absorption

Adverse Reactions
EENT: Altered taste, metallic taste
GI: Diarrhea, elevated liver function test results, nausea
GU: Nephrotoxicity
MS: Bone fractures, bone pain, jaw osteonecrosis
Other: Hypocalcemia

Nursing Considerations
• Anticipate beginning etidronate therapy as soon as possible after spinal cord injury, preferably before evidence of heterotopic ossification exists.
• Dilute parenteral form in at least 250 ml of normal saline solution.
• Give parenteral form slowly over at least 2 hours.
• Store diluted parenteral solution at room temperature for up to 48 hours.
• **WARNING** Monitor for hypocalcemia if patient receives parenteral form for more than 3 days.
• When treating hypercalcemia, expect to continue drug for up to 90 days if serum calcium level remains within acceptable range.
PATIENT TEACHING
• Instruct patient to notify prescriber if adverse reactions occur.

etoposide
Toposar, VePesid

etoposide phosphate
Etopophos

Class and Category
Chemical: Podophyllotoxin derivative
Therapeutic: Antineoplastic
Pregnancy category: D

Indications and Dosages
▶ *To treat germ cell testicular cancer*
I.V. INFUSION
Adults. 50 to 100 mg (base)/m^2 daily for 5 days to 100 mg/m^2 on days 1, 3, and 5. Course repeated every 3 to 4 wk.
▶ *To treat small-cell lung cancer*

I.V. INFUSION
Adults. 35 mg (base)/m^2 daily for 4 days to 50 mg/m^2 daily for 5 days. Course repeated every 3 to 4 wk.

Mechanism of Action

May act at the premitotic stage of cell division to inhibit DNA synthesis by blocking topoisomerase II, an enzyme responsible for uncoiling and repairing damaged DNA. Etoposide is cell-cycle dependent and cell-cycle–phase specific, exerting maximum effect on the S and G$_2$ phases of cell division.

Contraindications

Hypersensitivity to etoposide, etoposide phosphate, or their components

Interactions

DRUGS

blood-dyscrasia–causing drugs (such as cephalosporins and sulfasalazine): Increased risk of leukopenia and thrombocytopenia
bone marrow depressants (such as carboplatin and lomustine): Possibly additive bone marrow depression
cyclosporine: Possibly increased blood etoposide level and increased risk of adverse reactions
phosphatase activity inhibitors (such as levamisole): Possibly inhibition of etoposide phosphate
vaccines, killed virus: Possibly decreased antibody response to vaccine
vaccines, live virus: Possibly decreased antibody response to vaccine, increased adverse effects of vaccine, and severe infection

Adverse Reactions

CNS: CNS toxicity, neurotoxicity
CV: Hypotension, thrombophlebitis
EENT: Stomatitis
GI: Anorexia, diarrhea, hepatotoxicity, nausea, vomiting
HEME: Anemia, leukopenia, myelosuppression (dose-related), thrombocytopenia
SKIN: Alopecia, phlebitis, pruritus, rash
Other: Anaphylaxis-like reaction, metabolic acidosis

Nursing Considerations

- Follow facility protocols for preparing and handling antineoplastic drugs and for appropriate disposal of used equipment.
- Monitor CBC, including hematocrit, platelet count, and WBC

with differential, before and intermittently during therapy.

- Be aware that adverse reactions can vary when etoposide is administered in combination therapy. Review information for all drugs administered as part of a specific regimen, including drug interactions and adverse effects.
- Anticipate dosage adjustment in patients with impaired renal or hepatic function because they may experience decreased hepatic clearance or elimination of etoposide.
- Dilute etoposide injection with D_5W or normal saline solution to a concentration of 0.2 to 0.4 mg/ml (200 to 400 mcg/ml). Be aware that a precipitate may form if concentration exceeds 0.4 mg/ml. Use 0.2-mg/ml concentration within 96 hours and 0.4-mg/ml concentration within 24 hours when stored at 25° C (77° F) under normal fluorescent light. Be aware that cracking and leaking of container has been observed when *undiluted* etoposide is placed in a plastic container made of ABS (acrylonitrile, butadiene, and styrene).
- Reconstitute etoposide phosphate for injection using 5 or 10 ml of sterile water for injection, 5% dextrose injection, normal saline injection, bacteriostatic water for injection with benzyl alcohol, or bacteriostatic sodium chloride for injection with benzyl alcohol to a concentration of 20 mg/ml or 10 mg/ml, respectively. Drug may be administered as reconstituted or further diluted with D_5W or normal saline solution to a final concentration as low as 0.1 mg/ml. Use reconstituted or diluted solution within 24 hours when stored at 20° to 25° C (68° to 77° F) or 2° to 8° C (36° to 46° F). Allow refrigerated solution to warm to room temperature before use.
- Administer an antiemetic, as prescribed, before administering etoposide to minimize nausea and vomiting.
- Inspect patient's mouth for signs of stomatitis before giving each etoposide dose.
- To prevent hypotension, give etoposide slowly over 30 to 60 minutes (infusion). Give etoposide phosphate injection over 5 to 10 minutes.
- **WARNING** Monitor patient for hypotension, which can result from too-rapid infusion. If hypotension occurs, stop infusion and notify prescriber immediately. Expect to administer fluids and other supportive treatment and then resume etoposide infusion at a slower rate.
- If etoposide solution comes in contact with your skin or mucosa, wash it off thoroughly with warm water.

• Monitor serum albumin level, as ordered. Low serum albumin level increases the risk of drug-related toxicity.
• **WARNING** Monitor patient for hypersensitivity reactions, such as rash, pruritus, wheezing, and dysphagia from laryngeal edema. If such reactions occur, stop infusion and notify prescriber immediately. If anaphylaxis occurs, administer epinephrine, antihistamines, and corticosteroids, as prescribed.
• Monitor patients who have or have recently been exposed to chicken pox or who have herpes zoster for signs and symptoms of severe, generalized disease.
• Be aware that patients who are receiving concurrent or consecutive radiation therapy are at risk for additive bone marrow depression.
• If patient develops thrombocytopenia, implement protective precautions according to facility policy.
• Assess for signs of infection, such as fever, if patient develops leukopenia. Expect to obtain appropriate specimens for culture and sensitivity testing.
• Before diluting etoposide injection, store it at a controlled room temperature. Store etoposide phosphate for injection at 2° to 8° C (36° to 46° F); don't freeze.

PATIENT TEACHING

• Advise patient to have dental work completed before beginning etoposide treatment, if possible, or to defer needed dental work until blood counts return to normal because etoposide can delay healing and cause gingival bleeding. Teach patient to perform proper oral hygiene, and advise him to use a soft-bristled toothbrush.
• Advise patient to immediately report GI upset.
• Instruct patient who develops bone marrow depression to avoid people with infections. Advise him to report fever, chills, cough, hoarseness, lower back or side pain, or painful or difficult urination because these signs and symptoms may signal an infection.
• Advise patient to immediately report unusual bleeding or bruising, black or tarry stools, blood in urine or stool, or red pinpoint spots on skin.
• Stress the importance of avoiding accidental cuts from sharp objects, such as razor blades or fingernail clippers, because excessive bleeding or infection may occur.
• Caution patient to avoid contact sports and other activities that put him at risk for bruising or injury.

- Instruct patient to avoid touching his eyes or inside of his nose unless he washes his hands immediately beforehand.
- Advise patient with stomatitis to eat bland, soft foods served cold or at room temperature to decrease irritation.
- Advise patient to use contraception to avoid pregnancy during etoposide therapy and to notify prescriber immediately if pregnancy occurs.
- Stress the importance of complying with the dosage regimen and keeping follow-up medical appointments and appointments for laboratory tests.
- Caution patient to avoid receiving immunizations unless approved by prescriber. Instruct him to avoid people who have recently received vaccines or to wear a protective mask over his nose and mouth when in their presence.

famotidine

Pepcid

Class and Category

Chemical: Thiazole derivative
Therapeutic: Antiulcer agent, gastric acid secretion inhibitor
Pregnancy category: B

Indications and Dosages

▶ *To provide short-term treatment of active duodenal ulcer*
I.V. INFUSION, I.V. INJECTION
Adults and adolescents over age 16. 20 mg every 12 hr, infused over 15 to 30 min or injected over at least 2 min.
Children ages 1 to 16. *Initial:* 0.25 mg/kg every 12 hr, infused over 15 to 30 min or injected over at least 2 min. *Maximum:* 40 mg daily.
▶ *To provide short-term treatment for active, benign gastric ulcer*
I.V. INFUSION, I.V. INJECTION
Adults and adolescents over age 16. 20 mg every 12 hr.
Children ages 1 to 16. *Initial:* 0.25 mg/kg every 12 hr. *Maximum:* 40 mg daily.
▶ *To treat gastroesophageal reflux disease*
I.V. INFUSION, I.V. INJECTION
Children ages 1 to 16. *Initial:* 0.25 mg/kg every 12 hr. *Maximum:* 40 mg daily.
▶ *To treat gastric hypersecretory conditions, such as Zollinger-Ellison syndrome*

I.V. INFUSION, I.V. INJECTION
Adults and adolescents. 20 mg every 12 hr.
DOSAGE ADJUSTMENT Parenteral dosage reduced or interval increased (to 36 to 48 hr), if needed, in patients with renal insufficiency and creatinine clearance of 49 ml/min/1.73 m² or less.

Route	Onset	Peak	Duration
I.V.	In 30 min	30 min to 3 hr	10 to 12 hr

Mechanism of Action

In normal digestion, parietal cells in the gastric epithelium secrete hydrogen (H^+) ions, which combine with chloride ions (Cl^-) to form hydrochloric acid (HCl), as shown below left. However, HCl can inflame, ulcerate, and perforate the gastric and intestinal mucosa that's normally protected by mucus. Famotidine, an H_2-receptor antagonist, reduces HCl formation by preventing histamine from binding with H_2 receptors on the surface of parietal cells, as shown below right. By doing so, the drug helps prevent peptic ulcers from forming and helps heal existing ones.

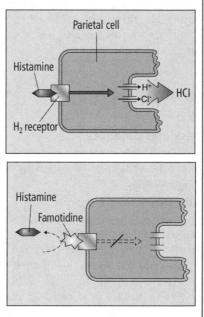

Contraindications

Hypersensitivity to famotidine, other H_2-receptor antagonists, or their components

Interactions
DRUGS

antacids, sucralfate: Possibly decreased absorption of famotidine
bone marrow depressants: Increased risk of blood dyscrasias
itraconazole, ketoconazole: Possibly decreased absorption of these drugs

ACTIVITIES
alcohol use: Possibly increased blood alcohol level

Adverse Reactions
CNS: Agitation (infants), dizziness, fever, headache, insomnia, mental or mood changes, seizures (in patients with impaired renal function)
CV: Arrhythmias, palpitations
EENT: Dry mouth, laryngeal edema, tinnitus
GI: Abdominal pain, anorexia, constipation, diarrhea, hepatitis, nausea, vomiting
HEME: Aplastic anemia, leukopenia, neutropenia, pancytopenia, thrombocytopenia
RESP: Bronchospasm, dyspnea, interstitial pneumonia, wheezing
SKIN: Alopecia, dry skin, erythema multiforme, exfoliative dermatitis, jaundice, pruritus, rash, Stevens-Johnson syndrome, toxic epidermal necrolysis, urticaria
Other: Anaphylaxis, angioedema, facial edema, hyperuricemia

Nursing Considerations
• Dilute injection form (2 ml) with normal saline or other solution to 5 to 10 ml; give I.V. injection over at least 2 minutes. Or dilute in 100 ml of D_5W and infuse over 15 to 30 minutes. Or infuse premixed injection (20 mg/50 ml normal saline solution) over 15 to 30 minutes.

PATIENT TEACHING
• Caution patient to avoid alcohol and smoking during famotidine therapy because they irritate the stomach and can delay ulcer healing.
• Encourage patient to notify prescriber if she develops pain or has trouble swallowing or if she has bloody vomit or black stools.
• Caution patient not to take famotidine with other acid-reducing products.

fenoldopam mesylate
Corlopam

Class and Category
Chemical: Dopamine agonist
Therapeutic: Antihypertensive
Pregnancy category: B

Indications and Dosages

▶ *To treat severe hypertension when rapid, but quickly reversible, emergency reduction of blood pressure is clinically indicated, including malignant hypertension with deteriorating end-organ function*

I.V. INFUSION

Adults. *Initial:* 0.025 to 0.3 mcg/kg/min, individualized according to patient weight and desired effect. *Usual:* 0.01 to 1.6 mcg/kg/min. *Maximum:* 1.6 mcg/kg/min for up to 48 hr.

Route	Onset	Peak	Duration
I.V.	Rapid	Unknown	Unknown

Mechanism of Action

Stimulates dopamine-1 postsynaptic receptors, which mediate renal and mesenteric vasodilation. Vasodilation lowers blood pressure and total peripheral resistance while increasing renal blood flow.

Contraindications

Hypersensitivity to fenoldopam or its components

Interactions

DRUGS

antihypertensives: Additive hypotensive effect
beta blockers: Increased risk of hypotension
dopamine antagonists, metoclopramide: Possibly decreased effects of fenoldopam

Adverse Reactions

CNS: Anxiety, headache, light-headedness
CV: Hypotension, ST- and T-wave changes, tachycardia
EENT: Increased intraocular pressure
GI: Abdominal pain, nausea
SKIN: Diaphoresis, flushing
Other: Hypokalemia, injection site pain

Nursing Considerations

• Reconstitute by adding 40 mg of fenoldopam (4 ml of concentrate) to 1,000 ml of normal saline solution or D_5W, or 20 mg of fenoldopam (2 ml of concentrate) to 500 ml of normal saline solution or D_5W, or 10 mg of fenoldopam (1 ml of concentrate) to 250 ml of normal saline solution or D_5W to produce a final fenoldopam concentration of 40 mcg/ml.
• Infuse through a mechanical infusion pump.

- Expect to titrate dosage in increments of 0.05 to 0.1 mcg/kg/min, as prescribed.
- Expect to monitor heart rate and blood pressure every 15 minutes during fenoldopam therapy because most of drug's effect on blood pressure occurs within 15 minutes of any dosage change.
- Be aware that patient may be started on oral antihypertensive therapy, as prescribed, any time after blood pressure is stable during fenoldopam infusion.
- Discard any reconstituted solution not used within 24 hours.
- **WARNING** Assess patient for signs of increased myocardial oxygen demand, especially if patient has heart failure or a history of angina, because fenoldopam may produce a rapid decline in blood pressure, resulting in symptomatic hypotension and a dose-dependent increase in heart rate.
- Monitor serum potassium level because fenoldopam decreases serum potassium concentrations, which may result in hypokalemia, exacerbate arrhythmias, or precipitate conduction abnormalities, especially in patients with cardiac disease.
- Monitor patients with glaucoma or increased intraocular pressure for changes in vision because fenoldopam may cause a dose-dependent increase in intraocular pressure.
- Be alert for possible allergic- or anaphylactic-type reaction to sodium metabisulfite, a component of fenoldopam injection, especially in patients with asthma.

PATIENT TEACHING
- Inform patient that she'll be switched to an oral antihypertensive once her blood pressure is controlled.
- Instruct patient to expect frequent monitoring of vital signs.

fentanyl citrate
Sublimaze

Class, Category, and Schedule
Chemical: Opioid, phenylpiperidine derivative
Therapeutic: Analgesic, anesthesia adjunct
Pregnancy category: C
Controlled substance schedule: II

Indications and Dosages
▶ *As adjunct to regional anesthesia*
I.V. INJECTION
Adults. 0.05 to 0.1 mg I.M. or slow I.V. over 1 to 2 min.

Route	Onset	Peak	Duration
I.V.	1 to 2 min	3 to 5 min	30 to 60 min

Mechanism of Action

Binds to opiate receptor sites in the CNS, altering perception of and emotional response to pain by inhibiting ascending pain pathways. Fentanyl may alter neurotransmitter release from afferent nerves responsive to painful stimuli, and it causes respiratory depression by acting directly on respiratory centers in the brain stem.

Contraindications

Asthma, children younger than age 2, hypersensitivity to opioids, myasthenia gravis, patients who aren't opioid-tolerant, significant respiratory depression, upper airway obstruction (I.V. or I.M. form); acute or chronic pain, body weight less than 10 kg (22 lb), doses above 5 mcg/kg in adults or 15 mcg/kg in children (transmucosal form); acute or postoperative pain, age less than 12 (or less than 18 if weight is less than 50 kg [110 lb]), dosage that exceeds 25 mcg/hr at the start of therapy, hypersensitivity to fentanyl (or alfentanil, sufentanil, or adhesives), treatment of mild to moderate pain responsive to nonopioid drugs (transdermal form)

Interactions

DRUGS

amprenavir, aprepitant, clarithromycin, diltiazem, erythromycin, fluconazole, fosamprenavir, itraconazole, ketoconazole, nefazodone, nelfinavir, ritonavir, troleandomycin, verapamil: Possibly increased opioid effect, leading to increased or prolonged adverse effects, including severe respiratory depression

anticholinergics, antidiarrheals (such as loperamide and paregoric): Increased risk of severe constipation

antihypertensives, diuretics: Possibly potentiated hypotension

benzodiazepines: Possibly reduced fentanyl dose required for anesthesia induction

buprenorphine: Possibly decreased effects of buprenorphine

CNS depressants: Possibly increased CNS and respiratory depression and hypotension

cytochrome P-450 inducers (such as rifampin, carbamazepine, phenytoin): Possibly induced metabolism and increased clearance of fentanyl

hydroxyzine: Possibly increased analgesic effect of fentanyl and increased CNS depression and hypotension

MAO inhibitors: Possibly unpredictable, even fatal, effects if taken within 14 days of fentanyl

metoclopramide: Possibly antagonized effect of metoclopramide on gastric motility

nalbuphine, pentazocine: Possibly antagonized analgesic, respiratory depressant, and CNS depressant effects of fentanyl; possibly additive hypotensive and CNS and respiratory depressant effects of both drugs

naloxone: Antagonized analgesic, hypotensive, CNS, and respiratory depressant effects of fentanyl

naltrexone: Possibly blocked therapeutic effects of fentanyl

neuromuscular blockers: Possibly prevention or reversal of muscle rigidity by fentanyl

ACTIVITIES

alcohol use: Increased CNS and respiratory depression and hypotension

Adverse Reactions

CNS: Agitation, amnesia, anxiety, asthenia, ataxia, confusion, delusions, depression, dizziness, drowsiness, euphoria, fever, hallucinations, headache, lack of coordination, light-headedness, nervousness, paranoia, sedation, seizures, sleep disturbance, slurred speech, syncope, tremor, weakness, yawning

CV: Asystole, bradycardia, chest pain, edema, hypotension, orthostatic hypotension, tachycardia

EENT: Blurred vision, dental caries, dry mouth, gum line erosion, laryngospasm, rhinitis, sneezing, tooth loss

GI: Anorexia, constipation, ileus, indigestion, nausea, vomiting

GU: Anorgasmia, decreased libido, ejaculatory difficulty, urinary hesitancy, urine retention

RESP: Apnea, depressed cough reflex, dyspnea, hypoventilation, respiratory depression

SKIN: Diaphoresis, exfoliative dermatitis, localized skin redness and swelling (with transdermal form), pruritus, rash

Other: Anaphylaxis, drug tolerance, physical or psychological dependence with long-term use, weight loss

Nursing Considerations

- **WARNING** Monitor patient's respiratory status closely, especially during the first 24 to 72 hours after therapy starts or dosage increases, because severe hypoventilation may occur without warning at any time during therapy.
- To prevent withdrawal symptoms after long-term use, expect to

taper drug dosage gradually, as prescribed.
- Assess patient for withdrawal symptoms after dosage reduction or conversion to another opioid analgesic.
- For patient with bradycardia, implement cardiac monitoring, as ordered, and assess heart rate and rhythm frequently during fentanyl therapy because drug may further slow heart rate.
- **WARNING** Expect respiratory depressant effects to last longer than analgesic effects. Also be prepared for residual drug to potentiate the effects of subsequent doses. Residual drug can be detected for at least 6 hours after I.V. dose. Monitor patient closely for at least 24 hours after therapy ends.

PATIENT TEACHING
- Reassure patient that he will be monitored closely throughout fentanyl therapy.

filgrastim
(granulocyte colony-stimulating factor, rG-CSF)
Neupogen

Class and Category
Chemical: Granulocyte colony-stimulating factor
Therapeutic: Antineutropenic, hematopoietic stimulator
Pregnancy category: C

Indications and Dosages
▶ *To prevent infection after myelosuppressive chemotherapy*
I.V. INFUSION
Adults. 5 mcg/kg daily over 15 to 30 min. Increased, if needed, by 5 mcg/kg with each chemotherapy cycle.
▶ *To reduce the duration of neutropenia after bone marrow transplantation*
I.V. INFUSION
Adults. 10 mcg/kg daily over 4 hr or as a continuous infusion over 24 hr.
DOSAGE ADJUSTMENT Dosage reduced for patients whose absolute neutrophil count remains above 10,000/mm^3.

Route	Onset	Peak	Duration
I.V.	In 5 min	Unknown	Unknown

Incompatibilities
Don't mix filgrastim in vial or syringe with normal saline solution because precipitate will form.

Mechanism of Action

Is pharmacologically identical to human granulocyte colony-stimulating factor, an endogenous hormone synthesized by monocytes, endothelial cells, and fibroblasts. Filgrastim induces the formation of neutrophil progenitor cells by binding directly to receptors on the surface of granulocytes, which then divide and differentiate. It also potentiates the effects of mature neutrophils, which reduces fever and the risk of infection raised by severe neutropenia.

Contraindications

Hypersensitivity to filgrastim, its components, or proteins derived from *Escherichia coli*

Interactions

DRUGS

lithium: Increased neutrophil production

Adverse Reactions

CNS: Fever, headache
CV: Transient supraventricular tachycardia
GI: Splenic rupture, splenomegaly
HEME: Leukocytosis
MS: Arthralgia; myalgia; pain in arms, legs, lower back, or pelvis
SKIN: Pruritus, rash
Other: Anaphylaxis, injection site pain and redness

Nursing Considerations

- Warm filgrastim to room temperature before injection. Discard drug if stored longer than 6 hours at room temperature or 24 hours in refrigerator.
- Withdraw only one dose from a vial; don't repuncture the vial.
- Don't shake the solution.
- For continuous infusion, dilute in D_5W (not normal saline solution) to produce less than 15 mcg/ml.
- After chemotherapy, give filgrastim over 15 to 30 minutes. Don't give within 24 hours before or after cytotoxic chemotherapy.
- Monitor CBC, hematocrit, and platelet count two or three times weekly, as appropriate.
- Inform prescriber and expect to stop drug if leukocytosis develops or absolute neutrophil count consistently exceeds 10,000/mm^3.
- Anticipate decreased response to drug if patient has received

extensive radiation therapy or long-term chemotherapy.

PATIENT TEACHING

- Provide patient with puncture-resistant container for needle and syringe disposal.
- Advise patient to promptly report left-upper-quadrant abdominal pain or shoulder-tip pain.
- Stress the importance of having follow-up laboratory tests.

fluconazole

Diflucan

Class and Category

Chemical: Triazole derivative
Therapeutic: Antifungal
Pregnancy category: C

Indications and Dosages

▶ *To treat oral and esophageal candidiasis*

I.V. INJECTION

Adults and adolescents. 200 mg on day 1 followed by 100 mg daily for at least 2 (oral) or 3 (esophageal) wk after symptoms resolve.

Children. 3 mg/kg daily for at least 2 (oral) or 3 (esophageal) wk and then for 2 wk after esophageal symptoms resolve.

▶ *To treat systemic candidiasis*

I.V. INJECTION

Adults and adolescents. 400 mg on day 1, followed by 200 mg daily for at least 4 wk and then for 2 wk after symptoms resolve.

▶ *To treat cryptococcal meningitis*

I.V. INJECTION

Adults and adolescents. 400 mg daily until patient responds to treatment; then 200 to 400 mg daily for 10 to 12 wk after CSF culture is negative. *Maintenance:* 200 mg daily to suppress relapse.

Children. 6 to 12 mg/kg daily for 10 to 12 wk after CSF culture is negative.

▶ *To prevent candidiasis after bone marrow transplantation*

I.V. INJECTION

Adults and adolescents. 400 mg daily starting several days before procedure if severe neutropenia is expected and continued for 7 days after absolute neutrophil count exceeds 1,000/mm^3.

DOSAGE ADJUSTMENT Dosage reduced for patients with hepatic or renal impairment. Dosage reduced by 50% for patients with creatinine clearance of 11 to 50 ml/min/1.73 m^2.

Mechanism of Action

Damages fungal cells by interfering with a cytochrome P-450 enzyme needed to convert lanosterol to ergosterol, an essential part of the fungal cell membrane.

Decreased ergosterol synthesis causes increased cell permeability, which allows cell contents to leak. Fluconazole also may inhibit endogenous respiration, interact with membrane phospholipids, inhibit transformation of yeasts to mycelial forms, inhibit purine uptake, and impair biosynthesis of triglycerides and phospholipids.

Incompatibilities

Don't add fluconazole to I.V. bag that contains any other drug.

Contraindications

Hypersensitivity to fluconazole or its components

Interactions

DRUGS

astemizole, terfenadine: Increased blood levels of these drugs
benzodiazepines (short-acting): Possibly increased blood benzodiazepine level and psychomotor effects
cimetidine: Decreased blood fluconazole level
cisapride: Possibly increased QT interval, leading to torsades de pointes
cyclosporine: Increased blood cyclosporine level
glipizide, glyburide, tolbutamide: Increased risk of hypoglycemia
hydrochlorothiazide: Increased blood fluconazole level from decreased excretion
isoniazid, rifampin: Decreased fluconazole effects
nonsedating antihistamines: Increased blood antihistamine level, increased risk of cardiotoxicity
oral anticoagulants: Increased anticoagulant effects
phenytoin: Increased blood phenytoin level
rifabutin: Increased blood rifabutin level
theophylline: Increased blood theophylline level
zidovudine: Increased blood zidovudine level

Adverse Reactions

CNS: Chills, dizziness, drowsiness, fever, headache, seizures
CV: Prolonged QT interval, torsades de pointes
GI: Abdominal pain, anorexia, constipation, diarrhea, hepatic failure, nausea, vomiting
HEME: Agranulocytosis, leukopenia, thrombocytopenia

SKIN: Exfoliative dermatitis, photosensitivity, pruritus, rash
Other: Anaphylaxis, angioedema

Nursing Considerations

- Use fluconazole cautiously in patients with potentially proar-rhythmic conditions because drug may prolong the QT interval, which can lead to life-threatening torsades de pointes.
- Expect to obtain BUN and serum creatinine levels, culture and sensitivity, and liver function test results before therapy starts.
- Discard cloudy or precipitated I.V. solution. Don't infuse more than 200 mg/hr or add supplemental drugs to infusion.
- Monitor hepatic and renal function periodically during therapy, and notify prescriber if you detect signs of dysfunction.
- Assess for rash every 8 hours during therapy, and notify pre-scriber if rash occurs.
- If patient receives an oral anticoagulant, monitor coagulation test results and assess patient for bleeding.
- Monitor patient for symptoms of overdose, such as hallucina-tions and paranoia. If they occur, provide supportive treatment, gastric lavage, and, possibly, hemodialysis, which can reduce blood fluconazole level by half after about 3 hours.

PATIENT TEACHING

- If patient takes an oral antidiabetic, tell her to monitor blood glucose level often because of increased risk of hypoglycemia.
- Alert patient that fluconazole may change the taste of food.
- Advise patient to notify prescriber immediately about diarrhea, headache, nausea, rash, right-upper-quadrant abdominal pain, yellow skin or whites of eyes, or vomiting.
- Suggest that breast-feeding patient consult prescriber because breast-feeding may need to be stopped during therapy.

flumazenil

Anexate (CAN), Romazicon

Class and Category

Chemical: Imidazobenzodiazepine derivative
Therapeutic: Benzodiazepine antidote
Pregnancy category: C

Indications and Dosages

▶ *To reverse sedation from benzodiazepine therapy*
I.V. INJECTION
Adults. 0.2 mg, repeated after 45 to 60 sec if response is inade-

quate and then repeated every 1 min, if needed. If sedation recurs, regimen is repeated every 20 min or more. *Maximum:* 1 mg
over 5 min or 3 mg in 1-hr period.

▶ *To reverse benzodiazepine toxicity or suspected overdose*
I.V. INJECTION
Adults. 0.2 mg followed by 0.3 mg 30 to 60 sec later if response
is inadequate and then 0.5 mg repeated every 1 min. If sedation
recurs, regimen is repeated every 20 min. *Maximum:* 3 mg in 1-hr
period.

Route	Onset	Peak	Duration
I.V.	1 to 2 min	6 to 10 min	Variable

Mechanism of Action
Antagonizes the CNS effects of benzodiazepines by competing for their binding sites.

Contraindications
Evidence of tricyclic antidepressant overdose; hypersensitivity to
flumazenil, benzodiazepines, or their components; use of benzodiazepine to control intracranial pressure, status epilepticus, or a
potentially life-threatening condition

Interactions
DRUGS
benzodiazepines: Benzodiazepine withdrawal, including seizures
nonbenzodiazepine agonists: Loss of effectiveness of these drugs
tetracyclic or tricyclic antidepressant overdose: High risk of seizures
FOODS
all foods: Increased flumazenil clearance (by half) with food ingestion during I.V. injection

Adverse Reactions
CNS: Agitation, anxiety, ataxia, confusion, dizziness, drowsiness,
emotional lability, fatigue, headache, hypoesthesia, insomnia,
paresthesia, resedation, seizures, tremor, vertigo
CV: Hot flashes, hypertension, palpitations
EENT: Blurred vision, diplopia, dry mouth
GI: Nausea, vomiting
RESP: Dyspnea, hyperventilation, hypoventilation
SKIN: Diaphoresis, flushing, rash
Other: Injection site pain and thrombophlebitis

Nursing Considerations

• Use flumazenil cautiously in patients with cardiac disease. Assess patient for increased stress or anxiety from benzodiazepine withdrawal because, in patient with cardiac disease, blood pressure may rise.

• Give flumazenil undiluted or diluted in a syringe with D_5W, normal saline solution, or lactated Ringer's solution. Give over 15 to 30 seconds directly into tubing of a free-flowing compatible I.V. solution. Use a large vein, if possible, to minimize pain at site. Avoid extravasation because drug may irritate tissue.

• Be aware that drug may cause benzodiazepine withdrawal in drug-dependent patient. Also, abrupt awakening from benzodiazepine overdose can cause agitation, dysphoria, and increased adverse reactions.

• Be aware that benzodiazepine reversal may cause an anxiety or a panic attack for patient with a history of them. Expect to adjust dosage carefully.

• Monitor for signs of resedation and hypoventilation for at least 2 hours after giving flumazenil because drug has a short half-life. Be aware that patient shouldn't be discharged until the risk of resedation has resolved.

PATIENT TEACHING

• Caution patient to avoid alcohol and OTC drugs for 10 to 24 hours after taking flumazenil.

• Advise patient to avoid hazardous activities for 18 to 24 hours after discharge.

• Inform patient and family that agitation, emotional lability, fear, and panic attack (if patient has a history of them) may occur. Tell them to seek medical care if patient develops depression, trouble breathing, flushing, hyperventilation, insomnia, palpitations, or tremor.

• Because drug doesn't always reverse postprocedure amnesia, provide written instructions or instructions to caregiver even if patient is alert.

fluorouracil
(5-FU)
Adrucil

Class and Category
Chemical: Pyrimidine analogue antimetabolite
Therapeutic: Antineoplastic

Pregnancy category: D

Indications and Dosages

▶ *To treat colorectal, breast, gastric, or pancreatic cancer*

I.V. INFUSION

Adults and adolescents. *Initial:* 7 to 12 mg/kg daily for 4 days; then, after 3 days, if no toxicity has occurred, 7 to 10 mg/kg every 3 days for a total course of 2 wk. Or, 12 mg/kg daily for 4 days; then, after 1 day, if no toxicity has occurred, 6 mg/kg every other day for 4 or 5 doses (days 6, 8, 10, and 12) for a total of 12 days. *Maintenance:* 7 to 12 mg/kg every 7 to 10 days or 300 to 500 mg/m^2 daily for 4 to 5 days, repeated monthly. *Maximum adult dose:* 800 mg daily (400 mg daily for poor-risk patients).

Adults and adolescents who have not received a loading dose. 15 mg/kg or 500 to 600 mg/m^2 every wk.

DOSAGE ADJUSTMENT For poor-risk patients, dosage adjusted to 3 to 6 mg/kg daily for 3 days; then, after 1 day, if no toxicity occurs, 3 mg/kg every other day for 3 doses. Dosage also may be adjusted for patients who have received cytotoxic drug therapy with alkylating agents or high-dose pelvic radiation and for patients with impaired renal or hepatic function.

Mechanism of Action

Inhibits the formation of thymidylate from uracil, which interferes with DNA synthesis and, to a lesser extent, RNA formation. This may create a thymine deficiency, which provokes unbalanced cell growth and death, most markedly in cells that grow rapidly and take up fluorouracil at a rapid rate. Fluorouracil is cell-cycle–phase specific; it's active during the S phase of cell division.

Contraindications

Bone marrow depression, hypersensitivity to fluorouracil, major surgery within 1 month before fluorouracil administration, poor nutritional status, potentially serious infection

Interactions

DRUGS

blood-dyscrasia–causing drugs (such as cephalosporins and sulfasalazine): Increased risk of leukopenia and thrombocytopenia

bone marrow depressants (such as carboplatin and lomustine): Possibly additive bone marrow depression

cimetidine: Possibly increased peak concentrations of fluorouracil *leucovorin:* Possibly increased therapeutic and toxic fluorouracil effects

vaccines, killed virus: Possibly decreased antibody response to vaccine

vaccines, live virus: Possibly decreased antibody response to vaccine, increased adverse effects of vaccine, and severe infection

warfarin and other coumarin-derived anticoagulants: Increased anticoagulant effect

Adverse Reactions

CNS: Acute cerebellar syndrome, confusion, disorientation, euphoria, headache, weakness

CV: Angina, myocardial ischemia, thrombophlebitis

EENT: Nystagmus, stomatitis

GI: Anorexia, diarrhea, esophogopharyngitis, GI ulceration, nausea, vomiting

HEME: Agranulocytosis, anemia, bone marrow depression, leukopenia, pancytopenia, thrombocytopenia

RESP: Pneumopathy

SKIN: Alopecia, dry skin and fissuring, maculopapular rash, palmar-plantar erythrodysesthesia syndrome, pruritus

Other: Anaphylaxis, infection

Nursing Considerations

- Follow facility protocols for preparation and handling of antineoplastic drugs and for appropriate disposal of used equipment.
- Be aware that fluorouracil should be administered only under the supervision of a qualifed physician. Expect patient to be hospitalized at least during the first course of therapy.
- Be aware that estimated lean body mass (dry weight) may be used to calculate dosage for obese patients and for those with weight gain secondary to abnormal fluid retention, ascites, or edema. Maximum fluorouracil daily dose for any patient should not exceed 800 mg.
- Monitor CBC, including hematocrit, platelet count, and WBC with differential, and liver function tests, including bilirubin and LDH values, before and intermittently during fluorouracil therapy, as ordered. Inspect patient's mouth for stomatitis before each dose.
- **WARNING** Be aware that adverse reactions can vary when fluorouracil is administered in combination therapy and that some reactions, such as severe diarrhea with dehydration and

electrolyte imbalances, may be life-threatening. Review information for all drugs given as part of a specific regimen, including drug their interactions and adverse effects. Expect increased patient evaluation and dosage adjustments based on combination used and incidence and severity of adverse reactions.

- Dilute fluorouracil with D_5W or normal saline solution. If using the 50-ml vial, don't use a syringe or needle to avoid leakage and contamination; instead, use a sterile dispensing device or a transfer set that accepts a syringe hub. Use proper aseptic technique under a laminar flow hood. Use diluted solution within 8 hours.

- Be aware that slight discoloration doesn't affect drug's potency or safety.

- **WARNING** Be aware that fluorouracil should not be administered intrathecally because of the increased risk of neurotoxicity.

- Infuse fluorouracil slowly, over 2 to 24 hours, to reduce the risk of toxicity. However, be aware that rapid injection (over 1 to 2 minutes) may be more effective.

- **WARNING** Because of fluorouracil's extremely toxic effects, expect to discontinue infusion if patient develops any of the following adverse reactions: diarrhea, esophagopharyngitis (heartburn with potential for sloughing and ulceration), GI bleeding or ulceration, hemorrhage (from any site), intractable vomiting, marked leukopenia or rapidly falling leukocyte count, stomatitis, or thrombocytopenia. Expect to restart fluorouracil infusion at a lower dose when adverse reactions subside.

- Monitor patients who have, or have recently been exposed to, chicken pox or who have herpes zoster for signs and symptoms of severe, generalized disease.

- Assess for signs of infection, such as fever, if patient develops leukopenia. Expect to obtain appropriate specimens for culture and sensitivity testing.

- **WARNING** Be aware that myocardial ischemia can occur several hours after a dose (even later doses). Continue to assess patient for signs of ischemia throughout the course of treatment.

- Be aware that patients who are receiving concurrent or consecutive radiation therapy are at risk for additive bone marrow depression.

- Assess patient for signs of palmar-plantar erythrodysesthesia syndrome (also known as hand-foot syndrome), characterized by tingling of hands and feet, followed by pain, erythema, and swelling. Expect symptoms to subside 5 to 7 days after interruption of therapy.
- Store drug at 15° to 30° C (59° to 86° F); protect from freezing and light. Heat solution to 60° C (140° F) and shake vigorously to dissolve precipitates formed at low temperatures. Allow solution to cool to body temperature before use.

PATIENT TEACHING
- Advise patient to have dental work completed before beginning fluorouracil treatment, if possible, or to defer such work until blood counts return to normal because drug can delay healing and cause gingival bleeding. Teach patient proper oral hygiene, and advise her to use a soft-bristled toothbrush.
- Instruct patient who develops bone marrow depression to avoid persons with infections. Advise her to report fever, chills, cough, hoarseness, lower back or side pain, or painful or difficult urination because these signs and symptoms may signal an infection.
- Advise patient to immediately report unusual bleeding or bruising, black or tarry stools, blood in urine or stool, or red pinpoint spots on skin.
- Stress the importance of avoiding accidental cuts from sharp objects, such as razor blades or fingernail clippers, because excessive bleeding or infection may occur.
- Urge patient to avoid contact sports or other activities that put her at risk for bruising or injury.
- Instruct patient to avoid touching her eyes or inside of her nose unless she washes her hands immediately beforehand.
- Advise patient to use contraception to avoid pregnancy during therapy and to notify prescriber immediately if pregnancy occurs.
- Advise patient with stomatitis to eat bland, soft foods served cold or at room temperature to decrease irritation.
- Stress the importance of complying with the dosage regimen and of keeping follow-up medical appointments and appointments for laboratory tests.
- Caution patient to avoid receiving immunizations unless approved by prescriber. Instruct her to avoid people who have recently received vaccines or to wear a protective mask over her nose and mouth when in their presence.

folic acid
(vitamin B₉)
Folvite

Class and Category
Chemical: Water-soluble B-complex vitamin
Therapeutic: Nutritional supplement
Pregnancy category: A

Indications and Dosages
▶ *To prevent deficiency based on U.S. and Canadian recommended daily allowances*
I.V INFUSION
Adults and children age 11 and over. Dosage individualized based on patient need and given as part of total parenteral nutrition solution.
▶ *To treat deficiency*
I.V. INFUSION
Adults and children age 11 and over. 0.25 to 1 mg daily until hematologic response occurs.

Mechanism of Action
Acts as a catalyst for normal production of RBCs, helping to prevent megaloblastic anemia, and helps maintain normal homocysteine levels. After being converted to tetrahydrofolic acid in the intestines, folic acid promotes synthesis of several enzymes, including purine and thymidylates; metabolism of amino acids, including glycine and methionine; and metabolism of histidine—all of which are essential for normal cell structure and growth.

Contraindications
Hypersensitivity to folic acid or its components

Interactions
DRUGS
analgesics, carbamazepine, estrogens (including oral contraceptives), phenobarbital, primidone: Possibly increased folic acid requirements
hydantoin anticonvulsants: Possibly decreased effectiveness of these drugs, possibly increased folic acid requirements
methotrexate, pyrimethamine, triamterene, trimethoprim: Possibly decreased effectiveness of folic acid
sulfasalazine: Possibly decreased folic acid absorption

Adverse Reactions

Other: Allergic reaction (bronchospasm, erythema, fever, malaise, rash, pruritus)

Nursing Considerations

- **WARNING** Don't administer injection form of folic acid containing benzyl alcohol to neonates or premature infants because they may develop a fatal toxic syndrome characterized by CNS, respiratory, circulatory, and renal impairment and metabolic acidosis.
- Be aware that although folic acid will correct hematologic disorders associated with pernicious anemia, neurologic problems will progressively worsen.
- Store drug at 15° to 30° C (59° to 86° F); protect from freezing and light.

PATIENT TEACHING

- Inform patient that folic acid supplements are not a substitute for proper diet. Teach her that the best sources of dietary folic acid are green vegetables, potatoes, cereals, and organ meats. Recommend that she eat raw green vegetables because cooking destroys up to 90% of folic acid found in food.
- Explain to patients with pernicious anemia that folic acid won't affect the neurologic symptoms associated with the disease.

fosaprepitant dimeglumine

Emend for Injection

Class and Category

Chemical: Prodrug of aprepitant (a substance P/neurokinin 1 [NK1] receptor antagonist)
Therapeutic: Antiemetic
Pregnancy category: B

Indications and Dosages

▶ *To prevent acute and delayed nausea and vomiting caused by highly emetogenic chemotherapy, including high-dose cisplatin; to prevent nausea and vomiting caused by initial and repeat courses of moderately emetogenic chemotherapy*

I.V. INFUSION

Adults. 115 mg over 15 min, infused 30 min before chemotherapy.

DOSAGE ADJUSTMENT Be aware that fosaprepitant for injection should only be used on day 1 of the CINV regimen

Mechanism of Action

Rapidly converted to aprepitant, which crosses the blood–brain barrier to occupy brain NK1 receptors. This prevents nerve transmission of signals that cause nausea and vomiting.

Incompatibilities

Do not mix or reconstitute with solutions containing divalent cations such as Ca2+ and Mg2+, including lactated Ringer's solution and Hartmann's solution.

Contraindications

Hypersensitivity to fosaprepitant, aprepitant, polysorbate 89 or any of its other components; use of astemizole, cisapride, pimozide, or terfenadine

Interactions

DRUGS

carbamazepine, phenytoin, rifampin: Possibly decreased blood aprepitant level

corticosteroids such as dexamethasone, methylprednisolone: Increased blood corticosteroid level

CYP2C9 metabolizers (such as phenytoin, tolbutamide, and warfarin): Decreased blood level and effectiveness of CYP2C9 metabolizers

CYP3A4 inhibitors (such as clarithromycin, diltiazem, itraconazole, ketoconazole, nefazodone, nelfinavir, and troleandomycin): Increased blood aprepitant level

CYP3A4 substrates (such as astemizole, benzodiazepines, cisapride, docetaxel, etoposide, ifosfamide, imatinib, irinotecan, paclitaxel, pimozide, terfenadine, vinblastine, vincristine, and vinorelbine): Increased blood level of CYP3A4 substrates, resulting in possibly serious or life-threatening adverse reactions

oral contraceptives: Possibly decreased effectiveness of oral contraceptives

paroxetine: Possibly decreased blood level of both drugs

Adverse Reactions

CNS: Anxiety, asthenia, confusion, depression, dizziness, fatigue, fever, headache, insomnia, malaise, peripheral or sensory neuropathy, somnolence

CV: Deep vein thrombosis, edema, hypertension, hypotension, tachycardia

EENT: Increased salivation, mucous membrane alteration, nasal

discharge, pharyngitis, taste perversion, tinnitus, vocal disturbance
ENDO: Hyperglycemia
GI: Abdominal pain, anorexia, constipation, diarrhea, dysphagia,
elevated liver function test results, epigastric discomfort, flatulence, gastritis, gastroesophageal reflux, heartburn, hiccups, nausea, obstipation, vomiting
GU: Dysuria, elevated BUN and serum creatinine levels, hematuria, leukocyturia, renal insufficiency
HEME: Anemia, febrile neutropenia, leukocytosis, thrombocytopenia
MS: Muscle weakness, myalgia, pelvic pain
RESP: Cough, dyspnea, non–small-cell lung carcinoma, pneumonitis, pulmonary embolism, respiratory insufficiency, respiratory tract infection
SKIN: Alopecia, diaphoresis, flushing, pruritus, rash, urticaria
Other: Anaphylaxis, dehydration, hypokalemia, hyponatremia,
infusion site pain or induration, malignant neoplasm, septic
shock, weight loss

Nursing Considerations

- Use caution when giving fosaprepitant to patients with severe
  hepatic insufficiency because drug's effects on such patients
  aren't known.
- To prepare fosaprepitant for injection, aseptically inject 5 ml of
  saline solution into the vial along the vial wall to prevent foaming. Swirl the vial gently. Avoid shaking and jetting saline into
  the vial. Withdraw the entire volume of solution from vial and
  transfer into infusion bag containing 110 ml of saline solution
  to yield a total volume of 115 ml and a final concentration of
  1 mg/1 ml. Gently invert the bag 2 to 3 times.
- Be aware that reconstituted final drug solution may be kept for
  24 hours at or below 25° C.
- For maximum antiemetic effects, expect to administer fosaprepitant with dexamethasone and a 5-HT$_3$ antagonist, such as
  dolasetron, granisetron, or ondansetron.

PATIENT TEACHING

- Urge women taking oral contraceptives to use a different or an
  additional contraceptive during and for 1 month after fosaprepitant therapy; drug reduces contraceptive effectiveness.
- Tell patient taking warfarin regularly to have his clotting status
  monitored closely for 2 weeks after the first dose of fosaprepitant, especially every 7 to 10 days during each chemotherapy

cycle in which the drug is used.
• Tell patient to report prescribed drugs, OTC drugs, and herbal supplements he takes; they may interact with fosaprepitant.

foscarnet sodium
Foscavir

Class and Category
Chemical: Organic pyrophosphate analogue
Therapeutic: Antiviral
Pregnancy category: C

Indications and Dosages
▶ *To treat cytomegalovirus retinitis*
I.V. INFUSION
Adults. *Induction:* 90 mg/kg over 1½ to 2 hr every 12 hr, or 60 mg/kg over 1 hr every 8 hr, for 14 to 21 days. *Maintenance:* 90 to 120 mg/kg over 2 hr daily.
DOSAGE ADJUSTMENT To achieve induction dose equivalent of 90 mg/kg every 12 hr in patients with impaired renal function, dosage reduced as follows: for creatinine clearance greater than 1 to 1.4 ml/min/kg, 70 mg/kg every 12 hr; for clearance greater than 0.8 to 1 ml/min/kg, 50 mg/kg every 12 hr; for clearance greater than 0.6 to 0.8 ml/min/kg, 80 mg/kg every 24 hr; for clearance greater than 0.5 to 0.6 ml/min/kg, 60 mg/kg every 24 hr; for clearance of 0.4 to 0.5 ml/min/kg or greater, 50 mg/kg every 24 hr; and for clearance less than 0.4 ml/min/kg, use not recommended.
To achieve induction dose equivalent of 60 mg/kg every 8 hr in patients with impaired renal function, dosage reduced as follows: for creatinine clearance greater than 1 to 1.4 ml/min/kg, 45 mg/kg every 8 hr; for clearance greater than 0.8 to 1 ml/min/kg, 50 mg/kg every 12 hr; for clearance greater than 0.6 to 0.8 ml/min/kg, 40 mg/kg every 12 hr; for clearance greater than 0.5 to 0.6 ml/min/kg, 60 mg/kg every 24 hr; for clearance greater than or equal to 0.4 to 0.5 ml/min/kg, 50 mg/kg every 24 hr; and for clearance less than 0.4 ml/min/kg, use not recommended.
DOSAGE ADJUSTMENT For patients with impaired renal function who are receiving 90-mg/kg daily maintenance dose, dosage reduced as follows: for creatinine clearance greater than 1 to 1.4 ml/min/kg, 70 mg/kg daily; for clearance greater than

0.8 to 1 ml/min/kg, 50 mg/kg daily; for clearance greater than 0.6 to 0.8 ml/min/kg, 80 mg/kg every 48 hr; for clearance greater than 0.5 to 0.6 ml/min/kg, 60 mg/kg every 48 hr; for clearance greater than or equal to 0.4 to 0.5 ml/min/kg, 50 mg/kg every 48 hr; and for clearance less than 0.4 ml/min/kg, use not recommended.

For patients with impaired renal function who are receiving 120-mg/kg daily maintenance dose, dosage reduced as follows: for creatinine clearance greater than 1 to 1.4 ml/min/kg, 90 mg/kg every day; for clearance greater than 0.8 to 1 ml/min/kg, 65 mg/kg every day; for clearance greater than 0.6 to 0.8 ml/min/kg, 105 mg/kg every 48 hr; for clearance greater than 0.5 to 0.6 ml/min/kg, 80 mg/kg every 48 hr; for clearance greater than or equal to 0.4 to 0.5 ml/min/kg, 65 mg/kg every 48 hr; and for clearance less than 0.4 ml/min/kg, use not recommended.

▶ *To treat acyclovir-resistant mucocutaneous herpes simplex*

I.V. INFUSION

Adults. 40 mg/kg over 1 hr every 8 or 12 hr for 14 to 21 days or until healed.

DOSAGE ADJUSTMENT For patients with impaired renal function who are receiving 40-mg/kg dose every 8 hr, dosage reduced as follows: for creatinine clearance greater than 1 to 1.4 ml/min/kg, 30 mg/kg every 8 hr; for clearance greater than 0.8 to 1 ml/min/kg, 35 mg/kg every 12 hr; for clearance greater than 0.6 to 0.8 ml/min/kg, 25 mg/kg every 12 hr; for clearance greater than 0.5 to 0.6 ml/min/kg, 40 mg/kg every 24 hr; for clearance greater than or equal to 0.4 to 0.5 ml/min/kg, 35 mg/kg every 24 hr; and for clearance less than 0.4 ml/min/kg, use not recommended.

For patients with impaired renal function who are receiving 40-mg/kg dose every 12 hr, dosage reduced as follows: for creatinine clearance greater than 1 to 1.4 ml/min/kg, 30 mg/kg every 12 hr; for clearance greater than 0.8 to 1 ml/min/kg, 20 mg/kg every 12 hr; for clearance greater than 0.6 to 0.8 ml/min/kg, 35 mg/kg every 24 hr; for clearance greater than 0.5 to 0.6 ml/min/kg, 25 mg/kg every 24 hr; for clearance greater than or equal to 0.4 to 0.5 ml/min/kg, 20 mg/kg every 24 hr; and for creatinine clearance less than 0.4 ml/min/kg, use not recommended.

Incompatibilities

Don't mix foscarnet through the same I.V. line or concurrently through the same catheter as any other solution or drug. Foscarnet is incompatible with solutions containing calcium, 30% dextrose solution, or lactated Ringer's solution. To avoid precipitation, don't mix foscarnet with acyclovir, amphotericin B, cotrimoxazole, dobutamine, droperidol, ganciclovir, haloperidol, pentamidine, trimetrexate, or vancomycin. To avoid gas production, don't mix foscarnet with diazepam, digoxin, lorazepam, midazolam, or promethazine hydrochloride. To avoid cloudiness or color change, don't mix foscarnet with diphenhydramine, leucovorin, or prochlorperazine.

Mechanism of Action

Inhibits replication of herpes simplex virus types 1 and 2, Epstein-Barr virus, cytomegalovirus, human herpes virus 6, and varicella-zoster virus by selectively inhibiting the pyrophosphate-binding site of viral DNA polymerase, an enzyme used in the viral DNA replication process. Viral replication resumes when drug therapy stops.

Contraindications

Clinically significant hypersensitivity to foscarnet sodium

Interactions

DRUGS

aminoglycosides, amphotericin B, cidofovir, and other nephrotoxic drugs: Increased risk of nephrotoxicity
calcium-altering drugs: Altered serum calcium level
pentamidine (I.V.): Hypocalcemia (possibly fatal), hypomagnesemia, and nephrotoxicity
ritonavir, saquinavir: Abnormal renal function
zidovudine: Possibly increased risk of anemia

Adverse Reactions

CNS: Headache, neurotoxicity (including dizziness, paresthesia, seizures)
CV: Phlebitis
EENT: Mouth or throat ulcers
GI: Abdominal pain, anorexia, diarrhea, nausea, vomiting
GU: Elevated serum creatinine level, genital ulcers, nephrotoxicity
HEME: Anemia, granulocytopenia, leukopenia
Other: Hypocalcemia, hypophosphatemia, hyperphosphatemia, hypomagnesemia, hypokalemia

Nursing Considerations

- Expect to hydrate patient with ½ to 1 L of normal saline solution or D_5W, as ordered, before first dose of foscarnet and with each subsequent dose to avoid nephrotoxicity.
- Prepare peripheral infusion by diluting foscarnet with an equal amount of D_5W or normal saline solution, which will result in a final concentration of 12 mg/ml. Use diluted drug within 24 hours, and discard any unused portion. Infuse undiluted foscarnet (24 mg/ml) by central line to prevent venous irritation.
- Administer 60-mg/kg doses over at least 1 hour and higher doses over at least 2 hours.
- **WARNING** Always administer foscarnet at a steady rate using an infusion pump; rapid infusion may result in increased blood level of foscarnet, which can lead to acute hypocalcemia or another toxicity.
- Monitor serum electrolyte levels, especially calcium, magnesium, phosphate, and potassium, 2 to 3 times a week during induction and weekly during maintenance therapy, as ordered. Be aware that patient may have decreased ionized calcium level even if serum calcium level seems to be normal. Assess patient for signs and symptoms of hypocalcemia, such as perioral tingling, numbness, and paresthesia. Be aware that electrolyte abnormalities can cause severe effects, such as arrhythmias, seizures, and tetany.
- Obtain patient's baseline BUN and serum creatinine levels; then monitor these levels 2 to 3 times a week during induction therapy and at least once a week during maintenance therapy, as ordered. Assess input and output of patients who are dehydrated, are using other nephrotoxic drugs, or have preexisting impaired renal function because foscarnet increases the risk of nephrotoxicity. Monitor elderly patients closely because they are more likely to have decreased renal function.
- Monitor CBC periodically during foscarnet therapy, especially in patients with anemia, because foscarnet may decrease hemoglobin level.
- Store drug at 15° to 30° C (59° to 86° F); don't freeze. Discard drug if it becomes frozen because a precipitate will form.

PATIENT TEACHING
- Advise patient receiving foscarnet to immediately report signs of hypocalcemia, such as tingling around mouth or numbness of arms or legs, as well as other adverse reactions, such as changes

in urination pattern or increased eye pain.
• Stress the importance of keeping follow-up medical appointments and appointments for laboratory tests.
• Explain that retinitis may progress and vision loss may occur
during foscarnet treatment. Encourage patient to undergo follow-up ophthalmic examinations, even after she has completed
treatment.

fosphenytoin sodium
Cerebyx

Class and Category
Chemical: Hydantoin derivative
Therapeutic: Anticonvulsant
Pregnancy category: D

Indications and Dosages
▶ *To treat status epilepticus*
I.V. INFUSION
Adults and adolescents. *Initial:* 15 to 20 mg of phenytoin
equivalent (PE)/kg at 100 to 150 PE/min. *Maintenance:* 4 to 6 mg
PE/kg daily in divided doses b.i.d. to q.i.d. *Maximum:* 30 mg PE/kg
as total loading dose.
Children. *Initial:* 15 to 20 mg PE/kg given at up to 3 mg PE/
kg/min. *Maintenance:* 4 to 6 mg PE/kg daily in divided doses b.i.d.
to q.i.d.
▶ *To prevent or treat seizures during and after neurosurgery*
I.V. INFUSION
Adults and adolescents. *Initial:* 10 to 20 mg PE/kg, not to exceed 150 mg PE/min. *Maintenance:* 4 to 6 mg PE/kg daily in divided doses b.i.d. to q.i.d. *Maximum:* 30 mg PE/kg as total loading
dose.

Mechanism of Action
Is converted from fosphenytoin (a prodrug) to phenytoin, which limits the
spread of seizure activity and the start of new seizures. Phenytoin does so by
regulating voltage-dependent sodium and calcium channels in neurons, inhibiting calcium movement across neuronal membranes, and enhancing the
sodium-potassium–adenosine triphosphatase activity in neurons and glial
cells. These actions may stem from phenytoin's ability to slow the recovery
rate of inactivated sodium channels.

Contraindications

Hypersensitivity to fosphenytoin, phenytoin, other hydantoins, or their components

Interactions

DRUGS

acetaminophen (long-term use): Increased risk of hepatotoxicity

acyclovir: Decreased blood phenytoin level and loss of seizure control

alfentanil: Increased clearance and decreased effectiveness of alfentanil

amiodarone, fluoxetine: Possibly increased blood phenytoin level and risk of toxicity

antacids: Possibly decreased phenytoin effectiveness

antineoplastics: Increased phenytoin metabolism

beta blockers: Increased myocardial depression

bupropion, clozapine, loxapine, MAO inhibitors, maprotiline, phenothiazines, pimozide, thioxanthenes: Possibly lowered seizure threshold and decreased therapeutic effects of phenytoin, possibly intensified CNS depressant effects of these drugs

calcium: Possibly impaired phenytoin absorption

calcium channel blockers: Possibly increased blood phenytoin level

carbamazepine: Decreased blood carbamazepine level, possibly increased blood phenytoin level and risk of toxicity

chloramphenicol, cimetidine, disulfiram, isoniazid, methylphenidate, metronidazole, phenylbutazone, ranitidine, salicylates, sulfonamides, trimethoprim: Possibly impaired metabolism of these drugs, increased risk of phenytoin toxicity

CNS depressants: Possibly increased CNS depression

corticosteroids, cyclosporine, digoxin, disopyramide, doxycycline, furosemide, levodopa, mexiletine, quinidine: Decreased therapeutic effects of these drugs

diazoxide: Possibly decreased therapeutic effects of both drugs

dopamine: Possibly sudden hypotension or cardiac arrest after I.V. fosphenytoin administration

estrogen- and progestin-containing contraceptives: Possibly breakthrough bleeding and decreased contraceptive effectiveness

estrogens, progestins: Decreased therapeutic effects, increased blood phenytoin level

felbamate: Possibly impaired metabolism and increased blood level of phenytoin

fluconazole, itraconazole, ketoconazole, miconazole: Increased blood phenytoin level *folic acid:* Increased phenytoin metabolism, decreased seizure control

haloperidol: Possibly lowered seizure threshold and decreased therapeutic effects of fosphenytoin; possibly decreased blood haloperidol level

insulin, oral antidiabetic drugs: Possibly increased blood glucose level and decreased therapeutic effects of these drugs

lamotrigine: Possibly decreased therapeutic effects of lamotrigine

lidocaine: Possibly decreased blood lidocaine level, increased myocardial depression

lithium: Increased risk of lithium toxicity

methadone: Possibly increased methadone metabolism, leading to withdrawal symptoms

molindone: Possibly lowered seizure threshold, impaired absorption, and decreased therapeutic effects of phenytoin

omeprazole: Possibly increased blood phenytoin level

oral anticoagulants: Possibly impaired metabolism of these drugs and increased risk of phenytoin toxicity; possibly increased anticoagulant effects initially and then decreased effects with prolonged therapy

rifampin: Possibly decreased therapeutic effects of phenytoin

streptozocin: Possibly decreased therapeutic effects of streptozocin

sucralfate: Possibly decreased phenytoin absorption

tricyclic antidepressants: Possibly lowered seizure threshold and decreased therapeutic effects of phenytoin; possibly decreased blood antidepressant level

valproic acid: Decreased blood phenytoin level, increased blood valproic acid level

vitamin D analogues: Decreased vitamin D analogue activity

xanthines: Possibly inhibited phenytoin absorption and increased clearance of xanthines

zaleplon: Increased clearance and decreased effectiveness of zaleplon

ACTIVITIES

alcohol use: Possibly decreased phenytoin effectiveness

Adverse Reactions

CNS: Agitation, amnesia, asthenia, ataxia, cerebral edema, chills, coma, confusion, CVA, delusions, depression, dizziness, emotional lability, encephalitis, encephalopathy, extrapyramidal reactions, fever, headache, hemiplegia, hostility, hypoesthesia, lack of coordination, malaise, meningitis, nervousness, neurosis, paralysis, personality disorder, positive Babinski's sign, seizures, somnolence, speech disorders, stupor, subdural hematoma, syncope, transient paresthesia, tremor, vertigo

CV: Atrial flutter, bradycardia, bundle-branch block, cardiac arrest, cardiomegaly, edema, heart failure, hypertension, hypotension, orthostatic hypotension, palpitations, PVCs, shock, tachycardia, thrombophlebitis

EENT: Amblyopia, conjunctivitis, diplopia, dry mouth, earache, epistaxis, eye pain, gingival hyperplasia, hearing loss, hyperacusis, increased salivation, loss of taste, mydriasis, nystagmus, pharyngitis, photophobia, rhinitis, sinusitis, taste perversion, tinnitus, tongue swelling, visual field defects

ENDO: Diabetes insipidus, hyperglycemia, ketosis

GI: Anorexia, constipation, diarrhea, dysphagia, elevated liver function test results, flatulence, gastritis, GI bleeding, hepatic necrosis, hepatitis, ileus, indigestion, nausea, vomiting

GU: Albuminuria, dysuria, incontinence, oliguria, polyuria, renal failure, urine retention, vaginal candidiasis

HEME: Anemia, easy bruising, leukopenia, thrombocytopenia

MS: Arthralgia, back pain, leg cramps, muscle twitching, myalgia, myasthenia, myoclonus, myopathy

RESP: Apnea, asthma, atelectasis, bronchitis, dyspnea, hemoptysis, hyperventilation, hypoxia, increased cough, increased sputum production, pneumonia, pneumothorax

SKIN: Contact dermatitis, diaphoresis, maculopapular or pustular rash, nodules, photosensitivity, skin discoloration, Stevens-Johnson syndrome, transient pruritus, urticaria

Other: Cachexia, cryptococcosis, dehydration, facial edema, flu-like symptoms, hyperkalemia, hypokalemia, hypophosphatemia, infection, injection site reaction, lymphadenopathy, sepsis

Nursing Considerations

- **WARNING** Express the dosage, concentration, and infusion rate of fosphenytoin in PE units. Misreading an order or a label could result in a massive overdose.
- Dilute drug in D₅W or normal saline solution to 1.5 to 25 mg PE/ml. Use within 8 hours if stored at room temperature or within 24 hours if refrigerated.
- Inspect parenteral solution before administration. Discard solution that contains particles or is discolored.
- Be aware that drug is also administered by I.M. injection for maintenance doses. I.M. injection shouldn't be given for status epilepticus because I.V. route allows faster onset and peak.

- Keep in mind that I.V. fosphenytoin administration doesn't require use of a filter, as does phenytoin administration.
- Don't administer fosphenytoin solution at a rate exceeding 150 mg PE/minute because of the risk of hypotension. For a 50-kg (110-lb) patient, infusion typically takes 5 to 7 minutes. Be aware that I.V. fosphenytoin may be administered more rapidly than I.V. phenytoin.
- Follow loading dose with maintenance dosage of oral or parenteral phenytoin or parenteral fosphenytoin, as prescribed.
- As prescribed, give an I.V. benzodiazepine (such as lorazepam or diazepam) with fosphenytoin; otherwise, drug's full antiepileptic effect won't be immediate.
- Monitor ECG, blood pressure, and respiratory function during fosphenytoin infusion and for 10 to 20 minutes afterward.
- Expect to obtain blood fosphenytoin (phenytoin) level 2 hours after infusion. Therapeutic level generally ranges from 10 to 20 mcg/ml; steady state may be reached after several days to several weeks.
- Be aware that fosphenytoin may be substituted for oral phenytoin sodium at same total daily dose and frequency. If prescribed, give daily amount in two or more divided doses to maintain seizure control.
- When switching between phenytoin and fosphenytoin, remember that small differences in phenytoin bioavailability can lead to significant changes in blood phenytoin level and an increased risk of toxicity.
- If drug causes transient, infusion-related paresthesia and pruritus, decrease dosage or discontinue infusion, as ordered.
- Monitor CBC for thrombocytopenia or leukopenia—signs of hematologic toxicity. Also monitor serum albumin level and results of renal and liver function tests.
- Anticipate increased frequency and severity of adverse reactions after I.V. administration in patients with hepatic or renal impairment or hypoalbuminemia.
- Discontinue drug, as ordered, if patient develops signs of hypersensitivity—such as acute hepatotoxicity (hepatic necrosis and hepatitis), fever, lymphadenopathy, and skin reactions—during first 2 months of therapy.
- Monitor blood phenytoin level to detect early signs of toxicity, such as diplopia, nausea, confusion, slurred speech, and vomiting. Expect to reduce dosage or stop drug if such signs occur.

- **WARNING** Monitor patient for seizures because phenytoin is excitatory at toxic levels.
- **WARNING** If patient has bradycardia or heart block rhythm, notify prescriber and expect to withhold drug because severe CV reactions and death have occurred.
- Expect to provide vitamin D supplement if patient has inadequate dietary intake and is receiving long-term anticonvulsant treatment.
- Document type, onset, and characteristics of seizures as well as response to treatment.
- Before diluting fosphenytoin, store it at 2° to 8° C (36° to 46° F); don't freeze.

PATIENT TEACHING
- Inform patient that fosphenytoin typically is used for short-term treatment.
- Instruct patient to immediately report bothersome symptoms, especially rash and swollen glands.
- Because gingival hyperplasia may develop during long-term therapy, emphasize the importance of good oral hygiene and gum massage.
- Urge patient to consume an adequate amount of vitamin D–rich foods.

furosemide

Lasix, Lasix Special (CAN), Uritol (CAN)

Class and Category

Chemical: Sulfonamide
Therapeutic: Antihypertensive, diuretic
Pregnancy category: C

Indications and Dosages

▶ *To reduce edema caused by cirrhosis, heart failure, and renal disease, including nephrotic syndrome*

I.V. INFUSION, I.V. INJECTION

Adults. 20 to 40 mg as a single dose, increased by 20 mg every 2 hr until desired response occurs.

Children. 1 mg/kg as a single dose, increased by 1 mg/kg every 2 hr until desired response occurs. *Maximum:* 6 mg/kg/dose.

DOSAGE ADJUSTMENT Initial single dose limited to 20 mg for elderly patients.

▶ *To manage mild to moderate hypertension, as adjunct to treat acute pulmonary edema and hypertensive crisis*
I.V. INFUSION, I.V. INJECTION
Adults with normal renal function. 40 to 80 mg as a single dose over several min.
Adults with acute renal failure or pulmonary edema. 100 to 200 mg as a single dose over several min.
DOSAGE ADJUSTMENT For patients with acute pulmonary edema without hypertensive crisis, dosage reduced to 40 mg, followed by 80 mg 1 hr later if therapeutic response doesn't occur.

Route	Onset	Peak	Duration
I.V.	5 min	30 min	2 hr

Mechanism of Action

Inhibits sodium and water reabsorption in the loop of Henle and increases urine formation. As the body's plasma volume decreases, aldosterone production increases, which promotes sodium reabsorption and the loss of potassium and hydrogen ions. Furosemide also increases the excretion of calcium, magnesium, bicarbonate, ammonium, and phosphate. By reducing intracellular and extracellular fluid volume, the drug reduces blood pressure and decreases cardiac output. Over time, cardiac output returns to normal.

Incompatibilities

Don't mix furosemide (a milky, buffered alkaline solution) with highly acidic solutions.

Contraindications

Anuria unresponsive to furosemide; hypersensitivity to furosemide, sulfonamides, or their components

Interactions

DRUGS
ACE inhibitors: Possibly first-dose hypotension
aminoglycosides, cisplatin: Increased risk of ototoxicity
amiodarone: Increased risk of arrhythmias from hypokalemia
chloral hydrate: Possibly diaphoresis, hot flashes, and hypertension
digoxin: Increased risk of digitalis toxicity associated with hypokalemia

insulin, oral antidiabetic drugs: Increased blood glucose level
lithium: Increased risk of lithium toxicity
NSAIDs: Possibly decreased diuresis
phenytoin, probenecid: Possibly decreased therapeutic effects of furosemide
propranolol: Possibly increased blood propranolol level
thiazide diuretics: Possibly profound diuresis and electrolyte imbalance
ACTIVITIES
alcohol use: Possibly increased hypotensive and diuretic effects of furosemide

Adverse Reactions

CNS: Dizziness, fever, headache, paresthesia, restlessness, vertigo, weakness
CV: Orthostatic hypotension, shock, thromboembolism, thrombophlebitis
EENT: Blurred vision, ototoxicity, stomatitis, tinnitus, transient hearing loss (rapid I.V. injection), yellow vision
ENDO: Hyperglycemia
GI: Abdominal cramps, anorexia, constipation, diarrhea, indigestion, nausea, pancreatitis, vomiting
GU: Bladder spasms, glycosuria
HEME: Agranulocytosis (rare), anemia, aplastic anemia (rare), azotemia, hemolytic anemia, leukopenia, thrombocytopenia
MS: Muscle spasms
SKIN: Erythema multiforme, exfoliative dermatitis, jaundice, photosensitivity, pruritus, purpura, rash, urticaria
Other: Allergic reaction (interstitial nephritis, necrotizing vasculitis, systemic vasculitis), dehydration, hyperuricemia, hypochloremia, hypokalemia, hyponatremia, hypovolemia

Nursing Considerations

- Obtain patient's weight before and periodically during furosemide therapy to monitor fluid loss.
- For once-a-day dosing, give furosemide in the morning so patient's sleep won't be interrupted by increased need to urinate during the night.
- Prepare drug for infusion with normal saline solution, lactated Ringer's solution, or D_5W. Use within 24 hours.
- Administer drug slowly over 1 to 2 minutes to prevent ototoxicity. Expect to administer high doses by controlled I.V. infusion

at a rate not exceeding 4 mg/minute.

• Expect patient to have periodic hearing tests during prolonged or high-dose I.V. therapy.

• Monitor blood pressure and hepatic and renal function as well as BUN, blood glucose, and serum creatinine, electrolyte, and uric acid levels, as appropriate.

• Be aware that elderly patients are more susceptible to drug's hypotensive and electrolyte-altering effects and thus are at greater risk for shock and thromboembolism.

• **WARNING** Be aware that administration of furosemide in patients with advanced hepatic cirrhosis, especially those who also have a history of electrolyte imbalance or hepatic encephalopathy, may lead to lethal hepatic coma. Assess patient with cirrhosis for signs of deteriorating hepatic function, such as confusion, decreasing mental alertness, lethargy, and asterixis.

• If patient is at high risk for hypokalemia, give potassium supplements along with furosemide, as prescribed.

• Expect to discontinue furosemide at maximum dosage if oliguria persists for longer than 24 hours.

• Be aware that furosemide therapy may worsen left ventricular hypertrophy and adversely affect glucose tolerance and lipid metabolism.

• Notify prescriber if patient experiences hearing loss, vertigo, or ringing, buzzing, or sense of fullness in her ears. Drug may need to be discontinued.

• Store drug at 15° to 30° C (59° to 86° F); protect from freezing and light.

PATIENT TEACHING

• Advise patient receiving furosemide therapy to change position slowly to minimize the effects of orthostatic hypotension, and to take furosemide with food or milk to reduce the risk of GI distress.

• Caution patient against drinking alcoholic beverages, standing for prolonged periods, and exercising in hot weather because these actions increase the hypotensive effect of furosemide.

• Emphasize the importance of controlling weight and diet, especially of limiting sodium intake.

• Unless contraindicated, urge patient to eat more high-potassium foods and to take a potassium supplement, if prescribed, to prevent hypokalemia.

- Instruct patient to keep follow-up appointments with prescriber to monitor progress. Urge her to report persistent, severe nausea, vomiting, and diarrhea because these reactions may cause dehydration.
- Inform diabetic patient that she should check her blood glucose level often.

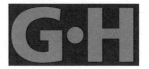

ganciclovir sodium

Cytovene (CAN), Cytovene-IV

Class and Category

Chemical: Acyclic guanosine analogue
Therapeutic: Antiviral
Pregnancy category: C

Indications and Dosages

▶ *To treat cytomegalovirus (CMV) retinitis in immunocompromised patients, including patients with AIDS*

I.V. INFUSION

Adults and adolescents. *Induction:* 5 mg/kg over at least 1 hr every 12 hr for 14 to 21 days. *Maintenance:* 5 mg/kg over at least 1 hr daily for 7 days/wk, or 6 mg/kg over at least 1 hr daily for 5 days/wk.

▶ *To prevent CMV disease in transplant recipients at risk for it*

I.V. INFUSION

Adults and adolescents. *Induction:* 5 mg/kg over at least 1 hr every 12 hr for 7 to 14 days. *Maintenance:* 5 mg/kg over at least 1 hr daily for 7 days/wk or 6 mg/kg over at least 1 hr daily for 5 days/wk.

DOSAGE ADJUSTMENT For patients with impaired renal function, dosage reduced as follows: for creatinine clearance of 50 to 69 ml/min/1.73 m^2, induction and maintenance dosages reduced to 2.5 mg/kg every 12 hr; for clearance of 25 to 49 ml/min/1.73 m^2, induction dosage reduced to 2.5 mg/kg every 24 hr and maintenance dosage reduced to 1.25 mg/kg every 24 hr; for clearance of 10 to 24 ml/min/1.73 m^2, induction dosage reduced to 1.25 mg/kg every 24 hr and maintenance dosage reduced to 0.625 mg/kg every 24 hr; and for clearance of less than 10 ml/min/1.73 m^2, induction dosage reduced to 1.25 mg/kg three times/wk after dialysis and maintenance dosage reduced to 0.625 mg/kg three times/wk after dialysis.

Mechanism of Action

Inhibits replication of CMV. Infected cells take up ganciclovir, which is then converted by cellular enzymes to ganciclovir triphosphate. Ganciclovir triphosphate is incorporated into the DNA chain and inhibits viral DNA polymerase, an enzyme used in the viral DNA replication process. This inhibits DNA synthesis by suppressing the ability of the DNA chain to elongate, which is part of the cellular replication process. Uninfected cells also take up ganciclovir and produce low levels of ganciclovir triphosphate, but the drug inhibits viral DNA polymerase more effectively than it inhibits cellular polymerase.

Incompatibilities

Don't mix ganciclovir with bacteriostatic water for injection containing parabens because a precipitate may form.

Contraindications

Hypersensitivity to ganciclovir or acyclovir

Interactions

DRUGS

blood-dyscrasia–causing drugs (such as cephalosporins and sulfasalazine), bone marrow depressants (such as carboplatin and lomustine): Possibly additive bone marrow depression

didanosine: Increased blood didanosine level, possibly increased blood ganciclovir level

imipenem and cilastatin: Possible risk of generalized seizures

nephrotoxic drugs (such as amphotericin B, cyclosporine, and tacrolimus): Possibly increased serum creatinine level, increased risk of impaired renal function, decreased ganciclovir elimination, and increased risk of ganciclovir toxicity

probenecid: Possibly decreased ganciclovir elimination and increased risk of ganciclovir toxicity

zidovudine: Possibly hematologic toxicity

Adverse Reactions

CNS: Fever, mental and mood changes, nervousness, neuropathy, tremors

GI: Abdominal pain, anorexia, diarrhea, elevated liver function test results, nausea, vomiting

HEME: Anemia, granulocytopenia, leukopenia, neutropenia, thrombocytopenia

SKIN: Rash

Other: Infusion site pain

Nursing Considerations

- Monitor CBC and platelet count before initiating ganciclovir therapy, every 2 days during induction, and at least once a week thereafter. Expect to perform daily neutrophil and platelet counts in patients undergoing hemodialysis, patients with neutrophil counts less than 1,000/mm^3 at beginning of treatment, and patients who have had leukopenia during previous treatment with ganciclovir or other nucleoside analogues.
- Be aware that ganciclovir shouldn't be given to patient with neutrophil count of less than 500/mm^3 or platelet count of less than 25,000/mm^3.
- Be aware that ganciclovir shares some mutagenic and carcinogenic properties of antineoplastics. Follow facility protocols for preparation and handling of such drugs and for appropriate disposal of used equipment.
- **WARNING** Avoid inhaling, ingesting, or coming in direct contact with ganciclovir. If ganciclovir solution comes in contact with your skin or mucosa, wash it off thoroughly with soap and water. If drug comes in contact with your eye, irrigate it thoroughly with plain water.
- To reconstitute ganciclovir, add 10 ml of sterile water for injection to 500-mg vial to yield a concentration of 50 mg/ml. Don't use bacteriostatic water for injection containing parabens to reconstitute ganciclovir because a precipitate may form. Shake vial until solution is clear. Store at room temperature and use within 12 hours.
- Further dilute reconstituted ganciclovir, typically with 100 ml of normal saline solution, D$_5$W, lactated Ringer's solution, or Ringer's solution, to a final concentration of 10 mg/ml or less. Refrigerate if not given immediately. Use within 24 hours.
- Infuse ganciclovir at a constant rate, over at least 1 hour, through a central or peripheral line. Ensure that patient is adequately hydrated, as ordered.
- Expect to administer no more than 1.25 mg/kg/24 hours if patient receives hemodialysis. Administer ganciclovir dose after hemodialysis to prevent decreased plasma ganciclovir level.
- Be aware that reinduction treatment may be ordered if CMV retinitis progresses while patient is on maintenance therapy.
- Monitor renal and liver function tests, as ordered. Anticipate a dosage adjustment or increased dosing intervals if renal function test results are elevated.

- Observe patient for fever, chills, pharyngitis, tiredness or weakness, or unusual bleeding or ecchymosis. Be aware that granulocytopenia typically occurs during the first week of treatment but may occur at any time.
- Be aware that patients receiving concurrent radiation therapy are at risk for additive bone marrow depression.
- Store unopened vials below 40° C (104° F).

PATIENT TEACHING

- Inform patient that ganciclovir is not a cure for CMV retinitis and that the disease may progress during or after treatment. Explain that maintenance therapy is used to help prevent relapse.
- Advise patient to contact prescriber immediately if he notices unusual bleeding or bruising, black or tarry stools, blood in urine or stool, or red pinpoint spots on skin.
- Teach patient proper oral hygiene and encourage him to use a soft-bristled toothbrush because ganciclovir can delay healing, increase the risk of infection, and cause gingival bleeding. Advise patient to check with prescriber before undergoing any dental work.
- Stress the importance of avoiding accidental cuts from sharp objects, such as razors or fingernail clippers, because excessive bleeding or infection may occur.
- Teach patient about the need for contraception during ganciclovir treatment because drug has caused birth defects in animals. Advise female patients to use effective contraceptive method during treatment and male patients to use barrier protection during treatment and for 90 days afterward. Inform patient that ganciclovir may cause infertility.
- Stress the importance of keeping follow-up appointments, including those for ophthalmic examinations, which may be scheduled weekly during induction and every 4 weeks during maintenance therapy.

gentamicin sulfate

Cidomycin (CAN), Garamycin, G-Mycin, Jenamicin

Class and Category

Chemical: Aminoglycoside derived from *Micromonospora purpurea*
Therapeutic: Antibiotic
Pregnancy category: D

Indications and Dosages

▶ *To treat serious bacterial infections caused by aerobic gram-negative organisms and some gram-positive organisms, including* Citrobacter *species,* Enterobacter *species,* Escherichia coli, Klebsiella *species,* Proteus *species,* Pseudomonas aeruginosa, Serratia *species,* Staphylococcus aureus, *and many strains of* Streptococcus *species*

I.V. INFUSION

Adults and adolescents. 1 to 1.7 mg/kg every 8 hr for 7 to 10 days.

Children. 2 to 2.5 mg/kg every 8 hr for 7 to 10 days.

Infants. 2.5 mg/kg every 8 to 16 hr for 7 to 10 days.

Premature or full-term neonates up to age 1 week. 2.5 mg/kg every 12 to 24 hr for 7 to 10 days.

▶ *To treat uncomplicated UTI*

I.V. INFUSION

Adults and adolescents weighing 60 kg (132 lb) or more. 160 mg daily or 80 mg every 12 hr.

Adults and adolescents weighing less than 60 kg. 3 mg/kg daily or 1.5 mg/kg every 12 hr.

DOSAGE ADJUSTMENT Supplemental dose of 1 to 1.7 mg/kg (2 to 2.5 mg/kg for children) given after hemodialysis, based on severity of infection.

Mechanism of Action

Binds to negatively charged sites on the outer cell membrane of bacteria, thereby disrupting the membrane's integrity. Gentamicin also binds to bacterial ribosomal subunits and inhibits protein synthesis. Both actions lead to cell death.

Incompatibilities

Don't administer gentamicin through same I.V. line as other drugs, especially beta-lactam antibiotics (penicillins and cephalosporins), because substantial mutual inactivation may occur. Give drugs through separate sites.

Contraindications

Hypersensitivity to gentamicin or its components, hypersensitivity or serious toxic reaction to other aminoglycosides

Interactions

DRUGS

aminoglycosides (concurrent use of two or more): Decreased bacterial uptake of each drug, increased risk of ototoxicity and nephro-toxicity

cephalosporins, enflurane, methoxyflurane, vancomycin: Increased risk of nephrotoxicity

loop diuretics: Increased risk of ototoxicity and nephrotoxicity

neuromuscular blockers: Prolonged respiratory depression, increased neuromuscular blockade

penicillins: Inactivation of gentamicin by certain penicillins, increased risk of nephrotoxicity

Adverse Reactions

CNS: Acute organic mental syndrome, confusion, depression, fever, headache, increased protein in cerebrospinal fluid, lethargy, myasthenia gravis–like syndrome, neurotoxicity (dizziness, hearing loss, tinnitus, vertigo), peripheral neuropathy or encephalopathy (muscle twitching, numbness, seizures, skin tingling), pseudotumor cerebri

CV: Hypertension, hypotension, palpitations

EENT: Blurred vision, increased salivation, laryngeal edema, ototoxicity, stomatitis, vision changes

GI: Anorexia, nausea, splenomegaly, transient hepatomegaly, vomiting

GU: Nephrotoxicity

HEME: Anemia, eosinophilia, granulocytopenia, increased or decreased reticulocyte count, leukopenia, thrombocytopenia

MS: Arthralgia, leg cramps

RESP: Pulmonary fibrosis, respiratory depression

SKIN: Alopecia, generalized burning sensation, pruritus, purpura, rash, urticaria

Other: Anaphylaxis, injection site pain, superinfection, weight loss

Nursing Considerations

- Before gentamicin therapy begins, expect to obtain a body fluid or tissue specimen for culture and sensitivity testing, as ordered.
- Dilute each dose with 50 to 200 ml of normal saline solution or D_5W to yield no more than 1 mg/ml. Be aware that no further dilution is needed if premixed flexible bags are used. Don't use an I.V. line with series connections when administering drug from a premixed flexible container to decrease the risk of air embolism. Don't administer if solution is discolored or contains precipitate. Administer slowly over 30 to 60 minutes.
- Expect to adjust dosage based on peak and trough blood drug levels drawn after third maintenance dose, as prescribed.

- Don't give gentamicin to pregnant women because drug can cause hearing loss in fetus.
- **WARNING** Be alert for allergic reactions—including anaphylaxis and, possibly, life-threatening asthmatic episodes—because some forms of drug contain sodium bisulfite.
- Assess for signs of other infections because gentamicin may cause overgrowth of nonsusceptible organisms.
- Be aware that premature infants, neonates, elderly patients, patients with impaired renal function, and dehydrated patients are at increased risk for nephrotoxicity.
- Be aware that premixed form contains 19.6 mEq of sodium per 50 ml. Take this into consideration if patient is on a sodium-restricted diet.
- Be aware that infants with botulism and patients with myasthenia gravis or Parkinson's disease may experience increased muscle weakness.
- Be aware that patients with impairment of cranial nerve VIII are at increased risk for ototoxicity or vestibular toxicity.
- Store vial at 15° to 30° C (59° to 86° F); store flexible bag at 2° to 30° C (36° to 86° F). Don't freeze gentamicin.

PATIENT TEACHING
- Stress the importance of completing the full course of gentamicin therapy.
- Instruct patient to immediately report adverse reactions, such as hearing loss, to avoid permanent effects.
- Emphasize the importance of keeping follow-up appointments and having diagnostic tests, such as audiometric tests and renal function tests, if ordered.

glucagon
Glucagon Diagnostic Kit, Glucagon Emergency Kit

Class and Category
Chemical: Synthetic hormone
Therapeutic: Antihypoglycemic, diagnostic aid adjunct
Pregnancy category: B

Indications and Dosages
▶ *To provide emergency treatment of severe hypoglycemia*
I.V. INJECTION
Adults and children weighing more than 20 kg (44 lb).
1 mg, repeated in 15 min if needed.

Children weighing 20 kg or less. 0.5 mg, or 0.02 to 0.03 mg/ kg, repeated in 15 min, if needed.

▶ *To provide diagnostic assistance by inhibiting bowel peristalsis in radiologic examination of GI tract*

I.V. INJECTION

Adults. 0.25 to 2 mg before procedure. Dose, route, and timing vary with segment of GI tract examined and length of procedure.

Route	Onset	Peak	Duration
I.V.	5 to 20 min*†	Unknown	90 min*‡

Mechanism of Action

Increases production of adenylate cyclase, which catalyzes the conversion of adenosine triphosphate to cAMP, a process that in turn activates phosphorylase. Phosphorylase promotes the breakdown of glycogen to glucose (glycogenolysis) in the liver. As a result, the blood glucose level increases and GI smooth muscles relax.

Incompatibilities

Don't mix glucagon with sodium chloride or solutions that have a pH of 3.0 to 9.5; use with dextrose solutions instead.

Contraindications

Hypersensitivity to glucagon or its components, pheochromocytoma

Interactions

DRUGS

oral anticoagulants: Possibly increased anticoagulant effects

Adverse Reactions

CV: Hypertension, hypotension (with hypersensitivity reaction), tachycardia

GI: Nausea, vomiting

RESP: Bronchospasm, respiratory distress

SKIN: Urticaria

Nursing Considerations

• Rouse patient as quickly as possible because prolonged hypoglycemia can cause cerebral damage.

---

* For antihypoglycemic action.
† 45 sec to 1 min for smooth-muscle relaxation.
‡ 9 to 25 min for smooth-muscle relaxation.

- For I.V. use, reconstitute a 1-mg vial of glucagon with 1 ml of diluent or a 10-mg vial with 10 ml of diluent. Don't give more than 1 mg/ml. For large doses, dilute with sterile water for injection.
- Before injecting glucagon, place unconscious patient on his side to prevent aspiration of vomitus when he regains consciousness.
- Administer by slow I.V. injection to decrease the risk of adverse reactions, such as tachycardia and vomiting.
- If patient doesn't respond to glucagon, expect to administer I.V. dextrose.
- When patient has regained consciousness or as soon as diagnostic procedure is completed, give him oral carbohydrates to restore hepatic glycogen stores and prevent secondary hypoglycemia.
- Keep in mind that glucagon isn't effective in patients with depleted hepatic glycogen stores caused by such conditions as adrenal insufficiency, chronic hypoglycemia, and starvation.

PATIENT TEACHING
- Instruct patient to monitor his blood glucose level, especially when signs of hypoglycemia occur.
- Teach patient and family members how to recognize signs of hypoglycemia and when to notify prescriber.
- Advise patient to carry candy or other simple sugars with him to treat early hypoglycemia.
- Emphasize the importance of a consistent diet, regular exercise, and proper use of insulin or an oral antidiabetic drug.
- Make sure unstable diabetic patients and family members know how to give glucagon subcutaneously in case of hypoglycemia. Instruct family members to keep patient on his side and give him a carbohydrate when he awakens. Advise against giving fluids by mouth until patient is fully conscious.
- Instruct patient and family members to call for emergency medical assistance after glucagon treatment, especially if patient can't ingest oral glucose or if he's taking the sulfonylurea chlorpropamide, in case secondary hypoglycemia occurs.

glycopyrrolate
Robinul

Class and Category
Chemical: Quaternary ammonium compound

Therapeutic: Antiarrhythmic, anticholinergic, cholinergic adjunct
Pregnancy category: B

Indications and Dosages

▶ *To treat peptic ulcer disease*
I.V, INJECTION
Adults and adolescents. 0.1 to 0.2 mg every 4 hr, p.r.n. *Maximum:* 4 doses daily.

▶ *To counteract intraoperative and anesthesia-induced arrhythmias*
I.V. INJECTION
Adults and adolescents. 0.1 mg, repeated every 2 to 3 min, if needed.
Children over age 2. 0.0044 mg/kg, repeated every 2 to 3 min, if needed. *Maximum:* 0.1 mg as a single dose.

▶ *As cholinergic adjunct in curariform block*
I.V. INJECTION
Adults and children over age 2. 0.2 mg glycopyrrolate for each 1 mg neostigmine or 5 mg pyridostigmine when given together.

Route	Onset	Peak	Duration
I.V.	1 min	Unknown	2 to 3 hr*

Mechanism of Action

Inhibits acetylcholine's action on postganglionic muscarinic receptors throughout the body. Depending on the receptors' location, glycopyrrolate produces various effects, such as:

• reducing the volume and acidity of gastric secretions
• controlling excessive bronchial, pharyngeal, and tracheal secretions and dilating the bronchi
• inhibiting vagal stimulation of the heart
• relaxing smooth muscle in the GI and GU tracts.

Incompatibilities

Don't mix glycopyrrolate with alkaline drugs or solutions with a pH over 6.0 because drug stability may be affected. A pH over 6.0 may occur if glycopyrrolate is mixed with dexamethasone sodium phosphate or LR solution. Gas or precipitate may form if glycopyrrolate is mixed in same syringe as chloramphenicol, diazepam,

---

* For vagal blocking effect.

dimenhydrinate, methohexital sodium, pentobarbital sodium, secobarbital sodium, sodium bicarbonate, or thiopental sodium.

Contraindications

Angle-closure glaucoma, asthma, hemorrhage with unstable cardiovascular status, hepatic disease, hypersensitivity to anticholinergics, ileus, intestinal atony, myasthenia gravis, obstructive GI or urinary disorders, severe ulcerative colitis, toxic megacolon

Interactions

DRUGS

anticholinergics, antiparkinsonian drugs, phenothiazines, tricyclic antidepressants: Possibly increased anticholinergic effects

antidiarrheals (adsorbent): Decreased glycopyrrolate absorption, leading to decreased therapeutic effectiveness

antimyasthenics: Possibly reduced intestinal motility

atenolol: Possibly potentiated atenolol effects

calcium- or magnesium-containing antacids, carbonic anhydrase inhibitors, citrates, sodium bicarbonate: Possibly reduced excretion of glycopyrrolate and increased therapeutic and adverse effects

cyclopropane: Possibly ventricular arrhythmias

digoxin: Possibly potentiated digoxin effects

haloperidol, phenothiazines: Possibly decreased effectiveness of these drugs

ketoconazole: Possibly decreased ketoconazole absorption

metoclopramide: Possibly antagonized effects of metoclopramide

opioids: Possibly severe constipation and urine retention, risk of ileus

potassium chloride: Possibly increased severity of potassium chloride–induced gastric lesions

Adverse Reactions

CNS: Confusion, dizziness, drowsiness, headache, insomnia, nervousness, weakness

CV: Bradycardia (low doses), heart block, palpitations, prolonged QT interval, tachycardia (high doses)

EENT: Blurred vision, cycloplegia, dilated pupils, dry mouth, increased intraocular pressure, loss of taste, mydriasis, nasal congestion, photophobia, taste perversion

GI: Abdominal distention, constipation, dysphagia, nausea, vomiting

GU: Impotence, urinary hesitancy, urine retention

RESP: Dyspnea

SKIN: Decreased sweating (heat exhaustion), dry skin, flushing, pruritus, urticaria
Other: Anaphylaxis

Nursing Considerations

- Use glycopyrrolate cautiously in patients with autonomic neuropathy, hepatic disease, mild to moderate ulcerative colitis, prostatic hypertrophy, or hiatal hernia because drug's anticholinergic effect can worsen these conditions; gastric ulcer because drug may delay gastric emptying; and renal disease because drug excretion may be altered.
- For I.V. use, administer by direct injection without diluting. Or inject into tubing of a flowing I.V. solution unless it contains an alkaline drug or sodium bicarbonate.
- Closure system contains dry natural rubber that may cause hypersensitivity reaction if handled by or used to inject someone with latex sensitivity.
- Use continuous cardiac monitoring, as ordered, to assess patient for arrhythmias during drug administration.
- **WARNING** Check all doses carefully because even a slight overdose can lead to toxicity.
- To prevent overheating caused by decreased sweating, adjust the room temperature and make sure patient is well hydrated.

PATIENT TEACHING

- Caution patient about possible drowsiness and dizziness and need to avoid hazardous activities until drug effects are known.
- Suggest that he use sugarless hard candy, ice, or saliva substitute to relieve dry mouth.
- Tell patient to notify prescriber about abdominal distention, trouble breathing or urinating, eye pain, irregular heartbeat, sensitivity to light, or severe constipation.
- Inform male patient that reversible impotence may occur during therapy.
- If urinary hesitancy occurs, advise patient to void before taking each dose.

granisetron hydrochloride
Kytril

Class and Category
Chemical: Carbazole
Therapeutic: Antiemetic
Pregnancy category: B

Indications and Dosages

▶ *To prevent nausea and vomiting caused by chemotherapy*
I.V. INFUSION

Adults and adolescents. 10 mcg/kg diluted and infused over 5 min, starting 30 min before chemotherapy; or 10 mcg/kg undiluted and infused over 30 sec, starting 30 min before chemotherapy.

▶ *To prevent or treat postoperative nausea and vomiting*
I.V. INJECTION

Adults and adolescents. For prevention, 1 mg given over 30 sec before anesthesia induction or immediately before anesthesia reversal. For treatment, 1 mg given over 30 sec after surgery.

Mechanism of Action

Has a high affinity for serotonin receptors along vagal nerve endings in the intestines. Because of this affinity, granisetron prevents the nausea and vomiting that usually result when serotonin is released by damaged enterochromaffin cells.

Incompatibilities

Don't mix granisetron in same solution as other drugs.

Contraindications

Hypersensitivity to granisetron or its components

Interactions

DRUGS

ketoconazole: May inhibit effectiveness of granisetron
phenobarbital: Increased total plasma clearance of I.V. granisetron

Adverse Reactions

CNS: Asthenia, chills, CNS stimulation, drowsiness, fever, headache, insomnia, somnolence
CV: Hypertension
EENT: Taste perversion
GI: Abdominal pain, anorexia, constipation, diarrhea, elevated liver function test results, nausea, vomiting
HEME: Anemia, leukopenia, thrombocytopenia
SKIN: Alopecia

Nursing Considerations

• For use with chemotherapy, dilute I.V. preparation of granisetron with normal saline solution or D_5W to a total volume of 20 to 50 ml. Mixture may be stored for up to 24 hours. Use only on days when chemotherapy is given.

PATIENT TEACHING
• Inform patient that granisetron is given I.V. before chemotherapy to help prevent nausea.
• Advise patient to report constipation, fever, severe diarrhea, or severe headache. Caution about possible drowsiness.

heparin calcium
Calcilean (CAN), Calciparine
heparin sodium
Hepalean (CAN), Heparin Leo (CAN), Heparin Lock Flush, Liquaemin

Class and Category
Chemical: Glycosaminoglycan
Therapeutic: Anticoagulant
Pregnancy category: C

Indications and Dosages
▶ *To prevent and treat deep vein thrombosis and pulmonary embolism, to treat peripheral arterial embolism, and to prevent thromboembolism before and after cardioversion of chronic atrial fibrillation*
I.V. INFUSION, I.V. INJECTION
Adults. *Loading:* 35 to 70 units/kg or 5,000 units by injection. Then 20,000 to 40,000 units infused over 24 hr.
Children. *Loading:* 50 units/kg by injection. Then 100 units/kg infused every 4 hr or 20,000 units/m^2 infused over 24 hr.
I.V. INJECTION
Adults. *Initial:* 10,000 units. *Maintenance:* 5,000 to 10,000 units every 4 to 6 hr.
Children. *Initial:* 50 units/kg. *Maintenance:* 100 units/kg/dose every 4 hr.
I.V. INJECTION
Adults. *Loading:* 5,000 units I.V.; then 10,000 to 20,000 units subcutaneously. *Maintenance:* 8,000 to 10,000 units subcutaneously every 8 hr or 15,000 to 20,000 units subcutaneously every 12 hr.
▶ *To diagnose and treat disseminated intravascular coagulation (DIC)*
I.V. INFUSION, I.V. INJECTION
Adults. 50 to 100 units/kg every 4 hr. Drug may be discontinued if no improvement occurs in 4 to 8 hr.

Children. 25 to 50 units/kg every 4 hr. Drug may be discontinued if no improvement occurs in 4 to 8 hr.

▶ *To prevent clots in patients undergoing open-heart and vascular surgery*

I.V. INFUSION, I.V. INJECTION

Adults. 300 units/kg for procedures that last less than 60 min; 400 units/kg for procedures that last longer than 60 min. *Minimum:* 150 units/kg.

Children. 300 units/kg for procedures that last less than 60 min. Then dosage is based on coagulation test results. *Minimum:* 150 units/kg.

▶ *To maintain heparin lock patency*

I.V. INJECTION

Adults. 10 to 100 units/ml heparin flush solution (enough to fill device) after each use of device.

Route	Onset	Peak	Duration
I.V.	Immediate	Minutes	Unknown

Mechanism of Action

Binds with antithrombin III, enhancing antithrombin III's inactivation of the coagulation enzymes thrombin (factor IIa) and factors Xa and XIa. At low doses, heparin inhibits factor Xa and prevents the conversion of prothrombin to thrombin. Thrombin is necessary for the conversion of fibrinogen to fibrin; without fibrin, clots can't form. At high doses, heparin inactivates thrombin, preventing fibrin formation and existing clot extension.

Incompatibilities

Don't mix heparin with any other drug unless you have an order to do so and have checked with pharmacist. Heparin is incompatible with many drugs and solutions, especially ones that contain a phosphate buffer, sodium bicarbonate, or sodium oxalate.

Contraindications

Hypersensitivity to heparin or its components; severe thrombocytopenia; uncontrolled bleeding, except in DIC

Interactions

DRUGS

antihistamines, digoxin, nicotine, tetracyclines: Decreased anticoagulant effect of heparin *aspirin, NSAIDs, platelet aggregation inhibitors, sulfinpyrazone:* Increased platelet inhibition and risk of bleeding

cefamandole, cefoperazone, cefotetan, methimazole, plicamycin, propylthiouracil, valproic acid: Possibly hypoprothrombinemia and increased risk of bleeding

chloroquine, hydroxychloroquine: Possibly thrombocytopenia and increased risk of hemorrhage

ethacrynic acid, glucocorticoids, salicylates: Increased risk of bleeding and GI ulceration and hemorrhage

nitroglycerin (I.V.): Possibly decreased anticoagulant effect of heparin

probenecid: Possibly increased anticoagulant effect of heparin

thrombolytics: Increased risk of hemorrhage

ACTIVITIES

smoking: Decreased anticoagulant effect of heparin

Adverse Reactions

CNS: Chills, dizziness, fever, headache, peripheral neuropathy

CV: Chest pain, thrombosis

EENT: Epistaxis, gingival bleeding, rhinitis

GI: Abdominal distention and pain, hematemesis, melena, nausea, vomiting

GU: Hematuria, hypermenorrhea

HEME: Easy bruising, excessive bleeding from wounds, thrombocytopenia

MS: Back pain, myalgia, osteoporosis

RESP: Dyspnea, wheezing

SKIN: Alopecia, cyanosis, petechiae, pruritus, urticaria

Other: Anaphylaxis; injection site hematoma, irritation, pain, redness, and ulceration

Nursing Considerations

- **WARNING** Be aware that heparin sodium injection is not recommended for use in neonates because it contains the preservative benzyl alcohol, which has been linked to fatal "gasping syndrome" when given intravenously to children less than 1 month old.
- Use drug cautiously in alcoholics; menstruating women; patients over age 60, especially women; and patients with mild hepatic or renal disease or a history of allergies, asthma, or GI ulcer.
- **WARNING** Give heparin only by subcutaneous or I.V routes.; I.M. use causes hematoma, irritation, and pain.
- Avoid injecting any drugs by I.M. route during heparin therapy to decrease the risk of bleeding and hematoma.

- **WARNING** Be vigilant when examining heparin sodium injection vials to make sure you have the correct strength. Children have died after heparin vials were confused with "catheter lock flush" vials.
- To prepare heparin for continuous infusion, invert container at least six times to prevent drug from pooling. Anticipate slight discoloration of prepared solution; it doesn't indicate a change in potency.
- During continuous I.V. therapy, expect to obtain APTT after 8 hours of therapy. Use the arm opposite the infusion site.
- For intermittent I.V. therapy, expect to adjust heparin dose based on coagulation test results performed 30 minutes earlier. Therapeutic range is typically 1.5 to 2.5 times the control.
- Take safety precautions to prevent bleeding, such as having patient use a soft-bristled toothbrush and an electric razor.
- Monitor blood test results and observe for signs of bleeding, such as ecchymosis, epistaxis, hematemesis, hematuria, melena, and petechiae. If a recurrent thrombosis develops, notify prescriber and expect heparin to be discontinued.
- Make sure all health care providers know that patient is receiving heparin.
- Keep protamine sulfate on hand to use as an antidote for heparin. Be aware that each milligram of protamine sulfate neutralizes 100 units of heparin.
- Be aware that prescriber may order oral anticoagulants before discontinuing heparin to avoid increased coagulation caused by heparin withdrawal. Heparin may be discontinued when full therapeutic effect of oral anticoagulant is achieved.
- Know that women over age 60 have the highest risk of hemorrhage during therapy.
- Be aware that heparin-induced thrombocytopenia may develop up to several weeks after heparin has been discontinued and may progress to venous and arterial thromboses.

PATIENT TEACHING
- Tell patient that heparin can't be taken orally.
- Explain the increased risk of bleeding; urge her to avoid injuries and to use a soft-bristled toothbrush and an electric razor.
- Advise patient to avoid drugs that interact with heparin, such as aspirin and ibuprofen.
- Instruct patient and family to report abdominal or lower back pain, black stools, bleeding gums, bloody urine, excessive menstrual bleeding, nosebleeds, and severe headaches.
- Inform patient that temporary hair loss may occur.

- Advise patient to wear or carry medical identification.
- Urge patient to report any abnormal sign or symptom to prescriber, even if it occurs weeks after heparin has been discontinued; delayed adverse reactions are possible.

hydralazine hydrochloride

Apresoline (CAN)

Class and Category

Chemical: Phthalazine derivative
Therapeutic: Antihypertensive, vasodilator
Pregnancy category: C

Indications and Dosages

▶ *To manage severe essential hypertension when drug can't be taken orally or when need to reduce blood pressure is urgent*

I.V. INJECTION

Adults. 5 to 40 mg, repeated as needed.
Children. 1.7 to 3.5 mg/kg daily in divided doses every 4 to 6 hr, as needed.

Route	Onset	Peak	Duration
I.V.	5 to 20 min	10 to 80 min	2 to 6 hr

Incompatibilities

Don't mix hydralazine in I.V. infusion solutions.

Contraindications

Coronary artery disease, hypersensitivity to hydralazine or its components, mitral valve disease

---

Mechanism of Action

May act in a manner that resembles organic nitrates and sodium nitroprusside, except that hydralazine is selective for arteries. This drug:

- exerts a direct vasodilating effect on vascular smooth muscle
- interferes with calcium movement in vascular smooth muscle by altering cellular calcium metabolism
- dilates arteries rather than veins, which minimizes orthostatic hypotension and increases cardiac output and cerebral blood flow
- causes a reflex autonomic response that increases heart rate, cardiac output, and left ventricular ejection fraction
- has a positive inotropic effect on the heart.

Interactions
DRUGS
beta blockers: Increased effects of both drugs
diazoxide, MAO inhibitors, other antihypertensives: Risk of severe hypotension
epinephrine: Possibly decreased vasopressor effect of epinephrine
NSAIDs: Decreased hydralazine effects
sympathomimetics: Possibly decreased antihypertensive effect of hydralazine

Adverse Reactions
CNS: Chills, fever, headache, peripheral neuritis
CV: Angina, edema, orthostatic hypotension, palpitations, tachycardia
EENT: Lacrimation, nasal congestion
GI: Anorexia, constipation, diarrhea, nausea, vomiting
RESP: Dyspnea
SKIN: Blisters, flushing, pruritus, rash, urticaria
Other: Lupuslike symptoms (especially with high doses), lymphadenopathy

Nursing Considerations
- Monitor CBC, lupus erythematosus cell preparation, and ANA titer before hydralazine therapy and periodically, as appropriate, during long-term treatment.
- Use drug immediately after opening ampule.
- Anticipate that drug may change color in solution. Consult pharmacist if color change occurs.
- Be aware that hydralazine also may undergo color changes when exposed to a metal filter.
- Monitor blood pressure and pulse rate regularly and weigh patient daily during therapy.
- Check blood pressure with patient in lying, sitting, and standing positions, and watch for signs of orthostatic hypotension. Expect orthostatic hypotension to be most common in the morning, during hot weather, and with exercise.
- **WARNING** Expect to discontinue drug immediately if patient experiences lupuslike symptoms, such as arthralgia, fever, myalgia, pharyngitis, and splenomegaly.
- Expect prescriber to withdraw drug gradually to avoid a rapid increase in blood pressure.
- Before opening ampule, store it at 15° to 30° C (59° to 86° F); don't freeze.
- Expect to treat peripheral neuritis with pyridoxine.

PATIENT TEACHING
- Advise patient to change position slowly, especially in the morning, while receiving hydralazine. Caution her that hot showers may increase hypotension.
- Instruct patient to immediately report fever, aching muscles and joints, and sore throat.
- Urge patient to report numbness and tingling in the limbs, which may require treatment with another drug.

hydrocortisone sodium phosphate
Hydrocortone Phosphate
hydrocortisone sodium succinate
A-hydroCort, Solu-Cortef

Class and Category
Chemical: Glucocorticoid
Therapeutic: Adrenocorticoid replacement, anti-inflammatory
Pregnancy category: Not rated

Indications and Dosages
▶ *To treat severe inflammation or acute adrenal insufficiency*
I.V. INFUSION, I.V. INJECTION (HYDROCORTISONE SODIUM PHOSPHATE)
Adults. 15 to 240 mg daily as a single dose or in divided doses.
Usual: One-half to one-third the oral dose.
DOSAGE ADJUSTMENT Dosage increased to more than 240 mg daily if needed to treat acute disease.
I.V. INFUSION, I.V. INJECTION (HYDROCORTISONE SODIUM SUCCINATE)
Adults. 100 to 500 mg every 2, 4, or 6 hr.

Route	Onset	Peak	Duration
I.V. (phosphate, succinate)	Rapid	Unknown	Unknown

Mechanism of Action
Binds to intracellular glucocorticoid receptors and suppresses the inflammatory and immune responses by:
- inhibiting neutrophil and monocyte accumulation at the inflammation site and suppressing their phagocytic and bactericidal activity
- stabilizing lysosomal membranes
- suppressing the antigen response of macrophages and helper T cells
- inhibiting the synthesis of cellular mediators of the inflammatory response, such as cytokines, interleukins, and prostaglandins.

Contraindications

Hypersensitivity to hydrocortisone or its components, recent vaccination with live-virus vaccine, systemic fungal infection

Interactions

DRUGS

acetaminophen: Increased risk of hepatotoxicity

amphotericin B, carbonic anhydrase inhibitors: Possibly severe hypokalemia

anabolic steroids, androgens: Increased risk of edema and severe acne

anticholinergics: Possibly increased intraocular pressure

anticoagulants, thrombolytics: Increased risk of GI ulceration and hemorrhage, possibly decreased therapeutic effects of these drugs

asparaginase: Increased risk of hyperglycemia and toxicity

aspirin, NSAIDs: Increased risk of GI distress and bleeding

digoxin: Possibly hypokalemia-induced arrhythmias and digitalis toxicity

ephedrine, phenobarbital, phenytoin, rifampin: Decreased blood hydrocortisone level

estrogens, oral contraceptives: Possibly increased therapeutic and toxic effects of hydrocortisone

isoniazid: Possibly decreased therapeutic effects of isoniazid

mexiletine: Possibly decreased blood mexiletine level

neuromuscular blockers: Possibly increased neuromuscular blockade, causing respiratory depression or apnea

potassium-depleting drugs (such as thiazide diuretics): Possibly severe hypokalemia

potassium supplements: Possibly decreased effects of these supplements

salicylates: Possibly decreased effectiveness and blood level of salicylates

somatrem, somatropin: Possibly decreased therapeutic effects of these drugs

streptozocin: Increased risk of hyperglycemia

vaccines: Decreased antibody response and increased risk of neurologic complications

ACTIVITIES

alcohol use: Increased risk of GI distress and bleeding

Adverse Reactions

CNS: Ataxia, behavioral changes, depression, dizziness, euphoria, fatigue, headache, increased ICP with papilledema, insomnia, malaise, mood changes, paresthesia, seizures, steroid psychosis, syncope, vertigo

CV: Arrhythmias (from hypokalemia), fat embolism, heart failure, hypertension, hypotension, thromboembolism, thrombophlebitis
EENT: Exophthalmos, glaucoma, increased intraocular pressure, nystagmus, posterior subcapsular cataracts
ENDO: Adrenal insufficiency during stress, cushingoid symptoms (buffalo hump, central obesity, moon face, supraclavicular fat pad enlargement), diabetes mellitus, growth suppression in children, hyperglycemia, negative nitrogen balance from protein catabolism
GI: Abdominal distention, hiccups, increased appetite, nausea, pancreatitis, peptic ulcer, ulcerative esophagitis, vomiting
GU: Amenorrhea, glycosuria, menstrual irregularities, perineal burning or tingling
HEME: Easy bruising, leukocytosis
MS: Arthralgia; aseptic necrosis of femoral and humeral heads; compression fractures; muscle atrophy, twitching, or weakness; myalgia; osteoporosis; spontaneous fractures; steroid myopathy; tendon rupture
SKIN: Acne; altered skin pigmentation; diaphoresis; erythema; hirsutism; necrotizing vasculitis; petechiae; purpura; rash; scarring; sterile abscess; striae; subcutaneous fat atrophy; thin, fragile skin; urticaria
Other: Anaphylaxis, hypocalcemia, hypokalemia, hypokalemic alkalosis, impaired wound healing, masking of signs of infection, metabolic alkalosis, suppressed skin test reaction, weight gain

Nursing Considerations

- Be aware that systemic hydrocortisone shouldn't be given to immunocompromised patients, such as those with fungal and other infections, including amebiasis, hepatitis B, tuberculosis, vaccinia, and varicella.
- **WARNING** Don't give hydrocortisone containing benzyl alcohol to neonates or premature infants because they may develop a fatal toxic syndrome characterized by CNS, respiratory, circulatory, and renal impairment and metabolic acidosis.
- Give daily dose of hydrocortisone in the morning to mimic the normal peak in adrenocortical secretion of corticosteroids.
- Don't give acetate injectable suspension by I.V. route. This form is used for intra-articular, intralesional, and soft-tissue injection.
- Give hydrocortisone sodium succinate as direct I.V. injection over 30 seconds to several minutes, or as intermittent or continuous infusion. For infusion, dilute to 1 mg/ml or less with D_5W, normal saline solution, or dextrose 5% in normal saline

solution. Use reconstituted hydrocortisone sodium succinate within 3 days. Protect reconstituted solution from light; discard if not clear.

• **WARNING** Avoid rapid admnistration of high hydrocortisone doses, which may cause anaphylaxis, angioedema, seizures, and possibly sudden death. Maintain ECG monitoring, as prescribed, and have emergency equipment and drugs readily available.

• Dilute hydrocortisone sodium phosphate with D_5W or normal saline solution, and use diluted solution within 24 hours.

• Be aware that high-dose therapy shouldn't be given for longer than 48 hours. Be alert for depression or psychotic episodes during high-dose therapy.

• Regularly monitor weight, blood pressure, and serum electrolyte levels during therapy.

• Expect hydrocortisone to exacerbate infections or mask their signs and symptoms.

• Monitor blood glucose level in diabetic patients, and increase insulin or oral antidiabetic drug dosage, as prescribed.

• Know that elderly patients are at high risk for osteoporosis during long-term therapy.

• Anticipate the possibility of acute adrenal insufficiency with stress, such as emotional upset, fever, surgery, and trauma. Increase hydrocortisone dosage, as prescribed.

• **WARNING** Avoid withdrawing drug suddenly after long-term use because adrenal crisis can result. Expect to reduce dosage gradually and to monitor patient's response.

• Store hydrocortisone at 15° to 30° C (59° to 86° F); don't freeze.

PATIENT TEACHING

• Instruct patient receiving hydrocortisone to report early signs of adrenal insufficiency: anorexia, difficulty breathing, dizziness, fainting, fatigue, joint pain, muscle weakness, and nausea.

• Inform patient that she may bruise easily.

• Advise patient on long-term therapy to have periodic ophthalmic examinations and to carry or wear medical identification.

hydromorphone hydrochloride
(dihydromorphinone)
Dilaudid, Dilaudid-HP

Class, Category, and Schedule
Chemical: Phenanthrene derivative, semisynthetic opioid derivative

Therapeutic: Opioid analgesic
Pregnancy category: C
Controlled substance schedule: II

Indications and Dosages

▶ *To relieve moderate to severe pain*
I.V. INJECTION
Adults. 1 mg every 3 hr, p.r.n.

Route	Onset	Peak	Duration
I.V.	10 to 15 min	15 to 30 min	2 to 3 hr

Mechanism of Action

May bind with opiate receptors in the spinal cord and higher levels in the CNS. In this way, hydromorphone is believed to stimulate mu and kappa receptors, thus altering the perception of, and emotional response to, pain.

Contraindications

Acute asthma; hypersensitivity to hydromorphone, other opioid analgesics, or their components; increased ICP; severe respiratory depression; upper respiratory tract obstruction

Interactions

DRUGS

anticholinergics: Increased risk of ileus, severe constipation, or urine retention

antihypertensives, diuretics, guanadrel, guanethidine, mecamylamine: Increased risk of orthostatic hypotension

barbiturate anesthetics: Increased sedative effect of hydromorphone

belladonna alkaloids, difenoxin and atropine, diphenoxylate and atropine, kaolin pectin, loperamide, paregoric: Increased risk of CNS depression and severe constipation

buprenorphine, butorphanol, dezocine, nalbuphine, pentazocine: Possibly potentiated or suppressed symptoms of spontaneous opioid withdrawal

CNS depressants, other opioid analgesics: Additive CNS depression and hypotension

hydroxyzine: Increased analgesia, CNS depression, and hypotension

metoclopramide: Decreased effect of metoclopramide on GI motility

naloxone: Possibly withdrawal symptoms in physically dependent patients

naltrexone: Possibly prolonged respiratory depression, cardiac arrest
neuromuscular blockers: Additive CNS depression
ACTIVITIES
alcohol use: Increased CNS depression

Adverse Reactions

CNS: Anxiety, confusion, dizziness, drowsiness, euphoria, hallucinations, headache, nervousness, restlessness, sedation, somnolence, tremor, weakness
CV: Hypertension, orthostatic hypotension, palpitations, tachycardia
EENT: Blurred vision, diplopia, dry mouth, laryngeal edema, laryngospasm, nystagmus, tinnitus
GI: Abdominal cramps, anorexia, biliary tract spasm, constipation, hepatotoxicity, nausea, vomiting
GU: Dysuria, urine retention
RESP: Dyspnea, respiratory depression, wheezing
SKIN: Diaphoresis, flushing
Other: Injection site pain, redness, and swelling; physical and psychological dependence

Nursing Considerations

- To improve analgesic action, give hydromorphone before pain becomes intense.
- Instruct patient to lie down during hydromorphone administration and for a period afterward to lessen dizziness, lightheadedness, nausea, and vomiting.
- **WARNING** Administer hydromorphone slowly over several minutes. Rapid administration may cause serious adverse reactions, including anaphylaxis, severe respiratory depression, hypotension, peripheral circulatory collapse, and cardiac arrest. Make sure emergency equipment and drugs are available.
- Administer hydromorphone by direct injection over at least 2 minutes. For infusion, mix drug with D_5W, normal saline solution, or Ringer's solution.
- Watch for respiratory depression, especially in patients who are having an acute asthma attack and those with chronic respiratory disease. Children, elderly patients, and debilitated or seriously ill patients are at increased risk for respiratory depression. Keep resuscitation equipment and naloxone nearby.
- Monitor patient for evidence of drug-induced CNS depression or increased CSF pressure, such as altered LOC, restlessness, and irritability, in patients with a head injury, intracranial lesions, or other conditions that could cause these effects. Patients

who are taking, or have recently taken, drugs that cause CNS depression are also more susceptible to these effects. Take appropriate safety precautions.

• Be aware that hydromorphone may induce or worsen arrhythmias or seizures in patients with a history of these conditions and may mask symptoms of acute abdominal conditions.

• Be aware that patients with a history of drug abuse (including acute alcoholism), emotional instability, or suicidal ideation or attempts are at increased risk for opioid abuse.

• Assess patient for constipation.

• Watch for signs of physical dependence or abuse.

• Anticipate that drug may mask or worsen gallbladder pain.

• Store drug at 15° to 30° C (59° to 86° F); protect from freezing and light.

PATIENT TEACHING

• Instruct patient receiving hydromorphone to report constipation, difficulty breathing, severe nausea, or vomiting.

• Inform patient that drug may cause drowsiness and sedation. Advise her to avoid potentially hazardous activities until drug's CNS effects are known.

• Advise patient to change position slowly to minimize effects of orthostatic hypotension.

• To prevent constipation, encourage patient to consume plenty of fluids and high-fiber foods, if not contraindicated by another condition.

• Instruct patient to report pain before it becomes severe.

• Caution patient to avoid alcohol and OTC drugs during therapy, unless prescriber approves.

hyoscyamine sulfate

Levsin

Class and Category

Chemical: Belladonna alkaloid, tertiary amine
Therapeutic: Antimuscarinic, antispasmodic
Pregnancy category: C

Indications and Dosages

▶ *To treat peptic ulcers and GI tract disorders caused by spasm*

I.V. INJECTION

Adults and adolescents. 0.25 to 0.5 mg every 4 to 6 hr.

Children. Dosage individualized by weight.

▶ *To control salivation and excessive secretions during surgical procedures*

I. V. INJECTION

Adults and adolescents. 0.5 mg 30 to 60 min before procedure.

Route	Onset	Peak	Duration
I.V.	2 to 3 min	15 to 30 min	4 hr

Mechanism of Action

Competitively inhibits acetylcholine at autonomic postganglionic cholinergic receptors. Because the most sensitive receptors are in the salivary, bronchial, and sweat glands, hyoscyamine acts mainly to reduce salivary, bronchial, and sweat gland secretions. It also causes GI smooth muscle to contract and decreases gastric secretion and GI motility. In addition, hyoscyamine causes the bladder detrusor muscle to contract; reduces nasal and oropharyngeal secretions; and decreases airway resistance from relaxation of smooth muscle in the bronchi and bronchioles.

Contraindications

Acute hemorrhage and hemodynamic instability; angle-closure glaucoma; hepatic disease; hypersensitivity to hyoscyamine, other anticholinergics, or their components; ileus; intestinal atony; myasthenia gravis; myocardial ischemia; obstructive GI disease; obstructive uropathy; renal disease; severe ulcerative colitis; tachycardia; toxic megacolon

Interactions

DRUGS

anticholinergics: Possibly increased anticholingeric effects

calcium- and magnesium-containing antacids, carbonic anhydrase inhibitors, citrates, sodium bicarbonate, urinary alkalinizers: Possibly potentiated therapeutic and adverse effects of hyoscyamine

haloperidol: Possibly decreased therapeutic effects of haloperidol

ketoconazole: Possibly reduced ketoconazole absorption

metoclopramide: Possibly antagonized therapeutic effects of metoclopramide

opioid analgesics: Increased risk of severe constipation and ileus

Adverse Reactions

CNS: Drowsiness, insomnia

EENT: Blurred vision; dry mouth, nose, and throat; photophobia

ENDO: Decreased lactation
GI: Constipation
GU: Impotence, urine retention
SKIN: Decreased sweating
Other: Heatstroke, injection site redness and urticaria

Nursing Considerations

• Give hyoscyamine 30 to 60 minutes before meals and at bedtime. Give bedtime dose at least 2 hours after last meal.
• **WARNING** Expect an increased risk of drug-induced heatstroke in hot or humid weather because hyoscyamine decreases sweating.
• **WARNING** Be aware that lower doses may paradoxically decrease the heart rate and that higher doses affect nicotinic receptors in autonomic ganglia, causing delirium, disorientation, hallucinations, and restlessness.
• Monitor patients with the following conditions for exacerbations caused by drug's anticholinergic effects: arrhythmias, coronary artery disease, heart failure, hiatal hernia with reflux esophagitis, hypertension, hyperthyroidism, or tachycardia. Also monitor blood pressure in patients with toxemia from pregnancy because they're at risk for aggravated hypertension.
• Monitor urine output, and be alert for urine retention, especially in patients with autonomic neuropathy.
• Be aware that infants, patients with Down syndrome, and children with brain damage or spastic paralysis may be more sensitive to drug's effects.
• Be aware that elderly patients and patients with impaired renal function are at increased risk for adverse reactions.
• Store drug at 15° to 30° C (59° to 86° F); don't freeze.

PATIENT TEACHING

• Instruct patient to void before receiving each dose of hyoscyamine and to report trouble urinating during hyoscyamine therapy.
• Inform patient that drug may cause drowsiness. Advise her to avoid potentially hazardous activities until drug's CNS effects are known.
• If patient reports dry mouth, suggest using sugarless hard candy or gum.
• Inform male patient that drug may cause impotence. If it occurs, suggest that he discuss it with prescriber.
• Advise patient to avoid exposure to high temperatures and to increase fluid intake, unless contraindicated.

ibandronate sodium
Boniva

Class and Category
Chemical: Nitrogen-containing bisphosphonate
Therapeutic: Bone resorption inhibitor
Pregnancy category: C

Indications and Dosages
▶ *To prevent or treat osteoporosis in postmenopausal women*
I.V. INJECTION
Adults. 3 mg over 15 to 30 sec every 3 mo.

Route	Onset	Peak	Duration
I.V.	Unknown	30 min to 2 hr	Unknown

Mechanism of Action
Binds to calcified bone matrix because of its affinity for hydroxyapatite in the mineral matrix, thus reducing bone solubility, inhibiting osteoclast activity, and reducing bone resorption and turnover. In postmenopausal women, ibandronate also reduces the elevated rate of bone turnover, leading to, on average, a net gain in bone mass. These activities help prevent or alleviate the loss of bone mass in osteoporosis.

Incompatibilities
Do not give with calcium-containing solutions or other intravenous drugs.

Contraindications
Esophageal stricture or achlasia, hypersensitivity to ibandronate or its components, hypocalcemia, inability to stand or sit upright for at least 60 minutes (oral form only), severe renal impairment (parenteral form only), untreated vitamin D deficiency

Interactions
DRUGS
aspirin, NSAIDs: Increased risk of GI irritation

calcium-containing preparations, including antacids containing calcium, aluminum, magnesium, or iron: Impaired absorption of ibandronate
FOODS
all foods: Decreased ibandronate bioavailability

Adverse Reactions

CNS: Asthenia, dizziness, headache, insomnia, vertigo
CV: Hypercholesterolemia, hypertension
EENT: Conjunctivitis, nasopharyngitis, ocular pain, scleritis, uveitis, visual impairment
GI: Abdominal pain, constipation, diarrhea, dyspepsia, gastritis, nausea, vomiting
GU: UTI
MS: Arthritis; back, bone, extremity, joint, or muscle pain; joint dysfunction; localized osteoarthritis; muscle cramps; myalgia
RESP: Bronchitis, pneumonia, bronchitis, upper respiratory tract infection
SKIN: Rash
Other: Allergic reaction, angioedema, flulike symptoms, infection

Nursing Considerations

- Use needle provided with the prefilled syringe when giving ibandronate intravenously. Know that parenteral form of drug should be given only as an I.V. bolus over 15 to 30 seconds.
- Give supplemental calcium and vitamin D, as prescribed, during ibandronate therapy if patient's dietary intake of these nutrients is inadequate.
- Separate calcium supplements and antacids from ibandronate to avoid impaired drug absorption and altered effectiveness.
- Monitor patient for hypersensitivity skin reactions such as generalized rash or angioedema because such reactions, although rare, can be severe.
- Be aware that although ibandronate has not been linked to osteonecrosis, biphosphates as a group have been, especially osteonecrosis affecting the jaw. Monitor patient for complaints of jaw or bone pain, and report to prescriber.
- Know that biphosphates but not specifically ibandronate have caused severe, sometimes incapacitating bone, joint, and muscle pain. If these symptoms occur, notify prescriber and expect drug to be discontinued.

PATIENT TEACHING

- Instruct patient to take ibandronate with 6 to 8 oz of water, in an upright position, at least 1 hour before first food or drink of the day. Tell patient to avoid mineral waters that contain a higher concentration of calcium. Caution against lying down for at least 60 minutes after taking drug to prevent it from lodging in esophagus and causing irritation.

- Advise patient to report symptoms of esophageal irritation, such as new or worsening dysphagia, pain on swallowing, retrosternal pain, or heartburn.
- Tell patient not to chew or suck on tablet because of risk of oropharyngeal ulcer.
- Instruct patient taking the 150-mg tablet to do so on the same date each month. If patient misses the monthly dose and the next scheduled dose is more than 7 days away, tell patient to take one 150-mg tablet the morning after she remembers the missed dose. She should then resume the normal schedule. Caution her never to take two 150-mg tablets in the same week.
- Advise patient to take calcium supplements or antacids at different time of day than ibandronate.
- Tell patient to stop taking ibandronate and notify prescriber immediately if she has skin reactions, such as a rash, or swelling, especially of the face or throat.
- Advise patient to report jaw discomfort to prescriber.
- Urge woman of childbearing age to tell prescriber if she is, could be, or is considering pregnancy while taking ibandronate because of risk to the fetus, especially the skeleton.

ibutilide fumarate
Corvert

Class and Category
Chemical: Methanesulfonanilide derivative
Therapeutic: Class III antiarrhythmic
Pregnancy category: C

Indications and Dosages
▶ *To rapidly convert recent-onset atrial flutter or fibrillation to sinus rhythm*
I.V. INFUSION
Adults weighing 60 kg (132 lb) or more. 1 mg over 10 min. Repeated 10 min after first dose is finished if arrhythmia persists.
Adults weighing less than 60 kg. 0.01 mg/kg over 10 min. Repeated 10 min after first dose is finished if arrhythmia persists.
DOSAGE ADJUSTMENT Infusion discontinued if arrhythmia is terminated or if sustained or nonsustained ventricular tachycardia or prolonged QT or QTc interval develops.

Mechanism of Action

May promote sodium movement through slow inward sodium channels in myocardial cell membranes. Ibutilide also may inhibit a component of potassium channels in myocardial cell membranes involved in cardiac repolarization. These actions prolong the cardiac action potential by delaying repolarization and increasing atrial and ventricular refractoriness. As a result, the sinus rate slows and AV conduction is delayed.

Contraindications

Hypersensitivity to ibutilide or its components

Interactions

DRUGS

amiodarone, astemizole, disopyramide, maprotiline, phenothiazines, procainamide, quinidine, sotalol, tricyclic antidepressants: Possibly prolonged QT interval, leading to increased risk of proarrhythmias

Adverse Reactions

CNS: Headache, syncope
CV: AV block, bradycardia, bundle-branch block, heart failure, hypertension, hypotension, idioventricular rhythm, orthostatic hypotension, palpitations, prolonged QT interval, sinus and supraventricular tachycardia, supraventricular arrhythmias, ventricular arrhythmias, ventricular tachycardia (sustained and nonsustained)
GI: Nausea
GU: Renal failure

Nursing Considerations

• Before giving ibutilide, check serum electrolyte levels and expect to correct abnormalities. Be especially alert for hypokalemia and hypomagnesemia, which can lead to arrhythmias.
• Give drug undiluted, or dilute it in 50 ml of normal saline solution or D_5W. Add contents of 10-ml vial (0.1 mg/ml) to 50 ml of solution to obtain 0.017 mg/ml. Use polyvinyl chloride plastic bags or polyolefin bags for ibutilide admixtures. Administer within 24 hours (48 hours if refrigerated).
• Infuse drug slowly over 10 minutes.
• As ordered, monitor cardiac rhythm continuously during drug infusion and for at least 4 hours afterward—longer if arrhythmias appear or if patient has abnormal hepatic function. Observe for ventricular ectopy.

- **WARNING** Be aware that ibutilide use is not recommended for patients with a history of prolonged QT interval or torsades de pointes. Also be aware that patients with bradycardia, heart failure, or a history of low left ventricular ejection fraction are at increased risk for torsades de pointes and those with a history of chronic atrial fibrillation are at increased risk for recurrence after conversion to sinus rhythm.
- Before preparing ibutilide, store it at 20° to 25° C (68° to 77° F).
- Make sure that a defibrillator and drugs to treat sustained ventricular tachycardia are available during therapy and when monitoring patient after therapy.

PATIENT TEACHING
- Inform patient that ibutilide will be given by I.V. infusion and that his heart rhythm will be monitored continuously.
- Ask patient to report chest pain, faintness, numbness, tingling, palpitations, and shortness of breath.
- Advise patient to keep appointments to monitor heart rhythm.

imipenem and cilastatin sodium

Primaxin (CAN), Primaxin ADD-Vantage, Primaxin IM, Primaxin IV

Class and Category

Chemical: Thienamycin derivative (imipenem), heptenoic acid derivative (cilastatin sodium)
Therapeutic: Antibiotic
Pregnancy category: C

Indications and Dosages

▶ *To treat severe or life-threatening bacterial infections (including endocarditis, pneumonia, and septicemia as well as bone, joint, intra-abdominal, skin, and soft-tissue infections) caused by gram-positive anaerobic organisms, such as most staphylococci and streptococci and some enterococci (including* Enterococcus faecalis*); most strains of* Enterobacteriaceae *(including* Citrobacter *species,* Enterobacter *species,* Escherichia coli, Klebsiella *species,* Morganella morganii, Proteus mirabilis, Providencia stuartii, *and* Serratia marcescens*); and many gram-negative aerobic and anaerobic species (including* Bacteroides *species,* Campylobacter *species,* Clostridium *species,* Haemophilus influenzae, Legionella *species,* Neisseria gonorrhoeae, *and* Pseudomonas aeruginosa*)*

I.V. INFUSION (DOSAGES BASED ON IMIPENEM CONTENT)
Adults and adolescents. 500 mg every 6 hr to 1,000 mg every 6 to 8 hr. *Maximum:* 50 mg/kg or 4 g daily, whichever is lower.

Children age 3 months and over. 15 to 25 mg/kg every 6 hr. *Maximum:* 2,000 to 4,000 mg daily.

Infants ages 4 weeks to 3 months weighing 1,500 g (3 lb, 3 oz) or more. 25 mg/kg every 6 hr. *Maximum:* 2,000 to 4,000 mg daily.

Neonates ages 1 to 4 weeks weighing 1,500 g or more. 25 mg/kg every 8 hr. *Maximum:* 2,000 to 4,000 mg daily.

Neonates under age 1 week weighing 1,500 g or more. 25 mg/kg every 12 hr. *Maximum:* 2,000 to 4,000 mg daily.

▶ *To treat moderate infections caused by the organisms listed above*
I.V. INFUSION (DOSAGES BASED ON IMIPENEM CONTENT)

Adults and adolescents. 500 mg every 6 to 8 hr up to 1,000 mg every 8 hr. *Maximum:* 50 mg/kg or 4 g daily, whichever is lower.

Children age 3 months and older. 15 to 25 mg/kg every 6 hr. *Maximum:* 2,000 to 4,000 mg daily.

Infants ages 4 weeks to 3 months weighing 1,500 g or more. 25 mg/kg every 6 hr. *Maximum:* 2,000 to 4,000 mg daily.

Neonates ages 1 to 4 weeks weighing 1,500 g or more. 25 mg/kg every 8 hr. *Maximum:* 2,000 to 4,000 mg daily.

Neonates under age 1 week weighing 1,500 g or more. 25 mg/kg every 12 hr. *Maximum:* 2,000 to 4,000 mg daily.

▶ *To treat mild infections caused by the organisms listed above*
I.V. INFUSION (DOSAGES BASED ON IMIPENEM CONTENT)

Adults and adolescents. 250 to 500 mg every 6 hr. *Maximum:* 50 mg/kg or 4 g daily, whichever is lower.

Children age 3 months and over. 15 to 25 mg/kg every 6 hr. *Maximum:* 2,000 mg (for fully susceptible organisms) to 4,000 mg (for moderately susceptible organisms) daily.

Infants ages 4 weeks to 3 months weighing 1,500 g or more. 25 mg/kg every 6 hr. *Maximum:* 2,000 to 4,000 mg daily.

Neonates ages 1 to 4 weeks weighing 1,500 g or more. 25 mg/kg every 8 hr. *Maximum:* 2,000 to 4,000 mg daily.

Neonates under age 1 week weighing 1,500 g or more. 25 mg/kg every 12 hr. *Maximum:* 2,000 to 4,000 mg daily.

▶ *To treat uncomplicated UTI caused by the organisms listed above*
I.V. INFUSION (DOSAGES BASED ON IMIPENEM CONTENT)

Adults and adolescents. 250 mg every 6 hr. *Maximum:* 50 mg/kg or 4 g daily, whichever is less.

▶ *To treat complicated UTI caused by the organisms listed above*
I.V. INFUSION (DOSAGES BASED ON IMIPENEM CONTENT)

Adults and adolescents. 500 mg every 6 hr. *Maximum:* 50 mg/kg or 4 g daily, whichever is less.

DOSAGE ADJUSTMENT Dosage reduced based on creatinine clearance for patients with impaired renal function.

Mechanism of Action

Produces two related actions. During bacterial cell wall synthesis, imipenem selectively binds to penicillin-binding proteins that are responsible for cell wall formation. This action causes bacterial cells to rapidly lyse and die. Cilastatin sodium inhibits imipenem's breakdown in the kidneys, thus maintaining a high imipenem level in the urinary tract.

Incompatibilities

Don't administer imipenem and cilastatin through same I.V. line as beta-lactam antibiotics or aminoglycosides.

Contraindications

Hypersensitivity to imipenem, its components, other beta–lactam antibiotics, or amide-type local anesthetics (I.M.); meningitis (I.V.); severe heart block or shock (I.M.)

Interactions

DRUGS

cyclosporine: Increased adverse CNS effects of both drugs
ganciclovir: Increased risk of seizures
probenecid: Slightly increased blood level and half-life of imipenem

Adverse Reactions

CNS: Confusion, dizziness, fever, seizures, somnolence, tremor, weakness
CV: Hypotension
EENT: Oral candidiasis
GI: Diarrhea, hepatic failure, hepatitis, nausea, pseudomembranous colitis, vomiting
RESP: Wheezing
SKIN: Diaphoresis, pruritus, rash, urticaria
Other: Anaphylaxis, injection site thrombophlebitis

Nursing Considerations

- Obtain specimens for culture and sensitivity testing, as ordered, before giving imipenem and cilastatin.
- For I.V. administration, add about 10 ml of diluent to each 250- or 500-mg vial and shake well. Transfer this reconstituted drug to at least 100 ml of prescribed I.V. solution. After the transfer, add another 10 ml of diluent to each vial, shake, and then

transfer to infusion container. Shake infusion container until clear. To reconstitute piggyback bottles, add 100 ml of diluent to each 250- or 500-mg infusion bottle, and shake well.

- Give reconstituted drug within 4 to 10 hours, depending on diluent used (24 to 48 hours if refrigerated). Color may range from clear to yellow; don't administer solution that contains particles.
- Infuse 500-mg or smaller dose over 20 to 30 minutes and 750- to 1,000-mg dose over 40 to 60 minutes.
- Expect increased risk of imipenem-induced seizures in patients with brain lesions, head trauma, or history of CNS disorders and in those receiving more than 2 g of drug daily.
- Assess patient for signs and symptoms of allergic reaction and bacterial or fungal superinfection.

PATIENT TEACHING
- Inform patient that drug must be given by infusion or injection.
- Instruct patient to report discomfort at I.V. insertion site.
- Advise patient to report itching, signs of superinfection (such as diarrhea and sore mouth), and hives.

immune globulin intravenous (human)
(IGIV, immune serum globulin, ISG, IVIG)

Gamimune N 5% S/D, Gamimune N 10% S/D, Gammagard Liquid, Gammagard S/D, Gammagard S/D 0.5 g, Gammar-P IV, Gamunex 10%, Iveegam EN, Octagam 5%, Polygam S/D, Rhophylac, Sandoglobulin, Venoglobulin-I, Venoglobulin-S 5%, Venoglobulin-S 10%, WinRho SDF

Class and Category

Chemical: Polyvalent antibody
Therapeutic: Antibacterial, anti–Kawasaki disease agent, antipolyneuropathy agent, antiviral, immunizing agent, platelet count stimulator
Pregnancy category: C

Indications and Dosages

▶ *To treat primary immunodeficiency*
I.V. INFUSION (GAMMAR-P IV)
Adults. 200 to 400 mg/kg every 3 to 4 wk.
Adolescents and children. 200 mg/kg every 3 to 4 wk.
I.V. INFUSION (IVEEGAM EN)
Adults. 200 mg/kg every mo.

I.V. INFUSION (SANDOGLOBULIN)

Adults and children. 200 mg/kg every mo. If response is inadequate, dose may be increased to 300 mg/kg or dosing frequency may be increased.

I.V. INFUSION (GAMIMUNE N 5% S/D OR 10% S/D)

Adults. 100 to 200 mg/kg every mo. If response is inadequate, dose may be increased to as high as 400 mg/kg or dosing frequency may be increased.

I.V. INFUSION (GAMMAGARD S/D, POLYGAM S/D)

Adults. 200 to 400 mg/kg initially, then at least 100 mg/kg every mo thereafter. If response is inadequate, dose or frequency may be adjusted.

I.V. INFUSION (OCTAGAM 5%)

Adults. *Initial:* 30 mg/kg/hr for first 30 minutes; increased, if tolerated, to 60 mg/kg/hr for second 30 minutes and, if tolerated, to 120 mg/kg/hr for another 30 minutes; followed by maintenance infusion of up to 200 mg/kg/hr.

I.V. INFUSION (GAMUNEX 10%)

Adults. 300 to 600 mg/kg every 3 or 4 wk.

I.V. INFUSION (VENOGLOBULIN-I)

Adults and children. 200 mg/kg every mo. If response is inadequate, dose may be increased to 300 to 400 mg/kg every mo or dosing frequency may be increased.

I.V. INFUSION (VENOGLOBULIN-S 5% OR 10%)

Adults and children. 200 mg/kg every mo. If response is inadequate, dose may be increased to as high as 400 mg/kg or dosing frequency may be increased.

▶ *To treat primary immunodeficiency disorders associated with defects in humoral immunity*

I.V. INFUSION (GAMMAGARD LIQUID)

Adults and children. 300 to 600 mg/kg daily every 3 to 4 wk.

▶ *To treat idiopathic thrombocytopenic purpura (ITP)*

I.V. INFUSION (GAMIMUNE N 5% S/D)

Adults and children. 400 mg/kg daily for 5 days. Or, 1,000 mg/kg for 1 or 2 days for patients not at risk for increased fluid volume.

I.V. INFUSION (GAMIMUNE N 10% S/D)

Adults and children. 1,000 mg/kg for 1 or 2 days for patients not at risk for increased fluid volume.

I.V. INFUSION (GAMUNEX 10%)

Adults. 1 g/kg daily for 2 consecutive days (second dose may be withheld if platelet count increases adequately 24 hours after first dose). Alternatively, 0.4 g/kg daily for 5 consecutive days.

DOSAGE ADJUSTMENT In acute ITP of childhood, I.V. Sandoglobulin therapy may be stopped after second day of 5-day course if initial platelet count response is adequate (30,000 to 50,000/mm³). In chronic ITP, an additional I.V. infusion of 400 mg/kg (of either Sandoglobulin or Gamimune) may be prescribed if platelet count falls below 30,000/mm³ or if patient develops significant bleeding. If response remains inadequate, an additional I.V. infusion of 800 to 1,000 mg/kg may be given.

I.V. INFUSION (GAMMAGARD S/D)

Adults. 1 g/kg. If response is inadequate, up to three separate doses may be administered on alternate days.

I.V. INFUSION (SANDOGLOBULIN)

Adults and adolescents. 400 mg/kg daily for 2 to 5 consecutive days.

I.V. INFUSION (VENOGLOBULIN-I)

Adults and children. *Induction:* Cumulative dose up to 2 g/kg over 2 to 7 consecutive days. *Maintenance (adults):* 2 g/kg as a single dose every 2 wk as needed to maintain platelet count above 30,000/mm³ or prevent bleeding episodes. *Maintenance (children):* 1 g/kg as a single dose every 2 wk as needed to maintain platelet count above 30,000/mm³ or prevent bleeding episodes.

I.V. INFUSION (VENOGLOBULIN-S 5% OR 10%)

Adults and children. Cumulative dose up to 2,000 mg/kg over 5 consecutive days.

DOSAGE ADJUSTMENT An additional I.V. infusion of 1,000 mg/kg may be given to maintain a platelet count of 30,000/mm³ in children or 20,000/mm³ in adults or to prevent bleeding episodes.

I.V. INFUSION (RHOPHYLAC)

Adults. 50 mcg/kg at 2 ml/15 to 60 sec.

▶ *To treat acute or chronic pediatric immune thrombocytopenia purpura; to treat chronic adult-onset immune thrombocytopenia purpura; to treat prediatric- and adult-onset immune thrombocytopenia purpura secondary to HIV infection*

I.V. INJECTION (WINRHO SDF)

Adults and children. *Initial:* 250 international units/kg given as a single injection over 3 to 5 min. Or 125 international units/kg given as a single injection over 3 to 5 min and repeated once on a separate day. *Maintenance:* Frequency and dosage highly individualized based on patient's hemoglobin and platelet levels.

DOSAGE ADJUSTMENT For patients with a hemoglobin level less than 10 g/dl, dose reduced to 125 to 200 international units/kg.

▶ *As adjunct to treat Kawasaki disease*
I.V. INFUSION (GAMMAGARD S/D)
Adults and adolescents. 1 g/kg as a single dose; or, 400 mg/kg daily for 4 consecutive days.
I.V. INFUSION (IVEEGAM EN, VENOGLOBULIN-S 5% OR 10%)
Adults and adolescents. 2 g/kg as a single dose; alternatively, Iveegam EN may be given at 400 mg/kg daily for 4 days.

▶ *To decrease the risk of graft-versus-host disease, interstitial pneumonia, septicemia, and other infections during first 100 days after bone marrow transplantation*
I.V. INFUSION (GAMIMUNE N 5% S/D OR 10% S/D)
Adults over age 20. 500 mg/kg on seventh and second days before transplantation (or at time conditioning therapy for transplantation begins), and then weekly through 90th day after transplant.

▶ *As adjunct to treat bacterial infections secondary to B-cell chronic lymphocytic leukemia*
I.V. INFUSION (GAMMAGARD S/D, POLYGAM S/D)
Adults and adolescents. 400 mg/kg every 3 to 4 wk.

▶ *To prevent bacterial infection in children with HIV who are immunosuppressed*
I.V. INFUSION (GAMIMUNE N 5% S/D OR 10% S/D)
Children. 400 mg/kg daily every 28 days.

▶ *To suppress Rh isoimmunization*
I.V. INJECTION (WINRHO SDF)
Adult pregnant women. 1,500 international units as a single dose infused over 3 to 5 min at 28 wk gestation followed by 600 international units infused over 3 to 5 min within 72 hr after delivery of an Rh-positive newborn.

DOSAGE ADJUSTMENT For patients who are at more than 34 wk gestation and are having an abortion, amniocentesis, or other manipulative procedure, 600 international units given within 72 hr but preferably immediately after procedure. For patients who are 34 wk gestation or less and are having amniocentesis or chorionic villus sampling, 1,500 international units given immediately after procedure and repeated every 12 wk for duration of pregnancy. For patients with a threatened abortion at any stage of pregnancy, 1,500 international units given immediately.

I.V. INFUSION (RHOPHYLAC)

Adult pregnant women. 1,500 international units as a single dose at 28 to 30 wk gestation, followed by 1,500 international units as a single dose within 72 hr after delivery of an Rh-positive newborn.

▶ *To treat incompatible blood transfusions*

I.V. INJECTION (WINRHO SDF)

Adults exposed to Rh-positive whole blood. 3,000 international units infused over 3 to 5 min every 8 hr until total dose (45 international units/ml of blood) is given.

Adults exposed to Rh-positive RBCs. 3,000 international units infused over 3 to 5 min every 8 hr until total dose (90 international units/ml of cells) is given.

I.V. INFUSION (RHOPHYLAC)

Adults exposed to Rh-positive RBCs. 100 international units/2 ml of transfused blood or per 1 ml erythrocyte concentrate within 72 hours of exposure.

▶ *To treat massive fetomaternal hemorrhage*

I.V. INFUSION (RHOPHYLAC)

Adults exposed to Rh-positive RBCs. If transplacental bleeding is quantified, 1,500 international units plus 100 international units for every 1 ml of fetal RBCs exceeding 15 ml. If transplacental bleeding can't be quantified within 72 hours of hemorrhage, additional 1,500 international units.

I.V. INJECTION (WINRHO SDF)

Adults exposed to Rh-positive whole blood. 3,000 international units infused over 3 to 5 min every 8 hr until total dose (45 international units/ml of blood) is given.

Adults exposed to Rh-positive RBCs. 3,000 international units infused over 3 to 5 min every 8 hr until total dose (90 international units/ml of cells) is given.

Route	Onset	Peak	Duration
I.V.	Unknown	Unknown	21 to 28 days

Incompatibilities

Don't mix immune globulin with any other drugs, including other immune globulins, or with any I.V. solutions other than D_5W or manufacturer's supplied diluent because effects of doing so are unknown.

Contraindications

Hypersensitivity to immune globulin (human) or its components, IgA deficiency in patients with known antibody to IgA

Mechanism of Action

Releases antibody-specific globulins to produce an antibody-antigen reaction that results in bacterial lysis and facilitates bacterial phagocytosis. In treatment of ITP, immune globulin blocks iron receptors on macrophages to increase immunoglobulin action. Immune globulin also increases cytokine production and improves B-cell immune function by regulating T-cell and macrophage activity. Newly formed antigen-antibody complexes produce split complement components that cause bacterial lysis.

In Kawasaki disease and bacterial infections secondary to B-cell chronic lymphocytic leukemia, immune globulin neutralizes bacterial and viral toxins that harm the immune and inflammatory responses.

Interactions

DRUGS

vaccines, live-virus: Possibly decreased response to vaccine

Adverse Reactions

CNS: Headache, malaise
CV: Tachycardia
GI: Nausea, vomiting
HEME: Disseminated intravascular coagulation, hemolysis
MS: Arthralgia, back pain, myalgia
RESP: Dyspnea

Nursing Considerations

- Before giving immune globulin, monitor patient's fluid volume and BUN and serum creatinine levels, as ordered, to determine if he's at risk for acute renal failure. Those at increased risk include patients with existing renal insufficiency, diabetes mellitus, volume depletion, sepsis, or paraproteinemia; those taking concomitant nephrotoxic drugs; and those over age 65. Expect drug to be discontinued if renal function deteriorates.
- When preparing drug for administration, verify that immune globulin intravenous for I.V. infusion is being used because the drug is also available as immune globulin intramuscular.
- To reconstitute drug (except Gammagard Liquid, which doesn't need reconstitution), follow manufacturer's guidelines and use only diluent recommended by manufacturer. Don't shake solution; excessive shaking causes foaming. If drug or diluent is cold, drug may take up to 20 minutes to dissolve.
- If drug is reconstituted outside of sterile laminar airflow conditions, administer it immediately and discard unused portions.

- Consult manufacturer's guidelines to determine appropriate flow rate for starting infusion. Expect to increase flow rate after 15 to 30 minutes, according to guidelines.
- **WARNING** Watch for an acute inflammatory reaction in patients who haven't received immune globulin before, in those whose last treatment was more than 8 weeks ago, and in those whose initial infusion rate exceeded 1 ml/minute. Within 30 minutes to 1 hour after infusion starts, assess patient for chills, fever, facial flushing, feeling of tightness in chest, dizziness, nausea and vomiting, diaphoresis, and hypotension. Notify prescriber immediately, and be prepared to stop infusion until symptoms have subsided.
- **WARNING** After administration, monitor patient closely for aseptic meningitis. Notify prescriber if patient develops drowsiness, fever, nausea and vomiting, nuchal rigidity, photophobia, painful eye movements, or severe headache.
- Be aware that immune globulin intravenous is made from human plasma and may contain infectious agents, such as viruses. However, the risk of transmitting a virus by infusion has been reduced by screening blood donors, testing donated blood, and inactivating or removing certain viruses from the product.
- For patient receiving WinRho SDF to treat immune thrombocytopenia purpura, assess clinical response by monitoring platelet count, RBC count, hemoglobin level, and reticulocyte level.
- For patient receiving WinRho SDF for exposure to incompatible blood transfusions or massive fetal hemorrhage, give drug within 72 hours of incident.

PATIENT TEACHING

- Instruct patient to immediately report any symptoms he experiences after receiving immune globulin.
- Inform patient that he'll need to postpone live-virus vaccinations for up to 11 months after receiving immune globulin because drug may delay or inhibit his response to vaccine.

inamrinone lactate
(amrinone lactate)
Inocor

Class and Category
Chemical: Bipyridine derivative
Therapeutic: Cardiac inotrope
Pregnancy category: C

Indications and Dosages

▶ *To treat heart failure in patients who haven't responded sufficiently to digoxin, diuretics, or vasodilators*

I.V. INFUSION

Adults. *Initial:* 0.75 mg/kg by bolus administered over 2 to 3 min and repeated after 30 min, if needed. *Maintenance:* 5 to 10 mcg/kg/min by infusion. *Maximum:* 10 mg/kg daily.

Route	Onset	Peak	Duration
I.V.	2 to 5 min	In 10 min	30 min to 2 hr

Mechanism of Action

Inhibits phosphodiesterase enzymes that normally degrade myocardial cAMP. This action increases intracellular levels of cAMP, which regulates intracellular and extracellular calcium balance. An increased intracellular cAMP level enhances the influx of calcium into the cell, thereby increasing the force of myocardial contractions. Inamrinone also acts directly on peripheral vascular smooth-muscle cells, causing relaxation and dilation. This action reduces preload and afterload.

Incompatibilities

Don't administer inamrinone through same I.V. line as furosemide to prevent precipitate formation. Don't dilute inamrinone in solution that contains dextrose because a chemical interaction occurs over 24 hours.

Contraindications

Hypersensitivity to inamrinone, bisulfites, or their components; severe aortic or pulmonary valvular disease

Interactions

DRUGS

disopyramide: Possibly severe hypotension

Adverse Reactions

CNS: Fever

CV: Chest pain, hypotension, pericarditis, supraventricular tachycardia, ventricular arrhythmias

GI: Abdominal pain, anorexia, elevated liver function test results, hepatotoxicity, nausea, vomiting

HEME: Elevated erythrocyte sedimentation rate, thrombocytopenia (especially with high-dose or long-term treatment)

MS: Myositis

RESP: Hypoxemia, pleuritis
SKIN: Jaundice
Other: Infusion site burning

Nursing Considerations

- **WARNING** Be aware that inamrinone may increase the risk of ventricular arrhythmias in patients with atrial flutter or fibrillation. To minimize this risk, expect to pretreat such patients with digoxin.
- Give inamrinone undiluted or diluted in normal saline solution or 0.45 normal saline solution to a concentration of 1 to 3 mg/ml, as prescribed. Use diluted solution within 24 hours. Don't use if solution is discolored or contains particles.
- **WARNING** Monitor vital signs regularly. If blood pressure falls significantly, slow or stop inamrinone infusion and notify prescriber.
- Monitor weight, cardiac index, central venous pressure, pulmonary artery wedge pressure, and fluid intake and output as appropriate to assess effectiveness of therapy.
- **WARNING** Assess often for signs of thrombocytopenia, such as bruising or bleeding and altered platelet count. If signs appear, expect to decrease inamrinone dose or discontinue drug.
- Store drug at 15° to 30° C (59° to 86° F), protected from light.

PATIENT TEACHING

- Instruct patient to report dizziness, which may indicate hypotension, or signs of an allergic reaction, such as a rash, facial swelling, or difficulty breathing or swallowing.

indomethacin sodium trihydrate

Indocid PDA (CAN), Indocin I.V.

Class and Category

Chemical: Indoleacetic acid derivative
Therapeutic: Antigout, anti-inflammatory, antirheumatic
Pregnancy category: Not rated

Indications and Dosages

▶ *To treat hemodynamically significant patent ductus arteriosus in premature infants weighing 500 to 1,750 g (1 to 3.9 lb)*

I.V. INJECTION

Infants over age 7 days. *Initial:* 200 mcg/kg (0.2 mg/kg) over 5 to 10 sec; 1 or 2 additional doses of 250 mcg/kg (0.25 mg/kg) given at 12- to 24-hr intervals, if needed.

Neonates ages 2 to 7 days. *Initial:* 200 mcg/kg (0.2 mg/kg) over 5 to 10 sec; 1 or 2 additional doses of 200 mcg/kg (0.2 mg/kg) given at 12- to 24-hr intervals, if needed.

Neonates under age 48 hours. *Initial:* 200 mcg/kg (0.2 mg/kg) over 5 to 10 sec; 1 or 2 additional doses of 100 mcg/kg (0.1 mg/kg) given at 12- to 24-hr intervals, if needed.

Mechanism of Action

Blocks the activity of cyclooxygenase, the enzyme needed to synthesize prostaglandins, which mediate the inflammatory response and cause local vasodilation, swelling, and pain. By blocking cyclooxygenase and inhibiting prostaglandins, this NSAID reduces inflammatory symptoms and helps relieve pain.

Incompatibilities

Don't give indomethacin suspension with alkaline antacids or liquids. Don't mix reconstituted indomethacin sodium with I.V. infusion solutions.

Contraindications

Allergy or hypersensitivity to aspirin, indomethacin, iodides, other NSAIDs, or their components; history of proctitis or recent rectal bleeding (suppositories)

Interactions

DRUGS

Note: All effects listed are for oral forms and suppositories unless indicated.

acetaminophen: Increased risk of adverse renal effects (with long-term use of both drugs)

aluminum- and magnesium-containing antacids: Possibly decreased blood indomethacin level

aminoglycosides: Increased risk of aminoglycoside toxicity

antihypertensives: Decreased effectiveness of these drugs

aspirin, other NSAIDs: Increased risk of adverse GI effects and non-GI bleeding

bone marrow depressants: Possibly increased leukopenic or thrombocytopenic effects of these drugs

cefamandole, cefoperazone, cefotetan: Increased risk of hypoprothrombinemia and bleeding

colchicine, platelet aggregation inhibitors: Increased risk of GI bleeding, hemorrhage, and ulcers *corticosteroids, potassium supplements:* Increased risk of adverse GI effects

cyclosporine: Increased risk of nephrotoxicity from both drugs, increased blood cyclosporine level

diflunisal: Increased blood indomethacin level and risk of GI bleeding

digoxin: Increased blood digoxin level and risk of digitalis toxicity (all forms)

diuretics (thiazide, loop, and potassium-sparing): Decreased diuretic and antihypertensive effects

gold compounds, nephrotoxic drugs: Increased risk of adverse renal effects

heparin, oral anticoagulants, thrombolytics: Possibly increased anticoagulant effects and risk of hemorrhage

lithium: Increased blood lithium level and risk of toxicity

methotrexate: Increased risk of methotrexate toxicity

plicamycin, valproic acid: Increased risk of hypoprothrombinemia and GI bleeding, hemorrhage, and ulcers

probenecid: Increased blood level and effectiveness of indomethacin, increased risk of indomethacin toxicity

zidovudine: Increased blood zidovudine level and risk of toxicity, increased risk of indomethacin toxicity

ACTIVITIES

alcohol use: Increased risk of adverse GI effects

Adverse Reactions

CNS: Confusion, depression, dizziness, drowsiness, fatigue, hallucinations, headache, intraventricular hemorrhage, peripheral neuropathy, seizures, stroke, syncope, vertigo

CV: Arrhythmias, chest pain, edema, fluid retention (all forms), heart failure, hypertension, MI, pulmonary hypertension, tachycardia

EENT: Blurred vision, corneal and retinal damage, epistaxis, hearing loss, tinnitus

ENDO: Hypoglycemia

GI: Abdominal cramps or pain, abdominal distention, anorexia, constipation, diarrhea, diverticulitis, dyspepsia, dysphagia, epigastric discomfort, esophagitis, gastric perforation, gastritis, gastroenteritis, gastroesophageal reflux disease, GI bleeding and ulceration (all forms), hemorrhoids, hepatic dysfunction, hepatic failure, hiatal hernia, ileus, indigestion, melena, nausea, necrotizing enterocolitis, pancreatitis, peptic ulcer, perforation of stomach or intestine, stomatitis, vomiting (all forms)

GU: Acute renal failure, hematuria, interstitial nephritis, nephrotic syndrome, oliguria, proteinuria, renal dysfunction, vaginal bleeding

HEME: Agranulocytosis, anemia, aplastic anemia, bone marrow depression, disseminated intravascular coagulation, hemolytic anemia, iron deficiency anemia, leukopenia, neutropenia, pancytopenia, thrombocytopenia, unusual bleeding or bruising (all forms)

RESP: Asthma, respiratory depression

SKIN: Ecchymosis, erythema multiforme, erythema nodosum, photosensitivity, pruritus, rash, Stevens-Johnson syndrome, toxic epidermal necrolysis, urticaria

Other: Anaphylaxis, angioedema, hyperkalemia, hyponatremia, injection site irritation

Nursing Considerations

- Use indomethacin cautiously in patients with hypertension, and monitor blood pressure closely throughout therapy. Drug may cause hypertension or worsen it.
- To reconstitute I.V. form, add 1 to 2 ml of preservative-free sodium chloride for injection or preservative-free sterile water to vial. Solution made with 1 ml of diluent contains 100 mcg (0.1 mg) of indomethacin/0.1 ml. Solution made with 2 ml of diluent contains 50 mcg (0.05 mg) of indomethacin/0.1 ml. Use solution immediately because it contains no preservatives. Discard unused portion.
- Be aware that scheduled I.V. doses may be withheld if infant or neonate has anuria or a significant decrease in urine output (less than 0.6 ml/kg/hr).
- When using I.V. form, avoid extravasation to protect surrounding tissue.
- Anticipate a second course (another 3 doses) of I.V. indomethacin if patent ductus arteriosus fails to close or reopens. After two courses, surgery may be performed.
- **WARNING** Monitor patient closely for thrombotic events, including MI and stroke, because NSAIDs increase the risk.
- Monitor infant for necrotizing entercolitis such as abdomen distention, severe abdominal pain, and fever.
- Monitor CBC for decreased hemoglobin and hematocrit because drug may worsen anemia.
- **WARNING** If patient has bone marrow suppression or is receiving an antineoplastic drug, monitor laboratory results (including WBC count), and watch for evidence of infection because anti-inflammatory and antipyretic actions of in-

domethacin may mask signs and symptoms, such as fever and pain.
- Assess patient's skin regularly for signs of rash or other hypersensitivity reaction because indomethacin is an NSAID and may cause serious skin reactions without warning, even in patients with no history of NSAID sensivitity. At first sign of reaction, stop drug and notify prescriber.
- Because indomethacin causes sodium retention, monitor weight and blood pressure, especially if patient has hypertension.

PATIENT TEACHING
- Reassure parents that infant will be monitored closely throughout course of therapy.

infliximab
Remicade

Class and Category
Chemical: Monoclonal antibody
Therapeutic: Anti-inflammatory
Pregnancy category: C

Indications and Dosages
▶ *To control moderate to severe Crohn's disease long term*
I.V. INFUSION
Adults and children. *Induction:* 5 mg/kg over 2 hr, repeated 2 and 6 wk after first infusion. *Maintenance:* 5 mg/kg over 2 hr every 8 wk.
DOSAGE ADJUSTMENT For adult patients who respond and then lose response, dosage may be increased up to 10 mg/kg.
▶ *To reduce number of draining enterocutaneous and rectovaginal fistulas and to maintain fistula closure in fistulizing Crohn's disease*
I.V. INFUSION
Adults. *Induction:* 5 mg/kg over 2 hr, repeated 2 and 6 wk after first infusion. *Maintenance:* 5 mg/kg over 2 hr every 8 wk.
DOSAGE ADJUSTMENT For patients who respond and then lose response, dosage may be increased up to 10 mg/kg.
▶ *To reduce signs and symptoms, to induce and maintain remission and mucosal healing, and eliminate corticosteroid use in patients with moderate to severe active ulcerative colitis who have had an inadequate response to conventional therapy*
I.V. INFUSION
Adults. 5 mg/kg over 2 hr, repeated 2 and 6 wk after infusion.

Maintenance: 5 mg/kg over 2 hr every 8 wk.

▶ *As adjunct to reduce signs and symptoms, inhibit progression of structural damage, and improve physical function in patients with moderate to severe active rheumatoid arthritis*

I.V. INFUSION

Adults. 3 mg/kg, with methotrexate, repeated 2 and 6 wk after first infusion and then every 8 wk thereafter.

DOSAGE ADJUSTMENT For patients with inadequate response to combination treatment, infliximab increased to 10 mg/kg or frequency increased to every 4 wk.

▶ *To treat active ankylosing spondylitis*

I.V. INFUSION

Adults. 5 mg/kg, repeated 2 and 6 wk after first infusion and then every 6 wk thereafter.

▶ *To reduce signs and symptoms, inhibit progression of structural damage, and improve physical function in patients with psoriatic arthritis*

I.V. INFUSION

Adults. 5 mg/kg, with or without methotrexate, repeated 2 and 6 wk after first infusion and then every 8 wk thereafter.

▶ *To treat chronic severe plaque psoriasis in patients who are candidates for systemic therapy when those therapies are medically less appropriate*

I.V. INFUSION

Adults. 5 mg/kg, repeated 2 and 6 wk after first infusion and then every 8 wk thereafter.

Mechanism of Action

Binds with cytokine tumor necrosis factor-alpha (TNF-alpha), preventing it from binding with its receptors. As a result, TNF-alpha can't produce proinflammatory cytokines and endothelial permeability. Infiltration of inflammatory cells into inflamed intestine and joints declines.

Incompatibilities

Don't infuse infliximab in same I.V. line with other drugs or through plasticized polyvinyl chloride infusion equipment or devices.

Contraindications

Breast-feeding, hypersensitivity to infliximab, murine proteins, or their components; moderate or severe (NYHA Class III or IV) heart failure

Interactions

DRUGS

anakinra, etanercept: Increased risk of neutropenia and serious infections

Adverse Reactions

CNS: Chills, CVA, dizziness, fatigue, fever, Guillain-Barré syndrome, headache, meningitis, neuritis, numbness, paresthesia, pericardial effusion, syncope, tingling

CV: Arrhythmias, chest pain, hypertension, hypotension, MI, myelitis, neuropathies, systemic and cutaneous vasculitis, thrombophlebitis

EENT: Oral candidiasis, pharyngitis, rhinitis, sinusitis, visual changes

GI: Abdominal hernia; abdominal pain; acute hepatic failure; cholecystitis; cholestasis; diarrhea; dyspepsia; elevated aminotransferases; gastrointestinal hemorrhage; hepatitis; hepatotoxicity; ileus; intestinal obstruction, perforation, or stenosis; melena; nausea; pancreatitis; splenic infarction; splenomegaly; vomiting

GU: Kidney infection, renal failure, ureteral obstruction, UTI, vaginal candidiasis, vaginitis

HEME: Anemia, leukopenia, neutropenia, pancytopenia, thrombocytopenia

MS: Arthralgia, back pain, extremity weakness, myalgia

RESP: Adult respiratory distress syndrome, bronchitis, cough, dyspnea, interstitial pneumonitis or fibrosis, pneumonia, pulmonary edema or embolism, tuberculosis, respiratory tract infection, wheezing

SKIN: Facial flushing, jaundice, pruritus, rash, urticaria

Other: Antibody formation to infliximab; bacterial, fungal or viral infections; infusion reactions; lupuslike symptoms; lymphadenopathy; lymphoma; sepsis

Nursing Considerations

- **WARNING** Avoid giving infliximab to patients with NYHA Class III or IV congestive heart failure (CHF) because it may worsen the condition or cause death. If patient does receive infliximab, expect to stop it if CHF worsens.
- Use cautiously in elderly patients because they are at higher risk for developing infections.
- **WARNING** Because infliximab increases the risk of developing tuberculosis or reactivating latent tuberculosis, expect prescriber to evaluate patient's risk and start tuberculosis treatment, as needed, before starting infliximab.

- **WARNING** Be aware that infliximab increases the risk of serious or fatal opportunistic infections, including histoplasmosis, listeriosis, and pneumocystosis. Expect prescriber to evaluate patient's risk before starting drug.
- To reconstitute infliximab, use a 21G (or smaller) needle to add 10 ml of sterile water for injection to each vial of drug. Swirl to mix; don't shake. Be aware that solution may foam and be clear or light yellow.
- Withdraw a volume equal to amount of reconstituted drug from a 250-ml glass bottle or polypropylene or polyolefin infusion bag of normal saline solution. Then add reconstituted infliximab to bottle to dilute to 250 ml. Use within 3 hours.
- Infuse over at least 2 hours using polyethylene-lined infusion set and in-line, sterile, nonpyrogenic, low–protein-binding filter with pores of 1.2 microns or less. Don't reuse.
- Be prepared to stop infusion if a hypersensitivity or CNS reaction occurs. Keep acetaminophen, antihistamines, corticosteroids, and epinephrine on hand. A reaction may occur 2 hours to 12 days after infusion.
- **WARNING** Watch for infection, especially if patient receives immunosuppressant therapy or has a chronic infection. Upper respiratory tract infections and UTIs are most common, but sepsis and fatal infections have occurred.
- Because severe hepatic reactions may occur, monitor liver function. Expect to stop infliximab if jaundice develops or liver enzymes are 5 times or more the upper limit of normal.

PATIENT TEACHING
- Explain that infliximab should take effect within 1 to 2 weeks.
- Urge patient to report signs of infection, such as painful urination, cough, and sore throat. Infusion reaction (chest pain, chills, dyspnea, facial flushing, fever, itching, headache, rash) may occur for up to 12 days.
- Explain that infliximab increases the risk of lymphoma; urge prompt medical attention for suspicious signs or symptoms.

insulin injection, regular
Regular Iletin II, Regular Insulin

insulin human injection, regular
Humulin R, Novolin ge Toronto (CAN), Novolin R

insulin human injection, buffered regular
Velosulin BR

Class and Category
Chemical: Polypeptide hormone
Therapeutic: Antidiabetic
Pregnancy category: B

Indications and Dosages
▶ *To treat diabetic ketoacidosis*
I.V. INJECTION OR INFUSION
Adults and adolescents. Loading dose of 0.15 USP Insulin Unit/kg, followed by 0.1 USP Insulin Unit/kg/hr by continuous infusion.

Route	Onset	Peak	Duration
I.V.*	10 to 30 min	15 to 30 min	30 to 60 min

Mechanism of Action
Controls the storage and metabolism of carbohydrates, proteins, and fats that bind to receptor sites on cellular plasma membranes, especially in the liver, muscle, and adipose tissues. In hyperglycemia, the body lacks sufficient insulin or is unable to use insulin to transport glucose through the cellular membranes. When this occurs, the body uses proteins and fats for energy. The liver produces excess ketone bodies, which accumulate in the blood; metabolic acidosis develops, resulting in diabetic ketoacidosis.

Insulin stimulates carbohydrate metabolism in skeletal and cardiac muscle and adipose tissue by facilitating transport of glucose into these cells. It also increases conversion of glucose to glycogen in the liver and suppresses hepatic glucose output.

Contraindications
Hypersensitivity to specific insulin preparation (animal or human)

Interactions
DRUGS
ACE inhibitors, anabolic steroids (such as stanozolol and oxandrolone), androgens, antidiabetic drugs, bromocriptine, clofibrate, ketoconazole, lithium, mebendazole, pyridoxine, sulfonamides, theophylline: Increased risk of hypoglycemia
beta blockers (systemic and oral), guanethidine, MAO inhibitors (such as furazolidone), procarbazine: Possibly hyperglycemia or hypoglycemia and masking of hypoglycemic adverse effects

---

*Individual responses vary.

calcium channel blockers, clonidine, corticosteroids, danazole, dextrothyroxine, diazoxide (parenteral), epinephrine, estrogen, glucagon, growth hormone, heparin, loop and thiazide diuretics, morphine, oral contraceptives (containing estrogen and progestin), phenytoin, sulfinpyrazone, thyroid hormones: Possibly hyperglycemia

carbonic anhydrase inhibitors (such as acetazolamide), sulfonylureas: Possibly increased hypoglycemic response

chloroquine, quinidine, quinine: Increased risk of hypoglycemia, increased blood insulin level

NSAIDs, salicylates (large doses): Increased hypoglycemic effect

octreotide: Possibly hyperglycemia or hypoglycemia

pentamidine: Possibly hyperglycemia, hypoglycemia, or hypoinsulinemia

tetracycline: Increased tissue sensitivity to insulin

ACTIVITIES

alcohol use: Increased hypoglycemic effect of insulin, increased risk of prolonged hypoglycemia

marijuana use, smoking: Possibly hyperglycemia

Adverse Reactions

CV: Edema
ENDO: Hypoglycemia
Other: Allergic reaction, weight gain

Nursing Considerations

- **WARNING** Be aware that the 100-USP unit concentration of regular insulin is the only type of insulin that should be used for I.V. infusion.
- Monitor patient's blood glucose level frequently, as ordered, before starting insulin infusion and at least hourly, as ordered, during the infusion.
- Don't use cloudy or viscous regular insulin. Use only clear, colorless solutions. In addition, use only syringes specifically calibrated to measure 100–USP unit concentrations when preparing for infusion.
- Be aware that insulin can be adsorbed to glass and plastic I.V. infusion containers and I.V. tubing. To minimize adsorption, allow 50 ml of diluted solution to run through the infusion apparatus before use and wait 30 minutes to administer a prepared solution. Follow facility protocols for preparing and administering insulin I.V. infusions.
- Monitor urine ketone and glucose levels, as ordered. Expect urine glucose level to return to normal more slowly than blood glucose level.

- Be aware that patients with impaired renal or hepatic function may require an increase or decrease in insulin dosage.
- Monitor blood pH and serum electrolyte levels, particularly potassium, sodium chloride, and phosphate, as ordered. After initially experiencing hyperkalemia due to decreased pH, patient may develop hypokalemia as potassium reenters cells with insulin administration.
- Expect to decrease infusion rate when blood glucose level is 300 mg/dl or less. Expect a separate infusion of D_5W to be ordered when blood glucose level is 250 mg/dl.
- Assess patient for signs and symptoms of hypoglycemia, including anxiety, behavioral changes, blurred vision, cold sweats, confusion, cool skin, decreased concentration, headache, hunger, nausea, nervousness, nightmares, restless sleep, pallor, shakiness, slurred speech, tachycardia, tiredness, and weakness. Severe hypoglycemia may also cause coma or seizures.
- Anticipate an order for an appropriate subcutaneous or I.M. dose of insulin 30 minutes before insulin infusion ends.
- Store regular insulin at 2° to 8° C (36° to 46° F); protect from freezing and sunlight.

PATIENT TEACHING
- Advise patient receiving insulin infusion to immediately report signs of abnormal blood glucose level, including anxiety, tachycardia, blurred vision, and tremors.
- Review with patient events that may trigger a change in insulin requirements, including fever, infection, injury, psychological or physical stress, surgery, and medical conditions affecting food intake or absorption, such as vomiting and diarrhea.
- Stress the need to keep follow-up appointments, to use insulin as prescribed, and to monitor blood glucose level.
- Refer patient to an outpatient diabetes education program, if needed, for additional information and support.

interferon alfa-2b, recombinant
Intron A

Class and Category
Chemical: Cytokine
Therapeutic: Antineoplastic, immunomodulator
Pregnancy category: C

Indications and Dosages
▶ *To treat malignant melanoma*

I.V. INFUSION, SUBCUTANEOUS INJECTION
Adults. *Initial:* 20 million international units/m^2 I.V. for 5 consecutive days/wk for 4 wk. *Maintenance:* 10 million international units/m^2 subcutaneously 3 times/wk for 48 wk.

Mechanism of Action

May exert a cytostatic effect, reducing the rate of cell proliferation by delaying RNA and protein production. This delay induces cells to enter a resting stage. Interferon alfa-2b also increases the action of human natural killer cells, which lyse certain tumor cells and normal targets. In addition, the drug selectively increases the number of cytotoxic T-cells, thereby affecting tumor growth, and increases phagocytic activity of macrophages.

Contraindications

Hypersensitivity to interferon alfa or its components

Interactions

DRUGS

barbiturates and other CNS depressants: Possibly increased CNS depression

blood-dyscrasia–causing drugs (such as cephalosporins and sulfasalazine): Increased risk of leukopenia and thrombocytopenia

bone marrow depressants (such as carboplatin and lomustine): Possibly increased bone marrow depression

theophylline: Risk of decreased theophylline clearance and increased blood theophylline level

vaccines, killed virus: Possibly decreased antibody response to vaccine

vaccines, live virus: Possibly decreased antibody response to vaccine, increased adverse effects of vaccine, and severe infection

ACTIVITIES

alcohol use: Increased risk of CNS depression

Adverse Reactions

CNS: Dizziness, fatigue, neurotoxicity, peripheral neuropathy
CV: Cardiotoxicity, hypotension
EENT: Altered taste, blurred vision, dry mouth, stomatitis
GI: Anorexia, diarrhea, hepatotoxicity, nausea, vomiting
HEME: Anemia, leukopenia, neutropenia, thrombocytopenia
MS: Leg cramps
SKIN: Alopecia, diaphoresis, dry skin, pruritus, rash
Other: Flulike symptoms, weight loss

Nursing Considerations

- **WARNING** Be aware that recombinant interferon alfa-2b is *not* interchangeable with other interferon preparations, including interferon alfa-2a, -n1, and -n3. Don't use interferon alfa-2b solution for injection for I.V. treatment of malignant melanoma; use the recombinant powder for injection.

- Monitor liver function tests, hematocrit, hemoglobin, platelet count, and total and differential leukocyte count before and periodically during therapy.

- Obtain an ECG before and during therapy, as ordered, in patients with a history of cardiac disease or advanced malignant melanoma.

- Anticipate the need to hydrate patient before therapy. Monitor blood pressure during therapy to detect hypotensive changes.

- Reconstitute interferon with appropriate amount of bacteriostatic water for injection provided. Agitate gently to dissolve. Expect liquid to be clear and colorless to light yellow. Use within 1 month if stored between 2° and 8° C (36° and 46° F).

- Be aware that patients receiving concurrent or consecutive radiation therapy and those who have received previous cytotoxic drug therapy are at risk for additive bone marrow depression. Expect prescriber to decrease dosage.

- If patient develops thrombocytopenia, implement protective precautions according to facility policy.

- Monitor patients with severe renal disease for exacerbation caused by fever and dehydrating effects of interferon alfa-2b. Monitor patients with cardiac disease (including recent MI), diabetes mellitus prone to ketoacidosis, or pulmonary disease for exacerbations of these conditions caused by interferon-induced fever and chills.

- Monitor patients with herpes zoster or recent or current chicken pox (including recent exposure) for signs and symptoms of severe generalized disease.

- Assess patients with a history of autoimmune disease for exacerbation of condition.

- Be aware that elderly patients may be more prone to adverse effects because of underlying CNS, cardiac, or renal disease.

- Be aware that patients with a history of compromised CNS function, severe psychiatric conditions, or seizure disorders are at risk for severe CNS adverse reactions. Neuropsychiatric follow-up may be ordered, especially for patients receiving high doses of drug.

- Administer acetaminophen, as ordered, to prevent or treat flu-like symptoms, such as fever or headache.
- Be aware that interferon alfa-2b is also given subcutaneously with ribavirin for treating chronic hepatitis. Consult manufacturer's insert for specific information, including contraindications, adverse reactions, and nursing considerations, relating to combination therapy.
- Store drug at 2° to 8° C (36° to 46° F).

PATIENT TEACHING

- Advise patient to avoid potentially hazardous activities until interferon alfa-2b's CNS effects are known.
- Instruct patient to avoid alcohol and CNS depressants during therapy.
- Advise patient to contact prescriber immediately if he notices unusual bleeding or bruising, black or tarry stools, blood in urine or stools, or red pinpoint spots on skin.
- Instruct patient to avoid touching his eyes or inside of nose unless he washes hands immediately beforehand.
- Urge patient to avoid people with infection if he develops bone marrow depression. Advise him to contact prescriber if he experiences fever, chills, cough, hoarseness, lower back or side pain, or painful or difficult urination because these signs and symptoms may signal an infection.
- Teach patient proper oral hygiene, and advise him to use a soft-bristled toothbrush because drug can delay healing, increase the risk of infection, and cause gingival bleeding. Advise patient to check with prescriber before undergoing any dental work.
- Stress the importance of avoiding accidental cuts from sharp objects, such as razors and fingernail clippers, because excessive bleeding or infection may occur. Also, caution patient to avoid contact sports and other activities that increase the risk of injury.
- If patient will self-administer interferon alpha-2b, teach him and his caregiver the proper administration technique, including bedtime administration to decrease effect of fatigue on daily activities.
- Caution patient and caregiver not to reuse needles or syringes, and teach them how to properly dispose of needles and syringes in puncture-resistant containers.
- Stress the importance of complying with the dosage regimen and of keeping follow-up medical appointments and appointments for laboratory tests.

irinotecan hydrochloride

Camptosar

Class and Category

Chemical: Synthetic camptothecin derivative
Therapeutic: Antineoplastic
Pregnancy category: D

Indications and Dosages

▶ *To treat colorectal cancer*

I.V. INFUSION

Adults receiving drug as a single agent. 125 mg/m^2 over
90 min every wk for 4 wk, followed by 2-wk rest period, then
subsequent courses. Alternatively, 240 to 350 mg/m^2 over 90 min
every 3 wk. *Maximum:* 150 mg/m^2/wk.

DOSAGE ADJUSTMENT Dosage is highly individualized,
ranging from 50 to 150 mg/m^2, and may be adjusted in increments—typically 25 to 50 mg/m^2. Doses may even be omitted,
based on severity of adverse reactions, according to the National Cancer Institute's (NCI) Common Toxicity Criteria. Expect initial dose to be decreased to 100 mg/m^2 or less for patients over age 65 with impaired hepatic function *and* a history
of pelvic or abdominal irradiation.

Adults receiving drug with fluorouracil and leucovorin. If
administering fluorouracil-leucovorin boluses, 125 mg/m^2 over
90 min on days 1, 8, 15, and 22, with next course beginning on
day 43. Alternatively, if administering fluorouracil-leucovorin infusions, 180 mg/m^2 over 90 min on days 1, 15, and 29, with next
course beginning on day 43. *Maximum:* 125 mg/m^2/wk.

DOSAGE ADJUSTMENT Dosage reduced or doses omitted
based on severity of adverse reactions, according to NCI's Common Toxicity Criteria.

Mechanism of Action

Inhibits the activity of topoisomerase I, an enzyme that allows single-strand
breaks in the double-stranded DNA chain. Single-strand breaks during DNA
replication, recombination, and repair decrease the torsional strain of the
DNA configuration. Irinotrecan and its metabolite, SN-38, bind to the topoisomerase I complex and prevent religation of the single-strand breaks, which
normally takes place after the DNA has relaxed. This action halts DNA replication, resulting in DNA damage and, eventually, in cell death.

Incompatibilities

Don't refrigerate irinotecan diluted with normal saline solution because a precipitate may form. Don't mix irinotecan with any other drugs.

Contraindications

Hypersensitivity to irinotecan

Interactions

DRUGS

blood-dyscrasia–causing drugs (such as cephalosporins and sulfasalazine): Increased risk of leukopenia and thrombocytopenia
bone marrow depressants (such as carboplatin and lomustine): Possibly additive bone marrow depression
corticosteroids, cyclosporine, and other immunosuppressive drugs: Increased risk of infection
dexamethasone: Possibly hyperglycemia, increased risk of lymphocytopenia
laxatives: Increased risk of severe diarrhea
vaccine, killed virus: Possibly decreased antibody response to vaccine
vaccine, live virus: Possibly decreased antibody response to vaccine, increased adverse effects of vaccine, and severe infection

Adverse Reactions

CNS: Asthenia, chills, fever, headache
CV: Bradycardia, edema, vasodilation (flushing)
EENT: Rhinitis, stomatitis
GI: Abdominal cramps or pain, abdominal distention, anorexia, bloating, constipation, diarrhea, indigestion, nausea, vomiting
HEME: Anemia, leukopenia, neutropenia, thrombocytopenia
RESP: Cough, dyspnea, upper respiratory tract infection
SKIN: Alopecia, diaphoresis, rash
Other: Allergic reaction, anaphylaxis, dehydration, infection (minor), weight loss

Nursing Considerations

- Be aware that irinotecan should be administered only under the supervision of a qualified physician and in a setting where appropriate diagnostic and treatment facilities are available.
- Expect to obtain hemoglobin level and leukocyte and platelet counts before beginning each course of therapy and periodically thereafter. Expect dosage to be adjusted if test results reveal hematologic toxicity—for example, a granulocyte count less than 1,500/mm^3 or a platelet count less than 100,000/mm^3.

- Follow facility policy for handling antineoplastic drugs and for appropriate disposal of used equipment. If irinotecan solution comes in contact with your skin, wash if off thoroughly with soap and water. If drug comes in contact with mucous membranes, irrigate the area thoroughly with water.
- Dilute irinotecan with D_5W (preferred) or normal saline solution to a concentration of 0.12 to 2.8 mg/ml. Discard unused portion in single-use vials (2 ml and 5 ml).
- Because drug contains no preservatives, use solutions prepared with D_5W within 6 hours if stored at room temperature or within 24 hours if refrigerated at 2° to 8° C (36° to 46° F).
- Use solutions made with normal saline solution within 6 hours if stored at room temperature. Don't refrigerate solutions diluted with normal saline solution because precipitate will form.
- Be aware that adverse reactions can vary when irinotecan is administered in combination therapy. Review information for all drugs administered as part of a specific regimen, including drug interactions and adverse effects. Expect dosage to be adjusted based on type of combination therapy used and on incidence and severity of adverse reactions.
- Assess patient often for diarrhea, which may occur immediately after or more than 24 hours after irinotecan dose. Expect to give loperamide at first sign of increased bowel movements.
- Monitor liver function test results periodically, as prescribed, to identify signs of hepatic function impairment.
- Monitor patients with herpes zoster or recent or current chicken pox (including recent exposure) for signs and symptoms of severe generalized disease.
- Assess for signs of infection, such as fever, if patient develops leukopenia. Expect to obtain appropriate specimens for culture and sensitivity testing. Be aware that patients with a preexisting infection may experience impaired recovery.
- Be aware that patients receiving concurrent or consecutive radiation therapy and those with preexisting bone marrow depression are at risk for increased bone marrow depression.
- If extravasation occurs, stop the infusion, flush the area with sterile water, and apply ice. Restart infusion in another vein.
- Monitor patients with drug-induced vomiting and diarrhea for signs of dehydration, such as decreased urine output, poor skin turgor, dry and furrowed tongue, and dry mucous membranes. Patients taking diuretics are at increased risk and may have diuretic withheld if vomiting or diarrhea occurs.

• Store drug at 15° to 30° C (59° to 86° F); protect from freezing and light.

PATIENT TEACHING

• Advise patient to have dental work completed before irinotecan treatment begins, if possible, or to defer such work until blood counts return to normal because drug can delay healing and cause gingival bleeding. Teach patient proper oral hygiene, and suggest that he use a toothbrush with soft bristles.

• Instruct patient to immediately report nausea, vomiting, or diarrhea during irinotecan therapy. Advise him to avoid foods that may irritate the GI system, including high-fiber foods (bran, whole grain breads, and raw fruits and vegetables) and fatty, spicy, or fried foods.

• Advise patient to report burning or other signs of extravasation, such as redness, at I.V. insertion site.

• Encourage patient to drink fluids as prescribed. Urge him to avoid alcohol and caffeinated beverages, such as coffee and cola, which can exacerbate dehydration.

• If patient develops thrombocytopenia, implement protective precautions according to facility policy.

• Urge patient to avoid people with infection if he develops bone marrow depression. Advise him to contact prescriber if he experiences fever, chills, cough, hoarseness, lower back or side pain, or painful or difficult urination because these signs and symptoms may signal an infection.

• Advise patient to contact prescriber immediately if he notices unusual bleeding or bruising, black or tarry stools, blood in urine or stools, or red pinpoint spots on skin.

• Instruct patient to avoid touching his eyes or inside of nose unless he washes hands immediately beforehand.

• Stress the importance of avoiding accidental cuts from sharp objects, such as razors or nail clippers, because excessive bleeding or infection may occur. Also, caution patient to avoid contact sports and other activities that increase the risk of injury.

• Caution patient to avoid receiving immunizations unless approved by prescriber. Instruct him to avoid people who have recently received vaccines or to wear a protective mask that covers his nose and mouth when he's around them.

• Advise patient with stomatitis to eat bland, soft foods served cold or at room temperature to decrease irritation.

• Stress the importance of complying with the dosage regimen and of keeping follow-up medical and laboraotry appointments.

iron dextran
(contains 50 mg of elemental iron per milliliter)
DexFerrum, DexIron (CAN), InFeD

Class and Category
Chemical: Iron salt, mineral
Therapeutic: Antianemic
Pregnancy category: C

Indications and Dosages
▶ *To treat iron deficiency anemia*
I.V. INFUSION
Adults and children weighing over 15 kg (33 lb). Dose (ml) = 0.0442 (desired hemoglobin − observed hemoglobin) × lean body weight (in kg) + (0.26 × lean body weight). Or, consult dosage table provided in package insert. *Maximum:* 2 ml (100 mg) daily.
Children over age 4 months weighing 5 to 15 kg (11 to 33 lb). Dose (ml) = 0.0442 (desired hemoglobin − observed hemoglobin) × weight (kg) + (0.26 × weight). Or, consult dosage table in package insert. *Maximum:* 1 ml (50 mg) daily.
▶ *To replace iron lost in blood loss*
I.V. INFUSION
Adults. Replacement iron (mg) = ml of blood loss × hematocrit.

Mechanism of Action
Restores hemoglobin and replenishes iron stores. Iron, an essential component of hemoglobin, myoglobin, and several enzymes (including cytochromes, catalase, and peroxidase), is needed for catecholamine metabolism and normal neutrophil function. In iron dextran therapy, iron binds to available protein parts after the drug has been split into iron and dextran by cells of the reticuloendothelial system. The bound iron forms hemosiderin or ferritin, physiologic forms of iron, and transferrin, which replenish hemoglobin and depleted iron stores. Dextran is metabolized or excreted.

Incompatibilities
Don't mix iron dextran with blood for transfusion, other drugs, or parenteral nutrition solutions for I.V. infusion.

Contraindications
Anemia other than iron deficiency, hypersensitivity to iron dextran or its components

Interactions
None known.

Adverse Reactions
CNS: Chills, disorientation, dizziness, fever, headache, malaise, paresthesia, seizures, syncope, unconsciousness, weakness
CV: Arrhythmias, bradycardia, chest pain, shock, hypotension, hypertension, tachycardia
EENT: Altered taste
GI: Abdominal pain, diarrhea, nausea, vomiting
GU: Hematuria
HEME: Leukocytosis
MS: Arthralgia, arthritis, backache, myalgia, rhabdomyolysis
RESP: Bronchospasm, dyspnea, respiratory arrest, wheezing
SKIN: Cyanosis, diaphoresis, rash, pruritus, purpura, urticaria
Other: Anaphylaxis, infusion site phlebitis

Nursing Considerations
- Expect oral iron therapy to be stopped before iron dextran therapy starts. Iron dextran is given only when oral therapy is not feasible; it also may be given by I.M. injection.
- Expect to monitor hemoglobin, hematocrit, serum ferritin, and transferrin saturation, as ordered, before, during, and after iron dextran therapy.
- **WARNING** Before starting therapy, administer a test dose of 0.5 ml of iron dextran gradually over 30 seconds, as prescribed, and watch closely for an anaphylactic reaction.
- Wait 1 to 2 hours before administering the remainder of the dose. Infuse undiluted iron dextran slowly, at a rate not to exceed 1 ml/minute (50 mg/minute).
- **WARNING** Monitor patient closely for signs and symptoms of anaphylaxis, such as severe hypotension, loss of consciousness, collapse, dyspnea, and seizures, during and after infusion. Patients with a history of asthma or known allergies are at increased risk for anaphylaxis and, possibly, death. Institute emergency resuscitation measures as needed, including epinephrine administration, as prescribed.
- **WARNING** Assess blood pressure frequently after drug administration because hypotension is a common adverse effect that may be related to infusion rate; avoid rapid infusion.
- Be aware that patient may exhibit adverse reactions, including arthralgia, backache, chills, and vomiting, 1 to 2 days after drug therapy. Symptoms should resolve within 3 to 4 days.

- Assess patients with a history of rheumatoid arthritis for exacerbation of joint pain and swelling.
- Monitor patients with cardiovascular disease for an exacerbation caused by drug's adverse effects.
- Assess patient for iron overload, characterized by sedation, decreased activity, pale eyes, and bleeding in GI tract and lungs.
- Store iron dextran at 15° to 30° C (59° to 86° F).

PATIENT TEACHING

- Instruct patient to immediately report adverse reactions, such as shortness of breath, wheezing, or rash, during iron dextran therapy.
- Advise patient not to take any oral iron preparations without first consulting prescriber.
- Inform patient that symptoms of iron deficiency may include decreased stamina, learning problems, shortness of breath, and fatigue. During periods of anemia, encourage patient to plan periods of activity and rest in order to avoid excessive fatigue.
- Stress the need to follow dosage regimen and keep follow-up medical and laboratory appointments.

iron sucrose
(contains 100 mg of elemental iron per 5 ml)
Venofer

Class and Category
Chemical: Iron salt, mineral
Therapeutic: Antianemic
Pregnancy category: B

Indications and Dosages
▶ *To treat iron deficiency anemia in hemodialysis patients receiving erythropoietin*

I.V. INJECTION

Adults. *Initial:* 100 mg of elemental iron injected undiluted over 2 to 5 min during dialysis. *Usual:* 100 mg of elemental iron every wk to three times/wk to a total dose of 1,000 mg. Dosage repeated as needed to maintain target levels of hemoglobin and hematocrit and acceptable blood iron level. *Maximum:* 100 mg/dose.

I.V. INFUSION

Adults. *Initial:* 100 mg of elemental iron infused diluted over 15 min during dialysis. *Usual:* 100 mg of elemental iron every wk to three times/wk to a total dose of 1,000 mg. Dosage repeated as needed to maintain target levels of hemoglobin and hematocrit and acceptable blood iron level. *Maximum:* 100 mg/dose.

▶ *To treat iron deficiency anemia in peritoneal dialysis patients receiving erythropoietin*

I.V. INFUSION

Adults. *Initial:* 300 mg of elemental iron infused diluted over 1.5 hr on days 1 and 14, followed by 400 mg of elemental iron infused over 2.5 hr on day 28. Dosage repeated as needed to maintain target levels of hemoglobin and hematocrit and acceptable blood iron level. *Maximum:* 1,000 mg/28 days.

▶ *To treat iron deficiency anemia in nondialysis patients with chronic renal disease regardless of whether they're receiving erythropoietin*

I.V. INJECTION

Adults. *Initial:* 200 mg of elemental iron injected undiluted over 2 to 5 min and repeated four more times over a 14-day period for a total dose of 1,000 mg. Dosage repeated as needed to maintain target levels of hemoglobin and hematocrit and acceptable blood iron level. *Maximum:* 1,000 mg/14 days.

I.V. INFUSION

Adults. 500 mg of elemental iron infused diluted over 3.5 to 5 hr on days 1 and 14. Dosage repeated as needed to maintain target levels of hemoglobin and hematocrit and acceptable blood iron level. *Maximum:* 1,000 mg/14 days.

Mechanism of Action

Acts to replenish iron stores lost during dialysis because of increased erythropoiesis and insufficient absorption of iron from the GI tract. Iron is an essential component of hemoglobin, myoglobin, and several enzymes, including cytochromes, catalase, and peroxidase, and is needed for catecholamine metabolism and normal neutrophil function. Iron sucrose injection also normalizes RBC production by binding with hemoglobin or being stored as ferritin in reticuloendothelial cells of the liver, spleen, and bone marrow.

Incompatibilities

Don't mix with other drugs or parenteral nutrition solutions for I.V. infusion.

Contraindications

Anemia other than iron deficiency, hypersensitivity to iron salts or their components, iron overload

Interactions
DRUGS

chloramphenicol: Possibly decreased effectiveness of iron sucrose

oral iron preparations: Possibly reduced absorption of oral iron supplements

Adverse Reactions

CNS: Asthenia, dizziness, fatigue, fever, headache, hypoesthesia, loss of consciousness or collapse, malaise, seizure

CV: Chest pain, heart failure, hypertension, hypotension, peripheral edema

EENT: Conjunctivitis, ear pain, nasal congestion, nasopharyngitis, rhinitis, sinusitis, taste perversion

ENDO: Hyperglycemia, hypoglycemia

GI: Abdominal pain, constipation, diarrhea, dysgeusia, elevated liver function test results, nausea, occult-positive feces, peritoneal infection, vomiting

GU: UTI

MS: Arthralgia, arthritis, back pain, leg cramps, muscle pain or weakness, myalgia

RESP: Bronchospasm, cough, dyspnea, pneumonia, upper respiratory tract infection, wheezing

SKIN: Pruritus, rash

Other: Anaphylaxis; fluid overload; gout; hypervolemia; infusion or injection site burning, pain, or redness; sepsis

Nursing Considerations

- To reconstitute iron sucrose injection for infusion, dilute 100 mg of elemental iron in no more than 100 ml (hemodialysis) or 250 ml (peritoneal or no dialysis) of normal saline solution immediately before infusion. Discard any unused diluted iron sucrose solution.
- Give drug directly into dialysis line by slow I.V. injection or infusion.
- **WARNING** Monitor patient closely for signs or symptoms of anaphylaxis, such as severe hypotension, loss of consciousness, collapse, dyspnea, or seizures, during and after iron sucrose therapy. Institute emergency resuscitation measures as needed.
- **WARNING** Assess patient's blood pressure often after giving iron sucrose. Hypotension is common and may be related to the infusion rate (avoid rapid infusion) or the total cumulative dose.

- Monitor hemoglobin, hematocrit, serum ferritin, and transferrin saturation, as ordered, before, during, and after iron sucrose therapy. Serum iron levels must be tested 48 hours after last dose. Notify prescriber and expect to stop therapy if blood iron levels are normal or elevated, to prevent iron toxicity.
- Watch for possible iron overload, characterized by sedation, decreased activity, pale eyes, and bleeding in GI tract and lungs.

PATIENT TEACHING

- Advise patient not to take any oral iron preparations during iron sucrose therapy without first consulting prescriber.
- Inform patient that iron deficiency may cause decreased stamina, learning problems, shortness of breath, and fatigue.

isoproterenol hydrochloride
Isuprel

Class and Category
Chemical: Catecholamine
Therapeutic: Antiarrhythmic, bronchodilator
Pregnancy category: C

Indications and Dosages
▶ *To manage bronchospasm during anesthesia*
I.V. INJECTION
Adults. 0.01 to 0.02 mg, repeated p.r.n.
▶ *To treat bradycardia with significant hemodynamic change, such as third-degree heart block or prolonged QT interval*
I.V. INFUSION
Adults. *Initial:* 2 mcg/min, titrated according to heart rate, as ordered. *Maximum:* 10 mcg/min.

Route	Onset	Peak	Duration
I.V.	In 5 min*	Unknown	10 min†

Contraindications
Angina pectoris, heart block or tachycardia from digitalis toxicity, hypersensitivity to isoproterenol or its components (such as sulfite in some preparations), tachyarrhythmias, ventricular arrhythmias that require inotropic therapy

---

* For treatment of bradycardia; unknown for treatment of bronchospasm.
† For treatment of bradycardia; 1 to 2 hr for treatment of bronchospasm.

Mechanism of Action

Stimulates beta$_1$ receptors in the myocardium and cardiac conduction system, resulting in positive inotropic and chronotropic effects. Isoproterenol also shortens the AV conduction time and refractory period in patients with AV block. This action increases the ventricular rate and halts bradycardia and associated syncope.

In addition, isoproterenol attaches to beta$_2$ receptors on bronchial cell membranes. This action stimulates the intracellular enzyme adenylate cyclase to convert adenosine triphosphate to cAMP. An increased intracellular level of cAMP relaxes bronchial smooth-muscle cells, stabilizes mast cells, and inhibits histamine release.

Interactions

DRUGS

alpha blockers, other drugs with alpha-blocking effects: Possibly decreased peripheral vasoconstricting and hypertensive effects of isoproterenol

astemizole, cisapride, drugs that prolong QTc interval, terfenadine: Possibly prolonged QTc interval

beta blockers (ophthalmic): Decreased effects of isoproterenol, increased risk of bronchospasm, wheezing, decreased pulmonary function, and respiratory failure

beta blockers (systemic): Increased risk of bronchospasm, decreased effects of both drugs

digoxin: Increased risk of arrhythmias, hypokalemia, and digitalis toxicity

diuretics, other antihypertensives: Possibly decreased antihypertensive effects

ergot alkaloids: Increased vasoconstriction and vasopressor effects

hydrocarbon inhalation anesthetics: Increased risk of atrial and ventricular arrhythmias

MAO inhibitors: Intensified and extended cardiac stimulation and vasopressor effects

quinidine, other drugs that affect myocardial reaction to sympathomimetics: Increased risk of arrhythmias

theophylline: Increased risk of cardiotoxicity, decreased blood theophylline level

thyroid hormones: Increased effects of both drugs, and increased risk of coronary insufficiency in patients with coronary artery disease

tricyclic antidepressants: Increased vasopressor response, increased risk of prolonged QTc interval and arrhythmias

Adverse Reactions

CNS: Dizziness, headache, insomnia, nervousness, syncope, tremor, weakness
CV: Adams-Stokes syndrome, angina, arrhythmias, bradycardia, hypertension, hypotension, palpitations, tachycardia, ventricular arrhythmias
EENT: Blurred vision, oropharyngeal edema
ENDO: Hyperglycemia
GI: Nausea, vomiting
MS: Muscle spasms and twitching
RESP: Bronchospasm, dyspnea, wheezing
SKIN: Diaphoresis, erythema multiforme, pallor, pruritus, rash, Stevens-Johnson syndrome, urticaria
Other: Angioedema, hypokalemia

Nursing Considerations

- Expect to give lowest possible dose of isoproterenol for shortest possible time to minimize tolerance.
- Don't give isoproterenol if it is pink or brown or contains precipitate.
- Inspect drug label carefully to verify correct concentration, which ranges from 0.02 mg/ml (1:50,000) to 0.2 mg/ml (1:5,000).
- Administer infusion through large vein, and watch for signs of extravasation.
- Monitor blood pressure, cardiac rhythm, central venous pressure, and urine output during administration. Adjust infusion rate to response, as ordered.
- Notify prescriber immediately if heart rate increases significantly or exceeds 110 beats/minute during infusion.
- Know that drug may increase pulse pressure and cause hypotension. Expect to reduce infusion slowly to decrease the risk of hypotension.
- **WARNING** Be aware that isoproterenol markedly increases the risk of arrhythmias. If an arrhythmia occurs, expect to give a cardioselective beta blocker, such as atenolol, as prescribed.
- Be aware that isoproterenol isn't used regularly to treat asthma, decreased cardiac output, hypotension, or shock because it increases the risk of arrhythmias, hypotension, and ischemia.

- **WARNING** If isoproterenol aggravates a ventilation-perfusion problem, expect patient's blood oxygen level to fall even as his breathing seems to improve.
- Consult manufacturer's guidelines for storage information. Recommended temperature varies with form used.

PATIENT TEACHING

- Instruct patient receiving isoproterenol to report chest pain, difficulty breathing, dizziness, hyperglycemic symptoms (such as abdominal cramps, lethargy, nausea, and vomiting), insomnia, irregular heartbeat, palpitations, tremor, and weakness.

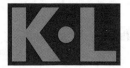

kanamycin sulfate
Kantrex

Class and Category
Chemical: Aminoglycoside
Therapeutic: Antibiotic
Pregnancy category: D

Indications and Dosages
▶ *To treat infections caused by gram-negative organisms (including* Acinetobacter *species,* Enterobacter aerogenes, Escherichia coli, Haemophilus influenzae, Klebsiella pneumoniae, Neisseria *species,* Proteus *species,* Providencia *species,* Salmonella *species,* Serratia marcescens, Shigella *species, and* Yersinia *species) and gram-positive organisms (including* Staphylococcus aureus *and* Staphylococcus epidermidis*)*

I.V. INFUSION

Adults and children. 5 mg/kg every 8 hr or 7.5 mg/kg every 12 hr for 7 to 10 days. *Maximum:* 1.5 g daily.

DOSAGE ADJUSTMENT For elderly patients and those with renal failure, dosage reduced and blood kanamycin level and renal function test results monitored.

Route	Onset	Peak	Duration
I.V.	Rapid	Unknown	Unknown

Mechanism of Action
Binds to negatively charged sites on bacterial outer cell membranes, which disrupts cell membrane integrity. Kanamycin also binds to bacterial ribosomal subunits and inhibits protein synthesis; these actions lead to cell death.

Contraindications
Hypersensitivity to kanamycin, other aminoglycosides, or their components

Incompatibilities

Don't mix kanamycin in same syringe or administer through same I.V. line as other antibiotics.

Interactions

DRUGS

cephalosporins, vancomycin: Increased risk of nephrotoxicity
digoxin, loop diuretics: Increased ototoxic and nephrotoxic effects of kanamycin
general anesthetics, neuromuscular blockers: Increased risk of neuromuscular blockade
penicillins: Inactivation of kanamycin or synergistic effects

Adverse Reactions

CNS: Ataxia, dizziness, headache
EENT: Hearing loss
GI: Diarrhea
GU: Elevated BUN and serum creatinine levels, oliguria, proteinuria
MS: Muscle paralysis
RESP: Apnea
SKIN: Injection site irritation or pain, rash, pruritus, urticaria

Nursing Considerations

- Obtain body fluid or tissue specimen for culture and sensitivity testing before kanamycin therapy begins, as indicated. Therapy may begin before test results are available.
- Dilute 500-mg vial with 100 to 200 ml normal saline solution or D_5W, or 1-g vial with 200 to 400 ml normnal saline solution or D_5W, and infuse over 30 to 60 minutes. Adjust amount of diluent proportionately for pediatric doses. Be aware that vial contents may darken during storage; potency isn't affected.
- Keep patient well hydrated before and during therapy.
- Check blood kanamycin level periodically during therapy, as appropriate.
- Be aware that prolonged treatment increases the risk of ototoxicity and nephrotoxicity. Monitor hearing and renal function if therapy lasts longer than 10 days.
- Store drug at 15° to 30° C (59° to 86° F); don't freeze.

PATIENT TEACHING

- Advise patient to report dizziness, hearing loss, and severe diarrhea or headache during kanamycin therapy.
- Explain the need to receive kanamycin at prescribed intervals around the clock until patient completes full course of therapy.

ketorolac tromethamine

Toradol

Class and Category

Chemical: Acetic acid derivative
Therapeutic: Analgesic, anti-inflammatory
Pregnancy category: C

Indications and Dosages

▶ *To treat moderate to severe pain*

I.V. INJECTION

Adults ages 16 to 64. *Initial:* 30 mg as a single dose or 30 mg every 6 hr p.r.n. *Maximum:* 120 mg daily for no more than 5 days.

DOSAGE ADJUSTMENT For patients weighing less than 50 kg, elderly patients, and patients with impaired renal function, initial dose reduced to 15 mg, followed by oral ketorolac if needed; or 15 mg every 6 hr p.r.n., up to maximum of 60 mg daily for no more than 5 days.

Route	Onset	Peak	Duration
I.V.	30 to 60 min	1 to 2 hr	4 to 6 hr

Mechanism of Action

Blocks the activity of cyclooxygenase, the enzyme needed to synthesize prostaglandins. Prostaglandins mediate the inflammatory response and cause local vasodilation, swelling, and pain. They also promote pain transmission from the periphery to the spinal cord. By blocking cyclooxygenase and inhibiting prostaglandins, this NSAID reduces inflammatory symptoms and relieves pain.

Contraindications

Advanced renal impairment or risk of renal impairment due to volume depletion; before or during surgery if hemostasis is critical; breast-feeding; cerebrovascular bleeding; concurrent use of aspirin or other salicylates, other NSAIDs, or probenecid; hemophilia or other bleeding problems, including coagulation or platelet function disorders; hemorrhagic diathesis; history of GI bleeding, GI perforation, or peptic ulcer disease; hypersensitivity to ketorolac tromethamine, aspirin, other NSAIDs, or their components; incomplete hemostasis; labor and delivery; treatment of perioperative pain in coronary artery bypass surgery

Interactions

DRUGS

ACE inhibitors: Increased risk of renal function impairment; decreased effectiveness of ACE inhibitors

acetaminophen, gold compounds: Increased risk of adverse renal effects

amphotericin, penicillamine, and other nephrotoxic drugs: Increased risk or severity of adverse renal effects

antihypertensives, diuretics: Possibly reduced effects of these drugs

aspirin and other salicylates, other NSAIDs: Additive toxicity

cefamandole, cefoperazone, cefotetan: Possibly hypoprothrombinemia

corticosteroids, potassium supplements: Increased risk of gastric ulceration or hemorrhage

furosemide: Decreased effects of furosemide

heparin, oral anticoagulants, platelet aggregation inhibitors, thrombolytics: Increased risk of GI bleeding

lithium: Possibly increased blood lithium level and increased risk of lithium toxicity

methotrexate: Possibly methotrexate toxicity

nondepolarizing muscle relaxants: Increased risk of apnea

pentoxifylline: Increased risk of bleeding

plicamycin, valproic acid: Possibly hypoprothrombinemia and increased risk of bleeding

probenecid: Decreased elimination of ketorolac, increased risk of adverse effects

selective serotonin reuptake inhibitors: Increased risk of GI bleeding

ACTIVITIES

alcohol use: Increased risk of adverse GI effects

Adverse Reactions

CNS: Cerebral hemorrhage, CVA, dizziness, drowsiness, headache

CV: Edema, fluid retention, hypertension

EENT: Stomatitis

GI: Abdominal pain; bloating; constipation; diarrhea; diverticulitis; flatulence; GI bleeding, perforation, or ulceration; hepatic failure; indigestion; nausea; perforation of stomach or intestine; vomiting; worsening of inflammatory bowel disease

GU: Interstitial nephritis

HEME: Anemia

SKIN: Diaphoresis, erythema multiforme, exfoliative dermatitis, pruritus, rash, Stevens-Johnson syndrome, toxic epidermal necrolysis

Other: Anaphylaxis, angioedema, injection site pain, unusual weight gain

Nursing Considerations

- Read ketorolac label carefully. Don't use I.M. form for I.V. administration. Be aware that ketorolac is not for intrathecal or epidural use.
- Administer drug over at least 15 seconds.
- Notify prescriber if pain relief is inadequate or if breakthrough pain occurs between doses because supplemental doses of an opioid analgesic may be required.
- Use ketorolac with extreme caution in patients with a history of inflammatory bowel disease (ulcerative colitis, Crohn's disease), GI ulcer disease, or GI bleeding because NSAIDs such as ketorolac may worsen inflammatory bowel disease and increase the risk of GI bleeding and ulceration. Ketorolac should be used for the shortest possible time in these patients.
- Be aware that serious GI tract ulceration, bleeding, and perforation may occur without warning or symptoms. Elderly patients are at greater risk. To minimize risk, give drug with food. If GI distress occurs, withhold drug and notify prescriber immediately.
- Use ketorolac cautiously in patients with hypertension, and monitor blood pressure closely during therapy because ketorolac may lead to or worsen hypertension.
- **WARNING** Monitor patient closely for thrombotic events, including MI and CVA, because use of NSAIDs such as ketorolac increases the risk.
- Monitor patient—especially if he's elderly—for less common but serious adverse GI reactions, including anorexia, constipation, diverticulitis, dysphagia, esophagitis, gastritis, gastroenteritis, gastroesophageal reflux disease, hemorrhoids, hiatal hernia, melena, stomatitis, and vomiting.
- Monitor liver function test results because elevations may rarely progress to severe hepatic reactions, including fatal hepatitis, liver necrosis, and hepatic failure.
- Monitor BUN and serum creatinine levels in patients with heart failure, impaired renal function, or hepatic dysfunction; those who take diuretics or ACE inhibitors; and the elderly because ketorolac may cause renal failure.
- Monitor CBC for decreased hemoglobin and hematocrit; ketorolac may worsen anemia.
- **WARNING** If patient has bone marrow suppression or is re-

ceiving antineoplastic therapy, monitor laboratory results (including WBCs) and watch for evidence of infection because ketorolac has anti-inflammatory and antipyretic actions that may mask signs and symptoms, such as fever and pain.

• Assess patient's skin routinely for evidence of rash or other hypersensitivity reactions because NSAIDs such as ketorolac may cause serious skin reactions without warning, even in patients with no history of NSAID hypersensitivity. Discontinue drug at first sign of reaction, and notify prescriber.

• **WARNING** Monitor patients with a history of peripheral edema, heart failure, or hypertension for adequate fluid balance because drug can promote fluid retention and exacerbate these conditions. Assess for dyspnea, edema, unexplained rapid weight gain, and decreased activity tolerance. Notify prescriber if such symptoms develop.

• Be aware that maximum duration of ketorolac therapy is 5 days.

• Store drug at 15° to 30° C (59° to 86° F), and protect from light.

PATIENT TEACHING

• Advise patient to avoid taking acetaminophen, aspirin, other salicylates, and other NSAIDs while receiving ketorolac unless prescriber approves.

• Instruct him to notify prescriber immediately if he experiences blood in urine, easy bruising, itching, rash, swelling, or yellow eyes or skin.

• Caution pregnant patient that NSAIDs such as ketolac should not be taken during the last trimester because drug may cause premature closure of the ductus arteriosus.

• Explain that ketorolac may increase the risk of serious adverse cardiovascular reactions; urge patient to seek immediate medical attention if he has such signs and symptoms as chest pain, shortness of breath, weakness, and slurring of speech.

• Tell patient that ketorolac may increase the risk of serious adverse GI problems; stress the need to seek immediate medical attention for such signs or symptoms as epigastric or abdominal pain, indigestion, black or tarry stools, and vomiting blood or matrial that looks like coffee grounds.

• Alert patient to the possibility of serious skin reactions, although rare, with ketorolac therapy. Urge patient to seek immediate medical attention for such signs and symptoms as a rash, blisters, fever, or other signs of hypersensitivity, such as itching.

- Caution patient to avoid potentially hazardous activities until drug's CNS effects are known.
- Urge patient to avoid alcohol during ketorolac therapy because of increased risk of adverse GI effects.
- Encourage patient to have dental procedures performed before starting drug therapy because of increased risk of bleeding.
- Teach patient proper oral hygiene measures, and encourage him to use a soft-bristled toothbrush during ketorolac therapy.

labetalol hydrochloride
Normodyne, Trandate

Class and Category
Chemical: Benzamine derivative
Therapeutic: Antihypertensive
Pregnancy category: C

Indications and Dosages
▶ *To manage severe hypertension and treat hypertensive emergencies*
I. V. INFUSION
Adults. 200 mg diluted in 160 ml of D_5W and infused at 2 mg/min until desired response occurs.
I.V. INJECTION
Adults. 20 mg given over 2 min; additional doses given in increments of 40 to 80 mg every 10 min as indicated until desired response occurs. *Maximum:* 300 mg.

Route	Onset	Peak	Duration
I.V.	2 to 5 min	5 to 15 min	2 to 4 hr

Mechanism of Action
Selectively blocks $alpha_1$ and $beta_2$ receptors in vascular smooth muscle and $beta_1$ receptors in the heart. These actions reduce peripheral vascular resistance and blood pressure. Potent beta blockade prevents reflex tachycardia, which commonly occurs when alpha blockers reduce the resting heart rate, cardiac output, or stroke volume.

Incompatibilities
Don't dilute labetalol in sodium bicarbonate solution or administer through same I.V. line as alkaline drugs, such as furosemide; doing so may cause a white precipitate to form.

Contraindications

Asthma, cardiogenic shock, heart failure, hypersensitivity to labetalol or its components, second- or third-degree heart block, severe bradycardia

Interactions

DRUGS

allergen immunotherapy, allergenic extracts for skin testing: Increased risk of serious systemic reaction or anaphylaxis

calcium channel blockers, clonidine, diazoxide, guanabenz, reserpine: Possibly hypotension

cimetidine: Possibly increased labetalol effects

estrogens, NSAIDs: Possibly reduced antihypertensive effect of labetalol

general anesthetics: Increased risk of hypotension and myocardial depression

insulin, oral antidiabetic drugs: Increased risk of hyperglycemia

nitroglycerin: Possibly hypertension

phenoxybenzamine, phentolamine: Possibly additive $alpha_1$-blocking effects

sympathomimetics with alpha- and beta-adrenergic effects (such as pseudoephedrine): Possibly hypertension, excessive bradycardia, or heart block

xanthines (aminophylline and theophylline): Possibly decreased therapeutic effects of both drugs

FOODS

all food: Increased blood labetalol level

ACTIVITIES

alcohol use: Increased labetalol effects

Adverse Reactions

CNS: Anxiety, confusion, depression, dizziness, drowsiness, fatigue, paresthesia, syncope, vertigo, weakness, yawning

CV: Bradycardia, chest pain, edema, heart block, heart failure, hypotension, orthostatic hypotension, ventricular arrhythmias

EENT: Nasal congestion, taste perversion

GI: Elevated liver function test results, hepatic necrosis, hepatitis, indigestion, nausea, vomiting

GU: Ejaculation failure, impotence

RESP: Dyspnea, wheezing

SKIN: Jaundice, pruritus, rash, scalp tingling

Nursing Considerations

• Dilute labetalol to a final concentration of 1 or 3 mg/ml. Administer infusion by infusion pump or another method that allows precise measurement.

- During labetalol administration, monitor blood pressure according to facility policy, usually every 5 minutes for 30 minutes, then every 30 minutes for 2 hours, and then every hour for 6 hours. Monitor ECG as ordered.
- Keep patient in supine position for 3 hours after I.V. administration.
- **WARNING** Be aware that labetalol masks common signs of shock.
- Monitor blood glucose level in diabetic patient because labetalol may conceal symptoms of hypoglycemia such as tachycardia.
- Expect to discontinue drug if patient's liver function test results are elevated. Monitor closely for signs of hepatotoxicity, such as jaundice and flulike symptoms.
- Monitor for signs of heart failure, such as dyspnea and crackles. Expect to administer a digitalis glycoside, a diuretic, or both at first sign of heart failure. If heart failure continues, expect to discontinue labetalol gradually, if possible.
- Monitor patients who are receiving other drugs with antihypertensive effects. Expect labetalol dosage to be adjusted if patient experiences adverse reactions, such as hypotension or bradycardia, or if prescriber adds or discontinues another drug.
- Store drug at 2° to 30° C (36° to 86° F); protect from freezing and light.

PATIENT TEACHING
- Advise patient to report confusion, difficulty breathing, rash, slow pulse, and swelling in arms or legs during labetalol therapy.
- Suggest that patient rise slowly and avoid sudden position changes to minimize effects of orthostatic hypotension.
- Inform diabetic patient that her blood glucose level will be monitored often; instruct her to report signs of hypoglycemia.
- Inform patient that transient scalp tingling may occur during early phase of treatment.

lansoprazole
Prevacid, Prevacid I.V., Prevacid SoluTab

Class and Category
Chemical: Substituted benzimidazole
Therapeutic: Antisecretory, antiulcer
Pregnancy category: B

Indications and Dosages

▶ *To treat erosive esophagitis short-term (up to 7 days) in patients unable to take oral medication*

I.V. INFUSION

Adults. 30 mg daily infused over 30 min for up to 7 days.

Route	Onset	Peak	Duration
P.O.	1 to 3 hr	Unknown	More than 24 hr

Mechanism of Action

Binds to and inactivates the hydrogen-potassium adenosine triphosphate enzyme system (also called the proton pump) in gastric parietal cells. This action blocks the final step of gastric acid production.

Incompatibilities

Don't give any other drugs with parenteral lansoprazole, and dilute only with solutions recommended by manufacturer (sterile water for initial reconstitution and normal saline solution, lactated Ringer's solution, or D_5W for further dilution).

Contraindications

Hypersensitivity to lansoprazole or its components

Interactions

DRUGS

ampicillin, digoxin, iron salts, ketoconazole, other drugs that depend on low gastric pH for bioavailability: Inhibited absorption of these drugs
atazanavir: Decreased plasma atazanavir level and possible loss of effectiveness
sucralfate: Delayed lansoprazole absorption
theophylline: Slightly decreased blood theophylline level
warfarin: Increased INR and PT with possible increased risk of serious bleeding

Adverse Reactions

CNS: Dizziness, headache
GI: Abdominal pain, anorexia, diarrhea, hepatotoxicity, increased appetite, nausea, pancreatitis, pseudomembranous colitis, vomiting
GU: Interstitial nephritis, urine retention
HEME: Agranulocytosis, aplastic anemia, hemolytic anemia, leukopenia, neutropenia, pancytopenia, thrombocytopenia,

thrombotic thrombocytopenic purpura
MS: Arthralgia, myositis
SKIN: Erythema multiforme, pruritus, rash, Stevens-Johnson syndrome, toxic epidermal necrolysis
Other: Anaphylaxis, injection site reaction

Nursing Considerations
• Reconstitute parenteral form by injecting 5 ml of sterile water into 30-mg vial of drug. Mix gently until powder dissolves. Use within 1 hour. After reconstitution, dilute with 50 ml of normal saline solution, lactated Ringer's solution, or D$_5$W. Give within 12 hours if mixed with D$_5$W or 24 hours if mixed with normal saline solution or lactated Ringer's solution.
• Give parenteral drug with a filter following manufacturer's guidelines. Change filter every 24 hours. Give as an I.V. infusion over 30 minutes. Flush the line with normal saline solution, lactated Ringer's solution, or D$_5$W before and after giving lansoprazole.
• Expect to use lansoprazole with antibiotics because decreased gastric acid secretion helps antibiotics eradicate *Helicobacter pylori.*
• If given with antibiotics, watch for diarrhea from possible pseudomembranous colitis.
PATIENT TEACHING
• Advise patient to report diarrhea, severe headache, or worsening of symptoms immediately to prescriber.

lepirudin
Refludan

Class and Category
Chemical: Yeast-derived recombinant form of hirudin
Therapeutic: Anticoagulant
Pregnancy category: B

Indications and Dosages
▶ *To prevent thromboembolic complications in patients with heparin-induced thrombocytopenia and associated thromboembolic disease*
I.V. INFUSION, I.V. INJECTION
Adults. *Initial:* 0.4 mg/kg, but no more than 44 mg, given by bolus over 15 to 20 sec, followed by continuous infusion of 0.15 mg/kg/ hr for 2 to 10 days or longer, as indicated. *Maximum:* 0.21 mg/kg/hr.

DOSAGE ADJUSTMENT For patients with renal insufficiency, bolus dose decreased to 0.2 mg/kg and infusion rate adjusted as follows: for creatinine clearance of 45 to 60 ml/min/1.73 m^2, 50% of standard infusion rate; for creatinine clearance of 30 to 44 ml/min/1.73 m^2, 30% of standard infusion rate; for creatinine clearance of 15 to 29 ml/min/1.73 m^2, 15% of standard infusion rate; for clearance of less than 15 ml/min/1.73 m^2, expect drug to be stopped.

Route	Onset	Peak	Duration
I.V.	Immediate	Unknown	Unknown

Mechanism of Action
Forms a tight bond with thrombin, neutralizing this enzyme's actions, even when the enzyme is trapped within clots. One molecule of lepirudin binds with one molecule of thrombin. Thrombin causes fibrinogen to convert to fibrin, which is essential for clot formation.

Incompatibilities
Don't mix lepirudin in same I.V. line with other drugs.

Contraindications
Hypersensitivity to lepirudin or other hirudins

Interactions
oral anticoagulants, platelet aggregation inhibitors, thrombolytics: Increased risk of bleeding complications and enhanced effects of lepirudin

Adverse Reactions
CNS: Chills, fever, intracranial hemorrhage
CV: Heart failure
EENT: Epistaxis
GI: GI or rectal bleeding, hepatic dysfunction
GU: Hematuria, vaginal bleeding
HEME: Anemia, easy bruising, hematoma
RESP: Hemoptysis, pneumonia
SKIN: Excessive bleeding from wounds, rash, pruritus, urticaria
Other: Anaphylaxis, injection site bleeding, sepsis

Nursing Considerations
• Be aware that patients with heparin-induced thrombocytopenia have low platelet counts, which can lead to severe bleeding and

even death. Lepirudin prevents clotting without further reducing platelet count.

- To reconstitute, mix drug with normal saline solution or sterile water for injection. Warm solution to room temperature before administering.
- For I.V. bolus, reconstitute 50 mg with 1 ml sterile water for injection or sodium chloride for injection. Further dilute by withdrawing reconstituted solution into a 10-ml syringe and adding enough sterile water for injection, sodium chloride for injection, or D_5W to produce a total volume of 10 ml, or 5 mg of lepirudin/ml. Administer prescribed dose over 15 to 20 seconds.
- For I.V. infusion, reconstitute 2 vials of drug and transfer to infusion bag that contains 250 or 500 ml of normal saline solution or D_5W. Concentration will be 0.4 or 0.2 mg/ml.
- Adjust infusion rate as prescribed, according to patient's APTT ratio, which is APTT divided by a control value. Target APTT ratio during treatment is 1.5 to 2.5.
- Expect to obtain first APTT 4 hours after starting infusion and to obtain follow-up APTT daily (more often for patients with hepatic or renal impairment).
- Stop infusion for 2 hours, as ordered, if APTT is above target range. Expect to decrease infusion rate by one-half when restarting. If APTT is below target range, expect to increase rate in 20% increments and recheck APTT in 4 hours.
- Avoid I.M. injections or needle sticks during therapy to minimize risk of hematoma.
- Observe I.M. injection sites, I.V. infusion sites, and wounds for bleeding.
- Monitor for ecchymoses on arms and legs, epistaxis, hematemesis, hematuria, melena, and vaginal bleeding.
- Be aware that when the patient is scheduled to switch to an oral anticoagulant, the lepirudin dosage may need to be tapered over some days, as ordered, until the APPT is just above 1.5 before starting the oral anticoagulant. In addition, the patient's INR and PT will need to be monitored closely, as ordered, to prevent adverse bleeding effects.

PATIENT TEACHING
- Tell patient to report unexpected bleeding: blood in urine, easy bruising, nosebleeds, tarry stools, and vaginal bleeding.
- Advise patient to avoid bumping arms and legs because of the risk of bruising.
- Encourage patient to use an electric razor and a soft toothbrush to reduce the risk of bleeding.

levetiracetam

Keppra

Class and Category

Chemical: Pyrrolidine derivative
Therapeutic: Anticonvulsant
Pregnancy category: C

Indications and Dosages

▶ *As adjunct to treat partial seizures in patients with epilepsy who are temporarily unable to take oral form*

I.V. INFUSION

Adults and adolescents over age 16. *Initial:* 500 mg b.i.d., over 15 min, increased by 1,000 mg daily every 2 wk if needed. *Maximum:* 3,000 mg daily.

DOSAGE ADJUSTMENT Maximum dosage reduced to 2,000 mg/day if creatinine clearance is 50 to 80 ml/min/ 1.73 m^2; reduced to 1,500 mg/day if clearance is 30 to 49 ml/ min/1.73 m^2; and reduced to 1,000 mg/day if clearance is less than 30 ml/min/1.73 m^2. For patients with end-stage renal disease who are receiving dialysis, expect to give another 250 to 500 mg/dose, as prescribed, after each session.

Mechanism of Action

May protect against secondary generalized seizure activity by preventing co-ordination of epileptiform burst firing. Levetiracetam doesn't seem to involve inhibitory and excitatory neurotransmission.

Contraindications

Hypersensitivity to levetiracetam or its components

Adverse Reactions

CNS: Aggression, agitation, anger, anxiety, apathy, asthenia, ataxia, confusion, depresson, dizziness, emotional lability, fatigue, headache, hostility, increased reflexes, irritability, mental or mood changes, nervousness, neurosis, paresthesia, personality disorder, somnolence, vertigo

EENT: Amblyopia, conjunctivitis, diplopia, ear pain, pharyngitis, rhinitis, sinusitis

GI: Anorexia, constipation, diarrhea, gastroenteritis, pancreatitis, vomiting

GU: Albuminuria

HEME: Leukopenia, neutropenia, pancytopenia, thrombocytopenia

MS: Neck pain

RESP: Asthma, cough

SKIN: Alopecia, ecchymosis, pruritus, skin discoloration, vesiculobullous rash

Other: Dehydration, facial edema, infection

Nursing Considerations

- Dilute levetiracetam (500 mg/5 ml) in 100 ml normal saline solution, lactated Ringer's solution, or D_5W before administration.
- Assess compliance during first 4 weeks of therapy, when adverse reactions are most common.
- Monitor patient for seizure activity during levetiracetam therapy. As appropriate, implement seizure precautions according to facility policy.
- Stopping drug may increase seizure activity. Expect to taper dosage gradually.

PATIENT TEACHING

- Caution patient that levetiracetam may cause dizziness and drowsiness, especially during first 4 weeks of therapy.
- Advise patient to avoid hazardous activities until drug's full CNS effects are known.
- Caution patient not to stop taking levetiracetam abruptly; inform her that drug dosage should be tapered under prescriber's direction to reduce the risk of breakthrough seizures.
- Advise patient to keep taking other anticonvulsants, as ordered, while taking levetiracetam.
- Encourage patient to avoid alcohol during therapy because alcohol can increase incidence of drowsiness and dizziness.
- Instruct patient to see prescriber regularly so that her progress can be monitored.

levofloxacin

Levaquin

Class and Category

Chemical: Fluoroquinolone

Therapeutic: Antibiotic

Pregnancy category: C

Indications and Dosages

▶ *To treat acute maxillary sinusitis caused by* Haemophilus influenzae, Moraxella catarrhalis, *or* Streptococcus pneumoniae

I.V. INFUSION

Adults. 500 mg daily (over 60 min) for 10 to 14 days.

▶ *To treat acute exacerbations of chronic bacterial bronchitis caused by* H. influenzae, Haemophilus parainfluenzae, M. catarrhalis, S. pneumoniae, *or* Staphylococcus aureus

I.V. INFUSION

Adults. 500 mg daily (over 60 min) for 7 days.

▶ *To treat community-acquired pneumonia caused by* Chlamydia pneumoniae, H. influenzae, H. parainfluenzae, Klebsiella pneumoniae, Legionella pneumophila, M. catarrhalis, Mycoplasma pneumoniae, S. aureus, *or* S. pneumoniae

I.V. INFUSION

Adults. 500 mg daily (over 60 min) for 7 to 14 days. Alternatively, for infection caused by *C. pneumoniae, H. influenzae, H. parainfluenzae, M. pneumoniae, or S. pneumoniae*, 750 mg daily (over 60 to 90 min) for 5 days.

▶ *To treat uncomplicated UTI caused by* Escherichia coli, K. pneumoniae, *or* Staphylococcus saprophyticus

I.V. INFUSION

Adults. 250 mg daily (over 60 min) for 3 days.

▶ *To treat acute pyelonephritis caused by* E. coli

I.V. INFUSION

Adults. 250 mg daily (over 60 min) for 10 days. Alternatively, 750 mg daily (over 90 min) for 5 days.

▶ *To treat mild to moderate complicated UTI caused by* Enterococcus faecalis, Enterobacter cloacae, E. coli, K. pneumoniae, Proteus mirabilis, *or* Pseudomonas aeruginosa

I.V. INFUSION

Adults. 250 mg daily (over 60 min) for 10 days.

▶ *To treat complicated UTI caused by* E. coli, K. pneumoniae, *or* P. mirabilis

I.V. INFUSION

Adults. 750 mg daily (over 90 min) for 5 days.

▶ *To treat mild to moderate skin and soft-tissue infections caused by* S. aureus *or* Streptococcus pyogenes

I.V. INFUSION

Adults. 500 mg daily (over 60 min) for 7 to 10 days.

▶ *To treat complicated skin and soft-tissue infections caused by methicillin-sensitive* Enterococcus faecalis, Proteus mirabilis, S. aureus, *or* S. pyogenes; *to treat nosocomial pneumonia caused by* S. aureus, Pseudomonas aeruginosa, Serratia marcescens, E. coli, K. pneumoniae, H. influenzae, *or* S. pneumoniae

I.V. INFUSION

Adults. 750 mg daily (over 60 min) for 7 to 14 days.

▶ *To treat chronic bacterial prostatitis caused by* E. coli, E. faecalis, *or* S. epidermidis

I.V. INFUSION

Adults. 500 mg daily (over 60 min) for 28 days.

DOSAGE ADJUSTMENT *For 750-mg dosage level:* If creatinine clearance is 20 to 49 ml/min, dosage reduced to 750 mg every 48 hr; if clearance is 10 to 19 ml/min or patient receives hemodialysis or chronic ambulatory peritoneal dialysis (CAPD), dosage reduced to 750-mg initial dose followed by 500 mg every 48 hr. *For 500-mg dosage level:* If creatinine clearance is 20 to 49 ml/min, dosage reduced to 500-mg initial dose followed by 250 mg every 24 hr; if clearance is 10 to 19 ml/min or patient receives hemodialysis or CAPD, dosage reduced to 500-mg initial dose followed by 250 mg every 48 hr. *For 250-mg dosage level:* If creatinine clearance is 20 to 49 ml/min, no dosage adjustment needed; if clearance is 10 to 19 ml/min, dosage reduced to 250 mg every 48 hr (except for uncomplicated UTI, which needs no dosage adjustment); no information available for patients receiving hemodialysis or CAPD.

Mechanism of Action

Interferes with bacterial cell replication by inhibiting the bacterial enzyme DNA gyrase, which is essential for replication and repair of bacterial DNA.

Contraindications

Hypersensitivity to levofloxacin, other fluoroquinolones, or their components

Interactions

DRUGS

aluminum-, calcium-, or magnesium-containing antacids; didanosine; iron; sucralfate; zinc: Reduced GI absorption of levofloxacin

antineoplastics: Decreased blood levofloxacin level

cimetidine: Increased blood levofloxacin level

cyclosporine: Increased risk of nephrotoxicity

NSAIDs: Possibly increased CNS stimulation and risk of seizures

oral anticoagulants: Increased anticoagulant effect and risk of bleeding

oral antidiabetic drugs: Possibly hyperglycemia or hypoglycemia

theophylline: Increased blood theophylline level and risk of toxicity

ACTIVITIES

sun exposure: Increased risk of photosensitivity

Adverse Reactions

CNS: Anxiety, CNS stimulation, dizziness, headache, increased ICP, light-headedness, nervousness, peripheral neuropathy, psychosis, seizures, sleep disturbance, suicidal ideation

CV: Arrhythmias, leukocytoclastic vasculitis, prolonged QT interval, torsades de pointes

EENT: Taste perversion

ENDO: Hyperglycemia, hypoglycemia

GI: Abdominal pain, acute hepatic necrosis or failure, anorexia, constipation, diarrhea, flatulence, hepatitis, indigestion, nausea, pseudomembranous colitis, vomiting

GU: Acute renal failure or insufficiency, crystalluria, interstitial nephritis, vaginal candidiasis

HEME: Agranulocytosis, aplastic anemia, eosinophilia, hemolytic anemia, leukopenia, pancytopenia, thrombocytopenia

MS: Back pain, rhabdomyolysis, tendon rupture

RESP: Allergic pneumonitis

SKIN: Photosensitivity, pruritus, rash, Stevens-Johnson syndrome, toxic epidermal necrolysis, urticaria

Other: Anaphylaxis, angioedema, serum sickness

Nursing Considerations

- Use levofloxacin cautiously in patients with renal insufficiency. Monitor renal function as appropriate during treatment.
- Use drug cautiously in patients with CNS disorders that may lower the seizure threshold, such as epilepsy.
- Use levofloxacin cautiously in elderly patients because they're more susceptible to a prolonged QT interval and are at increased risk of tendon disorders, including rupture, especially if also taking a corticorsteroid.
- Expect to obtain culture and sensitivity tests before levofloxacin treatment begins.
- Avoid giving drug within 2 hours of antacids.
- Give parenteral form over 60 to 90 minutes, depending on dosage, because bolus or rapid I.V. delivery may cause hypotension.
- **WARNING** Stop levofloxacin at the first sign of hypersensitivity, including rash, jaundice, or other signs, because it may lead to anaphylaxis. Reaction may occur after the first dose. Expect to give epinephrine, and provide supportive care.
- Monitor blood glucose level, especially in diabetic patient who

takes an oral antidiabetic or insulin, because levfloxacin may alter blood glucose levels. If so, notify prescriber, stop drug immediately for hypoglycemia, and provide prescribed treatment.

- Monitor patient's QT interval if needed. If it lengthens, notify prescriber immediately and stop drug. Patients with hypokalemia, significant bradycardia, or cardiomyopathy and those receiving a class Ia or III antiarrhythmic shouldn't receive levofloxacin.
- Notify prescriber if patient has symptoms of peripheral neuropathy (pain, burning, tingling, numbness, weakness, or altered sensations of light touch, pain, temperature, position sense, or vibration sense), which could be permanent; tendon rupture, which requires immediate rest; or CNS abnormalities (seizures, psychosis, increased ICP or CNS stimulation), which may lead to more serious adverse reactions, such as suicidal thoughts. In each case, expect to stop levofloxacin.
- Monitor patient's bowel elimination. If diarrhea develops, obtain stool culture to check for pseudomembranous colitis. If confirmed, expect to stop drug and give fluid, electrolytes, and antibiotics effective against *Clostridium difficile.*

PATIENT TEACHING

- Advise patient to increase fluid intake during levofloxacin therapy to prevent crystalluria.
- Advise patient to avoid excessive exposure to sunlight and to wear sunscreen because of increased risk of photosensitivity. Tell patient to notify prescriber at the first sign of photosensitivity.
- Caution patient to avoid hazardous activities until drug's CNS effects are known.
- Tell patient to stop drug and notify prescriber if he develops tendon pain or inflammation or abnormal changes in motor or sensory function.
- Urge patient to stop drug and tell prescriber if a rash or other allergic reaction develops.
- Advise diabetic patient to monitor blood glucose level and notify prescriber about changes.
- Advise patient to notify prescriber about heart palpitations or loss of consciousness because an ECG may be needed to determine whether drug is having adverse effects on the heart.
- Instruct patient to notify prescriber about severe diarrhea, even up to 2 months after levofloxacin therapy has ended; he may need additional treatment.

levorphanol tartrate
Levo-Dromoran

Class, Category, and Schedule
Chemical: Morphinan derivative
Therapeutic: Opioid analgesic
Pregnancy category: Not rated
Controlled substance schedule: II

Indications and Dosages
▶ *To relieve moderate to severe pain*
I.V. INJECTION
Adults. Up to 1 mg every 3 to 6 hr, p.r.n. *Maximum:* 8 mg daily for non–opioid-dependent patients.

Route	Onset	Peak	Duration
I.V.	Unknown	In 20 min	4 to 5 hr

Mechanism of Action
Decreases intracellular cAMP level by inhibiting adenylate cyclase, which regulates the release of pain neurotransmitters, such as substance P, gamma-aminobutyric acid, dopamine, acetylcholine, and noradrenaline. Levorphanol also stimulates mu and kappa opiate receptors, altering the perception of pain and, possibly, the emotional response to it.

Incompatibilities
Don't mix levorphanol tartrate with solutions that contain aminophylline, ammonium chloride, amobarbital sodium, chlorothiazide sodium, heparin sodium, methicillin sodium, nitrofurantoin sodium, novobiacin sodium, pentobarbital sodium, perphenazine, phenobarbital sodium, phenytoin, secobarbital sodium, sodium bicarbonate, sodium iodide, sulfadiazine sodium, sulfisoxazole diethanolamine, or thiopental sodium.

Contraindications
Acute alcoholism, acute or severe asthma, anoxia, hypersensitivity to levorphanol tartrate or its components, increased ICP, respiratory depression, upper airway obstruction

Interactions
DRUGS
alfentanil, CNS depressants, fentanyl, sufentanil: Possibly increased CNS and respiratory depression and hypotension

anticholinergics: Increased risk of severe constipation
antidiarrheals (such as difenoxin and atropine, kaolin, and loperamide): Possibly severe constipation and increased CNS depression
antihypertensives: Increased risk of hypotension
buprenorphine: Possibly decreased therapeutic effects of levorphanol and increased risk of respiratory depression
hydroxyzine: Increased risk of CNS depression and hypotension
metoclopramide: Possibly antagonized effects of metoclopramide
naloxone, naltrexone: Decreased therapeutic effects of levorphanol
neuromuscular blockers: Increased risk of prolonged CNS and respiratory depression
ACTIVITIES
alcohol use: Possibly increased CNS and respiratory depression and hypotension

Adverse Reactions

CNS: Amnesia, coma, confusion, delusions, depression, dizziness, drowsiness, dyskinesia, hypokinesia, insomnia, nervousness, personality disorder, seizures
CV: Bradycardia, cardiac arrest, hypotension, orthostatic hypotension, palpitations, shock, tachycardia
EENT: Abnormal vision, diplopia, dry mouth
GI: Abdominal pain, biliary tract spasm, constipation, hepatic failure, indigestion, nausea, vomiting
GU: Dysuria, urine retention
RESP: Apnea, hyperventilation
SKIN: Cyanosis, pruritus, rash, urticaria
Other: Injection site pain, redness, and swelling; physical and psychological dependence

Nursing Considerations

- **WARNING** Be aware that levorphanol may be habit-forming and that patients with a history of drug abuse (including acute alcoholism), emotional instability, or suicidal ideation or attempts are at increased risk for opioid abuse.
- **WARNING** Give levorphanol slowly, over several minutes, because rapid administration of other opioid analgesics has caused anaphylaxis, severe respiratory depression, hypotension, peripheral circulatory collapse, and cardiac arrest. Keep emergency equipment and drugs nearby.
- Assess patient's respiratory status closely, especially in patients having an acute asthma attack and those with adrenal insufficiency, chronic respiratory disease, hypothyroidism, myxedema, severe hepatic or renal impairment, or conditions that increase

CSF pressure, because drug causes respiratory depression. Elderly, extremely ill, or debilitated patients and patients who have recently taken, or are currently taking, drugs with respiratory depressant effects are also more sensitive to levorphanol's effects.

- Monitor supine and standing blood pressure periodically, and notify prescriber of orthostatic hypotension.
- Watch carefully for adverse reactions in elderly patients because they're especially sensitive to levorphanol and at increased risk for constipation.
- Monitor for signs of drug-induced CNS depression or increased CSF pressure, such as altered LOC, restlessness, and irritability, in patients with a coma, head injury, intracranial lesions, or other conditions that could cause these effects. Patients who are taking, or have recently taken, drugs that depress the CNS are also more susceptible to these effects.
- Be aware that opioids such as levorphanol may induce or worsen arrhythmias or seizures in patients with a history of these conditions. It also may mask acute abdominal conditions.
- Because levorphanol is metabolized in the liver, be aware of need to monitor patients with hepatic impairment and those taking drugs that decrease hepatic clearance for signs of increased sedation.
- Monitor patients with prostatic hypertrophy, renal function impairment, urethral stricture, or recent urinary tract surgery for signs of urine retention, such as difficulty voiding or feeling that the bladder isn't empty after voiding, peripheral edema, or weight gain. Impaired renal function can affect excretion of levorphanol, causing increased effects.
- Monitor patients with biliary tract disease for biliary colic (pain in upper midline area that may radiate to the back and right shoulder), which may be caused by drug-induced increase in intracholedochal pressure.
- Because levorphanol's effects on the heart aren't known, expect limited use of this drug in patients with acute MI, ventricular dysfunction, or coronary insufficiency.
- Store drug 15° to 30° C (59° and 86° F); don't freeze.

PATIENT TEACHING

- Instruct patient to lie down during levorphanol administration and for a period afterward to lessen drug's hypotensive effects (dizziness, light-headedness) and other adverse effects, such as nausea and vomiting.

- Advise patient to avoid potentially hazardous activities until drug's CNS effects are known.
- Instruct patient to avoid alcoholic beverages during therapy.
- Direct patient to change position slowly to minimize effects of orthostatic hypotension.
- Advise patient to report constipation, nausea, or vomiting to prescriber.
- Suggest that patient relieve dry mouth with sugarless candy or gum or ice chips.

levothyroxine sodium
(L-thyroxine sodium, T₄, thyroxine sodium)
Levothroid, Synthroid

Class and Category
Chemical: Synthetic thyroxine (T_4)
Therapeutic: Thyroid hormone replacement
Pregnancy category: A

Indications and Dosages
▶ *To treat severe hypothyroidism*
I.V. INJECTION
Adults. 50 to 100 mcg daily until therapeutic blood level is reached.
Children. 75% of usual P.O. dose daily until therapeutic blood level is reached.
▶ *To treat myxedema coma*
I.V. INJECTION
Adults. 200 to 500 mcg on day 1. If no significant improvement occurs, 100 to 300 mcg on day 2. Daily dose continued as prescribed until therapeutic blood level is reached and P.O. route is tolerated.
Children. 75% of usual P.O. dose daily until therapeutic blood level is reached and P.O. route is tolerated.

Route	Onset	Peak	Duration
I.V.	6 to 8 hr	24 hr	Unknown

Contraindications
Acute MI (unless caused or complicated by hyperthyroidism), hypersensitivity to levothyroxine or its components, uncorrected adrenal insufficiency, untreated thyrotoxicosis

Mechanism of Action

Replaces endogenous thyroid hormone, which may exert its physiologic effects by controlling DNA transcription and protein synthesis. Levothyroxine exhibits all of the following actions of endogenous thyroid hormone. The drug:

- increases energy expenditure
- accelerates the rate of cellular oxidation, which stimulates body tissue growth, maturation, and metabolism
- regulates differentiation and proliferation of stem cells
- aids in myelination of nerves and development of synaptic processes in the nervous system
- regulates growth
- decreases blood and hepatic cholesterol concentrations
- enhances carbohydrate and protein metabolism, increasing gluconeogenesis and protein synthesis.

Interactions

DRUGS

adrenocorticoids: Possibly adrenocorticoid dosage adjustments as thyroid status changes

aluminum- and magnesium-containing antacids, bile acid sequestrants, calcium carbonate, cation exchange resins, cholestyramine, colestipol, ferrous sulfate, kayexalate, sucralfate: Possibly reduced effects of levothyroxine

amiodarone, iodide: Possibly hyperthyroidism

beta blockers: Possibly impaired action of beta blockers and decreased conversion of T_4 to triiodothyronine (T_3)

cholestyramine, colestipol: Delayed or inhibited levothyroxine absorption

digoxin: Reduced therapeutic effects of digoxin

estrogen, phenylbutazone, phenytoin: Reduced binding of levothyroxine to protein, possibly requiring increased levothyroxine dosage

insulin, oral antidiabetic drugs: Possibly uncontrolled diabetes mellitus, requiring increased dosage of insulin or oral antidiabetic drug

ketamine: Possibly hypertension and tachycardia

maprotiline: Increased risk of arrhythmias

oral anticoagulants: Altered anticoagulant activity, possibly need for anticoagulant dosage adjustment

selective serotonin reuptake inhibitors, tricyclic and tetracyclic antidepressants: Increased therapeutic and toxic effects of both drugs

sympathomimetics: Increased risk of coronary insufficiency in pa-

tients with coronary artery disease
theophylline: Decreased theophylline clearance
FOODS
dietary fiber, soybean flour (infant formula), walnuts: Possibly decreased absorption of levothyroxine from GI tract

Adverse Reactions

CNS: Fatigue, headache, insomnia, somnolence
ENDO: Hyperthyroidism (with overdose)
GI: Dysphagia
MS: Muscle weakness, myalgia, slipped capital femoral epiphysis
SKIN: Alopecia (transient), rash, urticaria
Other: Weight gain

Nursing Considerations

- Expect to give drug I.V. if patient can't take tablets. Be aware that drug shouldn't be given subcutaneously.
- For I.V. use, reconstitute drug by adding 5 ml of normal saline solution.
- Monitor PT of patient who is receiving anticoagulants; she may require a dosage adjustment.
- Monitor blood glucose level of diabetic patient. Prescriber may reduce antidiabetic drug dosage as thyroid hormone level enters therapeutic range.
- Expect patient to undergo regular thyroid function tests during levothyroxine therapy.

PATIENT TEACHING

- Inform patient that levothyroxine replaces a hormone that is normally produced by the thyroid gland and that she'll probably need to take drug for life.
- Inform patient that drug may require a few weeks to take effect.
- Instruct patient to report signs of hyperthyroidism, such as diarrhea, excessive sweating, heat intolerance, insomnia, palpitations, weight loss, chest pain, shortness of breath, leg cramps, headache, nervousness, irritability, tremors, changes in appetite, vomiting, fever, and changes in menstrual periods.
- Tell patient to notify prescriber if rash or hives develop during drug use.
- Inform patient that transient hair loss may occur during first few months of therapy.
- Instruct female patient of childbearing age to notify prescriber immediately if she becomes pregnant because levothyroxine dosage may need to be increased.

lidocaine hydrochloride
(lignocaine hydrochloride)
Xylocaine, Xylocard (CAN)

Class and Category
Chemical: Aminoacyamide
Therapeutic: Class IB antiarrhythmic
Pregnancy category: B

Indications and Dosages
▶ *To treat ventricular tachycardia or ventricular fibrillation*
I.V. INFUSION, I.V. INJECTION
Adults. *Loading:* 50 to 100 mg (or 1 to 1.5 mg/kg), administered at 25 to 50 mg/min. If desired response isn't achieved after 5 to 10 min, second dose of 25 to 50 mg (or 0.5 to 0.75 mg/kg) is given every 5 to 10 min until maximum loading dose (300 mg in 1 hr) has been given. *Maintenance:* 20 to 50 mcg/kg/min (1 to 4 mg/min) gven by continuous infusion. Smaller bolus dose repeated 15 to 20 min after start of infusion if needed to maintain therapeutic blood level. *Maximum:* 300 mg (or 3 mg/kg) over 1 hr.
Children. *Loading:* 1 mg/kg. *Maintenance:* 30 mcg/kg/min by continuous infusion. *Maximum:* 3 mg/kg.
DOSAGE ADJUSTMENT For elderly patients receiving lidocaine to treat arrhythmias and for patients with acute hepatitis or decompensated cirrhosis, loading dose and continuous infusion rate reduced by 50%.

Route	Onset	Peak	Duration
I.V.	45 to 90 sec	Immediate	10 to 20 min

Mechanism of Action
Combines with fast sodium channels in myocardial cell membranes, which inhibits sodium influx into cells and decreases ventricular depolarization, automaticity, and excitability during diastole.

Contraindications
Adams-Stokes syndrome; hypersensitivity to lidocaine, amide anesthetics, or their components; severe heart block (without artificial pacemaker); Wolff-Parkinson-White syndrome

Interactions
DRUGS

beta blockers, cimetidine: Increased blood lidocaine level and risk of toxicity

MAO inhibitors, tricyclic antidepressants: Risk of severe, prolonged hypertension

mexiletine, tocainide: Additive cardiac effects

neuromuscular blockers: Possibly increased neuromuscular blockade

phenytoin, procainamide: Increased cardiac depression

Adverse Reactions
CNS: Anxiety, confusion, difficulty speaking, dizziness, hallucinations, lethargy, paresthesia, seizures

CV: Bradycardia, cardiac arrest, hypotension, new or worsening arrhythmias

EENT: Blurred vision, diplopia, tinnitus

GI: Nausea

MS: Muscle twitching

RESP: Respiratory arrest or depression

Other: Allergic reaction; injection site burning, irritation, stinging, swelling, or tenderness

Nursing Considerations
- Carefully check prefilled lidocaine syringes before using. Use only syringes labeled "FOR CARDIAC ARRHYTHMIAS."
- Check label to verify that you're using a lidocaine preparation that does *not* contain preservatives or other drugs. Dilute drug with D_5W, typically to a final concentration of 1 or 2 mg/ml. Consult manufacturer's guidelines for alternative dilution information. Include final concentration on label. Administer drug using an infusion pump or another device that allows precise measurement.
- Observe for respiratory depression after bolus injection and during I.V. infusion of lidocaine.
- Keep life-support equipment and vasopressors nearby during administration in case respiratory depression or other reactions occur.
- Titrate dosage, as prescribed, to minimum amount needed to prevent arrhythmias.
- During administration, place patient on cardiac monitor, as ordered, and closely observe her at all times. Monitor for worsening arrhythmias, widening QRS complex, and prolonged PR interval—possible signs of drug toxicity.

- Monitor blood lidocaine level, as ordered. Check for therapeutic level of 2 to 5 mcg/ml.
- If signs of toxicity, such as dizziness, occur, notify prescriber and expect to discontinue or slow infusion.
- Monitor vital signs as well as BUN and serum creatinine and electrolyte levels during and after therapy.
- Store drug at 15° to 30° C (59° to 86° F).

PATIENT TEACHING
- Advise patient who receives lidocaine to report difficulty speaking, dizziness, injection site pain, nausea, numbness or tingling, or vision changes.

lincomycin hydrochloride

Lincocin

Class and Category

Chemical: Lincosamide
Therapeutic: Bacteriostatic or bactericidal antibiotic
Pregnancy category: C

Indications and Dosages

▶ *To treat serious respiratory, skin, and soft-tissue infections caused by susceptible strains of streptococci, pneumococci, and staphylococci*

I.V. INFUSION

Adults. 600 mg to 1 g every 8 to 12 hr. *Maximum:* 8 g daily in divided doses for life-threatening infection.

Children over age 1 month. 10 to 20 mg/kg daily in divided doses every 8 to 12 hr, depending on severity of infection.

DOSAGE ADJUSTMENT Dosage reduced by 25% to 30% in patients with severely impaired renal function.

Mechanism of Action

Inhibits protein synthesis in susceptible bacteria by binding to the 50S sub-unit of bacterial ribosomes and preventing peptide bond formation, thus causing bacterial cells to die.

Incompatibilities

Don't administer lincomycin with novobiocin or kanamycin.

Contraindications

Hypersensitivity to lincomycin or clindamycin

Interactions

DRUGS

antimyasthenic drugs: Possibly antagonized antimyasthenic effects
chloramphenicol, clindamycin, erythromycin: Possibly blocked access
of lincomycin to its site of action
hydrocarbon inhalation anesthetics, neuromuscular blockers: Increased
neuromuscular blockade, possibly severe respiratory depression
opioid analgesics: Increased risk of prolonged or increased respiratory depression

Adverse Reactions

CNS: Fever, vertigo
CV: Cardiac arrest and hypotension (with rapid administration)
EENT: Glossitis, stomatitis, tinnitus
GI: Abdominal cramps, colitis, diarrhea, nausea, pseudomembranous colitis, rectal candidiasis, vomiting
GU: Vaginal candidiasis
HEME: Agranulocytosis, eosinophilia, leukopenia, neutropenia, thrombocytopenic purpura
SKIN: Erythema multiforme, rash, Stevens-Johnson syndrome, urticaria
Other: Anaphylaxis, angioedema, superinfection

Nursing Considerations

- Expect to obtain a specimen for culture and sensitivity testing before administering first dose of lincomycin.
- **WARNING** Some preparations of lincomycin contain benzyl alcohol, which can cause a fatal toxic syndrome in neonates or premature infants, characterized by CNS, respiratory, circulatory, and renal impairment and metabolic acidosis. Because drug may appear in breast milk, breast-feeding patient may need to stop drug or stop breast-feeding.
- Dilute 600-mg dose in at least 100 ml of D_5W, $D_{10}W$, normal saline solution, dextrose 5% in normal saline solution, or other compatible diluent identified on manufacturer's insert. Dilute higher doses with 100 ml of a compatible diluent for each gram being administered—for example, you'd dilute a 3-g dose in at least 300 ml of diluent. Use diluted solution within 24 hours if stored at room temperature.
- **WARNING** Administer lincomycin over at least 1 hour for each gram being administered. For example, you'd infuse 1 g over 1 hour and 3 g over 3 hours. Too-rapid infusion may result in cardiac arrest or hypotension.

- **WARNING** Watch for hypersensitivity reactions, such as rash, pruritus, wheezing, and dysphagia from laryngeal edema. If such reactions occur, stop infusion and notify prescriber immediately. If anaphylaxis occurs, administer epinephrine, antihistamines, oxygen, and corticosteroids, as prescribed. Be aware that patients with a history of asthma or significant allergies are at increased risk for a hypersensitivity reaction.
- Observe patient for signs of superinfection, such as vaginal itching and sore mouth.
- Monitor patient for signs of pseudomembranous colitis, such as watery, loose stools. Patients with a history of GI disease, particularly colitis or regional enteritis, are at increased risk for colitis. Be aware that antibiotic-related diarrhea may be more severe and less well tolerated in elderly patients. Expect to discontinue lincomycin if diarrhea occurs.
- Monitor results of liver and renal function tests, CBC, and platelet counts periodically during lincomycin therapy.
- Before diluting drug, store it at a controlled room temperature of 20° to 25° C (68° to 77° F).

PATIENT TEACHING
- Review with patient possibly serious adverse reactions associated with lincomycin use, such as difficulty breathing, rash, and chest tightness, and tell him to report any that occur.
- Inform him that yogurt or buttermilk can help maintain intestinal flora and may decrease the risk of diarrhea.
- Stress the importance of following dosage regimen and keeping follow-up medical and laboratory appointments.

linezolid

Zyvox

Class and Category

Chemical: Oxazolidinone
Therapeutic: Antibiotic
Pregnancy category: C

Indications and Dosages

▶ *To treat vancomycin-resistant* Enterococcus faecium *infections, including bacteremia*

I.V. INFUSION

Adults and adolescents. 600 mg every 12 hr for 14 to 28 days.
Infants and children. 10 mg/kg every 8 hr for 14 to 28 days.

▶ *To treat nosocomial pneumonia caused by* Staphylococcus aureus

Mechanism of Action

Inhibits bacterial protein synthesis by interfering with translation of ribonucleic acid (RNA) to protein. In bacteria, protein synthesis begins with binding of a 30S ribosomal subunit and a 50S ribosomal subunit to a messenger RNA (mRNA) molecule to form a 70S initiation complex, as shown in the top illustration. The 50S ribosomal subunit consists of 23S ribosomal RNA (rRNA) and other ribosomal subunits. Then translation begins. Transfer RNA (tRNA) attaches to the 50S subunit and brings specific amino acids into place. As the

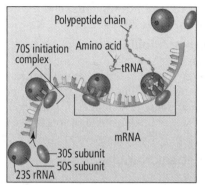

tRNA and amino acids fall into place, they are joined together by peptide bonds and elongate to form a polypeptide chain. This chain eventually combines with other polypeptide chains to form a complete protein molecule. After translation is complete, the ribosomal subunits fall away and are ready to combine with more mRNA to start the translation process over again.

Linezolid binds to a site on the bacterial 23S rRNA of the 50S subunit, as shown in the bottom illustration. This action prevents formation of a func-

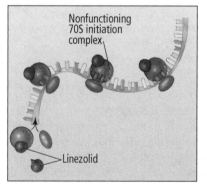

tional 70S initiation complex, an essential component of the bacterial translation. Without proper protein production, susceptible bacteria can't multiply. Linezolid is bacteriostatic against staphylococci and enterococci and bactericidal against most streptococci.

(methicillin-susceptible and -resistant strains) or Streptococcus pneumoniae *(penicillin-susceptible strains only) and community-acquired pneumonia, including accompanying bacteremia, caused by* S. aureus *(methicillin-susceptible strains only) or* S. pneumoniae *(penicillin-susceptible strains only); to treat complicated skin and soft-*

tissue infections, including diabetic foot infections without concomitant osteomyelitis, caused by S. aureus *(methicillin-susceptible and -resistant strains),* Streptococcus pyogenes, *or* Streptococcus agalactiae

I.V. INFUSION

Adults and adolescents. 600 mg every 12 hr for 10 to 14 days.

Infants and children. 10 mg/kg every 8 hr for 10 to 14 days.

Incompatibilities

Don't add other drugs to linezolid solution. Don't infuse linezolid in the same I.V. line as amphotericin B, chlorpromazine hydrochloride, co-trimoxazole, diazepam, erythromycin lactobionate, pentamidine isethionate, or phenytoin sodium because they're physically incompatible. Don't infuse linezolid with ceftriaxone sodium because these two drugs are chemically incompatible.

Contraindications

Hypersensitivity to linezolid or its components; phenylketonuria (oral suspension)

Interactions

DRUGS

adrenergics, including pseudoephedrine and phenylpropanolamine: Enhanced vasopressor response of adrenergics, resulting in increased blood pressure

serotonergics: Possibly serotonin syndrome

FOODS

tyramine-containing foods and beverages: Possibly hypertension

Adverse Reactions

CNS: Dizziness, fever, headache, insomnia, optic and peripheral neuropathy, serotonin syndrome

CV: Hypertension

EENT: Oral candidiasis, tongue discoloration

GI: Abdominal pain, constipation, diarrhea, indigestion, nausea, pseudomembranous colitis, vomiting

GU: Vaginal candidiasis

HEME: Anemia, leukopenia, pancytopenia, thrombocytopenia

SKIN: Pruritus, rash

Other: Lactic acidosis

Nursing Considerations

• Obtain body tissue and fluid specimens for culture and sensitivity tests, as ordered, before giving first dose of linezolid. Expect to begin drug before test results are known.

• **WARNING** Be aware that linezolid shouldn't be used to treat catheter-related bloodstream infections, catheter-site infections, or infections caused by gram-negative bacteria because of an increased risk of death.

- Infuse I.V. solution over 30 to 120 minutes with D_5W, normal saline solution, or lactated Ringer's solution.
- **WARNING** Monitor CBC weekly, as ordered, to detect or track worsening myelosuppression in patients who need more than 2 weeks of therapy, who have preexisting myelosuppression and are receiving drugs that produce bone marrow suppression, or who have chronic infection and are receiving or have received antibiotic therapy.
- Notify prescriber if patient develops visual impairment that suggests optic neuropathy, such as changes in visual acuity or color vision, blurred vision, lost vision, or visual field defect. If optic or peripheral neuropathy develops, the drug may need to be stopped.
- Monitor bowel pattern daily. Assess patient for secondary infection, including oral candidiasis and profuse, watery diarrhea.

PATIENT TEACHING

- Advise patient not to take OTC cold remedies without consulting prescriber because medications that contain psedoephedrine or propanolamine may cause or worsen hypertension.
- Instruct patient to avoid foods and beverages that contain large amounts of tyramine, including aged cheese, fermented or air-dried meats, sauerkraut, soy sauce, tap beers, red wines, and protein-rich foods that have been stored for long periods or poorly refrigerated.
- Instruct patient to notify prescriber immediately about severe diarrhea, vision changes, or changes in limb sensation (such as pins and needles, numbness, or tingling) because drug may need to be stopped.

liothyronine sodium
(L-triiodothyronine, sodium L-triiodothyronine, T_3, thyronine sodium)

Triostat

Class and Category
Chemical: Synthetic triiodothyronine (T_3)
Therapeutic: Thyroid hormone replacement
Pregnancy category: A

Indications and Dosages

▶ *To treat myxedema coma or premyxedema coma (severe hypothyroidism)*

I.V. INJECTION

Adults. *Initial:* 25 to 50 mcg; repeated every 4 to 12 hr, depending on patient's response.

DOSAGE ADJUSTMENT Initial dose decreased to 10 to 20 mcg for patients with known or suspected cardiovascular disease who are being treated for myxedema coma.

Route	Onset	Peak	Duration
I.V.	2 to 4 hr	2 days	Unknown

Mechanism of Action

Replaces endogenous thyroid hormone, which may exert its physiologic effects by controlling DNA transcription and protein synthesis. Liothyronine exhibits all of the following actions of endogenous thyroid hormone:

- increases energy expenditure
- accelerates the rate of cellular oxidation, which stimulates body tissue growth, maturation, and metabolism
- regulates differentiation and proliferation of stem cells
- aids in myelination of nerves and development of synaptic processes in the nervous system
- regulates growth
- decreases blood and hepatic cholesterol concentrations
- enhances carbohydrate and protein metabolism, increasing gluconeogenesis and protein synthesis.

Contraindications

Acute MI (unless caused or complicated by hypothyroidism), hypersensitivity to liothyronine or its components, uncorrected adrenal insufficiency, untreated thyrotoxicosis

Interactions

DRUGS

adrenocorticoids: Possibly need for adrenocorticoid dosage adjustments as thyroid status changes

beta blockers: Possibly impaired action of beta blockers

cholestyramine, colestipol: Decreased liothyronine absorption

digoxin: Reduced therapeutic effects of digoxin

estrogen, phenylbutazone, phenytoin: Reduced binding of liothyronine

to protein, possibly requiring increased liothyronine dosage
insulin, oral antidiabetic drugs: Possibly uncontrolled diabetes mellitus, requiring increased dosage of insulin or oral antidiabetic drug
ketamine: Possibly hypertension and tachycardia
maprotiline: Increased risk of arrhythmias
oral anticoagulants: Altered anticoagulant activity, possibly need for anticoagulant dosage adjustment
sympathomimetics: Increased risk of coronary insufficiency in patients with coronary artery disease
theophylline: Decreased theophylline clearance
tricyclic antidepressants: Increased therapeutic and toxic effects of both drugs

Adverse Reactions
CNS: Insomnia
ENDO: Hyperthyroidism (with overdose)
SKIN: Alopecia (transient), rash, urticaria

Nursing Considerations
- Be aware that liothyronine is used most often when the patient needs rapid-onset or rapidly reversible thyroid hormone replacement.
- Give I.V. injections more than 4 hours but less than 12 hours apart.
- Evaluate response to therapy by monitoring pulse rate and blood pressure.
- Expect patient to undergo regular thyroid function tests during liothyronine therapy.
- Monitor PT of patient receiving anticoagulants; she may require a dosage adjustment.
- Monitor patients with a history of cardiovascular disease for signs of ischemia or tachyarrhythmias. If such signs occur, notify prescriber and expect to adjust liothyronine dosage.
- Frequently monitor blood glucose level of diabetic patient. Prescriber may reduce antidiabetic drug dosage as thyroid hormone level enters therapeutic range.
- Expect oral thyroid hormone replacement therapy to be initiated or resumed as soon as possible. Expect to discontinue infusion gradually if patient is switched to levothyroxine tablets because of levothyroxine's delayed onset of action.
- Be aware that patients with myxedema coma may also be prescribed corticosteroids; those with pituitary myxedema may also receive adrenocortical hormone replacement before or at begin-

ning of liothyronine therapy; and those with primary myxedema may receive adrenocortical hormone replacement to prevent adrenocortical insufficiency and shock.
• Store drug at 2° to 8° C (36° to 46° F).

PATIENT TEACHING
• Advise patient receiving liothyronine to report signs or symptoms of hyperthyroidism, such as chest pain, excessive sweating, heat intolerance, increased pulse rate, nervousness, and palpitations.
• Tell diabetic patient that her blood glucose level will be tested often because her antidiabetic dosage may need to be reduced.
• Inform patient of need for periodic blood tests to monitor drug's effectiveness.

lorazepam
Ativan

Class, Category, and Schedule
Chemical: Benzodiazepine
Therapeutic: Amnestic, antianxiety, anticonvulsant, sedative
Pregnancy category: D
Controlled substance schedule: IV

Indications and Dosages
▶ *To provide preoperative sedation*
I.V. INJECTION
Adults and adolescents. 0.044 mg/kg or 2 mg, whichever is less, given 2 hr before procedure. *Maximum:* 0.05 mg/kg or total of 4 mg.
▶ *To treat status epilepticus*
I.V. INJECTION
Adults and adolescents. *Initial:* 4 mg at 2 mg/min; if seizures don't subside, repeat in 10 to 15 min. *Maximum:* 8 mg/24 hr.

Route	Onset	Peak	Duration
I.V.	5 min	Unknown	12 to 24 hr

Incompatibilities
Don't mix I.V. lorazepam in same syringe as buprenorphine.

Contraindications
Acute angle-closure glaucoma; hypersensitivity to lorazepam, its components, or to benzodiazepines; intra-arterial administration; psychosis

Mechanism of Action
May potentiate the effects of gamma-aminobutyric acid (GABA) and other inhibitory neurotransmitters by binding to specific benzodiazepine receptors in the limbic and cortical areas of the CNS. GABA inhibits excitatory stimulation, which helps control emotional behavior. The limbic system contains a highly dense area of benzodiazepine receptors, which may explain the drug's antianxiety effects. Also, lorazepam hyperpolarizes neuronal cells, thereby interfering with their ability to generate seizures.

Interactions
DRUGS

aminophylline, theophylline: Possibly reduced sedative effects of lorazepam

clozapine: Increased risk of marked sedation, excessive salivation, hypotension, ataxia, delirium, and respiratory arrest

CNS depressants: Additive CNS depression, including potentially fatal respiratory depression

digoxin: Possibly increased blood digoxin level and risk of digitalis toxicity

fentanyl: Possibly decreased therapeutic effects of fentanyl

probenecid: Possibly increased therapeutic and adverse effects of lorazepam

valproate: Increased plasma lorazepam level

ACTIVITIES

alcohol use: Increased CNS depression

Adverse Reactions
CNS: Amnesia, anxiety, ataxia, coma, confusion, delusions, depression, dizziness, drowsiness, euphoria, extrapyramidal symptoms, headache, hypokinesia, irritability, malaise, nervousness, seizures, slurred speech, suicidal ideation, tremor

CV: Chest pain, palpitations, tachycardia

EENT: Blurred vision, diplopia, dry mouth, increased salivation, photophobia

ENDO: Syndrome of inappropriate antidiuretic hormone secretion

GI: Abdominal pain, constipation, diarrhea, increased liver enzyme levels, jaundice, nausea, thirst, vomiting

GU: Libido changes

HEME: Agranulocytosis, pancytopenia, thrombocytopenia

RESP: Apnea, respiratory depression, worsening of apnea or obstructive pulmonary disease

SKIN: Diaphoresis
Other: Anaphylaxis, injection site phlebitis, physical and psychological dependence, withdrawal symptoms

Nursing Considerations

- Use extreme caution when giving lorazepam to elderly patients because it may cause hypoventilation, sedation, and unsteadiness. Also use caution in patients with compromised respiratory function because drug may cause respiratory depression.
- Use cautiously in patients with a history of alcohol or drug abuse or a personality disorder because of higher risk of physical and psychological dependence. Also use cautiously in patients with severe hepatic insufficiency or encephalopathy because drug may worsen hepatic encephalopathy.
- Dilute drug with equal amount of sterile water for injection, sodium chloride for injection, or D$_5$W. Discard solution if you observe particles or discoloration. Give diluted drug slowly, at no more than 2 mg/minute.
- **WARNING** Monitor respirations every 5 to 15 minutes, and keep emergency resuscitation equipment readily available. Lorazepam may cause life-threatening respiratory depression.
- Because abrupt drug discontinuation increases the risk of withdrawal symptoms, expect to taper dosage gradually, especially in epileptic patients.
- Store drug at 2° to 8° C (36° to 46° F); protect from freezing and light.

PATIENT TEACHING
- Instruct patient to report excessive drowsiness and nausea during lorazepam therapy.
- Advise patient to avoid potentially hazardous activities until drug's CNS effects are known.
- Urge patient to avoid alcohol because it increases drug's CNS depressant effects.
- Inform pregnant patient that she'll need to stop lorazepam therapy early in the third trimester to avoid withdrawal symptoms in the newborn.

magnesium chloride
(contains 200 mg of elemental magnesium per 1 ml of injection)
Chloromag

magnesium sulfate
(contains 100 to 500 mg of elemental magnesium per 1 ml of injection and 1 to 5 g of elemental magnesium per 10 ml of injection)

Class and Category
Chemical: Cation, electrolyte
Therapeutic: Antiarrhythmic, anticonvulsant, electrolyte replacement
Pregnancy category: A

Indications and Dosages
▶ *To treat severe hypomagnesemia*
I.V. INFUSION (MAGNESIUM CHLORIDE)
Adults. 4 g diluted in 250 ml of D$_5$W and infused at no more than 3 ml/min. *Maximum:* 40 g daily.
I.V. INFUSION (MAGNESIUM SULFATE)
Adults and adolescents. 5 g diluted in 1 L of I.V. solution and infused over 3 hr.
▶ *To provide supplemental magnesium in total parenteral nutrition*
I.V. INFUSION (MAGNESIUM SULFATE)
Adults. 1 to 3 g daily.
Children. 0.25 to 1.25 g daily.
DOSAGE ADJUSTMENT Adult dosage may be increased to 6 g daily for certain conditions, such as short-bowel syndrome.
▶ *To prevent and control seizures in preeclampsia or eclampsia as well as seizures caused by epilepsy, glomerulonephritis, or hypothyroidism*
I.V. INFUSION, I.V. INJECTION (MAGNESIUM SULFATE)
Adults. *Loading:* 4 g diluted in 250 ml of compatible solution and infused over 30 min. *Maintenance:* 1 to 2 g/hr by continuous infusion.

Route	Onset	Peak	Duration
I.V. *	Immediate	Unknown	About 30 min

*For anticonvulsant effect.

473

> ## Mechanism of Action
>
> Assists all enzymes involved in phosphate transfer reactions that use ATP. Magnesium is required for normal function of the ATP-dependent sodium-potassium pump in muscle membranes. It may effectively treat digitalis glycoside–induced arrhythmias because correction of hypomagnesemia improves the sodium-potassium pump's ability to distribute potassium into intracellular spaces and because magnesium decreases calcium uptake and potassium outflow through myocardial cell membranes.
>
> As an anticonvulsant, magnesium depresses the CNS and blocks peripheral neuromuscular impulse transmission by decreasing the amount of available acetylcholine.

Incompatibilities

Don't combine magnesium sulfate with alkali carbonates or bicarbonates, alkali hydroxides, arsenates, calcium, clindamycin phosphate, dobutamine, fat emulsions, heavy metals, hydrocortisone sodium succinate, phosphates, polymyxin B, procaine hydrochloride, salicylates, sodium bicarbonate, strontium, and tartrates.

Contraindications

Hypersensitivity to magnesium salts or any component of magnesium-containing preparations
Magnesium chloride: Coma, heart disease, renal impairment
Magnesium sulfate: Heart block, MI, preeclampsia 2 hours or less before delivery

Interactions
DRUGS
amphotericin B, cisplatin, cyclosporine, gentamicin: Possibly magnesium wasting and need for magnesium dosage adjustment
calcium salts (I.V.): Possibly neutralization of magnesium sulfate's effects
CNS depressants: Possibly increased CNS depression
digoxin: Possibly heart block and conduction changes, especially when calcium salts are also administered
diuretics (loop or thiazide): Possibly hypomagnesemia
misoprostol: Increased misoprostol-induced diarrhea
neuromuscular blockers: Possibly increased neuromuscular blockade
nifedipine: Possibly increased hypotensive effects when taken with magnesium sulfate
potassium-sparing diuretics: Increased risk of hypermagnesemia

streptomycin, tetracycline, tobramycin: Possibly decreased therapeutic effectiveness of these drugs
FOODS
high-glucose intake: Increased urinary excretion of magnesium
ACTIVITIES
alcohol use: Increased urinary excretion of magnesium

Adverse Reactions

CNS: Decreased reflexes, dizziness, syncope
CV: Arrhythmias, hypotension
GI: Vomiting
MS: Muscle cramps
RESP: Dyspnea, respiratory depression or paralysis
SKIN: Diaphoresis
Other: Allergic reaction, hypermagnesemia, magnesium toxicity

Nursing Considerations

- **WARNING** Observe for early signs of hypermagnesemia: bradycardia, diminished deep tendon reflexes, diplopia, dyspnea, flushing, hypotension, nausea, slurred speech, vomiting, and weakness. Notify prescriber immediately if patient displays any of these signs.
- **WARNING** Be aware that magnesium may precipitate myasthenic crisis by decreasing patient's sensitivity to acetylcholine.
- Frequently assess cardiac status of patient taking drugs that lower heart rate, such as beta blockers, because magnesium may aggravate symptoms of heart block.
- **WARNING** Be aware that magnesium chloride for injection contains the preservative benzyl alcohol, which may cause a fatal toxic syndrome in neonates and premature infants, characterized by CNS, respiratory, circulatory, and renal impairment and metabolic acidosis.
- Monitor serum electrolyte levels in patients with renal insufficiency because they're at risk for magnesium toxicity.
- Be aware that magnesium salts aren't intended for long-term use.
- Store drug at 15° to 30° C (59° to 86° F); don't freeze.

PATIENT TEACHING

- Instruct patient to report signs of hypermagnesemia, such as shortness of breath, flushing, dizziness, and nausea.
- Inform patient that magnesium supplements used to replace electrolytes can cause diarrhea.

mannitol
Osmitrol, Resectisol

Class and Category
Chemical: Hexahydroxy alcohol
Therapeutic: Antiglaucoma, diagnostic agent, osmotic diuretic, urinary irrigant
Pregnancy category: B

Indications and Dosages
▶ *To reduce intracranial or intraocular pressure*
I.V. INFUSION
Adults and adolescents. 0.25 to 2 g/kg as 15% to 25% solution given over 30 to 60 min. If used before eye surgery, 1.5 to 2 g/kg 60 to 90 min before procedure. *Maximum:* 6 g/kg daily.
DOSAGE ADJUSTMENT For small or debilitated patients, dosage reduced to 0.5 g/kg.

▶ *To diagnose oliguria or inadequate renal function*
I.V. INFUSION
Adults and adolescents. 200 mg/kg or 12.5 g as 15% to 20% solution given over 3 to 5 min. Second dose given only if patient fails to excrete 30 to 50 ml of urine in 2 to 3 hr. Drug discontinued if no response after second dose. Or, 100 ml of 20% solution diluted in 180 ml of normal saline solution (forming 280 ml of 7.2% solution) and infused at 20 ml/min; followed by measurement of urine output. *Maximum:* 6 g/kg daily.

▶ *To prevent oliguria or acute renal failure*
I.V. INFUSION
Adults and adolescents. 50 to 100 g as 5% to 25% solution. *Maximum:* 6 g/kg daily.

▶ *To treat oliguria*
I.V. INFUSION
Adults and adolescents. 50 to 100 g as 15% to 25% solution given over 90 min to several hr. *Maximum:* 6 g/kg daily.

▶ *To promote diuresis in drug toxicity*
I.V. INFUSION
Adults and adolescents. *Loading:* 25 g. *Maintenance:* Up to 200 g as 5% to 25% solution given continuously to maintain urine output of 100 to 500 ml/hr with positive fluid balance of 1 to 2 L. *Maximum:* 6 g/kg daily.

▶ *To promote diuresis in hemolytic transfusion reaction*
I.V. INFUSION
Adults. 20 g over 5 min. Repeat if needed. *Maximum:* 6 g/kg daily.

Route	Onset	Peak	Duration
I.V.*	1 to 3 hr	Unknown	Up to 8 hr
I.V.†	30 to 60 min	Unknown	4 to 8 hr
I.V.‡	In 15 min	Unknown	3 to 8 hr

Mechanism of Action

Elevates plasma osmolality, causing water to flow from tissues, such as the brain and eyes, and from CSF, into extracellular fluid, thereby decreasing intracranial and intraocular pressure.

As an osmotic diuretic, mannitol increases the osmolarity of glomerular filtrate, which decreases water reabsorption. This leads to increased excretion of water, sodium, chloride, and toxic substances.

As an irrigant, mannitol minimizes hemolytic effects of water as an irrigant and reduces movement of hemolyzed blood from the urethra to the systemic circulation, preventing hemoglobinemia and serious renal complications.

Incompatibilities

Don't administer mannitol through same I.V. line as blood or blood products.

Contraindications

Active intracranial bleeding (except during craniotomy), anuria, hepatic failure, hypersensitivity to mannitol or its components, pulmonary edema, severe dehydration, severe heart failure, severe pulmonary congestion, severe renal insufficiency

Interactions

DRUGS

digoxin: Increased risk of digitalis toxicity from hypokalemia
diuretics: Possibly increased therapeutic effects of mannitol

Adverse Reactions

CNS: Chills, dizziness, fever, headache, seizures
CV: Chest pain, heart failure, hypertension, tachycardia, thrombophlebitis
EENT: Blurred vision, dry mouth, rhinitis
GI: Diarrhea, nausea, thirst, vomiting
GU: Polyuria, urine retention

---

* To produce diuresis.
† To decrease intraocular pressure.
‡ To decrease ICP.

RESP: Pulmonary edema
SKIN: Extravasation with edema and tissue necrosis, rash, urticaria
Other: Dehydration, hyperkalemia, hypernatremia, hypervolemia, hypokalemia, hyponatremia (dilutional), metabolic acidosis, water intoxication

Nursing Considerations

- If crystals form in mannitol solution exposed to low temperature, place solution in hot-water bath to redissolve crystals.
- Use a 5-micron in-line filter when administering drug solution of 15% or greater.
- Do not piggyback connections, pressurize intravenous mannitol solutions contained in flexible plastic containers, or use a vented intravenous administration set with the vent in the open position when administering drug solution because air embolism may occur because of residual air being drawn from one container before administration of the fluid from a secondary container is finished.
- Be aware that electrolyte-free mannitol should not be given simultaneously with blood without adding at least 20 mEq of sodium chloride to each liter of mannitol solution, as prescribed, to prevent pseudoagglutination.
- During I.V. infusion of mannitol, monitor patient's vital signs, central venous pressure, and fluid intake and output every hour. Measure urine output with indwelling urinary catheter, as appropriate.
- Check weight and monitor BUN and serum creatinine electrolyte levels daily.
- Provide frequent mouth care to relieve thirst and dry mouth.

PATIENT TEACHING
- Inform patient that he may experience dry mouth and thirst during mannitol therapy.
- Instruct patient to report chest pain, difficulty breathing, or pain at I.V. site.

meperidine hydrochloride
(pethidine hydrochloride)
Demerol

Class, Category, and Schedule
Chemical: Phenylpiperidine derivative opioid
Therapeutic: Analgesic

Pregnancy category: C
Controlled substance schedule: II

Indications and Dosages

▶ *To provide preoperative sedation*
I.V. INJECTION
Adults. 15 to 35 mg/hr, p.r.n.
▶ *As adjunct to anesthesia*
I.V. INFUSION, I.V. INJECTION
Adults. Individualized. Repeated slow injections of 10 mg/ml solution or continuous infusion of dilute solution (1 mg/ml) titrated as needed.
DOSAGE ADJUSTMENT For patients with creatinine clearance of 10 to 50 ml/min/1.73 m^2, 75% of usual dose is used; with creatinine clearance of less than 10 ml/min/1.73 m^2, 50% of usual dose is used.

Route	Onset	Peak	Duration
I.V.	1 min	5 to 7 min	2 to 4 hr

Mechanism of Action

Binds with opiate receptors in the spinal cord and higher levels of the CNS. In this way, meperidine stimulates mu and kappa receptors, which alters the perception of and emotional response to pain.

Incompatibilities

Don't mix meperidine in same syringe with aminophylline, barbiturates, heparin, iodides, methicillin, morphine sulfate, phenytoin, sodium bicarbonate, sulfadiazine, or sulfisoxazole.

Contraindications

Acute asthma; hypersensitivity to meperidine, narcotics, or their components; increased intracranial pressure; severe respiratory depression; upper respiratory tract obstruction; use within 14 days of MAO inhibitor therapy

Interactions

DRUGS
acyclovir, ritonavir: Possibly increased blood meperidine level
alfentanil, CNS depressants, fentanyl, sufentanil: Increased risk of CNS and respiratory depression and hypotension
amphetamines, MAO inhibitors: Risk of increased CNS excitation or depression with possibly fatal reactions

anticholinergics: Increased risk of severe constipation
antidiarrheals (such as loperamide and difenoxin and atropine): Increased risk of severe constipation and increased CNS depression
antihypertensives: Increased risk of hypotension
buprenorphine: Possibly decreased therapeutic effects of meperidine and increased risk of respiratory depression
cimetidine: Reduced clearance and volume of distribution of meperidine
hydroxyzine: Increased risk of CNS depression and hypotension
metoclopramide: Possibly decreased effects of metoclopramide
naloxone, naltrexone: Decreased pharmacologic effects of meperidine
neuromuscular blockers: Increased risk of prolonged respiratory and CNS depression
oral anticoagulants: Possibly increased anticoagulant effect and risk of bleeding
phenytoin: Possibly enhanced hepatic metabolism of meperidine
ACTIVITIES
alcohol use: Possibly increased CNS and respiratory depression and hypotension

Adverse Reactions

CNS: Confusion, depression, dizziness, drowsiness, euphoria, headache, increased intracranial pressure, lack of coordination, malaise, nervousness, nightmares, restlessness, seizures, syncope, tremor
CV: Hypotension, orthostatic hypotension, tachycardia
EENT: Blurred vision, diplopia, dry mouth
GI: Abdominal cramps or pain, anorexia, constipation, ileus, nausea, vomiting
GU: Dysuria, urinary frequency, urine retention
RESP: Dyspnea, respiratory arrest or depression, wheezing
SKIN: Diaphoresis, flushing, pruritus, rash, urticaria
Other: Injection site pain, redness, and swelling; physical and psychological dependence

Nursing Considerations

- Use meperidine with extreme caution in patients who have acute abdominal conditions, hepatic or renal disorders, hypothyroidism, prostatic hyperplasia, seizures, or supraventricular tachycardia.
- To minimize local anesthetic effect, dilute syrup with water before administration.

- Give I.V. dose slowly by direct injection or as a slow continuous infusion. Mix with D$_5$W, normal saline solution, or Ringer's or lactated Ringer's solution.
- Keep naloxone available when giving I.V. meperidine.
- Monitor patient's respiratory and cardiovascular status during treatment. Notify prescriber immediately and expect to discontinue drug if respiratory rate falls to less than 12 breaths/minute or if respiratory depth decreases.
- Monitor bowel function to detect constipation, and assess the need for stool softeners.
- Assess for signs of physical dependence and abuse.
- Expect withdrawal symptoms to occur if drug is abruptly withdrawn after long-term use.

PATIENT TEACHING
- Inform patient that meperidine is a controlled substance and that he'll need identification to purchase it.
- Advise patient to take drug exactly as prescribed.
- Instruct patient to report constipation, severe nausea, and shortness or breath.
- Advise patient to avoid potentially hazardous activities until drug's CNS effects are known.
- Instruct patient to prevent postoperative atelectasis by turning, coughing, and deep-breathing.
- Urge patient to avoid alcohol, sedatives, and tranquilizers during meperidine therapy.

mephentermine sulfate
Wyamine

Class and Category
Chemical: Sympathomimetic amine
Therapeutic: Vasopressor
Pregnancy category: C

Indications and Dosages
▶ *To treat hypotension secondary to spinal anesthesia*
I.V. INJECTION
Adults. 30 to 45 mg (15 mg for obstetrical patients); may be repeated as needed to maintain blood pressure.
I.V. INFUSION
Adults. Dosage individualized based on patient response to therapy. Average dose is 1 to 5 mg/min.

Route	Onset	Peak	Duration
I.V.	Almost immediate	Unknown	15 to 30 min

Mechanism of Action

Stimulates alpha-adrenergic receptors directly and indirectly, resulting in positive inotropic and chronotropic effects. Indirect stimulation occurs by the release of norepinephrine from its storage sites in the heart and other tissues. By enhancing cardiac contraction, mephentermine improves cardiac output, thereby increasing blood pressure. Increased peripheral resistance from peripheral vasoconstriction may also contribute to increased blood pressure. Mephentermine can affect the heart rate but the change is variable, based on vagal tone. It may also stimulate beta-adrenergic receptors.

Contraindications

Hypersensitivity to mephentermine, phenothiazine-induced hypotension, use within 14 days of MAO inhibitor therapy

Interactions

DRUGS

alpha blockers, other drugs with alpha-blocking effects: Possibly decreased peripheral vasoconstrictive and hypertensive effects of mephentermine

beta blockers (ophthalmic): Decreased effects of mephentermine; increased risk of bronchospasm, wheezing, decreased pulmonary function, and respiratory failure

beta blockers (systemic): Increased risk of bronchospasm, decreased effects of both drugs

diuretics and other antihypertensives: Possibly reduced effectiveness of these drugs

doxapram: Possibly increased vasopressor effects of either drug

ergot alkaloids: Increased vasopressor effects

guanadrel, guanethidine, mecamylamine, methyldopa, reserpine: Possibly decreased effects of these drugs and increased risk of adverse effects

hydrocarbon inhalation anesthetics: Increased risk of atrial and ventricular arrhythmias

MAO inhibitors: Intensified and extended cardiac stimulation and vasopressor effects, possibly severe headache and hypertensive crisis

maprotiline, tricyclic antidepressants: Increased vasopressor response;

increased risk of prolonged QTc interval, arrhythmias, hypertension, and hyperpyrexia

methylphenidate: Possibly increased vasopressor effect of mephentermine

nitrates: Possibly reduced antianginal effects of nitrates and decreased vasopressor effect

other sympathomimetics (such as dopamine): Possibly increased cardiac effects and adverse reactions

oxytocin: Possibly severe hypertension

thyroid hormones: Increased effects of both drugs, increased risk of coronary insufficiency in patients with coronary artery disease

Adverse Reactions

CNS: Anxiety, dizziness, drowsiness, euphoria, headache, incoherence, nervousness, psychosis, restlessness, seizures, weakness
CV: Angina, arrhythmias (including bradycardia, tachycardia, and ventricular arrhythmias), hypertension, hypotension, palpitations, peripheral vasoconstriction
GI: Nausea, vomiting
RESP: Dyspnea
SKIN: Peripheral necrosis

Nursing Considerations

- Before administering mephentermine, expect to intervene, as ordered, to correct hemorrhage, hypovolemia, metabolic acidosis, or hypoxia.
- Discard vial if you observe discoloration or precipitate.
- Using D_5W or normal saline solution, prepare a 1-mg/ml solution for infusion.
- Administer drug using an infusion pump to provide a controlled rate.
- Monitor blood pressure, cardiac rate and rhythm, central venous pressure (if appropriate), and urine output during administration. Adjust infusion rate according to patient response, as ordered. Be aware that patients with a history of cardiovascular disease (including hypertension) or hyperthyroidism and chronically ill patients are at increased risk for mephentermine's adverse cardiovascular effects.
- Assess patients with angle-closure glaucoma for signs of an exacerbation, such as eye pain or blurred vision.
- Assess circulation in patients with a history of occlusive vascular disease, such as atherosclerosis and Raynaud's disease, because mephentermine may cause decreased circulation and

increase the risk of necrosis or gangrene. Inspect I.V. site periodically for signs of extravasation.

- **WARNING** Be aware that weeping, excitability, seizures, and hallucinations are some of the symptoms of mephentermine overdose. Contact prescriber immediately if patient experiences such symptoms, and expect to provide supportive treatment.
- Be aware that mephentermine can increase contractions in pregnant women, especially during the third trimester. Expect drug to be prescribed only when benefits outweigh potential adverse effects.
- Store drug at 15° to 30° C (59° to 86° F); don't freeze.

PATIENT TEACHING

- Instruct patient receiving mephentermine to report adverse reactions, including chest pain, difficulty breathing, dizziness, irregular heartbeat, headache, and weakness.

meropenem

Merrem I.V.

Class and Category

Chemical: Carbapenem
Therapeutic: Antibiotic
Pregnancy category: B

Indications and Dosages

▶ *To treat complicated appendicitis and peritonitis caused by susceptible strains of alpha-hemolytic streptococci,* Bacteroides fragilis, Bacteroides thetaiotaomicron, Escherichia coli, Klebsiella pneumoniae, Peptostreptococcus *species, or* Pseudomonas aeruginosa

I.V. INFUSION, I.V. INJECTION

Adults and children weighing more than 50 kg (110 lb). 1 g every 8 hr infused over 15 to 30 min or given as a bolus over 3 to 5 min.

Children over age 3 months weighing less than 50 kg. 20 mg/kg every 8 hr infused over 15 to 30 min or given as a bolus over 3 to 5 min. *Maximum:* 1 g every 8 hr.

DOSAGE ADJUSTMENT For patients with creatinine clearance of 26 to 50 ml/min/1.73 m^2, dosage reduced to 1 g every 12 hr. For those with creatinine clearance of 10 to 25 ml/min/1.73 m^2, dosage reduced to 500 mg every 12 hr. For those with creatinine clearance of less than 10 ml/min/1.73 m^2, dosage reduced to 500 mg every 24 hr.

▶ *To treat complicated skin and skin structure infections caused by* Staphylococcus aureus, Streptococcus agalactiae, Streptococcus pyogenes, *viridans group streptococci,* Enterococcus faecalis *(excluding vancomycin-resistant isolates),* Pseudomonas aeruginosa, Escherichia coli, Proteus mirabilis, Bacteroides fragilis, *and* Peptostreptococcus *species*

I.V. INFUSION

Adults and children weighing more than 50 kg (110 lb). 500 mg every 8 hr infused over 15 to 30 min.

Children older than age 3 months weighing less than 50 kg. 10 mg/kg every 8 hr infused over 15 to 30 min. *Maximum:* 500 mg every 8 hr.

DOSAGE ADJUSTMENT For patients with creatinine clearance of 26 to 50 ml/min/1.73 m^2, dosage reduced to 500 mg every 12 hr. For those with creatinine clearance of 10 to 25 ml/min/1.73 m^2, dosage reduced to 250 mg every 12 hr. For those with creatinine clearance of less than 10 ml/min/1.73 m^2, dosage reduced to 250 mg every 24 hr.

▶ *To treat bacterial meningitis caused by* Haemophilus influenzae, Neisseria meningitidis, *or* Streptococcus pneumoniae *in children*

I.V. INFUSION, I.V. INJECTION

Children weighing more than 50 kg. 2 g every 8 hr infused over 15 to 30 min or given as a bolus over 3 to 5 min.

Children over age 3 months weighing less than 50 kg. 40 mg/kg every 8 hr infused over 15 to 30 min or given as a bolus over 3 to 5 min. *Maximum:* 2 g every 8 hr.

Mechanism of Action

Penetrates cell walls of most gram-negative and gram-positive bacteria, inactivating penicillin-binding proteins. This action inhibits bacterial cell wall synthesis and causes cell death.

Incompatibilities

Don't mix meropenem in same solution with other drugs.

Contraindications

Hypersensitivity to meropenem, other carbapenem drugs, beta lactams, or their components

Interactions

DRUGS

probenecid: Inhibited renal excretion of meropenem

valproic acid: Possibly reduced blood level of valproic acid to subtherapeutic level

Adverse Reactions

CNS: Headache, seizures

CV: Shock

EENT: Epistaxis, glossitis, oral candidiasis

GI: Anorexia, constipation, diarrhea, elevated liver function test results, nausea, pseudomembranous colitis, vomiting

GU: Elevated BUN and serum creatinine levels, hematuria, renal failure

HEME: Agranulocytosis, leukopenia, neutropenia

RESP: Apnea, dyspnea

SKIN: Diaper rash from candidiasis (children), erythema multiforme, pruritus, rash, Stevens-Johnson syndrome, toxic epidermal necrolysis

Other: Anaphylaxis; angioedema; injection site inflammation, pain, phlebitis, or thrombophlebitis; sepsis

Nursing Considerations

- Obtain body fluid and tissue samples, as ordered, for culture and sensitivity testing. Expect to review test results, if possible, before giving first dose of meropenem.
- For I.V. bolus, add 10 ml sterile water for injection to 500 mg/20-ml vial, or 20 ml of diluent to 1 g/30-ml vial of drug. Shake to dissolve.
- **WARNING** Be aware that fatal hypersensitivity reactions have occurred with meropenem administration. Determine whether patient has had previous reactions to antibiotics or other allergens.
- Be prepared to administer emergency treatment for anaphylaxis.
- Institute seizure precautions, according to facility policy, for patients with bacterial meningitis or CNS or renal disorders because these patients are at increased risk of seizures with meropenem.
- Monitor patient with creatinine clearance of 10 to 26 ml/min/1.73 m^2 for signs and symptoms of seizures, heart failure, renal failure, or shock.

PATIENT TEACHING

- Tell patient to report trouble breathing, diarrhea, injection site pain, or mouth soreness.

metaraminol bitartrate
Aramine

Class and Category
Chemical: Sympathomimetic amine
Therapeutic: Vasopressor
Pregnancy category: C

Indications and Dosages
▶ *To treat hypotension secondary to spinal anesthesia or as adjunct to treat hypotension caused by hemorrhage, adverse drug reactions, surgical complications, or shock resulting from brain damage secondary to trauma or tumor*

I.V. INFUSION

Adults. 15 to 100 mg (base) mixed in 500 ml of normal saline solution or D_5W; dosage individualized to maintain desired blood pressure.

▶ *To treat severe shock*

I.V. INJECTION

Adults. 500 mcg (0.5 mg) to 5 mg (base), followed by I.V. infusion individualized to maintain desired blood pressure.

Route	Onset	Peak	Duration
I.V.	1 to 2 min	Unknown	20 to 60 min

Mechanism of Action
May directly stimulate alpha-adrenergic receptors and inhibit activity of the intracellular enzyme adenyl cyclase, which then inhibits production of cAMP. Inhibition of cAMP causes arterial and venous constriction and increases peripheral vascular resistance and systolic blood pressure. Metaraminol also directly stimulates beta-adrenergic receptors in the myocardium and increases adenyl cyclase activity, producing positive inotropic and chronotropic effects.

Incompatibilities
Don't mix metaraminol with barbiturates, penicillins, phenytoin, sodium salts, or other drugs that have poor solubility in acidic solutions.

Contraindications
Hypersensitivity to metaraminol or its components, including sulfites; use with cyclopropane or halothane anesthesia unless clinically warranted

Interactions
DRUGS

alpha blockers, other drugs with alpha-blocking effects: Possibly decreased peripheral vasoconstrictive and hypertensive effects of metaraminol

beta blockers (ophthalmic): Decreased effects of metaraminol; increased risk of bronchospasm, wheezing, decreased pulmonary function, and respiratory failure

beta blockers (systemic): Increased risk of bronchospasm, decreased effects of both drugs

digoxin: Increased risk of arrhythmias

diuretics and other antihypertensives: Possibly reduced effectiveness of these drugs

doxapram: Possibly increased vasopressor effects of both drugs

ergot alkaloids: Increased vasopressor effects

guanadrel, guanethidine, mecamylamine, methyldopa: Possibly decreased effects of these drugs and increased risk of adverse effects

hydrocarbon inhalation anesthetics: Increased risk of atrial and ventricular arrhythmias

MAO inhibitors: Intensified and extended cardiac stimulation and vasopressor effects; possibly severe hypertension

maprotiline, tricyclic antidepressants: Increased vasopressor response; increased risk of prolonged QTc interval, arrhythmias, hypertension, and hyperpyrexia

methylphenidate: Possibly increased vasopressor effect of metaraminol

nitrates: Possibly reduced antianginal effects of nitrates, decreased vasopressor effect

other sympathomimetics (such as dopamine): Possibly increased cardiac effects and adverse reactions

oxytocin: Possibly severe hypertension

thyroid hormones: Increased effects of both drugs, increased risk of coronary insufficiency in patients with coronary artery disease

Adverse Reactions
CNS: Anxiety, dizziness, headache, nervousness, seizures, weakness

CV: Angina, arrhythmias (including bradycardia, tachycardia, and ventricular arrhythmias), hypertension, hypotension, palpitations, peripheral vasoconstriction

GI: Nausea, vomiting

RESP: Dyspnea

SKIN: Extravasation with tissue necrosis and sloughing

Other: Injection site abscess

Nursing Considerations

- Before starting metaraminol therapy, expect to administer blood, plasma volume expanders, I.V. fluids, and electrolyte replacement therapy, as ordered, to correct conditions that caused hypotension, such as hemorrhage or hypovolemia.
- Discard vial if you observe discoloration or precipitates.
- To prepare an I.V. infusion, add 15 to 100 mg of metaraminol to 500 ml of appropriate solution, such as normal saline soluion or D₅W. (You may use a smaller or larger amount of solution, depending on patient's fluid needs.) Use within 24 hours.
- Expect to use large veins for I.V. administration, such as antecubital fossa or a vein in the thigh. Administer infusion using an infusion pump to provide a controlled rate.
- Monitor blood pressure, cardiac rate and rhythm, central venous pressure, and urine output during administration. Be aware that vasoconstrictive effects of prolonged metaraminol administration may prevent volume expansion and prolong shock state. If this occurs, expect to administer blood and plasma volume expanders, as ordered.
- Allow at least 10 minutes to pass between dosage adjustments to let dose achieve maximum effect. Adjust infusion rate to patient response, as ordered.
- **WARNING** Assess patient for allergic reactions—including anaphylaxis and, possibly, life-threatening asthmatic episodes—because drug contains sodium bisulfite.
- Expect to discontinue metaraminol infusion gradually. Continue to monitor patient's blood pressure after infusion has stopped; elevated blood pressure may persist from drug's cumulative effects. Expect to restart metaraminol, as prescribed, if hypotension recurs.
- Be aware that patients with a history of cardiovascular disease (including hypertension) or hyperthyroidism and chronically ill patients are at increased risk for drug's adverse cardiovascular effects. Monitor patients with acute MI for worsening of condition because metaraminol can intensify or prolong myocardial ischemia.
- Monitor patients with cirrhosis for arrhythmias and diuresis. Expect to administer electrolytes, as prescribed, if diuresis occurs.
- Assess patients with angle-closure glaucoma for signs of an exacerbation, such as eye pain or blurred vision.
- Assess circulation in patients with a history of occlusive vascular disease, such as atherosclerosis, diabetic endarteritis, and

Raynaud's disease, because metaraminol may cause decreased circulation and increase the risk of necrosis or gangrene. Inspect I.V. site periodically for signs of extravasation.

• **WARNING** Be aware that metaraminol overdose may cause headache, euphoria, arrhythmias, severe hypertension, and MI. Contact prescriber immediately if patient experiences such symptoms, and expect to provide supportive treatment.

• Monitor patients with a history of malaria for evidence of a metaraminol-induced relapse, such as fever, chills, or muscle aches.

• Store drug at 15° to 30° C (59° to 86° F); protect from freezing and light.

PATIENT TEACHING

• Advise patient to immediately report any discomfort at metaraminol infusion site, such as pain, swelling, or redness.

• Instruct patient to report adverse reactions, including chest pain, difficulty breathing, dizziness, irregular heartbeat, headache, and weakness.

methicillin sodium
Staphcillin

Class and Category
Chemical: Penicillinase-resistant penicillin
Therapeutic: Antibiotic
Pregnancy category: B

Indications and Dosages
▶ *To treat general infections, such as sepsis, sinusitis, and skin and soft-tissue infections, caused by susceptible organisms (including penicillinase-producing and non–penicillinase-producing strains of* Staphylococcus epidermidis, Staphylococcus saprophyticus, *and* Streptococcus pneumoniae*)*

I.V. INFUSION

Adults and children weighing 40 kg (88 lb) or more. 1 g every 6 hr. *Maximum:* 24 g daily.

Children weighing less than 40 kg. 25 mg/kg every 6 hr.

DOSAGE ADJUSTMENT For adults and children with cystic fibrosis, dosage decreased to 50 mg/kg every 6 hr.

▶ *To treat bacterial meningitis*

I.V. INFUSION

Neonates weighing 2 kg (4.4 lb) or more. 50 mg/kg every 8 hr for first wk after birth and then 50 mg/kg every 6 hr.

Neonates weighing less than 2 kg. 25 to 50 mg/kg every 12 hr for first wk after birth and then 50 mg/kg every 8 hr.

Mechanism of Action

Kills bacterial cells by inhibiting bacterial cell wall synthesis. In susceptible bacteria, the rigid, cross-linked cell wall is assembled in several steps. In the final stage of cross-linking, methicillin binds with and inactivates penicillin-binding proteins (enzymes responsible for linking cell wall strands), resulting in bacterial cell lysis and death. *Staphylococcus aureus* has developed resistance to methicillin by altering its penicillin-binding proteins.

Incompatibilities

Don't mix methicillin in same syringe or I.V. solution with other drugs. Don't mix methicillin with dextrose solutions because their low acidity may damage drug. Administer methicillin at least 1 hour before or after aminoglycosides and at different sites to prevent mutual inactivation.

Contraindications

Hypersensitivity to methicillin sodium, other penicillins, or their components

Interactions

DRUGS

aminoglycosides: Substantial aminoglycoside inactivation
chloramphenicol, erythromycins, sulfonamides, tetracyclines: Possibly decreased therapeutic effects of methicillin
methotrexate: Increased risk of methotrexate toxicity
probenecid: Possibly decreased renal clearance, increased blood level, and increased risk of toxicity of methicillin

Adverse Reactions

CNS: Aggressiveness, agitation, anxiety, confusion, depression, headache, seizures
EENT: Oral candidiasis
GI: Abdominal pain, diarrhea, hepatotoxicity, nausea, pseudomembranous colitis, vomiting
GU: Interstitial nephritis, vaginitis
HEME: Leukopenia, neutropenia, thrombocytopenia
SKIN: Exfoliative dermatitis, pruritus, rash, urticaria
Other: Anaphylaxis; infusion site redness, swelling, and tenderness; serum-sicknesslike reaction

Nursing Considerations

- **WARNING** Be aware that methicillin is not a first-line treatment for the indications listed previously because of the prevalence of methicillin-resistant *Staphylococcus aureus*.
- Before giving first dose, obtain appropriate body fluid or tissue specimens for culture and sensitivity tests, as ordered, and review test results if available.
- Add 1.5 ml, 5.7 ml, or 8.6 ml of sterile water for injection or 0.9% sodium chloride injection to 1-g, 4-g, or 6-g vial, respectively, to yield a concentration of 500 mg/ml. Dilute further with 25 ml of normal saline solution for each 500 mg (1 ml) of drug. Use concentrations of 2 to 20 mg/ml within 8 hours if stored at room temperature.
- Observe infusion site closely during administration for redness, swelling, and tenderness.
- Monitor fluid intake and output and renal function test results during methicillin therapy.
- Observe for signs of superinfection, such as diarrhea, vaginal itching, and white patches or sores in mouth or on tongue. Notify prescriber if they occur.
- Closely monitor renal function test results, including serum creatinine level; about one-third of patients experience interstitial nephritis after 10 days of methicillin therapy.
- Monitor liver function test results, and observe for signs of hepatotoxicity, such as fever and nausea. Notify prescriber if such signs occur.
- When calculating sodium intake for patients on a sodium-restricted diet, keep in mind that each gram of methicillin contains approximately 2.24 mEq of sodium.
- Store drug at 15° to 30° C (59° to 86° F).

PATIENT TEACHING
- Unless contraindicated, instruct patient to drink extra fluids during methicillin therapy.
- Advise patient to report diarrhea, infusion site pain, mouth sores, or rash.

methocarbamol

Carbacot, Robaxin, Skelex

Class and Category

Chemical: Carbamate derivative of guaifenesin
Therapeutic: Skeletal muscle relaxant

Pregnancy category: C
Indications and Dosages
▶ *To relieve discomfort caused by acute, painful musculoskeletal conditions*
I.V. INJECTION (100 MG/ML)
Adults and adolescents. Up to 3,000 mg daily given at 8-hr intervals for 3 consecutive days. Regimen repeated as prescribed after patient is drug-free for 48 hr.
▶ *To provide supportive therapy for tetanus*
I.V. INFUSION, I.V. INJECTION (100 MG/ML)
Adults and adolescents. 1,000 to 3,000 mg by infusion or 1,000 to 2,000 mg by direct injection every 6 hr. *Maximum:* 300 mg (3 ml)/min.
Children. 15 mg/kg every 6 hr.

Route	Onset	Peak	Duration
I.V.	Immediate	Unknown	Unknown

Mechanism of Action
May depress the CNS, which leads to sedation and reduced skeletal muscle spasms. Methocarbamol also alters the perception of pain.

Contraindications
Hypersensitivity to methocarbamol or its components, renal disease (injectable form)

Interactions
DRUGS
CNS depressants: Increased CNS depression
ACTIVITIES
alcohol use: Increased CNS depression

Adverse Reactions
CNS: Dizziness, drowsiness, fever, headache, light-headedness, seizures (I.V.), syncope, vertigo, weakness
CV: Bradycardia, hypotension, and thrombophlebitis (parenteral)
EENT: Blurred vision, conjunctivitis, diplopia, metallic taste, nasal congestion, nystagmus
GI: Nausea
GU: Black, brown, or green urine
SKIN: Flushing, pruritus, rash, urticaria
Other: Anaphylaxis, angioedema, injection site sloughing

Nursing Considerations

- Administer I.V. form directly through infusion line at 3 ml/min. To prepare solution, add 10 ml to no more than 250 ml of D_5W or normal saline solution. Infuse at no more than 300 mg (3 ml)/minute to avoid hypotension and seizures.
- Keep patient recumbent during I.V. administration and for at least 15 minutes afterward. Then have him rise slowly.
- Monitor I.V. site regularly for signs of phlebitis.
- Keep epinephrine, antihistamines, and corticosteroids available in case patient experiences anaphylactic reaction.
- Be aware that the parenteral dosage form shouldn't be used in patients with renal dysfunction because the polyethylene glycol 300 vehicle is nephrotoxic.

PATIENT TEACHING

- Inform patient that urine may turn green, black, or brown until drug is discontinued.
- Advise patient to avoid potentially hazardous activities until drug's CNS effects are known.
- Instruct patient to avoid alcohol and other CNS depressants during therapy.

methotrexate (amethopterin)

Rheumatrex

methotrexate sodium

Folex, Folex PFS, Mexate, Mexate-AQ

Class and Category

Chemical: Folic acid analogue
Therapeutic: Antipsoriatic, antirheumatic
Pregnancy category: X

Indications and Dosages

▶ *To treat severe psoriasis unresponsive to other therapy*
I.V. (methotrexate sodium)
Adults. 10 mg/wk. *Maximum:* 25 mg/wk.

Route	Onset	Peak	Duration
I.V.	3 to 6 wk	Unknown	Unknown

Contraindications

Breast-feeding, hypersensitivity to methotrexate or its components, pregnancy

Mechanism of Action

May exert immunosuppressive effects by inhibiting replication and function of T and possibly B lymphocytes. Methotrexate also slows the growth of rapidly proliferating cells, such as epithelial skin cells associated with psoriasis. This action may result from the drug's ability to inhibit dihydrofolate reductase, the enzyme that reduces folic acid to tetrahydrofolic acid. Inhibition of tetrahydrofolic acid interferes with DNA synthesis and cell reproduction in rapidly proliferating cells.

Interactions

DRUGS

bone marrow depressants: Possibly increased bone marrow depression
co-trimoxazole: Possibly increased bone marrow suppression
folic acid: Possibly decreased effectiveness of methotrexate
hepatotoxic drugs: Increased risk of hepatotoxicity
chloramphenicol, neomycin, tetracycline: Possibly decreased absorption of methotrexate
NSAIDs, penicillins, phenylbutazone, phenytoin, probenecid, salicylates, sulfonamides: Increased risk of methotrexate toxicity
oral anticoagulants: Increased risk of bleeding
sulfonamides: Increased risk of hepatotoxicity
theophylline: Possibly increased risk of theophylline toxicity
trimethoprim and sulfamethoxazole: Possibly increased bone marrow suppression
vaccines: Risk of disseminated infection with live-virus vaccines, risk of suppressed response to killed-virus vaccines

ACTIVITIES

alcohol use: Increased risk of hepatotoxicity

Adverse Reactions

CNS: Aphasia, cerebral thrombosis, chills, dizziness, drowsiness, fatigue, fever, headache, hemiparesis, leukoencephalopathy, malaise, paresis, seizures
CV: Chest pain, deep vein thrombosis, hypotension, pericardial effusion, pericarditis, thromboembolism
ENDO: Gynecomastia
EENT: Blurred vision, conjunctivitis, gingivitis, glossitis, pharyngitis, stomatitis, transient blindness, tinnitus
GI: Abdominal pain, anorexia, cirrhosis, diarrhea, elevated liver function test results, enteritis, GI bleeding and ulceration, hepatitis, hepatotoxicity, nausea, pancreatitis, vomiting

GU: Cystitis, hematuria, infertility, menstrual dysfunction, nephropathy, renal failure, tubular necrosis, vaginal discharge
HEME: Anemia, aplastic anemia, leukopenia, neutropenia, pancytopenia, thrombocytopenia
MS: Arthralgia, dysarthia, myalgia, stress fracture
RESP: Dry nonproductive cough, dyspnea, interstitial pneumonitis, pneumonia, pulmonary fibrosis or failure, pulmonary infiltrates
SKIN: Acne, alopecia, altered skin pigmentation, ecchymosis, erythema multiforme, exfoliative dermatitis, furunculosis, necrosis, photosensitivity, pruritus, psoriatic lesions, rash, Stevens-Johnson syndrome, telangiectasia, toxic epidermal necrolysis, ulceration, urticaria
Other: Anaphylaxis, increased risk of infection, lymphadenopathy, lymphoproliferative disease

Nursing Considerations

- Follow facility policy for preparing and handling drug; parenteral form poses a risk of carcinogenicity, mutagenicity, and teratogenicity. Avoid skin contact.
- Monitor results of CBC, chest X-ray, liver and renal function tests, and urinalysis before and during treatment.
- Unless contraindicated, increase patient's fluid intake to 2 to 3 L daily to reduce the risk of adverse GU reactions.
- Assess patient for signs of bleeding and infection.
- **WARNING** Expect renal impairment to severely alter drug elimination.
- Be aware that high doses of methotrexate can impair renal elimination by forming crystals that obstruct urine flow. To prevent drug precipitation, alkalinize patient's urine with sodium bicarbonate tablets, as ordered.
- Follow standard precautions because drug can cause immunosuppression.
- If patient becomes dehydrated from vomiting, notify prescriber and expect to withhold drug until patient recovers.
- If patient receives high doses of drug, keep leucovorin readily available to use as antidote.
- Be aware that methotrexate resistance may develop with prolonged use.

PATIENT TEACHING

- Instruct patient to avoid alcohol during methotrexate therapy.
- Encourage frequent mouth care to reduce the risk of mouth sores.

- Instruct patient to use sunblock when exposed to sunlight.
- Advise patient to notify prescriber about bruising, chills, cough, fever, dark or bloody urine, mouth sores, shortness of breath, sore throat, and yellow skin or eyes.
- Urge women of childbearing age to use contraception during methotrexate therapy.

methoxy polyethylene glycol-epoetin beta

Mircera

Class and Category

Chemical: 165-amino acid glycoprotein identical to human erythropoietin
Therapeutic: Antianemic
Pregnancy category: C

Indications and Dosages

▶ *To treat anemia from chronic renal failure regardless of dialysis use for patients not currently receiving an erythropoiesis stimulating agent (ESA)*

I.V. OR SUBCUTANEOUS INJECTION

Adults. *Initial:* 0.6 mcg/kg every 2 wk. *Maintenance:* Dose individualized and increased 25% once monthly, as needed, to maintain a hemoglobin level greater than 10 g/dl but less than 12 g/dl. Once hemoglobin level stabilizes between 10 g/dl and 12 g/dl, dose may continue to be given every 2 wk. Alternatively, the previous every-2-week dose may be doubled and given monthly.

▶ *To treat anemia from chronic renal failure regardless of dialysis use for patients currently stabilized with an ESA*

I.V. OR SUBCUTANEOUS INJECTION

Adults. Dose given every 2 wk or monthly based on previous total weekly dose of darbepoetin alfa or epoetin alfa at time of conversion, beginning with the next scheduled dose of the previously administered ESA.

DOSAGE ADJUSTMENT Dose reduced by about 25% if hemoglobin level increases more than 1 g/dl in any 2-week period or if hemoglobin level increases and approaches 12 g/dl. If hemoglobin level continues to increase, doses temporarily withheld until hemoglobin level begins to decrease; then therapy restarted at about 25% below previous dose. Dose increased by about 25% of previous dose if hemoglobin level increases less than 1 g/dl over a month, but only if serum ferritin level is 100 mcg/mcg/L or greater and serum transferring saturation made at 4-week intervals until specified hemoglobin level is obtained.

Mechanism of Action
Stimulates the release of reticulocytes from the bone marrow into the bloodstream, where they develop into mature RBCs.

Contraindications
Hypersentivity to methoxy polyethylene glycol-epoetin beta or its components; uncontrolled hypertension

Interactions
DRUGS
None known.

Adverse Reactions
CNS: CVA, headache, seizures
CV: Arteriovenous fistular thrombosis, congestive heart failure, hypertension, hypotension, MI, tachycardia
EENT: Nasopharyngitis
GI: Constipation, diarrhea, vomiting
GU: UTI
HEME: Anti-erythropoietin antibody–associated anemia
MS: Back or limb pain, muscle spasms
RESP: Cough, upper respiratory tract infection
SKIN: Pruritus, rash
Other: Anaphylaxis, development of neutralizing antibodies to erythropoietin

Nursing Considerations
- Be aware that drug vial or prefilled syringe is for single use only. Don't use the vial or prefilled syringe more than one time, and don't pool unused portions from vials or prefilled syringes.
- Store drug in original cartons, and avoid vigorous shaking or prolonged exposure to light.
- Don't dilute drug before giving it.
- To use prefilled syringe, fully depress the plunger during injection to activate the needle guard. After administration, remove needle from the injection site and release the plunger, allowing the needle guard to move up until the entire needle is covered.

- Check patient's hemoglobin level every 2 weeks, as ordered, until hemoglobin stabilizes and maintenance dosage has been achieved. Then check it level every 2 to 4 weeks, as ordered.
- **WARNING** Be aware that the risk of cardiac arrest, seizures, CVA, worsening hypertension, congestive heart failure, vascular thrombosis, vascular ischemia, vascular infarction, acute MI, and fluid overload with peripheral edema increases if hemoglobin level increases more than about 1 g/dl during any 2-week period or if it exceeds 12 g/dl. Expect to decrease dosage if this occurs.
- Institute seizure precautions according to facility policy.
- Check blood pressure for hypertension often during therapy. If blood pressure is poorly controlled with antihypertensive and dietary measures, expect to reduce dosage or withhold drug.
- Evaluate patient's response to drug. If patient suddenly stops responding and develops severe anemia and low reticulocyte count, notify prescriber because the underlying cause will need to be investigated. If an anti-erythropoietin antibody–associated anemia occurs or is suspected, withhold drug and other erythropoietic proteins, as ordered.

PATIENT TEACHING
- Explain that drug may increase the risk of seizures, and advise against engaging in hazardous activities during therapy.
- Stress the need to comply with dosage regimen and keep follow-up medical and laboratory appointments.
- Advise patient to follow up with her prescriber for blood pressure monitoring.
- Encourage patient to eat adequate quantities of iron-rich foods.
- Review possible adverse reactions, and urge patient to notify prescriber if she has chest pain, headache, rash, seizures, shortness of breath, or swelling.

methyldopate hydrochloride
Aldomet

Class and Category
Chemical: 3,4-dihydroxyphenylalanine (DOPA) analogue
Therapeutic: Antihypertensive
Pregnancy category: C

Indications and Dosages
▶ *To manage hypertension, to treat hypertensive crisis*

I.V. INFUSION
Adults. 250 to 500 mg diluted in D₅W and infused over 30 to
60 min every 6 hr. *Maximum:* 1,000 mg every 6 hr.
Children. 20 to 40 mg/kg infused over 30 to 60 min every 6 hr.
Maximum: 65 mg/kg or 3,000 mg daily.

Route	Onset	Peak	Duration
I.V.	Unknown	4 to 6 hr	10 to 16 hr

Mechanism of Action
Is decarboxylated in the body to produce alpha-methylnorepinephrine, a metabolite that stimulates central inhibitory alpha-adrenergic receptors. This action may reduce blood pressure by decreasing sympathetic stimulation of the
heart and peripheral vascular system.

Incompatibilities
Don't administer methyldopate through same I.V. line as barbiturates or sulfonamides.

Contraindications
Active hepatic disease; hypersensitivity to methyldopa, methyldopate, or their components; impaired hepatic function from previous methyldopa or methyldopate therapy; use within 14 days of
MAO inhibitor therapy

Interactions
DRUGS
antihypertensives: Increased hypotension
appetite suppressants, NSAIDs, tricyclic antidepressants: Possibly decreased therapeutic effects of methyldopate
central anesthetics: Possibly need for reduced anesthetic dosage
CNS depressants: Possibly increased CNS depression
haloperidol: Increased risk of adverse CNS effects
levodopa: Possibly decreased therapeutic effects of levodopa and
increased risk of adverse CNS effects
lithium: Increased risk of lithium toxicity
MAO inhibitors: Possibly hallucinations, headaches, hyperexcitabil-
ity, and severe hypertension
oral anticoagulants: Possibly increased therapeutic effects of anticoagulants
sympathomimetics: Possibly decreased therapeutic effects of methyldopate and increased vasopressor effects of sympathomimetics

ACTIVITIES

alcohol use: Possibly increased CNS depression

Adverse Reactions

CNS: Decreased concentration, depression, dizziness, drowsiness, fever, headache, involuntary motor activity, memory loss (transient), nightmares, paresthesia, parkinsonism, sedation, vertigo, weakness

CV: Angina, bradycardia, edema, heart failure, myocarditis, orthostatic hypotension

EENT: Black or sore tongue, dry mouth, nasal congestion

ENDO: Gynecomastia

GI: Constipation, diarrhea, flatulence, hepatic necrosis, hepatitis, nausea, pancreatitis, vomiting

GU: Decreased libido, impotence

HEME: Agranulocytosis, hemolytic anemia, leukopenia, positive Coombs' test, positive tests for ANA and rheumatoid factor, thrombocytopenia

SKIN: Eczema, rash, urticaria

Other: Weight gain

Nursing Considerations

- Expect to monitor CBC and differential results before and periodically during methyldopate therapy.
- Add drug to 100 ml of D₅W, and give over 30 to 60 minutes.
- Monitor blood pressure regularly during therapy.
- Monitor results of Coombs' test; a positive result after several months of treatment indicates that patient has hemolytic anemia. Expect prescriber to discontinue drug.
- Assess for weight gain and edema. If they occur, administer a diuretic, as prescribed.
- Notify prescriber if patient experiences abnormal liver function test results, signs of heart failure (dyspnea, edema, hypertension), jaundice, fever, or involuntary jerky movements.
- Be aware that hypertension may return within 48 hours after drug is discontinued. Expect prescriber to convert patient to oral methyldopa, typically at same dosage as parenteral form. Maximum adult oral dosage is 3,000 mg daily.
- Store drug at 15° to 30° C (59° to 86° F); don't freeze.

PATIENT TEACHING

- Instruct patient to avoid hazardous activities until drug's CNS effects are known.
- Advise patient to change position slowly to minimize effects of orthostatic hypotension.

- Direct patient to report bruising, chest pain, fever, involuntary jerky movements, prolonged dizziness, rash, or yellow eyes or skin.

methylprednisolone sodium succinate
A-methaPred, Solu-Medrol

Class and Category
Chemical: Synthetic glucocorticoid
Therapeutic: Anti-inflammatory, immunosuppressant
Pregnancy category: Not rated

Indications and Dosages
▶ *To treat ulcerative colitis*
I.V. INFUSION
Adults. 40 to 120 mg 3 to 7 times/wk for 2 or more wk. Later doses based on patient's condition and response.
Children. 0.14 to 0.84 mg/kg daily in divided doses every 12 to 24 hr.
▶ *To treat many immune and inflammatory disorders, including allergic rhinitis, asthma, Crohn's disease, and systemic lupus erythematosus*
I.V. INFUSION
Adults. *Initial:* 10 to 40 mg infused over several min. Later doses based on patient's condition and response.
Children. 0.14 to 0.84 mg/kg every 12 to 24 hr.
▶ *To treat acute exacerbations of multiple sclerosis*
I.V. INJECTION
Adults. 160 mg daily for 1 wk, followed by 64 mg every other day for 1 mo.

Route	Onset	Peak	Duration
I.V.	Rapid	30 min	Unknown

Mechanism of Action
Binds to intracellular glucocorticoid receptors and suppresses inflammatory and immune responses by:
- inhibiting accumulation of neutrophils and monocytes at inflamed sites
- stabilizing lysosomal membranes
- suppressing the antigen response of macrophages and helper T cells
- inhibiting the synthesis of inflammatory response mediators, such as cytokines, interleukins, and prostaglandins.

Incompatibilities
Don't mix methylprednisolone with any drug without first consulting pharmacist.

Contraindications
Fungal infection, hypersensitivity to methylprednisolone or its components

Interactions
DRUGS

acetaminophen: Increased risk of hepatotoxicity

amphotericin B, carbonic anhydrase inhibitors: Possibly severe hypokalemia

anabolic steroids, androgens: Increased risk of edema and worsening of acne

anticholinergics: Possibly increased intraocular pressure

asparaginase: Increased risk of hyperglycemia and toxicity

aspirin, NSAIDs: Increased risk of adverse GI effects and bleeding

cyclosporine: Increased risk of seizures

digoxin: Possibly hypokalemia-induced arrhythmias and digitalis toxicity

ephedrine, phenobarbital, phenytoin, rifampin: Decreased blood methylprednisolone level

estrogens, oral contraceptives: Possibly increased therapeutic and toxic effects of methylprednisolone

isoniazid: Possibly decreased therapeutic effects of isoniazid

mexiletine: Possibly decreased blood mexiletine level

neuromuscular blockers: Possibly increased neuromuscular blockade, causing respiratory depression or apnea

oral anticoagulants, thrombolytics: Increased risk of GI ulceration and hemorrhage, possibly decreased therapeutic effects of these drugs

potassium-depleting drugs (such as thiazide diuretics): Possibly severe hypokalemia

potassium supplements: Possibly decreased effects of these supplements

somatrem, somatropin: Possibly decreased therapeutic effects of these drugs

streptozocin: Increased risk of hyperglycemia

troleandomycin: Increased blood methylprednisolone level

vaccines: Decreased antibody response and increased risk of neurologic complications

ACTIVITIES

alcohol use: Increased risk of adverse GI effects and bleeding

Adverse Reactions

CNS: Ataxia, behavioral changes, depression, dizziness, euphoria, fatigue, headache, increased ICP with papilledema, insomnia, malaise, mood changes, paresthesia, restlessness, seizures, steroid psychosis, syncope, vertigo

CV: Arrhythmias (from hypokalemia), edema, fat embolism, heart failure, hypertension, hypotension, thromboembolism, thrombophlebitis

EENT: Exophthalmos, glaucoma, increased intraocular pressure, nystagmus, posterior subcapsular cataracts

ENDO: Adrenal insufficiency, cushingoid symptoms (moon face, buffalo hump, central obesity, supraclavicular fat pad enlargement), diabetes mellitus, growth suppression in children, hyperglycemia, negative nitrogen balance from protein catabolism

GI: Abdominal distention, hiccups, increased appetite, melena, nausea, pancreatitis, peptic ulcer, ulcerative esophagitis, vomiting

GU: Amenorrhea, glycosuria, menstrual irregularities, perineal burning or tingling

HEME: Easy bruising, leukocytosis

MS: Arthralgia; aseptic necrosis of femoral and humeral heads; compression fractures; muscle atrophy, twitching, or weakness; myalgia; osteoporosis; spontaneous fractures; steroid myopathy; tendon rupture

SKIN: Acne; altered skin pigmentation; diaphoresis; erythema; hirsutism; necrotizing vasculitis; petechiae; purpura; rash; scarring; sterile abscess; striae; subcutaneous fat atrophy; thin, fragile skin; urticaria

Other: Anaphylaxis, hypocalcemia, hypokalemia, hypokalemic alkalosis, impaired wound healing, masking of infection, metabolic alkalosis, suppressed skin test reaction, weight gain

Nursing Considerations

- **WARNING** Don't administer methylprednisolone preparations that contain benzyl alcohol to neonates or premature infants because this preservative has been linked to a fatal toxic syndrome characterized by CNS, respiratory, circulatory, and renal impairment and metabolic acidosis.
- Don't give acetate injectable form by I.V. route; it's used for intra-articular, intralesional, I.M., and soft-tissue injections.
- After reconstituting drug according to manufacturer's directions, use it within 48 hours.
- Discard parenteral products if you observe discoloration or particles.

- Provide a low-sodium diet with added potassium, as prescribed.
- Protect patient from falling, especially elderly patient at risk for fractures from osteoporosis.
- Closely monitor patient for signs of infection because drug may mask them.
- Assess for possible depression or psychotic episodes during therapy.
- Monitor blood glucose level; dosage of insulin or oral antidiabetic drug may need to be adjusted for diabetic patient.
- **WARNING** To avoid possibly fatal acute adrenocortical insufficiency, expect to taper long-term therapy when it must be discontinued.
- Store drug at a controlled room temperature of 20° to 25° C (68° to 77° F), and protect from light.

PATIENT TEACHING

- Urge patient receiving methylprednisolone to immediately report dark or tarry stools; signs of impending adrenocortical insufficiency, such as anorexia, dizziness, fainting, fatigue, fever, joint pain, muscle weakness, or nausea; and sudden weight gain or swelling.
- Inform patient with diabetes that his blood glucose level will be checked frequently during therapy because methylprednisolone may affect glucose level.
- Advise patient to notify prescriber if he develops another illness or requires surgery during therapy or if his condition recurs or worsens after dosage is reduced or methylprednisolone therapy is discontinued.
- Instruct patient not to obtain vaccinations unless approved by prescriber.
- Urge patient to take vitamin D, calcium supplements, or both if recommended by prescriber.
- Instruct patient on long-term therapy to follow a low-sodium, high-potassium, high-protein diet, if prescribed, to help minimize weight gain. Advise him to inform prescriber if he's on a special diet.
- Inform patient that insomnia and restlessness usually resolve after 1 to 3 weeks of therapy.
- Caution patient to avoid people with contagious diseases, such as chicken pox or measles.
- Discuss the need for regular exercise or physical therapy to maintain muscle mass.
- Urge patient to avoid alcoholic beverages during therapy because alcohol increases the risk of GI bleeding.

- Encourage patient to keep regularly scheduled follow-up medical appointments, even after therapy stops.
- Instruct patient to undergo periodic ophthalmic examinations.
- Advise patient to carry medical identification that documents his need for long-term corticosteroid therapy.

metoclopramide hydrochloride
Reglan

Class and Category
Chemical: Benzamide
Therapeutic: Antiemetic, upper GI stimulant
Pregnancy category: B

Indications and Dosages
▶ *To treat diabetic gastroparesis*
I.V. INJECTION
Adults and adolescents. 10 mg t.i.d. or q.i.d. for severe symptoms; dosage adjusted as needed.
▶ *To prevent chemotherapy-induced vomiting*
I.V. INFUSION
Adults and adolescents. 3 mg/kg before chemotherapy and then 0.5 mg/kg/hr for 8 hr.
I.V. INJECTION
Adults and adolescents. 1 to 2 mg/kg 30 min before chemotherapy and then repeated every 2 to 3 hr, as needed.
Children. 1 mg/kg as a single dose, repeated in 1 hr. *Maximum:* 2 mg/kg.

Route	Onset	Peak	Duration
I.V.	1 to 3 min	Unknown	1 to 2 hr

Mechanism of Action
May enhance gastric motility by antagonizing the inhibitory neurotransmitter effect of dopamine on GI smooth muscle. This results in gastric contraction, which promotes gastric emptying and peristalsis, thereby reducing gastroesophageal reflux. Metoclopramide also blocks dopaminergic receptors in the chemoreceptor trigger zone, preventing nausea and vomiting.

Incompatibilities
Don't administer metoclopramide through same I.V. line as cal-

cium gluconate, cephalothin sodium, chloramphenicol sodium, cisplatin, erythromycin lactobionate, furosemide, methotrexate, penicillin G potassium, or sodium bicarbonate.

Contraindications

Concurrent use of butyrophenones, phenothiazines, or other drugs that may cause extrapyramidal reactions; GI hemorrhage, mechanical obstruction, or perforation; hypersensitivity to metoclopramide or its components; pheochromocytoma; seizure disorders

Interactions

DRUGS

anticholinergics, opioid analgesics: Possibly decreased therapeutic effects of metoclopramide
apomorphine: Possibly decreased antiemetic effect of apomorphine, possibly increased CNS depression
bromocriptine, pergolide: Possibly decreased therapeutic effects of these drugs
cimetidine: Possibly decreased cimetidine absorption and effects
CNS depressants: Possibly increased CNS depression
cyclosporine: Increased blood cyclosporine level
digoxin: Decreased gastric absorption of digoxin
levodopa: Possibly decreased levodopa effectiveness
MAO inhibitors: Increased risk of severe hypertension if patient has essential hypertension
mexiletine: Possibly faster mexiletene absorption
succinylcholine: Possibly prolonged therapeutic action of succinylcholine

ACTIVITIES

alcohol use: Increased risk of excessive sedation

Adverse Reactions

CNS: Agitation, anxiety, depression, dizziness, drowsiness, extrapyramidal reactions (motor restlessness, parkinsonism, tardive dyskinesia), fatigue, headache, insomnia, irritability, lassitude, neuroleptic malignant syndrome, panic reaction, restlessness
CV: AV block, fluid retention, heart failure, hypertension, hypotension, supraventricular tachycardia
EENT: Dry mouth
ENDO: Galactorrhea, gynecomastia
GI: Constipation, diarrhea, nausea
GU: Menstrual irregularities
HEME: Agranulocytosis

SKIN: Rash
Other: Restless leg syndrome

Nursing Considerations

- Use metoclopramide cautiously in patients with hypertension because it may increase catecholamine levels.
- Use drug cautiously in elderly patients because they have an increased risk of tardive dyskinesia and parkinsonian effects. Expect to stop drug if these symptoms develop.
- Monitor patient with NADH-cytochrome b5 reductase deficiency because metoclopramide increases the risk of methemoglobinemia and sulfhemoglobinemia and patient can't receive methylene blue.
- Assess patient for evidence of intestinal obstruction, such as abnormal bowel sounds, diarrhea, nausea, and vomiting, before giving metoclopramide. Notify prescriber if you detect them.
- For I.V. administration, you needn't dilute doses of 10 mg or less. Give drug over 1 to 2 minutes. For doses larger than 10 mg, dilute in 50 ml of normal saline solution, half-normal (0.45) saline solution, D_5W, or lactated Ringer's solution and infuse over at least 15 minutes.
- Avoid rapid I.V. delivery because it may cause anxiety, restlessness, and drowsiness.
- **WARNING** Notify prescriber about signs of toxicity, such as disorientation, drowsiness, and extrapyramidal reactions.
- Monitor patient, especially one with heart failure or cirrhosis, for possible signs of fluid retention or volume overload due to transient increase in plasma aldosterone level.
- Monitor patient closely for neuroleptic malignant syndrome, a rare but potentially fatal disorder causing hyperthermia, muscle rigidity, altered level of consciousness, irregular pulse or blood pressure, tachycardia, diaphoresis, and arrhythmias.
- Store drug in a light-resistant container; discard if discolored or contains particulate.

PATIENT TEACHING

- Advise against activities that require alertness for about 2 hours after each dose.
- Urge patient to avoid alcohol and CNS depressants while taking metoclopramide because they may increase CNS depression.
- Tell patient to immediately report involuntary movements of face, eyes, tongue, or hands.
- Alert patient that dizziness, nervousness, and headaches may occur after metoclopramide is discontinued.

metoprolol succinate

Toprol-XL

metoprolol tartrate

Apo-Metoprolol (CAN), Betaloc (CAN), Lopresor (CAN), Lopressor, Novometoprol (CAN)

Class and Category

Chemical: Beta$_1$-adrenergic antagonist
Therapeutic: Antianginal, antihypertensive, MI prophylaxis and treatment
Pregnancy category: C

Indications and Dosages

▶ *To treat acute MI or evolving acute MI*

I.V. INJECTION (METOPROLOL TARTRATE)

Adults. *Initial:* 5 mg by I.V. bolus every 2 min for 3 doses followed by 50 mg P.O. for patients who tolerate total I.V. dose (or 25 to 50 mg P.O. for patients who can't tolerate total I.V. dose) every 6 hr for 48 hr, starting 15 min after final I.V. dose; after 48 hr, 100 mg b.i.d. followed by maintenance dosage. *Maintenance:* 100 mg P.O. b.i.d. for at least 3 mo.

Route	Onset	Peak	Duration
I.V.	Unknown	20 min	Unknown

Mechanism of Action

Inhibits stimulation of beta$_1$-receptor sites, located mainly in the heart, resulting in decreased cardiac excitability, cardiac output, and myocardial oxygen demand. These effects help relieve angina. Metoprolol also helps reduce blood pressure by decreasing renal release of renin.

Contraindications

Acute heart failure, bradycardia of less than 45 beats/minute, cardiogenic shock, hypersensitivity to metoprolol, or its components, hypersensitivity to other beta blockers, pheochromocytoma, second- or third-degree AV block, severe peripheral arterial circulatory disorder, sick sinus syndrome

Interactions

DRUGS

aluminum salts, barbiturates, calcium salts, cholestyramine, colestipol,

NSAIDs, rifampin, salicylates, sulfinpyrazone: Decreased therapeutic effects of metoprolol

amiodarone, digoxin, diltiazem, verapamil: Increased risk of complete AV block

calcium channel blockers: Increased risk of heart failure, increased effects of both drugs

cimetidine: Increased blood metoprolol level

clonidine: Increased risk of hypotension; increased risk of rebound hypertension when clonidine is discontinued

CYP2D6 inhibitors: May increase plasma metoprolol levels

digoxin: Decreased heart rate and atrioventricular conduction

estrogens: Possibly decreased antihypertensive effect of metoprolol

general anesthetics: Increased risk of hypotension and heart failure

insulin, oral antidiabetic drugs: Decreased blood glucose control, possibly masked evidence of hypoglycemia (by metoprolol)

lidocaine: Increased risk of lidocaine toxicity

MAO inhibitors: Increased risk of hypertension

neuromuscular blockers: Possibly enhanced and prolonged neuromuscular blockade

other antihypertensives: Additive hypotensive effect

phenothiazines: Possibly increased blood levels of both drugs

propafenone: Increased blood level and half-life of metoprolol

sympathomimetics, xanthines: Possibly decreased therapeutic effects of these drugs or metoprolol

FOODS

all foods: Increased bioavailability of metoprolol

Adverse Reactions

CNS: Anxiety, confusion, depression, dizziness, drowsiness, fatigue, hallucinations, headache, insomnia, weakness

CV: Angina, arrhythmias (including AV block and bradycardia), chest pain, heart failure, hypertension, orthostatic hypotension

EENT: Nasal congestion, taste disturbance

GI: Constipation, diarrhea, hepatitis, nausea, vomiting

GU: Impotence

HEME: Leukopenia, thrombocytopenia

MS: Arthralgia, back pain, gangrene of extremity, myalgia

RESP: Bronchospasm, dyspnea

SKIN: Diaphoresis, photosensitivity, rash, urticaria

Nursing Considerations

• For patient with acute MI who can't tolerate initial dosage or who delays treatment, start with maintenance dosage, as prescribed and tolerated.

- **WARNING** If dosage exceeds 400 mg daily, monitor patient for bronchospasm and dyspnea because metoprolol competitively blocks beta$_2$-adrenergic receptors in bronchial and vascular smooth muscles.
- **WARNING** When substituting metoprolol for clonidine, expect to gradually reduce clonidine dosage and increase metoprolol dosage over several days. Giving these drugs together causes additive hypotensive effects.
- Be aware that patients who take metoprolol may be at risk for AV block. If AV block results from depressed AV node conduction, prepare to administer appropriate drug, as prescribed, or assist with insertion of temporary pacemaker.
- Check for signs and symptoms of poor glucose control in patient with diabetes mellitus. Metoprolol may interfere with therapeutic effects of insulin and oral antidiabetic drugs. It also may mask evidence of hypoglycemia, such as palpitations, tachycardia, and tremor.
- Monitor patient with peripheral vascular disease for signs and symptoms of arterial insufficiency (pain, pallor, and coldness in affected extremity) because metoprolol can precipitate or aggravate peripheral vascular disease.
- Be aware that abrupt withdrawal of drug can precipitate thyroid storm in patient with hyperthyroidism or thyrotoxicosis.
- **WARNING** Expect to taper metoprolol dosage when drug is discontinued; abrupt discontinuation can cause myocardial ischemia, MI, ventricular arrhythmias, or severe hypertension, especially in patients with cardiac disease.

PATIENT TEACHING
- Advise patient to notify prescriber if pulse rate falls below 60 beats/minute or is significantly lower than usual.
- Urge diabetic patient to check blood glucose level frequently during metoprolol therapy.

metronidazole
Flagyl, Flagyl I.V. RTU, Metro I.V.
metronidazole hydrochloride
Flagyl I.V.

Class and Category
Chemical: Nitroimidazole derivative
Therapeutic: Antibiotic, antiprotozoal
Pregnancy category: B

Indications and Dosages

▶ *To treat systemic anaerobic infections caused by* Bacteroides fragilis, Clostridium difficile, Clostridium perfringens, Eubacterium, Fusobacterium, Peptococcus, Peptostreptococcus, *and* Veillonella *species*

I.V. INFUSION

Adults and adolescents. *Initial:* 15 mg/kg and then 7.5 mg/kg up to 1,000 mg every 6 hr for 7 days or longer. *Maximum:* 4,000 mg daily.

Children. 7.5 mg/kg every 6 hr or 10 mg/kg every 8 hr.

▶ *To prevent perioperative bowel infection*

I.V. INFUSION

Adults and adolescents. 15 mg/kg 1 hr before surgery and then 7.5 mg/kg 6 and 12 hr after initial dose.

Mechanism of Action

Undergoes intracellular chemical reduction during anaerobic metabolism. After metronidazole is reduced, it damages DNA's helical structure and breaks its strands, which inhibits bacterial nucleic acid synthesis and causes cell death.

Incompatibilities

Don't administer I.V. metronidazole with aluminum needles or hubs or through same I.V. line as other drugs.

Contraindications

Breast-feeding, hypersensitivity to metronidazole or its components, trichomoniasis during first trimester of pregnancy

Interactions

DRUGS

cimetidine: Possibly delayed elimination and increased blood level of metronidazole

disulfiram: Possibly combined toxicity, resulting in confusion and psychotic reactions

neurotoxic drugs: Increased risk of neurotoxicity

oral anticoagulants: Possibly increased anticoagulant effect

phenobarbital: Increased metabolism and decreased blood level and half-life of metronidazole

phenytoin: Decreased phenytoin clearance

ACTIVITIES

alcohol use: Possibly disulfiram-like effects

Adverse Reactions

CNS: Ataxia, dizziness, encephalopathy, fever, headache, light-headedness, peripheral neuropathy, seizures (high doses)
EENT: Dry mouth, lacrimation (topical form), metallic taste, pharyngitis
GI: Abdominal cramps or pain, anorexia, diarrhea, nausea, pancreatitis, vomiting
GU: Darkened urine, vaginal candidiasis (oral, parenteral, and topical forms); burning or irritation of sexual partner's penis, candidal cervicitis or vaginitis, dysuria, urinary frequency, vulvitis (vaginal form)
HEME: Leukopenia
MS: Back pain
SKIN: Burning sensation, stinging sensation, dry skin (topical form); erythema, pruritus, rash, urticaria (oral and parenteral forms)
Other: Injection site edema, pain, or tenderness

Nursing Considerations

- Give by slow I.V. infusion (not direct injection) over 1 hour.
- Stop primary I.V. infusion during metronidazole infusion.
- **WARNING** If patient has adverse CNS reactions, such as seizures or peripheral neuropathy, tell prescriber and stop drug immediately.
- Monitor patient with severe liver disease because slowed metronidazole metabolism may cause drug to accumulate in body and increase the risk of adverse effects.
- Monitor CBC and culture and sensitivity tests if therapy lasts longer than 10 days or if second course of treatment is needed.

PATIENT TEACHING

- Instruct female patient to notify prescriber if she is pregnant, intends to get pregnant, or is breast-feeding.
- Caution patient to avoid alcohol during therapy and for at least 1 day afterward.
- Advise patient to avoid hazardous activities until drug's CNS effects are known.
- If patient reports dry mouth, suggest ice chips or sugarless hard candy or gum; suggest a dental visit if dryness lasts longer than 2 weeks.
- Instruct patient to notify prescriber if no improvement occurs within a few days of taking tablets or capsules.
- Urge patient to follow up with prescriber to make sure infection is gone.

mezlocillin sodium

Mezlin

Class and Category

Chemical: Acyclaminopenicillin
Therapeutic: Antibiotic
Pregnancy category: B

Indications and Dosages

▶ *To treat moderate to severe infections, including bacteremia, bone and joint infections, gynecologic infections (such as endometritis, pelvic cellulitis, and pelvic inflammatory disease), intra-abdominal infections (such as cholangitis, cholecystitis, hepatic abscess, intra-abdominal abscess, and peritonitis), lower respiratory tract infections (such as pneumonia and lung abscess), meningitis, septicemia caused by susceptible bacteria, or skin and soft-tissue infections (such as cellulitis and diabetic foot ulcer); to manage febrile neutropenia*

I.V. INFUSION

Adults and adolescents. 3 g every 4 hr or 4 g every 6 hr.

▶ *To treat life-threatening infections of the types listed above*

I.V. INFUSION

Adults and adolescents. Up to 350 mg/kg daily. *Maximum:* 24,000 mg daily.

Children and infants. 50 mg/kg every 4 hr.

Neonates over age 7 days weighing 2,000 g (4 lb, 6 oz) or less. 75 mg/kg every 8 hr.

Neonates age 7 days or less weighing 2,000 g or less. 75 mg/kg every 12 hr.

Neonates age 7 days or less weighing more than 2,000 g. 75 mg/kg every 6 hr.

▶ *To treat uncomplicated UTI*

I.V. INFUSION

Adults. 1.5 to 2 g every 6 hr.

▶ *To treat complicated UTI*

I.V. INFUSION

Adults. 3 g every 6 hr.

DOSAGE ADJUSTMENT Dosing interval extended to every 6 to 8 hr, if needed, for patients with creatinine clearance of 10 to 30 ml/min/1.73 m^2. Dosing interval extended and dosage reduced to 1.5 to 2 g for patients with creatinine clearance of less than 10 ml/min/1.73 m^2.

▶ *To treat uncomplicated gonorrhea caused by susceptible strains of* Neisseria gonorrhoeae

I.V. INFUSION
Adults. 1 to 2 g as a single dose given with 1 g of probenecid
P.O. (or probenecid given up to 30 min before mezlocillin).
▶ *To prevent infection from potentially contaminated surgical procedures*
I.V. INFUSION
Adults. 4 g 30 min before surgery and then 4 g every 6 hr for
2 more doses.
▶ *To prevent infection in cesarean section*
I.V. INFUSION
Adults. 4 g as soon as umbilical cord is clamped; then 4 g every
4 hr for 2 more doses, starting 4 hr after initial dose.

Mechanism of Action

Inhibits bacterial cell wall synthesis. In susceptible bacteria, the rigid, cross-linked cell wall is assembled in several steps. Mezlocillin exerts its effects in the final stage of the cross-linking process by binding with and inactivating penicillin-binding proteins (enzymes responsible for linking cell wall strands). This action causes bacterial cell lysis and death.

Incompatibilities
Administer mezlocillin at separate sites and at least 1 hour before
or after aminoglycosides. Don't mix mezlocillin in same I.V. bag,
bottle, or tubing as other drugs.

Contraindications
Hypersensitivity to mezlocillin, other penicillins, or their components

Interactions
DRUGS
aminoglycosides: Substantial aminoglycoside inactivation
chloramphenicol, erythromycins, sulfonamides, tetracyclines: Possibly decreased therapeutic effects of mezlocillin
methotrexate: Increased risk of methotrexate toxicity
probenecid: Increased blood level and prolonged half-life of mezlocillin

Adverse Reactions
CNS: Depression, headache, seizures
EENT: Oral candidiasis
GI: Abdominal pain, diarrhea, pseudomembranous colitis, nausea,
vomiting
GU: Vaginitis

HEME: Leukopenia, neutropenia
SKIN: Exfoliative dermatitis, pruritus, rash, urticaria
Other: Anaphylaxis; hypokalemia; injection site pain, redness, and swelling; serum sickness–like reaction

Nursing Considerations

• **WARNING** Before administering first dose of mezlocillin, make sure patient has had no previous hypersensitivity reactions to penicillins.

• Expect mezlocillin therapy to continue for at least 2 days after signs and symptoms have resolved—typically 7 to 10 days, depending on severity of infection. Complicated infections may need longer treatment. Group A beta-hemolytic streptococcal infections usually are treated for at least 10 days to reduce the risk of rheumatic fever or glomerulonephritis.

• Reconstitute each gram of mezlocillin with 10 ml of sterile water for injection, D_5W, or sodium chloride for injection and shake vigorously. Don't exceed a concentration of 100 mg/ml (10%). Be aware that stability of reconstituted solution varies, depending on type of diluent used, concentration, and storage temperature. Consult manufacturer's insert for specific storage guidelines. If a precipitate forms during refrigeration, warm solution to 37° C (98.6° F) using a water bath for 20 minutes. Shake well. Inject slowly, directly into I.V. tubing, over 3 to 5 minutes.

• For intermittent infusion, further dilute to desired volume (50 to 100 ml) with an appropriate I.V. solution and administer over 30 minutes. Discontinue other infusions during mezlocillin administration.

• Be aware that mezlocillin powder and reconstituted solution may darken slightly but that potency isn't affected.

• Periodically monitor serum potassium level of patients receiving long-term therapy, as appropriate.

• When calculating sodium intake for patients on a sodium-restricted diet, keep in mind that each gram of mezlocillin contains approximately 1.9 mEq of sodium.

• During long-term therapy, monitor for signs and symptoms of superinfection, such as oral candidiasis and vaginitis.

• Before reconstituting drug, store it at less than 30° (86° F).

PATIENT TEACHING

• Instruct patient receiving mezlocillin to immediately report increased bruising or other bleeding tendencies.

• Advise patient to report diarrhea and to check with prescriber before taking an antidiarrheal because it may mask symptoms of pseudomembranous colitis.

micafungin sodium
Mycamine

Class and Category
Chemical: Semisynthetic lipopeptide echinocandin
Therapeutic: Antifungal
Pregnancy category: C

Indications and Dosages
▶ *To treat esophageal candidiasis*
I.V. INFUSION
Adults. 150 mg infused over 1 hr daily.
▶ *To treat candidemia, acute disseminated candidiasis, and* Candida *peritonitis and abscesses*
I.V. INFUSION
Adults. 100 mg infused over 1 hr daily.
▶ *To prevent* Candida *infection in patients undergoing hematopoietic stem cell transplantation*
I.V. INFUSION
Adults. 50 mg infused over 1 hr daily.

Route	Onset	Peak	Duration
I.V.	Unknown	Unknown	Unknown

Mechanism of Action
Inhibits synthesis of 1,3-beta-D-glucan, which is an essential component of the *Candida* fungal cell wall. Without 1,3-beta-D-glucan, the fungal cell dies.

Contraindications
Hypersensitivity to micafungin, its components, or other echinocandins

Incompatibilities
Mixing or infusing with other drugs may cause micafungin to precipitate.

Interactions
DRUGS
immunosuppressants: Possibly additive adverse hematologic effects

nifedipine, sirolimus: Increased plasma nifedipine and sirolimus levels

Adverse Reactions

CNS: Delirium, dizziness, dysgeusia, fatigue, fever, headache, rigors, somnolence

CV: Hypertension, hypotension, shock, vasodilation

EENT: Mucosal inflammation

GI: Abdominal pain, anorexia, constipation, diarrhea, dyspepsia, elevated liver enzyme levels, hepatic dysfunction, hiccups, hyperbilirubinemia, nausea, vomiting

GU: Acute renal failure, elevated serum creatinine and blood urea levels

HEME: Anemia, eosinophilia, hemolytic anemia, leukopenia, lymphopenia, neutropenia, pancytopenia, thrombocytopenia

SKIN: Flushing, pruritus, rash, urticaria

Other: Anaphylaxis, angioedema, hypocalcemia, hypokalemia, hypomagnesemia, hypophosphatemia, injection site reactions including phlebitis and thrombophlebitis

Nursing Considerations

- Use cautiously in patients with hepatic or renal insufficiency.
- Reconstitute micafungin by adding 5 ml of normal saline solution to each 50-mg vial, yielding 10 mg micafungin/ml. Swirl vial gently to minimize excessive foaming. Add reconstituted solution to 100 ml of normal saline solution, and administer over 1 hour. Protect diluted solution from light, although you need not cover the infusion drip chamber or tubing.
- Always flush an existing intravenous line with normal saline solution before administering micafungin through that line.
- Monitor infusion rate carefully because infusions that took less than 1 hour to infuse have been associated with more frequent hypersensitivity reactions.
- WARNING Monitor patient closely for hypersensitivity reactions including anaphylaxis and angioedema. Discontinue micafungin infusion immediately if present, notify prescriber, and provide supportive care, as prescribed.
- Monitor patient's liver and renal function closely throughout therapy because liver and renal abnormalities may occur in patients receiving micafungin.
- Monitor patient's hematologic status closely because a variety of hematologic abnormalities may occur. If abnormalities are detected, monitor patient closely. If condition worsens, expect micafungin to be discontinued.

PATIENT TEACHING
• Instruct patient to report any infusion site discomfort immediately.
• Tell patient to report any unusual or persistent signs and symptoms to prescriber.

midazolam hydrochloride
Versed

Class, Category, and Schedule
Chemical: Benzodiazepine
Therapeutic: Sedative-hypnotic
Pregnancy category: D
Controlled substance schedule: IV

Indications and Dosages
▶ *To induce preoperative sedation or amnesia, to control preoperative anxiety*
I.V. INJECTION
Adults age 60 and over. 1.5 mg over 2 min given immediately before procedure. After 2-min waiting period, dosage adjusted to desired level in 25% increments, as ordered. *Maximum:* 1 mg in 2 min.
Adults under age 60 and adolescents. Up to 2.5 mg over 2 min immediately before procedure. After 2-min waiting period, dosage adjusted to desired level in 25% increments, as ordered. *Maximum:* 5 mg.
Children ages 6 to 12. *Initial:* 0.025 to 0.05 mg/kg, up to 0.4 mg/kg, if needed. *Maximum:* 10 mg.
Children ages 6 months to 5 years. *Initial:* 0.05 to 0.1 mg/kg, up to 0.6 mg/kg, if needed. *Maximum:* 6 mg.
▶ *To relieve agitation and anxiety in mechanically ventilated patients*
I.V. INFUSION
Adults. *Initial:* 0.01 to 0.05 mg/kg infused over several min, repeated at 10- to 15-min intervals until adequate sedation occurs. *Maintenance:* 0.02 to 0.1 mg/kg/hr initially, adjusted to desired level in 25% to 50% increments, as ordered. After achieving desired level of sedation, infusion rate decreased by 10% to 25% every few hr, as ordered, until minimum effective infusion rate is determined.
Children. *Initial:* 50 to 200 mcg/kg over 2 to 3 min followed by 1 to 2 mcg/kg/min by continuous infusion. *Maintenance:* 0.4 to 6 mcg/kg/min.

Infants age 32 weeks or over. 1 mcg/kg/min by continuous infusion.
Infants under age 32 weeks. 0.5 mcg/kg/min by continuous infusion.

Route	Onset	Peak	Duration
I.V.*	1.5 to 5 min	Rapid	2 to 6 hr

Mechanism of Action
May exert its sedating effect by increasing the activity of gamma-aminobutyric acid, a major inhibitory neurotransmitter in the brain. As a result, midazolam produces a calming effect, relaxes skeletal muscles, and—at high doses—induces sleep.

Contraindications
Acute angle-closure glaucoma; alcohol intoxication; coma; hypersensitivity to midazolam, other benzodiazepines, or their components; shock

Interactions
DRUGS
antihypertensives: Increased risk of hypotension
cimetidine, diltiazem, erythromycin, fluconazole, indinavir, itraconazole, ketoconazole, ranitidine, ritonavir, roxithromycin, saquinavir, verapamil: Prolonged sedation caused by reduced midazolam metabolism
CNS depressants: Possibly increased CNS and respiratory depression and hypotension
rifampin: Decreased blood midazolam level
FOODS
grapefruit, grapefruit juice: Possibly increased blood midazolam level and risk of toxicity
ACTIVITIES
alcohol use: Possibly increased CNS and respiratory depression and hypotension

Adverse Reactions
CNS: Agitation, delirium, or dreaming during emergence from anesthesia; anxiety; ataxia; chills; combativeness; confusion; dizziness; drowsiness; euphoria; excessive sedation; headache; insomnia; lethargy; nervousness; nightmares; paresthesia; prolonged

---

* For sedation.

emergence from anesthesia; restlessness; retrograde amnesia; sleep disturbance; slurred speech; weakness; yawning

CV: Cardiac arrest, hypotension, nodal rhythm, PVCs, tachycardia, vasovagal episodes

EENT: Blurred vision, diplopia, or other vision changes; increased salivation; laryngospasm; miosis; nystagmus; toothache

GI: Hiccups, nausea, retching, vomiting

RESP: Airway obstruction, bradypnea, bronchospasm, coughing, decreased tidal volume, dyspnea, hyperventilation, respiratory arrest, shallow breathing, tachypnea, wheezing

SKIN: Pruritus, rash, urticaria

Other: Infusion site burning, edema, induration, pain, redness, and tenderness

Nursing Considerations

- **WARNING** Be aware that I.V. midazolam is given only in hospitals or ambulatory care settings that allow continuous monitoring of respiratory and cardiac function. Keep resuscitative drugs and equipment readily available.
- As needed, combine midazolam injection with D$_5$W, normal saline solution, or lactated Ringer's solution. Solutions mixed with D$_5$W or normal saline solution are stable 24 hours; those mixed with lactated Ringer's solution are stable 4 hours.
- As needed, mix injection in same syringe with atropine sulfate, meperidine hydrochloride, morphine sulfate, or scopolamine hydrobromide. The resulting solution is stable for 30 minutes.
- Expect child's dosage to be based on ideal body weight. This is especially important for an obese child.
- **WARNING** Be aware that midazolam contains the preservative benzyl alcohol, which may cause a fatal toxic syndrome in neonates and premature infants, characterized by CNS, respiratory, circulatory, and renal impairment and metabolic acidosis. Because the 5-mg/ml and 1-mg/ml vials contain the same amount of benzyl alcohol, using the 5-mg/ml vial to prepare neonatal doses may decrease the amount of benzyl alcohol the patient receives.
- Be aware that neonates have a higher risk of respiratory depression than other pediatric or adult patients.
- Assess LOC frequently because the range between sedation and unconsciousness or disorientation is narrower with midazolam than with other benzodiazepines.
- Be aware that recovery time is usually 2 hours but may take up to 6 hours.

• Store drug at 15° to 30° C (59° to 86° F); don't freeze.
PATIENT TEACHING
• Inform patient that he may not remember procedure because midazolam produces amnesia.
• Advise patient to avoid hazardous activities until drug's adverse CNS effects, such as dizziness and drowsiness, have worn off.
• Instruct patient to avoid alcohol and other CNS depressants for 24 hours after receiving drug unless prescriber directs otherwise.

milrinone lactate
Primacor

Class and Category
Chemical: Bipyridine derivative
Therapeutic: Inotropic, vasodilator
Pregnancy category: C

Indications and Dosages
▶ *To provide short-term treatment of acute heart failure*
I.V. INFUSION
Adults. *Loading:* 50 mcg/kg over 10 min (at least 0.375 mcg/kg/min). *Usual:* 0.375 to 0.75 mcg/kg/min. *Maximum:* 1.13 mg/kg daily.
DOSAGE ADJUSTMENT Dosage adjusted according to cardiac output, pulmonary artery wedge pressure, and clinical response. For patients with creatinine clearance of 30 to 39 ml/min/1.73 m^2, infusion rate reduced to 0.33 mcg/kg/min; of 20 to 29 ml/min/1.73 m^2, to 0.28 mcg/kg/min; of 10 to 19 ml/min/1.73 m^2, to 0.23 mcg/kg/min; and of less than 9 ml/min/1.73 m^2, to 0.20 mcg/kg/min.

Route	Onset	Peak	Duration
I.V.	5 to 15 min	Unknown	3 to 6 hr

Incompatibilities
Don't administer milrinone through same I.V. line as furosemide because precipitate will form. Don't add other drugs to premixed milrinone flexible containers.

Contraindications
Hypersensitivity to milrinone or its components

Interactions
DRUGS
antihypertensives: Possibly hypotension

Mechanism of Action

An inotropic drug, milrinone increases the force of myocardial contraction—and cardiac output—by blocking the enzyme phosphodiesterase. Normally, this enzyme is activated by hormones binding to cell membrane receptors. As shown at top, phosphodiesterase degrades intracellular cAMP, which restricts calcium movement into myocardial cells. By inhibiting phosphodiesterase, as shown at bottom, milrinone slows cAMP degradation, increasing intracellular cAMP and the amount of calcium that enters myocardial cells. In blood vessels, increased cAMP causes smooth-muscle relaxation, which improves cardiac output by reducing preload and afterload.

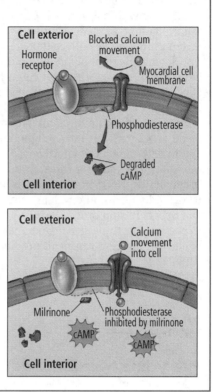

Adverse Reactions

CNS: Headache, tremor
CV: Angina, hypotension, supraventricular arrhythmias, ventricular ectopic activity, ventricular fibrillation, ventricular tachycardia, torsades de pointes
GI: Liver function test abnormalities
HEME: Thrombocytopenia
RESP: Bronchospasm
SKIN: Rash
Other: Anaphylactic shock, hypokalemia

Nursing Considerations

• Make sure ECG equipment is available for continuous monitoring during milrinone therapy.
• Discard drug if it's discolored or contains particles.
• For loading dose, directly infuse undiluted drug into I.V. line

with a compatible infusing solution. For continuous infusion, dilute drug with half-normal (0.45) saline solution, normal saline solution, or D₅W. Dilution isn't needed when using premixed milrinone flexible containers.

- Check platelet count before and during infusion, as ordered. Expect to stop drug if platelet count falls below 150,000/mm³.
- Give loading dose using a controlled-rate infusion device. For continuous infusion, use a calibrated electronic infusion device.
- Monitor cardiac output, pulmonary artery wedge pressure, blood pressure, heart rate, weight, and fluid status during therapy to determine drug effectiveness.
- Monitor renal and liver function test results and serum electrolyte levels. Notify prescriber of abnormalities.
- If severe hypotension develops, notify prescriber immediately and expect to stop drug.
- Expect patient to receive digoxin before starting milrinone, which can increase ventricular response rate.

PATIENT TEACHING
- Reassure patient that you'll be present and he'll be monitored constantly during therapy.

minocycline
Minocin

minocycline hydrochloride
Alti-Minocycline (CAN), Apo-Minocycline (CAN), Dynacin, Gen-Minocycline (CAN), Minocin, Novo-Minocycline (CAN), Vectrin

Class and Category
Chemical: Tetracycline
Therapeutic: Antibiotic, antiprotozoal
Pregnancy category: D

Indications and Dosages
▶ *To treat bartonellosis, brucellosis, chancroid, granuloma inguinale, inclusion conjunctivitis, lymphogranuloma venereum, nongonococcal urethritis, plague, psittacosis, Q fever, relapsing fever, respiratory tract infections (including pneumonia), rickettsial pox, Rocky Mountain spotted fever, tularemia, typhus, and UTI caused by gram-negative organisms (including* **Bartonella bacilliformis, Brucella** *species,* Haemophilus ducreyi, Haemophilus influenzae, Vibrio cholerae, *and* Yersinia pestis*), susceptible gram-positive organisms (including certain strains of* Streptococcus pneumoniae*), and other organisms (including* Actinomyces *species,* Bacillus anthracis, Borrelia recurrentis, Chlamydia

species, Mycoplasma pneumoniae, *and* Rickettsiae*); adjunct to treat intestinal amebiasis; alternative to treat listeriosis caused by* Listeria monocytogenes, *syphilis caused by* Treponema pallidum, *and yaws caused by* Treponema pertenue *for nonpregnant patients allergic to penicillin*

I.V. INJECTION

Adults and adolescents. *Initial:* 200 mg. *Maintenance:* 100 mg every 12 hr. *Maximum:* 400 mg daily.

Children over age 8. *Initial:* 4 mg/kg. *Maintenance:* 2 mg/kg every 12 hr.

DOSAGE ADJUSTMENT If patient has renal impairment, don't exceed 200 mg daily.

Route	Onset	Peak	Duration
I.V.	Unknown	Unknown	6 to 12 hr

Mechanism of Action

Inhibits bacterial protein synthesis by competitively binding to the 30S ribosomal subunit of the mRNA-ribosome complex of certain organisms.

Incompatibilities

Don't mix minocycline in same syringe with solution that contains calcium because precipitate will form.

Contraindications

Hypersensitivity to minocycline, other tetracyclines, or their components

Interactions

DRUGS

aluminum-, calcium-, or magnesium-containing antacids; calcium supplements; choline and magnesium salicylates; iron-containing preparations; magnesium-containing laxatives; sodium bicarbonate: Possibly formation of nonabsorbable complex, impaired minocycline absorption

cholestyramine, colestipol: Possibly impaired cholestyramine or colestipol absorption

cimetidine: Possibly decreased GI absorption and effectiveness of minocycline

digoxin: Possibly increased blood digoxin level and risk of digitalis toxicity

ergot alkaloids and derivatives: Increased risk of ergotism

insulin: Possibly decreased need for insulin

iron salts: Possibly decreased GI absorption and antimicrobial effect of minocycline

lithium: Possibly altered blood lithium level

methoxyflurane: Increased risk of nephrotoxicity

oral anticoagulants: Possibly potentiated anticoagulant effects

oral contraceptives containing estrogen: Decreased contraceptive effectiveness, increased risk of breakthrough bleeding

penicillin: Interference with bactericidal action of penicillin

vitamin A: Possibly benign intracranial hypertension

Adverse Reactions

CNS: Dizziness, fever, headache, light-headedness, unsteadiness, vertigo

CV: Pericarditis

EENT: Blurred vision, darkened or discolored tongue, glossitis, papilledema, tooth discoloration, vision changes

GI: Abdominal cramps or pain, anorexia, diarrhea, dysphagia, enterocolitis, esophageal irritation and ulceration, hepatitis, hepatotoxicity, indigestion, nausea, pancreatitis, pseudomembranous colitis, vomiting

GU: Genital candidiasis, nephrotoxicity

HEME: Eosinophilia, hemolytic anemia, neutropenia, thrombocytopenia, thrombocytopenic purpura

MS: Arthralgia, myopathy (transient)

RESP: Pulmonary infiltrates (with eosinophilia)

SKIN: Erythema multiforme, exfoliative dermatitis, brown pigmentation of skin and mucous membranes, erythematous and maculopapular rash, jaundice, onycholysis, photosensitivity, pruritus, purpura (anaphylactoid), Stevens-Johnson syndrome, urticaria

Other: Anaphylaxis, angioedema, serum sickness-like reaction, systemic lupus erythematosus exacerbation

Nursing Considerations

- Administer minocycline cautiously in patients who have renal or hepatic dysfunction and in patients who take other hepatotoxic drugs because minocycline may cause nephrotoxicity or hepatotoxicity.
- **WARNING** Notify prescriber if patient is breast-feeding because minocycline appears in breast milk and may have toxic effects.
- Monitor blood, renal, and hepatic tests before and during long-term therapy.
- To prepare drug for I.V. use, reconstitute each 100-mg vial with

5 to 10 ml of sterile water for injection. Further dilute in 500 to 1,000 ml of normal saline solution, D_5W, dextrose 5% in normal saline solution, or Ringer's or lactated Ringer's solution. Give final dilution immediately, but avoid giving it rapidly.

- Store reconstituted drug at room temperature and use within 24 hours.
- Assess patient for signs of superinfection; if they appear, notify prescriber, discontinue minocycline, and start appropriate therapy, as ordered.
- Monitor PT in patient who also takes an anticoagulant during minocycline therapy.
- Monitor patient for diarrhea during and up to 2 months after minocycline therapy; diarrhea may signal pseudomembranous colitis. If diarrhea occurs, notify prescriber and expect to obtain stool specimen for testing, withhold minocycline, and treat diarrhea with fluids, electrolytes, and antibiotics effective against *Clostridium difficile*.

PATIENT TEACHING

- Instruct patient to notify prescriber if no improvement occurs in a few days.
- Advise patient to avoid prolonged exposure to sun or sunlamps during therapy.
- Counsel female patient to avoid becoming pregnant because minocycline should be avoided, if possible, during tooth development (last half of gestation up to age 8). Drug may permanently turn teeth yellow, gray, or brown and cause enamel hypoplasia. It also may slow skeletal growth and cause congenital anomalies, including limb reduction.
- If patient takes an oral contraceptive, urge her to use an additional method during minocycline therapy.
- Instruct patient to notify prescriber immediately about blurred vision, dizziness, headache, known or suspected pregnancy, and unsteadiness.
- Urge patient to report watery, bloody stools to prescriber immediately, even up to 2 months after drug therapy has ended.

mitoxantrone hydrochloride
Novantrone

Class and Category
Chemical: Anthracenedione
Therapeutic: Antineoplastic
Pregnancy category: D

Indications and Dosages

▶ *To reduce neurologic disability and frequency of relapses in patients with secondary (chronic) progressive, progressive relapsing, or worsening relapsing-remitting multiple sclerosis (patients whose neurologic status is significantly abnormal between relapses)*

I.V. INFUSION

Adults. 12 mg/m^2 over 5 to 15 min every 3 mo. *Maximum:* Cumulative dose of 140 mg/m^2.

▶ *As adjunct to treat pain related to advanced hormone-refractory prostate cancer*

I.V. INFUSION

Adults. 12 to 14 mg/m^2 over 5 to 15 min every 21 days.

▶ *As adjunct to treat acute nonlymphocytic leukemia (ANLL)*

I.V. INFUSION

Adults. *Initial:* 12 mg/m^2 over at least 3 min on days 1 to 3 with 100 mg/m^2 of cytarabine as a continuous 24-hr infusion on days 1 to 7. If patient's antileukemic response is inadequate or incomplete, a second induction course is given at the same dosage. *Maintenance:* 6 wk after induction, 12 mg/m^2 over at least 3 min on days 1 and 2 with 100 mg/m^2 of cytarabine as a continuous 24-hr infusion on days 1 to 5. A second maintenance course is given 4 wk after the first if needed and tolerated.

Mechanism of Action

Binds to DNA, causing cross-linkage and strand breakage, interfering with RNA synthesis, and inhibiting topoisomerase II, an enzyme that uncoils and repairs damaged DNA. Mitoxantrone produces a cytocidal effect on proliferating and nonproliferating cells and doesn't appear to be cell-cycle specific. It's known to inhibit B-cell, T-cell, and macrophage proliferation and impair antigen function.

Incompatibilities

Don't mix mitoxantrone in the same infusion as heparin (because a precipitate may form); don't mix with any other drugs.

Contraindications

Hypersensitivity to mitoxantrone or its components

Interactions

DRUGS

allopurinol, colchicine, probenecid, sulfinpyrazone: Possibly interference with antihyperuricemic action of these drugs

blood-dyscrasia–causing drugs, such as cephalosporins and sulfasalazine: Increased risk of leukopenia and thrombocytopenia
bone marrow depressants, such as carboplatin and lomustine: Possibly additive bone marrow depression
daunorubicin, doxorubicin: Increased risk of cardiotoxicity
methotrexate and other antineoplastics: Risk of developing leukemia
vaccines, killed virus: Decreased antibody response to vaccine
vaccines, live virus: Increased risk of replication of and adverse effects of vaccine virus, decreased antibody response to vaccine

Adverse Reactions

CNS: Headache, seizures
CV: Arrhythmias, chest pain, congestive heart failure, decreased left ventricular ejection fraction, ECG changes
EENT: Blue-colored cornea, conjunctivitis, mucositis, stomatitis
GI: Abdominal pain, diarrhea, GI bleeding, nausea, vomiting
GU: Blue-green urine, renal failure
HEME: Acute myelogenous leukemia, leu-kopenia, other leukemias, thrombocytopenia
MS: Myelodysplasia
RESP: Cough, dyspnea
SKIN: Alopecia, extravasation, jaundice
Other: Allergic reaction, anaphylaxis, hyperuricemia, infection, infusion site pain or redness

Nursing Considerations

- Before and during therapy, expect patient to have an echocardiogram, ECG, and radionuclide angiography to evaluate cardiac status. Expect to obtain hematocrit, hemoglobin level, and CBC with platelet count.
- Be aware that drug shouldn't be given to patient with multiple sclerosis whose neutrophil count is less than $1,500/mm^3$.
- Obtain liver function test results, as ordered, before each course of therapy. Expect that drug won't be given to patient with multiple sclerosis and abnormal liver function.
- Anticipate obtaining pregnancy test before each course of therapy for women of childbearing age who have multiple sclerosis.
- Follow facility policy for handling antineoplastics. Be aware that manufacturer recommends goggles, gloves, and a gown during drug preparation and administration.
- Before infusing drug, dilute it in at least 50 ml of normal saline solution or D_5W.
- **WARNING** Be aware that drug shouldn't be given intrathecally because paralysis may occur.

- If mitoxantrone solution contacts your skin or mucosa, wash thoroughly with warm water. If it contacts your eyes, irrigate them thoroughly with water or normal saline solution.
- Discard unused diluted solution because it contains no preservatives. After penetration of the stopper, store undiluted drug for up to 7 days at room temperature or 14 days under refrigeration. Avoid freezing drug.
- If extravasation occurs, stop the infusion immediately and notify prescriber. Reinsert the I.V. line in another vein and resume the infusion. Although mitoxantrone is a nonvesicant, observe the extravasation site for signs of necrosis or phlebitis.
- Monitor patients with chickenpox or recent exposure to it and patients with herpes zoster for severe, generalized disease.
- Watch for evidence of cardiotoxicity, such as arrhythmias and chest pain, in patient with heart disease. Risk increases when cumulative dose reaches 140 mg/m^2 in cancer patient, 100 mg/m^2 in multiple sclerosis patient.
- Monitor blood uric acid level for hyperuricemia in patients with a history of gout or renal calculi. Expect to give allopurinol, as prescribed, to patients with leukemia or lymphoma who have elevated blood uric acid level to prevent uric acid nephropathy.
- **WARNING** If severe or life-threatening nonhematologic or hematologic toxicity occurs during the first induction course, expect to withhold the second course until it resolves.
- If patient develops thrombocytopenia, take precautions according to facility policy.
- Assess patient for evidence of infection, such as fever, if leukopenia occurs. Expect to obtain appropriate specimens for culture and sensitivity testing.
- Be aware that patients receiving mitoxantrone in combination with other antineoplastics or radiation therapy are at risk for developing secondary leukemia, including acute myelogenous leukemia.

PATIENT TEACHING
- Advise patient to complete dental work, if possible, before treatment begins or defer it until blood counts return to normal; drug may delay healing and cause gingival bleeding. Teach proper oral hygiene, and advise using a soft toothbrush.
- Urge patient to drink plenty of fluid to increase urine output and uric acid excretion.
- Advise patient to contact prescriber immediately if GI upset occurs, but to continue taking drug unless otherwise directed.

- Stress the importance of complying with the dosage regimen and keeping follow-up medical and laboratory appointments.
- Explain that urine may appear blue-green for 24 hours after treatment and that whites of eyes may appear blue. Stress that these effects are temporary and harmless. Explain that hair loss is possible, but that hair should return after therapy ends.
- Caution patient not to receive immunizations unless approved by prescriber. Also, advise persons who live in same household as patient to avoid receiving immunization with oral polio vaccine. Tell patient to avoid persons who recently received the oral polio vaccine or to wear a mask over his nose and mouth.
- Instruct patient to avoid persons with infections if bone marrow depression occurs. Advise patient to contact prescriber if fever, chills, cough, hoarseness, lower back or side pain, or painful or difficult urination occurs; these changes may signal an infection.
- Tell patient to contact prescriber immediately if he notices unusual bleeding or bruising, black or tarry stools, blood in urine or stool, or pinpoint red spots on his skin.
- Urge patient not to touch his eyes or inside his nose unless he has just washed his hands.
- Stress the need to avoid accidental cuts, as from a razor or fingernail clippers, because they may cause excessive bleeding or infection.
- Caution patient to avoid contact sports or activities that may cause bruising or injury.

morphine sulfate

Astramorph PF, Duramorph, Epimorph (CAN), Morphine Extra-Forte (CAN), Morphine Forte (CAN), Morphine H.P. (CAN)

Class, Category, and Schedule

Chemical: Phenanthrene derivative
Therapeutic: Analgesic
Pregnancy category: C
Controlled substance schedule: II

Indications and Dosages

▶ *To relieve acute or chronic moderate to severe pain; as adjunct to treat pulmonary edema caused by left-sided heart failure; to supplement general, local, or regional anesthesia*

I.V. INFUSION

Adults. *Initial:* 15 mg (or more) followed by 0.8 to 10 mg/hr, increased as needed for effectiveness. *Maintenance:* 0.8 to 80 mg/hr.

Children. 0.01 to 0.04 mg/kg/hr postoperatively, 0.025 to 2.6 mg/kg/hr for severe chronic cancer pain, or 0.03 to 0.15 mg/kg/hr for sickle cell crisis.

Neonates. *Initial:* 0.010 mg/kg/hr (10 mcg/kg/hr) postoperatively. *Maintenance:* 0.015 to 0.02 mg/kg/hr (15 to 20 mcg/kg/hr).

I.V. INJECTION

Adults. 2.5 to 15 mg injected slowly.

Children. 0.5 to 0.1 mg/kg administered slowly.

▶ *To relieve MI pain*

I.V. INJECTION

Adults. 1 to 4 mg by slow I.V. injection. Repeated up to every 5 min, if needed. *Maximum:* 2 to 15 mg.

Route	Onset	Peak	Duration
I.V.	Unknown	20 min	4 to 5 hr

Mechanism of Action

Binds with and activates opiate receptors (mainly mu receptors) in brain and spinal cord to produce analgesia and euphoria.

Contraindications

Acute alcoholism, alcohol withdrawal syndrome, arrhythmias, asthma, brain tumor, heart failure caused by chronic lung disease, hypersensitivity to morphine or its components, labor (premature delivery), prematurity (in infants), respiratory depression, seizure disorders, upper airway obstruction.

Interactions

DRUGS

amitriptyline, clomipramine, nortriptyline: Increased CNS and respiratory depression

anticholinergics: Possibly severe constipation leading to ileus, urine retention

antidiarrheals, such as loperamide and paregoric: CNS depression, possibly severe constipation

antihistamines, chloral hydrate, glutethimide, MAO inhibitors, methocarbamol: Increased CNS and respiratory depressant effects of morphine

antihypertensives, hypotension-producing drugs: Increased hypotension, risk of orthostatic hypotension

buprenorphine: Decreased therapeutic effects of morphine, in-

creased respiratory depression, possibly withdrawal symptoms
cimetidine: Increased analgesic and CNS and respiratory depressant effects of morphine
CNS depressants (antiemetics, general anesthetics, hypnotics, phenothiazines, sedatives, tranquilizers): Possibly coma, hypotension, respiratory depression, severe sedation
diuretics: Decreased diuretic efficacy
hydroxyzine: Increased analgesic, CNS depressant, and hypotensive effects of morphine
metoclopramide: Possibly antagonized metoclopramide effect on GI motility
mixed agonist-antagonist analgesics: Possibly withdrawal symptoms
naloxone: Antagonized analgesic and CNS and respiratory depressant effects of morphine, possibly withdrawal symptoms
naltrexone: Possibly induction or worsening of withdrawal symptoms if morphine given within 7 to 10 days before naltrexone
neuromuscular blockers: Increased or prolonged respiratory depression
opioid analgesics, such as alfentanil and sufentanil: Increased CNS and respiratory depression, increased hypotension
OTC preparations containing alcohol: Increased CNS and respiratory depression and hypotension
zidovudine: Decreased zidovudine clearance

ACTIVITIES
alcohol use: Increased CNS and respiratory depression, increased hypotension

Adverse Reactions

CNS: Amnesia, anxiety, coma, confusion, decreased concentration, delirium, delusions, depression, dizziness, drowsiness, euphoria, fever, hallucinations, headache, insomnia, lethargy, lightheadedness, malaise, psychosis, restlessness, sedation, seizures, syncope, tremor, unarousable state, unresponsive state
CV: Bradycardia, cardiac arrest, hypotension, orthostatic hypotension, palpitations, shock, tachycardia
EENT: Blurred vision, diplopia, dry mouth, laryngeal edema or laryngospasm (allergic), miosis, nystagmus, rhinitis
GI: Abdominal cramps or pain, anorexia, biliary tract spasm, constipation, diarrhea, dysphagia, elevated liver function test results, gastroesophageal reflux, hiccups, ileus and toxic megacolon (in patients with inflammatory bowel disease), intestinal obstruction, indigestion, nausea, vomiting
GU: Decreased ejaculate potency, decreased libido, difficult ejacu-

lation, impotence, menstrual irregularities, oliguria, prolonged labor, urinary hesitancy, urine retention

HEME: Anemia, leukopenia, thrombocytopenia

MS: Arthralgia

RESP: Apnea, asthma exacerbation, atelectasis, bronchospasm, depressed cough reflex, hypoventilation, pulmonary edema, respiratory arrest and depression, wheezing

SKIN: Diaphoresis, flushing, pallor, pruritus, urticaria

Other: Allergic reaction; anaphylaxis; facial edema; injection site edema, pain, rash, or redness; physical and psychological dependence; withdrawal symptoms

Nursing Considerations

- Store morphine sulfate at room temperature.
- Before giving morphine, make sure opioid antagonist and equipment for giving oxygen and controlling respiration are available.
- Before therapy, assess patient's drug use, including all prescription and OTC drugs.
- Discard injection solution that is discolored or darker than pale yellow or that contains precipitates that don't dissolve with shaking.
- **WARNING** Don't use highly concentrated morphine solutions (such as 10 to 25 mg/ml) for single-dose I.V. administration. These solutions are intended for use in continuous, controlled microinfusion devices.
- For direct I.V. injection, dilute appropriate dose with 4 to 5 ml of sterile water for injection. Inject 2.5 to 15 mg directly into tubing of free-flowing I.V. solution over 4 to 5 minutes. Rapid I.V. injection may increase adverse reactions.
- For continuous I.V. infusion, dilute drug in D_5W and administer with infusion-control device. Adjust dose and rate based on patient response, as prescribed.
- **WARNING** Monitor respiratory and cardiovascular status carefully and frequently during morphine therapy. Be alert for respiratory depression and hypotension.
- Monitor patient for excessive or persistent sedation; dosage may need to be adjusted.
- If patient is receiving a continuous morphine infusion, watch for and notify prescriber about new neurologic signs or symptoms. Inflammatory masses (such as granulomas) have caused serious neurologic reactions, including paralysis.
- Monitor patient with seizure disorder closely because morphine

may aggravate the disorder, increasing the risk of seizures.

• Expect morphine to cause physical and psychological dependence; watch for drug tolerance and withdrawal symptoms, such as body aches, diaphoresis, diarrhea, fever, piloerection, rhinorrhea, sneezing, and yawning.

• If tolerance to morphine develops, expect prescriber to increase dosage.

• Morphine may have a prolonged duration and cumulative effect in patients with impaired hepatic or renal function. It also may prolong labor by reducing strength, duration, and frequency of uterine contractions.

• When discontinuing morphine in patients receiving more than 30 mg daily, expect prescriber to reduce daily dose by about one-half for 2 days and then by 25% every 2 days thereafter until total dose reaches initial amount recommended for patients who haven't received opioids (15 to 30 mg daily). This regimen minimizes the risk of withdrawal symptoms.

PATIENT TEACHING

• Urge patient to avoid alcohol including OTC preparations containing alcohol and other CNS depressants during morphine therapy.

• Advise patient to avoid potentially hazardous activities during morphine therapy.

• Tell patient to change positions slowly to minimize the effects of orthostatic hypotension.

• Instruct patient to notify prescriber about worsening or breakthrough pain.

• Inform patient that morphine may be habit-forming. Urge him to notify prescriber if he experiences anxiety, decreased appetite, excessive tearing, irritability, muscle aches or twitching, rapid heart rate, or yawning.

• Advise female patient to notify prescriber if she becomes pregnant. Regular morphine use during pregnancy may cause physical dependence in fetus and withdrawal in neonate.

moxifloxacin hydrochloride
Avelox, Avelox IV

Class and Category
Chemical: Fluoroquinolone
Therapeutic: Antibiotic
Pregnancy category: C

Indications and Dosages

▶ *To treat acute sinusitis caused by* Haemophilus influenzae, Moraxella catarrhalis, *or* Streptococcus pneumoniae; *to treat mild to moderate community-acquired pneumonia caused by* Chlamydia pneumoniae, H. influenzae, M. catarrhalis, Mycoplasma pneumoniae, *or* S. pneumoniae *(including penicillin- or multi-drug–resistant strains)*

I.V. INFUSION

Adults. 400 mg every 24 hr for 10 days.

▶ *To treat acute exacerbation of chronic bronchitis caused by* H. influenzae, H. parainfluenzae, Klebsiella pneumoniae, M. catarrhalis, S. pneumoniae, *or* Staphylococcus aureus

I.V. INFUSION

Adults. 400 mg every 24 hr for 5 days.

▶ *To treat uncomplicated skin and soft-tissue infections caused by* S. aureus *or* Streptococcus pyogenes

I.V. INFUSION

Adults. 400 mg every 24 hr for 7 days.

▶ *To treat complicated skin and skin structure infections caused by* S. aureus, E. coli, K. pneumoniae, *or* Enterobacter cloacae

I.V. INFUSION

Adults. 400 mg every 24 hr for 7 to 21 days.

▶ *To treat complicated intra-abdominal infections, including polymicrobial infections such as abscesses caused by* E. coli, Bacteroides fragilis, Streptococcus anginosus, Streptococcus constellatus, Enterococcus faecalis, Proteus mirabilis, Clostridium perfringens, Bacteroides thetaiotaomicron, *or* Peptostreptococcus *species*

I.V. INFUSION

Adults. 400 mg every 24 hr for 5 to 14 days with initial dosage given as I.V. infusion.

Mechanism of Action

Inhibits synthesis of the bacterial enzyme DNA gyrase by counteracting the excessive supercoiling of DNA during replication or transcription. Inhibition of DNA gyrase causes rapid- and slow-growing bacterial cells to die.

Incompatibilities

Do not infuse I.V. form of moxifloxacin simultaneously through the same I.V. line with other I.V. substances, additives, or drugs.

Contraindications

Hypersensitivity to moxifloxacin, other fluoroquinolones, or their components

Interactions

DRUGS

aluminum- or magnesium-containing antacids; drug formulations with divalent or trivalent cations, such as didanosine chewable buffered tablets or powder for oral solution; metal cations, such as iron; multivitamins containing iron or zinc; sucralfate: Possibly substantial interference with moxifloxacin absorption, causing low blood moxifloxacin level

class Ia antiarrhythmics, such as quinidine; class III antiarrhythmics, such as sotalol; other drugs known to prolong QTc interval, such as disopyramide and pentamidine: Possibly prolonged QTc interval

corticosteroids: Increased risk of Achilles and other tendon ruptures

NSAIDs: Increased risk of CNS stimulation and seizures

warfarin: Possibly increased anticoagulation

Adverse Reactions

CNS: Dizziness, headache, psychosis, psychotic reaction, seizures, syncope

CV: Hypertension, hypotension, palpitations, peripheral edema, tachycardia, vasculitis, vasodilation, ventricular tachyarrhythmias

EENT: Altered taste

GI: Abdominal pain, abnormal liver function test results, acute hepatic necrosis or failure, cholestatic hepatitis, diarrhea, dyspepsia, hepatitis, jaundice, nausea, pseudomembranous colitis, vomiting

GU: Acute renal insufficiency or failure, interstitial nephritis

HEME: Agranulocytosis, anemia, aplastic and hemolytic anemia, eosinophilia, leukopenia, pancytopenia, prolonged PT, thrombocytopenia

MS: Tendon inflammation, pain, or rupture

RESP: Allergic peumonitis

Skin: Stevens-Johnson syndrome, toxic epidermal necrolysis

Other: Anaphylaxis, anaphylactic shock, angioedema, serum sickness

Nursing Considerations

- Obtain a fluid or tissue specimen for culture and sensitivity, as ordered. Expect to begin therapy before results are available.
- **WARNING** Before starting therapy, determine if patient receives a class Ia antiarrhythmic, such as quinidine; a class III antiarrhythmic, such as sotalol; or other drugs that prolong the QTc interval. Be aware that these drugs should be avoided in patients taking moxifloxacin because they may

prolong the QTc interval and lead to life-threatening ventricular tachycardia or torsades de pointes.

- Infuse over 60 minutes with ready-to-use flexible bags with 400 mg of moxifloxacin in 250 ml of 0.8% saline solution. Don't dilute further.
- If giving through Y-type tubing or piggyback method, stop other solutions during moxifloxacin infusion, and flush the line before and after infusion with a compatible solution, such as normal saline solution, 1M sodium chloride, 5% dextrose, sterile water for injection, 10% dextrose, or lactated Ringer's. Also flush before and after giving other drugs in the same I.V. line.
- Don't refrigerate I.V. moxifloxacin ready-to-use bags because precipitation will occur. Discard any unused portion; premixed bags are for single-use only.
- Expect to obtain a 12-lead ECG to check for a prolonged QTc interval. Ask patient if he or a blood relative has a history of prolonged QTc interval. Monitor elderly patients closely because they may be more susceptible to prolonged QT interval.
- If patient has hypokalemia, expect to correct it before beginning moxifloxacin therapy to prevent arrhythmias.
- Determine if patient has a history of a CNS disorder, such as cerebral arteriosclerosis or epilepsy, because drug may lower the seizure threshold. Notify prescriber before therapy starts, and take seizure precautions.
- If profuse, watery diarrhea develops, notify prescriber. Expect to obtain a stool specimen to test for pseudomembranous colitis and, if confirmed, withhold moxifloxacin and give fluids, electrolytes, and antibiotics effective against *Clostridium difficile*.
- Monitor serum potassium level, as ordered, during therapy to assess for hypokalemia.
- Keep emergency resuscitation equipment readily available, and watch for evidence of hypersensitivity, such as angioedema, dyspnea, and urticaria. If you suspect anaphylaxis, expect to give epinephrine, corticosteroids, and diphenhydramine.

PATIENT TEACHING
- Advise patient to notify prescriber immediately about palpitations or fainting; they may indicate a serious arrhythmia.
- Urge patient to drink plenty of fluids while taking moxifloxacin.
- Caution patient to stop taking drug and notify prescriber if he has trouble breathing, a rash, or other signs of allergic reaction.
- Urge patient to stop any exercise and contact prescriber immediately if he develops tendon inflammation, pain, or rupture.

- Caution patient to avoid activities of mental alertness until adverse CNS effects are known.
- Urge patient to report watery, bloody stools to prescriber immediately, even up to 2 months after drug therapy has ended.
- Caution patient to complete the prescribed course of therapy even if he feels better.

mycophenolate mofetil hydrochloride
CellCept Intravenous

Class and Category
Chemical: 2-morpholinoethyl ester of mycophenolic acid
Therapeutic: Immunosuppressant
Pregnancy category: D

Indications and Dosages
▶ *To prevent organ rejection in patients receiving allogenic kidney transplants*
I.V. INFUSION
Adults. 1 g (over 2 hr for I.V. infusion) b.i.d.
▶ *To prevent organ rejection in patients receiving allogenic heart transplants*
I.V. INFUSION
Adults. 1.5 g (over 2 hr for I.V. infusion) b.i.d.
▶ *To prevent organ rejection in patients receiving allogenic liver transplants*
I.V. INFUSION
Adults. 1 g infused over 2 hr b.i.d.

Mechanism of Action
Hydrolyzes to form mycophenolic acid (MPA), which inhibits guanosine nucleotide synthesis and proliferation of T and B lymphocytes. MPA also suppresses antibody formation by B lymphocytes and prevents glycosylation of lymphocyte and monocyte glycoproteins involved in adhesion to endothelial cells. MPA also may inhibit leukocytes from sites of inflammation and graft rejection, which may explain how mycophenolate mofetil prolongs allogeneic transplant survival.

Incompatibilities
Don't mix or administer mycophenolate mofetil hydrochloride in the same infusion catheter with other I.V. drugs or admixtures.

Contraindications

Hypersensitivity to mycophenolate mofetil hydrochloride or any of its components; hypersensitivity to polysorbate 80

Interactions

DRUGS

acyclovir, ganciclovir, probenecid: Increased plasma levels of both drugs

azathioprine: Increased bone marrow suppression

cyclosporine: Decreased plasma level of mycophenolate mofetil hydrochloride in renal transplant patients

live vaccines: Decreased effectiveness of live vaccines

oral contraceptives: Possibly decreased effectiveness of oral contraceptives

Adverse Reactions

CNS: Agitation, anxiety, chills, confusion, delirium, depression, dizziness, emotional lability, fever, hallucinations, headache, hypertonia, hypesthesia, insomnia, malaise, nervousness, neuropathy, paresthesia, psychosis, seizure, somnolence, syncope, thinking abnormality, tremor, vertigo

CV: Angina pectoris, arrhythmias, arterial thrombosis, atrial fibrillation or flutter, bradycardia, cardiac arrest, CV disorder, congestive heart failure, extrasystole, generalized edema, hemorrhage, hypercholesterolemia, hyperlipemia, hypertension, hypotension, increased lactic dehydrogenase, increased SGOT and SGPT, increased venous pressure, orthostatic hypotension, palpitations, pericardial effusion, peripheral edema, peripheral vascular disorder, pulmonary edema or hypertension, supraventricular tachycardia, thrombosis, vasodilation, vasospasm, ventricular extrasystole, ventricular tachycardia

EENT: Amblyopia, cataract, conjunctivitis, deafness, dry mouth, ear disorder or pain, epistaxis, eye hemorrhage, gingivitis, gum hyperplasia, lacrimation disorder, mouth ulceration, oral candidiasis, pharyngitis, rhinitis, sinusitis, stomatitis, tinnitus, vision abnormality, voice alteration

ENDO: Cushing's syndrome, diabetes mellitus, hypercalcemia, hypocalcemia, hypoglycemia, hypothyroidism, parathyroid disorder

GI: Abdomen enlargement or pain, anorexia, ascites, cholangitis, cholestatic colitis, jaundice, constipation, diarrhea, dyspepsia, dysphagia, esophagitis, flatulence, gastritis, gastroenteritis, GI hemorrhage, GI infection, GI candidiasis, hepatitis, hernia, ileus, jaundice, liver damage, liver function test abnormalities, melena, nausea, pancreatitis, peritonitis, rectal disorder, stomach ulcer, vomiting

GU: Albuminuria; bilirubinemia; dysuria; hematuria; hydronephrosis; impotence; increased BUN or creatinine levels; kidney tubular necrosis; nocturia; oliguria; pain; prostatic disorder; pyelonephritis; renal failure; scrotal edema, urinary tract disorder or infection; urinary abnormality, frequency, or incontinence; urine retention

HEME: Anemia, coagulation disorder, hypochromic anemia, increased prothrombin time or thromboplastin time, leukocytosis, leukopenia, polyhemia, thrombocytopenia

MS: Arthralgia; back, neck, or pelvic pain; joint disorder; leg cramps; myalgia; myasthenia; osteoporosis

RESP: Apnea; asthma; atelectasis; bronchitis; cough; dyspnea; hemoptysis; hyperventilation; hypoxia; life-threatening pulmonary fibrosis, lung edema; pleural effusion; pneumonia; pneumothorax; respiratory acidosis, candidiasis, neoplasm, or pain; sputum increase

SKIN: Abscess; acne; cellulite; ecchymosis; fungal dermatitis; pallor; petechia; pruritus; rash; benign neoplasm, carcinoma, hypertrophy, or ulcer; sweating; vesiculobullous rash

Other: Abnormal healing, accidental injury, acidosis, alkalosis, alopecia, cyst, dehydration, facial edema, flulike syndrome, gout, hiccups, hirsutism, hyperkalemia, hyperuricemia, hypervolemia, hypochloremia, hypokalemia, hypomagnesemia, hyponatremia, hypophosphatemia, hypoproteinemia, increased alkaline phosphatase, increased gamma glutamyl transpeptidase, infection, sepsis, thirst, weight gain or loss

Nursing Considerations

- Before starting mycophentolate in a woman of childbearing potential, make sure she has a confirmed negative pregnancy test within 1 week of starting therapy, using a test with a sensitivity of at least 25 mIU/ml.
- Expect to give I.V. form within 24 hours of transplantation and for no longer than 14 days. Expect to switch patient to oral form as soon as possible, as ordered.
- When preparing I.V. form, avoid inhalation or direct contact with skin or mucous membranes. If contact occurs, wash area thoroughly with soap and water and rinse eyes with water.
- Handle I.V. form similarly to a chemotherapeutic drug because mycophenolate mofetil hydrochloride is genotoxic and embryotoxic and may have mutagenic properties.

- Know that I.V. form must be reconstituted and diluted to 6 mg/ml using 5% dextrose injection USP. Inject 14 ml of 5% dextrose injection USP into each vial (2 vials will be needed for each 1-g dose; 3 vials for each 1.5-g dose), then shake gently. Further dilute a 1-g dose by adding 2 reconstituted vials to 140 ml of 5% dextrose injection USP; dilute a 1.5-g dose by adding 3 reconstituted vials to 210 ml of 5% dextrose injection USP.
- Be aware that I.V. infusion should be delivered over at least 2 hours, within 4 hours of constitution. Never administer by rapid or bolus I.V. injection.
- Know that cyclosporine and corticosteroids should be used with mycophenolate mofetil therapy.
- Obtain CBC weekly during first month of therapy, twice monthly for the second and third months of therapy, and then monthly through the first year, as ordered.
- Monitor patient closely for adverse reactions because drug has many adverse effects, some of which can be serious or severe.
- Expect to stop drug or reduce the dose and provide supportive care, as ordered, if neutropenia develops.

PATIENT TEACHING
- Advise women of childbearing age to use two forms of contraception before starting mycophenolate mofetil therapy and for 6 weeks afterward because of potential for fetal harm. Inform women who use oral contraceptives that mycophenolate mofetil may decrease their effectiveness. Urge patient to notify prescriber immediately if she becomes pregnant.
- Urge patient not to receive live vaccines during therapy and to either avoid people who have received such vaccines or to wear a protective mask when he's around them.
- Caution patient to avoid contact with people who have infections because drug causes immunosuppression.
- Tell patient to report any evidence of infection, unexpected bruising or bleeding, or any other sign of bone marrow depression immediately.
- Advise patient to avoid exposure to direct sunlight and UV light and to wear sunscreen when outdoors because of increased risk of skin cancer.
- Stress importance of follow-up care to monitor drug's effectiveness and possible adverse effects because of the increased risk of cancer and infections as a result of immunosuppression. Inform patient of the need for periodic laboratory tests.

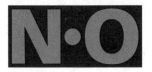

nafcillin sodium

Nafcil, Nallpen, Unipen

Class and Category

Chemical: Penicillin
Therapeutic: Antibiotic
Pregnancy category: B

Indications and Dosages

▶ *To treat infections caused by penicillinase-producing* Staphylococcus aureus

I.V. INFUSION

Adults and adolescents. 500 to 1,500 mg every 4 hr. *Maximum:* 20,000 mg daily.

Children from birth to age 12. 10 to 20 mg/kg every 4 hr, or 20 to 40 mg/kg every 8 hr.

▶ *To treat bone and joint infections, endocarditis, meningitis, and pericarditis caused by susceptible organisms*

I.V. INFUSION

Adults and adolescents. 1,500 to 2,000 mg every 4 to 6 hr. *Maximum:* 20,000 mg daily.

I.V. INFUSION

Children from birth to age 12. 10 to 20 mg/kg every 4 hr or 20 to 40 mg/kg every 8 hr. For meningitis in neonates weighing up to 2 kg (4.4 lb), 25 to 50 mg/kg every 12 hr for first week after birth and then 50 mg/kg every 8 hr. For neonates weighing 2 kg or more, 50 mg/kg every 8 hr during first week after birth and then 50 mg/kg every 6 hr.

Incompatibilities

Don't mix nafcillin in same I.V. bag as aminoglycosides; they're chemically incompatible.

Contraindications

Hypersensitivity to nafcillin, other penicillins, their components, or to corn or corn-containing products

Mechanism of Action

Binds to certain penicillin-binding proteins in bacterial cell walls, thereby inhibiting the final stage of bacterial cell wall synthesis. The result is cell lysis. Nafcillin's action is bolstered by its chemical composition; its unique side chain resists destruction by beta-lactamases.

Interactions

DRUGS

aminoglycosides: Substantial mutual inactivation
chloramphenicol, erythromycins, sulfonamides, tetracyclines: Possibly decreased therapeutic effects of nafcillin
hepatotoxic drugs: Increased risk of hepatotoxicity
methotrexate: Increased risk of methotrexate toxicity
probenecid: Increased blood nafcillin level

FOODS

all foods: Decreased nafcillin absorption

Adverse Reactions

CNS: Depression, headache, seizures
EENT: Oral candidiasis
GI: Abdominal pain, diarrhea, nausea, pseudomembranous colitis, vomiting
GU: Vaginitis
HEME: Leukopenia, neutropenia
SKIN: Exfoliative dermatitis, pruritus, rash, urticaria
Other: Anaphylaxis; hypokalemia; injection site pain, redness, and swelling; serum sickness–like reaction

Nursing Considerations

- Obtain body fluid or tissue samples for culture and sensitivity testing, as prescribed, and obtain test results, if possible, before giving nafcillin, as ordered.
- For intermittent I.V. infusion, infuse over 30 to 60 minutes.
- Give nafcillin at least 1 hour before or after aminoglycosides, especially if patient has renal disease.
- When giving nafcillin to patient at risk for hypertension or fluid overload, be aware that each gram contains 2.5 mEq of sodium.
- **WARNING** Avoid giving nafcillin to premature neonate if drug was reconstituted with bacteriostatic water that contains benzyl alcohol. Doing so can cause potentially fatal metabolic acidosis and circulatory, CNS, renal, and respiratory dysfunction.

- Monitor serum nafcillin levels closely in children, as ordered, because the liver and biliary tract, principal routes of nafcillin elimination, function immaturely in children.
- Monitor for signs of superinfection, such as oral candidiasis and pseudomembranous colitis, especially in elderly, immunocompromised, or debilitated patients who receive large doses of nafcillin.

PATIENT TEACHING
- Advise patient to notify prescriber if she experiences chills, fever, GI distress, or rash.

nalbuphine hydrochloride
Nubain

Class and Category
Chemical: Phenanthrene derivative
Therapeutic: Analgesic, anesthesia adjunct
Pregnancy category: B

Indications and Dosages
▶ *To relieve moderate to severe pain*
I.V. INJECTION
Adults weighing 70 kg (154 lb). 10 mg every 3 to 6 hr, p.r.n. Dosage adjusted for patients weighing more or less.
▶ *As adjunct to anesthesia*
I.V. INJECTION
Adults. 0.3 to 3 mg/kg over 10 to 15 min followed by 0.25 to 0.5 mg/kg, as needed.
DOSAGE ADJUSTMENT For patients who have repeatedly received an opioid agonist, initial dose possibly reduced to 25% of usual dosage. For patients in whom tolerance to drug's effects hasn't developed, maximum usually is 20 mg/dose or 160 mg daily.

Route	Onset	Peak	Duration
I.V.	2 to 3 min	30 min	3 to 4 hr

Mechanism of Action
Binds with and stimulates mu and kappa opiate receptors in the spinal cord and higher levels in the CNS. In this way, nalbuphine alters the perception of and emotional response to pain.

Incompatibilities

Don't give nalbuphine with diazepam or pentobarbital. Use separate I.V. line or flush line well before and after administration.

Contraindications

Hypersensitivity to nalbuphine or its components

Interactions

DRUGS

alfentanil, CNS depressants, fentanyl, sufentanil: Increased risk of hypotension and CNS and respiratory depression

anticholinergics: Increased risk of severe constipation and urine retention

antidiarrheals, such as difenoxin and atropine, loperamide, and paregoric: Increased risk of severe constipation and increased CNS depression

antihypertensives: Increased risk of hypotension

buprenorphine: Possibly decreased therapeutic effects of nalbuphine and increased risk of respiratory depression

hydroxyzine: Increased risk of CNS depression and hypotension

MAO inhibitors: Risk of possibly fatal increased CNS excitation or depression

metoclopramide: Possibly antagonized effects of metoclopramide

naloxone, naltrexone: Decreased pharmacologic effects of nalbuphine

neuromuscular blockers: Increased risk of prolonged CNS and respiratory depression

ACTIVITIES

alcohol use: Increased risk of coma, hypotension, profound sedation, and respiratory depression

Adverse Reactions

CNS: Anxiety, confusion, decreased or loss of consciousness, depression, dizziness, euphoria, fatigue, fever, hallucinations, headache, nervousness, restlessness, seizures, somnolence, syncope, tiredness, tremor, weakness

CV: Bradycardia, cardiac arrest, edema, hypertension, hypotension, tachycardia

EENT: Blurred vision, diplopia, dry mouth, laryngeal edema, stridor

GI: Abdominal cramps, anorexia, constipation, nausea, vomiting

GU: Decreased urine output, ureteral spasm

RESP: Dyspnea, pulmonary edema, respiratory depression, wheezing

SKIN: Diaphoresis, flushing, pruritus, rash, sensation of warmth, urticaria

Other: Anaphylaxis, injection site burning, pain, redness, swelling, and warmth

Nursing Considerations

- Use nalbuphine cautiously in patients taking other drugs that can cause respiratory depression.
- Be aware that nalbuphine is not recommended for use during labor and delivery because placental transfer of nalbuphine is high, increasing risk of fetal neurological damage or death.
- Keep resuscitation equipment and naloxone readily available to reverse nalbuphine's effects, if needed.
- For direct I.V. injection through an I.V. line with a compatible infusing solution, give drug slowly—no more than 10 mg over 3 to 5 minutes. Inject into free-flowing normal saline solution, D_5W, or lactated Ringer's solution.
- During prolonged use, expect to give a stool softener to minimize constipation.
- If patient is opioid-dependent, expect drug to cause withdrawal symptoms, such as abdominal cramps, anorexia, anxiety, backache, bone or joint pain, confusion, depression, diaphoresis, dysphoria, erythema, fear, fever, irritability, labile blood pressure and pulse, lacrimation, muscle spasms, myalgia, mydriasis, nasal congestion, nausea, opioid craving, piloerection, restlessness, rhinorrhea, sensation of crawling skin, sleep disturbances, tremor, uneasiness, vomiting, and yawning.
- **WARNING** Be aware that drug may obscure neurologic assessment findings if patient has a cerebral aneurysm, head injury, or increased intracranial pressure.

PATIENT TEACHING

- Advise patient to avoid potentially hazardous activities until nalbuphine's CNS effects are known.
- Counsel patient against making important decisions while receiving drug because it may cloud her judgment.

nalmefene hydrochloride

Revex

Class and Category

Chemical: 6-Methylene analogue of naltrexone
Therapeutic: Opioid antagonist
Pregnancy category: B

Indications and Dosages

▶ *To treat known or suspected opioid overdose*
I.V. INJECTION

Adults. 500 mcg/70 kg (154 lb) of body weight, followed by second dose of 1,000 mcg/70 kg in 2 to 5 min, as indicated. *Maximum:* 1,500 mcg/70 kg.

▶ *To treat postoperative opioid-induced respiratory depression*
I.V. INJECTION

Adults. *Initial:* 0.25 mcg/kg every 2 to 5 min until desired degree of reversal is achieved. *Maximum:* 1 mcg/kg.

DOSAGE ADJUSTMENT Initial and subsequent doses possibly reduced to 0.1 mcg/kg for patients at increased risk for CV complications.

Route	Onset	Peak	Duration
I.V.	2 to 5 min	Unknown	30 to 60 min*

Mechanism of Action

Antagonizes mu, kappa, and sigma opiate receptors in the CNS, thus reversing the analgesia, hypotension, respiratory depression, and sedation caused by most opioids. Mu receptors are responsible for analgesia, euphoria, miosis, and respiratory depression. Kappa receptors are responsible for analgesia and sedation. Sigma receptors control dysphoria and other delusional states.

Contraindications

Hypersensitivity to nalmefene or its components

Interactions

DRUGS

opioid analgesics (including alfentanil, fentanil, and sufentanil): Reversal of these drugs' analgesic and adverse effects, possibly withdrawal symptoms in opioid-dependent patients

Adverse Reactions

CNS: Agitation, chills, confusion, depression, dizziness, fever, hallucinations, headache, nervousness, somnolence, tremor
CV: Arrhythmias, hypertension, hypotension, tachycardia, vasodilation
EENT: Dry mouth, pharyngitis
GI: Diarrhea, nausea, vomiting

---

* For partial reversal of opioid effects; up to several hr for full reversal.

GU: Urine retention
SKIN: Pruritus
Other: Withdrawal symptoms

Nursing Considerations

- **WARNING** Read the label carefully before administering nalmefene because drug comes in concentrations of 100 mcg/ml and 1 mg/ml.
- Monitor patients with hepatic or renal dysfunction for signs of increased nalmefene effects because drug is metabolized by liver and excreted by kidneys.
- Monitor heart rate, respiratory rate, and blood pressure to detect CV complications. Patients who have received a cardiotoxic drug and those with cardiac disease are at increased risk.
- Continue to monitor patient after nalmefene administration because symptoms of opioid toxicity may return if opioid's duration of action is longer than that of nalmefene.
- **WARNING** Monitor for withdrawal symptoms, especially in opioid-dependent patients. Symptoms include abdominal cramps, anorexia, anxiety, backache, bone or joint pain, confusion, depression, diaphoresis, dysphoria, erythema, fear, fever, irritability, labile blood pressure and pulse, lacrimation, muscle spasms, myalgia, mydriasis, nasal congestion, nausea, opioid craving, piloerection, restlessness, rhinorrhea, sensation of crawling skin, sleep disturbances, tremor, uneasiness, vomiting, and yawning.
- Be prepared to administer mechanical or assisted ventilation if reversal of opioid-induced respiratory depression is incomplete.
- Store drug at 15° to 30° C (59° to 86° F).

PATIENT TEACHING
- Inform patient or family members that nalmefene is administered to reverse opioid-induced adverse reactions.
- Urge opioid-dependent patient to seek out a drug rehabilitation program.

naloxone hydrochloride
Narcan

Class and Category
Chemical: Thebaine derivative
Therapeutic: Opioid antagonist
Pregnancy category: B

Indications and Dosages

▶ *To treat known or suspected opioid overdose*
I.V. INJECTION
Adults, children age 5 and over, and children under age 5 weighing more than 20 kg (44 lb). 0.4 to 2 mg repeated every 2 to 3 min, p.r.n. If no response after 10 mg, patient may not have narcotic-induced respiratory depression.
Infants and children under age 5 weighing less than 20 kg. 0.01 mg/kg as a single dose; if no improvement, another 0.1 mg/kg, as prescribed. Alternatively, 0.1 mg/kg repeated every 2 to 3 min, as needed.
I.V. INJECTION
Neonates. 0.01 mg/kg repeated every 2 to 3 min, as prescribed, until desired response occurs. Or, initial dose of 0.1 mg/kg.
▶ *To treat postoperative opioid-induced respiratory depression*
I.V. INJECTION
Adults and adolescents. *Initial:* 0.1 to 0.2 mg every 2 to 3 min until desired response occurs. Additional doses given every 1 to 2 hr, if needed, based on patient response.
Children. *Initial:* 0.005 to 0.01 mg every 2 to 3 min until desired response occurs. Additional doses given every 1 to 2 hr, if needed, based on patient response.
▶ *To reverse opioid-induced asphyxia*
I.V. INJECTION
Neonates. *Initial:* 0.01 mg/kg every 2 to 3 min until desired response occurs. Additional doses given every 1 to 2 hr, if needed, based on patient response.
▶ *As adjunct to treat hypotension caused by septic shock*
I.V. INFUSION, I.V. INJECTION
Adults. 0.03 to 0.2 mg/kg over 5 min, followed by continuous infusion of 0.03 to 0.3 mg/kg/hr for 1 to 24 hr, as needed, based on patient response.

Route	Onset	Peak	Duration
I.V.	1 to 2 min	5 to 15 min	45 min or longer

Incompatibilities

Don't mix naloxone with any other solution unless you verify that drugs are compatible; drug is incompatible with alkaline, bisulfite, and metabisulfite solutions.

Contraindications

Hypersensitivity to naloxone or its components

Mechanism of Action

Briefly and competitively antagonizes mu, kappa, and sigma opiate receptors in the CNS, thus reversing the analgesia, hypotension, respiratory depression, and sedation caused by most opioids. Mu receptors are responsible for analgesia, euphoria, miosis, and respiratory depression. Kappa receptors are responsible for analgesia and sedation. Sigma receptors control dysphoria and other delusional states.

Interactions

DRUGS

butorphanol, nalbuphine, pentazocine: Reversal of these drugs' analgesic and adverse effects

opioid analgesics: Reversal of these drugs' analgesic and adverse effects, possibly withdrawal symptoms in opioid-dependent patients

Adverse Reactions

CNS: Excitement, irritability, nervousness, restlessness, seizures, tremor, violent behavior

CV: Hypertension (severe), hypotension, ventricular fibrillation, ventricular tachycardia

GI: Nausea, vomiting

RESP: Pulmonary edema

SKIN: Diaphoresis

Other: Withdrawal symptoms

Nursing Considerations

- Keep resuscitation equipment readily available during naloxone administration.
- If needed, dilute naloxone with sterile water before administering I.V. injection. To prepare a continuous infusion, add 2 mg of naloxone to 500 ml of normal saline solution or D$_5$W to yield 4 mcg/ml. Use within 24 hours.
- Give repeat doses as prescribed, depending on patient's response. Continue to monitor patient after naloxone administration because symptoms of opioid toxicity may return if opioid's duration of action is longer than that of naloxone.
- Be aware that rapid reversal of opioid effects can cause diaphoresis, nausea, and vomiting.
- **WARNING** Monitor for withdrawal symptoms, especially in opioid-dependent patients. Symptoms may include abdominal cramps, anorexia, anxiety, backache, bone or joint pain, confusion, depression, diaphoresis, dysphoria, erythema, fear,

fever, irritability, labile blood pressure and pulse, lacrimation, muscle spasms, myalgia, mydriasis, nasal congestion, nausea, opioid craving, piloerection, restlessness, rhinorrhea, sensation of crawling skin, sleep disturbances, tremor, uneasiness, vomiting, and yawning.
- Monitor cardiac and respiratory status of patients with a history of CV or pulmonary disease for signs of exacerbation.
- Expect patient with hepatic or renal dysfunction to have increased circulating blood naloxone level.
- Store naloxone at 15° to 30° C (59° to 86° F); protect from freezing and light.

PATIENT TEACHING
- Inform patient or family that naloxone is administered to reverse opioid-induced adverse reactions.
- Urge opioid-dependent patient to seek drug rehabilitation.

natalizumab

Tysabri

Class and Category

Chemical: Recombinant humanized IgG4k monoclonal antibody
Therapeutic: Immune modulator
Pregnancy category: C

Indications and Dosages

▶ *To delay physical disability and reduce the frequency of exacerbations in relapsing forms of multiple sclerosis; to induce and maintain remission in patients with moderate to severe active Crohn's disease with evidence of inflammation*

I.V. INFUSION
Adults. 300 mg infused over 60 min every 4 wk.

Route	Onset	Peak	Duration
I.V.	Unknown	24 wk	Unknown

Contraindications

History or presence of progressive multifocal leukoencephalopathy (PML), hypersensitivity to natalizumab or its components

Interactions

DRUGS
corticosteroids, immunosuppressants, immunomodulating agents, other antineoplastics: Increased risk of infection

Mechanism of Action

Inhibits migration of leukocytes out of the vascular space, increasing the number of circulating leukocytes, by binding to select integrins on the surface of all leukocytes except neutrophils. Also inhibits adhesion of leukocytes to their counter-receptors. In multiple sclerosis, lesions are believed to occur when activated inflammatory cells, including T-lymphocytes, cross the blood-brain barrier.

Adverse Reactions

CNS: Depression, dizziness, fatigue, headache, PML, rigors, somnolence, suicidal ideation, vertigo
CV: Chest discomfort, peripheral edema
EENT: Tonsillitis, tooth infections
GI: Abdominal discomfort, abnormal liver function test results, cholelithiasis, diarrhea, gastroenteritis, hepatotoxicity
GU: Amenorrhea, dysmenorrhea, irregular menstruation, ovarian cyst, UTI, urinary incontinence, urinary frequency or urgency, vaginitis
MS: Arthralgia, extremity pain, joint swelling, muscle cramps
RESP: Pneumonia
SKIN: Dermatitis, night sweats, pruritus, rash, urticaria
Other: Acute hypersensitivity reaction, anaphylaxis, antibody formation, herpes, infection, weight gain or loss

Nursing Considerations

- Determine that patient has enrolled in the TOUCH Prescribing Program before administering natalizumab. Once patient's signature and initials have been obtained on the TOUCH program enrollment form, place the original signed form in the patient's medical record, send a copy to Biogen Idec, and give a copy to the patient.
- Be aware that all serious opportunistic and atypical infections need to be reported to Biogen Idec at 1-800-456-2255 and to the FDA MedWatch Program at 1-800-FDA-1088.
- Make sure that patient has had a brain MRI before starting natalizumab therapy to help distinguish evidence of multiple sclerosis from PML if they arise after therapy has begun.
- Dilute natalizumab concentrate 300 mg/15 ml in 100 ml of normal saline solution. Gently invert the solution to mix completely. Do not shake.
- Following dilution, infuse drug immediately over 1 hour. After

infusion, flush line with normal saline solution injection.

- Do not administer as an I.V. push or bolus injection.
- If administration is delayed after dilution, refrigerate drug and use within 8 hours.
- Observe patient during and for 1 hour after infusion for evidence of a hypersensitivity reaction. If present, notify prescriber, expect to withhold drug, and provide supportive care.
- **WARNING** Monitor patient closely for evidence of PML because natalizumab increases the risk of this opportunistic viral brain infection. PML can lead to severe disability or death. If any unexplained neurological signs and symptoms occur, notify prescriber, withhold natalizumab, and prepare patient for a gadolinium-enhanced MRI of the brain and possible cerebrospinal fluid analysis, as ordered.
- Know that the patient should be reevaluated 3 months after the first infusion, 6 months after the first infusion, and every 6 months thereafter.
- Assess patient for signs of infection, such as fever, if leukopenia develops. Expect to obtain appropriate specimens for culture and sensitivity testing.
- Be aware that patients with Crohn's disease who take both a corticosteroid and natalizumab should begin corticosteroid withdrawal as soon as a therapeutic effect has occurred. If patient can't stop corticosteroid therapy within 6 months, expect natalizumab to be discontinued.

PATIENT TEACHING

- Explain the benefits and risks of natalizumab therapy, and provide patient with medication guide.
- Encourage patient to ask questions before signing the enrollment form.
- Emphasize importance of reporting any symptoms that persist or worsen over several days to the prescriber.
- Tell patient to inform all physicians that he is receiving natalizumab therapy.
- Stress importance of follow-up visits 3 months after the first infusion, 6 months after the first infusion, and at least every 6 months thereafter.
- Instruct patient to report signs and symptoms of an allergic reaction, such as urticaria, dizziness, fever, rash, rigors, pruritus, nausea, flushing, hypotension, dyspnea, and chest pain.
- Instruct patient to avoid people with infections. Advise him to report fever, cough, lower back or side pain, or other unexplained signs and symptoms. They may indicate infection.

neostigmine methylsulfate
Prostigmin

Class and Category
Chemical: Quaternary ammonium compound
Therapeutic: Anticholinesterase, curare antidote
Pregnancy category: C

Indications and Dosages
▶ *To reverse nondepolarizing neuromuscular blockade*
I.V. INJECTION
Adults. 0.5 to 2 mg by slow push, repeated as needed up to
5 mg; 0.6 to 1.2 mg of atropine or 0.2 to 0.6 mg of glycopyrrolate
is given with or a few minutes before neostigmine, as ordered.
Children. 0.04 mg/kg by slow push; 0.02 mg/kg of atropine is
given I.M. or subcutaneously with each dose or every other dose.

Route	Onset	Peak	Duration
I.V.	4 to 8 min	30 min	2 to 4 hr

Mechanism of Action
Inhibits the action of cholinesterase, an enzyme that destroys acetylcholine at
myoneuronal junctions, thereby increasing acetylcholine accumulation at
myoneuronal junctions and facilitating nerve impulse transmission. This action reverses the effects of nondepolarizing neuromuscular blockers.

Contraindications
Hypersensitivity to neostigmine, other anticholinesterases, bro-
mides, or their components; mechanical obstruction of intestinal
or urinary tract; peritonitis

Interactions
DRUGS
*aminoglycosides, anesthetics, capreomycin, colistimethate, colistin, lido-
caine, lincomycins, polymyxin B, quinine:* Increased risk of neuromuscular blockade
anticholinergics: Possibly masked signs of cholinergic crisis
guanadrel, guanethidine, mecamylamine, trimethaphan: Possibly antagonized effects of neostigmine, possibly decreased antihypertensive
effects
neuromuscular blockers: Possibly prolonged action of depolarizing
neuromuscular blockers and antagonized action of nondepolariz-

ing neuromuscular blockers

procainamide, quinidine: Possibly antagonized effects of neostigmine

quinine: Decreased neostigmine effectiveness

Adverse Reactions

CNS: Dizziness, drowsiness, headache, seizures, syncope, weakness

CV: Arrhythmias (AV block, bradycardia, nodal rhythm, tachycardia), cardiac arrest, ECG changes, hypotension

EENT: Increased salivation, lacrimation, miosis, vision changes

GI: Abdominal cramps, diarrhea, flatulence, increased peristalsis, nausea, vomiting

GU: Urinary frequency

MS: Arthralgia, dysarthria, muscle spasms

RESP: Bronchospasm, dyspnea, increased bronchial secretions, respiratory arrest or depression

SKIN: Flushing, diaphoresis, rash, urticaria

Nursing Considerations

- If also giving atropine, be sure to administer it with or before neostigmine, as prescribed.
- Make sure patient is well ventilated and airway remains patent until normal respiration is assured.
- **WARNING** Monitor for signs of neostigmine overdose, which can cause life-threatening cholinergic crisis (increased muscle weakness, including respiratory muscles). Expect to stop neostigmine and atropine, as ordered.
- Be aware that patients with postoperative atelectasis, pneumonia, UTI, or asthma may experience an exacerbation of their condition if given neostigmine.
- Store drug at 15° to 30° C (59° to 86° F); protect from freezing and light.

PATIENT TEACHING

- Instruct patient to report muscle weakness, excessive salivation, dizziness, urinary frequency, or other adverse reactions after receiving neostigmine.

nesiritide

Natrecor

Class and Category

Chemical: Human B-type natriuretic peptide

Therapeutic: Arterial and venous smooth-muscle cell relaxant

Pregnancy category: C

Indications and Dosages

▶ *To reduce dyspnea at rest or with minimal activity in patients with acute decompensated heart failure*

I.V. INJECTION, I.V. INFUSION

Adults. 2-mcg/kg bolus, followed by a continuous infusion of 0.01 mcg/kg/min for up to 48 hr.

Route	Onset	Peak	Duration
I.V.	In 15 min	1 hr	3 hr

Mechanism of Action

Binds to the guanylate cyclase receptor of vascular smooth-muscle and endothelial cells. This action increases intracellular levels of cGMP, which leads to arterial and venous smooth-muscle cell relaxation. Ultimately, nesiritide reduces pulmonary artery wedge pressure and systemic arterial pressure in patients with heart failure, thereby decreasing the heart's workload and subsequently relieving dyspnea.

Incompatibilities

Don't infuse nesiritide through the same I.V. line as bumetanide, enalaprilat, ethacrynate sodium, furosemide, heparin, hydralazine, or insulin because these drugs are chemically and physically incompatible with nesiritide. Don't infuse drugs that contain the preservative sodium metabisulfite through the same I.V. line as nesiritide because they're incompatible.

Contraindications

Hypersensitivity to nesiritide or its components, patients with a systolic blood pressure less than 90 mm Hg, primary therapy for cardiogenic shock

Interactions

DRUGS

ACE inhibitors: Increased risk of symptomatic hypotension

Adverse Reactions

CNS: Anxiety, dizziness, headache, insomnia

CV: Angina, bradycardia, hypotension, PVCs, ventricular tachycardia

GI: Abdominal pain, nausea, vomiting

GU: Elevated serum creatinine level

MS: Back pain

Nursing Considerations

- **WARNING** Be aware that nesiritide is not recommended for patients for whom vasodilating drugs are inappropriate, such as those with significant valvular stenosis, restrictive or obstructive cardiomyopathy, constrictive pericarditis, pericardial tamponade, or other conditions in which cardiac output is dependent upon venous return, or for patients suspected of having low cardiac filling pressures.

- Reconstitute 1.5-mg vial by adding 5 ml of diluent from a 250-ml plastic I.V. bag containing preservative-free D_5W, normal saline solution, dextrose 5% half-normal (0.45) saline solution, or dextrose 5% in quarter-normal (0.2) saline solution.

- Don't shake vial. To ensure complete reconstitution, rock vial gently so that all surfaces, including the stopper, come in contact with diluent. Inspect drug for particles and discoloration; if present, discard drug.

- Withdraw entire contents of reconstituted solution and add it to the same 250-ml plastic I.V. bag used to withdraw the diluent to yield a solution of approximately 6 mcg/ml. Invert I.V. bag several times to ensure that solution is completely mixed.

- After preparing infusion bag, withdraw bolus volume from infusion bag and give over approximately 60 seconds. Immediately after giving bolus, infuse drug at a flow rate of 0.1 ml/kg/hour, which will deliver a dose of 0.01 mcg/kg/minute.

- Prime I.V. tubing with 25 ml of solution before connecting to I.V. line and before administering bolus dose or starting infusion.

- Flush I.V. line between administering nesiritide and incompatible drugs.

- Because nesiritide binds to heparin and could bind to heparin lining of a heparin-coated catheter, don't administer drug through a central heparin-coated catheter.

- Store reconstituted vials at room temperature (20° to 25° C [68° to 77° F]) or refrigerate (2° to 8° C [36° to 46° F]) for up to 24 hours.

- Because nesiritide contains no antimicrobial preservatives, discard reconstituted solution after 24 hours.

- Monitor blood pressure and heart rate and rhythm frequently during drug therapy. If hypotension occurs, notify prescriber and expect dosage to be reduced or drug to be discontinued. Implement measures to support blood pressure, as prescribed.

- Assess breath sounds and respiratory rate, rhythm, depth, and quality frequently during nesiritide therapy.

- Monitor serum creatinine level during therapy and notify prescriber of abnormal results.
- Store unopened drug at controlled room temperature or refrigerate. Keep in carton until time of use.

PATIENT TEACHING

- Instruct patient to report dizziness during nesiritide therapy because this may indicate hypotension.
- Reassure patient that her blood pressure, heart rate, and breathing will be monitored frequently.

netilmicin sulfate

Netromycin

Class and Category

Chemical: Aminoglycoside
Therapeutic: Antibiotic
Pregnancy category: D

Indications and Dosages

▶ *To treat serious systemic infections, such as intra-abdominal infections, lower respiratory tract infections, septicemia, and skin and soft-tissue infections, caused by* Enterobacter aerogenes, Escherichia coli, Klebsiella pneumoniae, Proteus mirabilis, Pseudomonas aeruginosa, Serratia *species, and* Staphylococcus aureus

I.V. INFUSION

Adults and children age 12 and over. 1.3 to 2.2 mg/kg every 8 hr or 2 to 3.25 mg/kg every 12 hr for 7 to 14 days. *Maximum:* 7.5 mg/kg daily.

Children ages 6 weeks to 12 years. 1.8 to 2.7 mg/kg every 8 hr or 2.7 to 4 mg/kg every 12 hr for 7 to 14 days.

Infants up to age 6 weeks. 2 to 3.25 mg/kg every 12 hr for 7 to 14 days.

▶ *To treat complicated UTI caused by* Citrobacter *species,* Enterobacter *species,* E. coli, K. pneumoniae, P. mirabilis, P. aeruginosa, Serratia *species, and* Staphylococcus *species*

I.V. INFUSION

Adults and adolescents. 1.5 to 2 mg/kg every 12 hr for 7 to 14 days. *Maximum:* 7.5 mg/kg daily.

Incompatibilities

Don't mix netilmicin with beta-lactam antibiotics (penicillins and cephalosporins) because substantial mutual inactivation may result. If they're prescribed together, give them at separate sites.

Mechanism of Action

Is transported into bacterial cells, where it competes with messenger RNA to bind with a specific receptor protein on the 30S ribosomal subunit of DNA. This action causes abnormal, nonfunctioning proteins to form. A lack of functional proteins causes bacterial cell death.

Contraindications

Hypersensitivity to netilmicin, other aminoglycosides, or their components

Interactions

DRUGS

capreomycin, other aminoglycosides: Increased risk of nephrotoxicity, neuromuscular blockade, and ototoxicity

cephalosporins, nephrotoxic drugs: Increased risk of nephrotoxicity

loop diuretics, ototoxic drugs: Increased risk of ototoxicity

methoxyflurane, polymyxins (parenteral): Increased risk of nephrotoxicity and neuromuscular blockade

neuromuscular blockers: Increased neuromuscular blockade

Adverse Reactions

CNS: Disorientation, dizziness, encephalopathy, headache, myasthenia gravis–like syndrome, neuromuscular blockade (acute muscle paralysis and apnea), paresthesia, peripheral neuropathy, seizures, vertigo, weakness

CV: Hypotension, palpitations

EENT: Blurred vision, hearing loss, nystagmus, tinnitus

GI: Diarrhea, elevated liver function tests results, nausea, vomiting

GU: Elevated BUN and serum creatinine levels, nephrotoxicity, oliguria, proteinuria

HEME: Anemia, eosinophilia, leukopenia, prolonged PT, thrombocytopenia, thrombocytosis

MS: Muscle twitching

RESP: Apnea

SKIN: Allergic dermatitis, erythema, pruritus, rash

Other: Angioedema; hyperkalemia; injection site hematoma, induration, and pain

Nursing Considerations

- To prepare netilmicin for I.V. use, dilute each dose in 50 to 200 ml of suitable diluent, such as normal saline solution, D_5W, or lactated Ringer's solution, and administer slowly over 30 to

60 minutes. When giving drug to children, adjust amount of diluent proportionately, as required. Prepared solution typically may be stored for up to 72 hours at room temperature; however, storage times vary, depending on type of diluent used, type of container, concentration, and storage method. Consult manufacturer's insert for specific stability and storage information.

- Ensure adequate hydration during therapy to maintain adequate renal function.
- Monitor blood netilmicin level; optimum peak level is 6 to 10 mcg/ml and trough level is 0.5 to 2 mcg/ml.
- Check BUN and serum creatinine levels, urine specific gravity, and creatinine clearance during netilmicin therapy, as ordered.
- Anticipate higher risk of nephrotoxicity in infants, elderly patients, those with impaired renal function or dehydration, and those receiving high-dose or prolonged netilmicin therapy.
- Decrease dosage or discontinue drug, as ordered, if signs of drug-induced ototoxicity or vestibular toxicity occur, to reduce the risk of permanent damage. Patients with cranial nerve VIII impairment are at increased risk for both types of toxicity.
- Be aware that infants with botulism and patients with myasthenia gravis or Parkinson's disease may experience increased muscle weakness.
- Store drug at 15° to 30° C (59° to 86° F); don't freeze.

PATIENT TEACHING
- Urge patient to drink plenty of fluids during netilmicin therapy.
- Instruct patient to immediately report dizziness, hearing loss, muscle twitching, nausea, numbness and tingling, ringing or buzzing in ears, seizures, significant changes in amount of urine or frequency of urination, and vomiting.
- Urge patient to keep follow-up appointments—for example, for audiometric and renal function tests—to monitor progress.

niacin
niacinamide
(nicotinic acid, vitamin B$_3$)

Class and Category
Chemical: B complex vitamin
Therapeutic: Antihyperlipidemic (niacin), nutritional supplement
Pregnancy category: C (for doses above the RDA)

Indications and Dosages

▶ *To prevent niacin deficiency based on U.S. and Canadian recommended daily allowances*

I.V. INFUSION

Adults and children. Dosage individualized based on severity of deficiency, as prescribed, and given as part of total parenteral nutrition solution.

▶ *To treat niacin deficiency*

I.V. INJECTION

Adults and children age 11 and over. 25 to 100 mg at least b.i.d.

Children. Up to 300 mg daily.

Mechanism of Action

Acts as dietary supplement for vitamin B_3. After conversion to niacinamide, niacin becomes a compound of two coenzymes needed for tissue respiration, glycogenolysis, and metabolism of lipids, amino acids, proteins, and purines. Niacin also lowers serum cholesterol and triglyceride levels by inhibiting synthesis of very-low-density lipoproteins, which are needed to form low-density lipoproteins, the primary carrier of blood cholesterol.

Contraindications

Active peptic ulcer disease; arterial bleeding; hepatic impairment (significant or unexplained); hypersensitivity to niacin, niacinamide, or their components

Interactions

DRUGS

chenodiol, ursodiol: Decreased antihyperlipidemic effects of niacin

HMG-CoA reductase inhibitors: Increased risk of rhabdomyolysis and acute renal failure

Adverse Reactions

CNS: Asthenia, chills, dizziness, headache (niacin), insomnia, nervousness, paresthesia, syncope

CV: Arrhythmias, hypotension, palpitations, peripheral edema, peripheral vasodilation (niacin), syncope, tachycardia

EENT: Dry eyes, macular edema, rhinitis, toxic amblyopia

ENDO: Hyperglycemia

GI: Abdominal pain, cholestasis (E.R. niacin), diarrhea, dyspepsia, epigastric pain, eructation, flatulence, hepatotoxicity (E.R. niacin), jaundice, nausea, peptic ulceration, vomiting

GU: Hyperuricemia
MS: Leg cramps, myalgia, myasthenia
RESP: Dyspnea
SKIN: Acanthosis nigricans, dry skin, flushing (niacin), hyperpigmentation, maculopapular rash, pruritus, rash, sensation of warmth (niacin), urticaria
Other: Anaphylaxis (injection), angioedema, facial edema, gout

Nursing Considerations

- Dilute injection solution to a concentration of 2 mg/ml for direct I.V. injection and administer at a rate not exceeding 2 mg/min.
- For intermittent or continuous infusion, dilute appropriate dose in 500 ml of normal saline solution or other compatible solution and administer at no more than 2 mg/minute.
- Monitor patient for "niacin flush," a reaction caused by dilation of peripheral cutaneous blood vessels, which increases blood flow and causes redness, mainly in the face, neck, and chest. Expect patient to develop tolerance to this effect after 2 weeks of therapy. Notify prescriber of persistent flushing; effects may be controlled with aspirin, as prescribed, taken before each niacin dose.
- Expect to monitor liver function tests every 6 months during therapy or as clinically indicated. Expect niacin to be discontinued if serum transaminase levels rise to 3 times the upper limit of normal or if patient exhibits clinical symptoms of hepatic dysfunction.
- Monitor patients with peptic ulcer disease for possible worsened symptoms because nicotinic acid can stimulate histamine release, leading to increased gastric acid production.
- Monitor patients with or predisposed to gout for worsening of symptoms because drug can cause hyperuricemia at high doses.
- In patients taking statins and niacin for hyperlipidemia, stay alert for rhabdomyolysis (muscle pain, tenderness, or weakness), especially early in therapy or when the dosage of either drug increases. Be prepared to stop therapy if rhabdomyolysis occurs.
- Monitor patients with diabetes mellitus for altered glucose control because high doses of niacin may cause hyperglycemia.
- Monitor complete blood count, especially if patient has thrombocytopenia or coagulopathy or takes an anticoagulant, because niacin may cause slight decrease in platelet count or increased prothrombin time.

PATIENT TEACHING
- Instruct patient to avoid activities requiring mental alertness, such as driving or operating machinery, until full effects of drug are known because vasodilatory response to niacin may be dramatic at start of treatment.
- Inform patient that she may experience skin flushing, mainly in the face, neck, and chest, but that she may develop a tolerance to this effect after 2 weeks of therapy. Advise her to notify prescriber of persistent or intolerable flushing because prescriber may adjust drug dosage or recommend that patient take aspirin before each niacin dose to control flushing.

nicardipine hydrochloride
Cardene, Cardene I.V., Cardene SR

Class and Category
Chemical: Dihydropyridine derivative
Therapeutic: Antianginal, antihypertensive
Pregnancy category: C

Indications and Dosages
▶ *To manage angina pectoris and Prinzmetal's angina, to manage hypertension*
I.V. INFUSION
Adults. 0.5 to 2.2 mg/hr by continuous infusion.
▶ *To control acute hypertension*
I.V. INFUSION
Adults. *Initial:* 5 mg/hr by continuous infusion; increased by 2.5 mg/hr every 5 to 15 min, as prescribed. *Maximum:* 15 mg/hr.

Route	Onset	Peak	Duration
I.V.	Immediate	Unknown	Unknown

Mechanism of Action
May slow extracellular calcium movement into myocardial and vascular smooth-muscle cells by deforming calcium channels in cell membranes, inhibiting ion-controlled gating mechanisms, and interfering with calcium release from the sarcoplasmic reticulum. By decreasing the intracellular calcium level, nicardipine inhibits smooth-muscle–cell contraction and dilates coronary and systemic arteries. As with other calcium channel blockers, these actions lead to decreased myocardial oxygen requirements and reduced peripheral resistance, blood pressure, and afterload.

Incompatibilities
Don't mix nicardipine with, or administer through same I.V. line as, sodium bicarbonate or LR solution.

Contraindications
Advanced aortic stenosis, hypersensitivity to any calcium channel blocker, second- or third-degree AV block in patient without artificial pacemaker

Interactions
DRUGS
anesthetics (hydrocarbon inhalation): Possibly hypotension
beta blockers, other antihypertensives, prazosin: Increased risk of hypotension
calcium supplements: Possibly impaired action of nicardipine
cimetidine: Increased nicardipine bioavailability
digoxin: Transiently increased blood digoxin level, increased risk of digitalis toxicity
disopyramide, flecainide: Increased risk of bradycardia, conduction defects, and heart failure
estrogens: Possibly increased fluid retention and decreased therapeutic effects of nicardipine
lithium: Increased risk of neurotoxicity
NSAIDs, sympathomimetics: Possibly decreased effects of nicardipine
procainamide, quinidine: Possibly prolonged QT interval
FOODS
grapefruit, grapefruit juice: Possibly increased drug bioavailability
high-fat meals: Decreased blood nicardipine level
ACTIVITIES
alcohol use: Increased hypotensive effect

Adverse Reactions
CNS: Anxiety, asthenia, ataxia, confusion, dizziness, drowsiness, headache, nervousness, paresthesia, psychiatric disturbance, syncope, tremor, weakness
CV: Bradycardia, chest pain, heart failure, hypotension, orthostatic hypotension, palpitations, peripheral edema, tachycardia
EENT: Altered taste, blurred vision, dry mouth, epistaxis, gingival hyperplasia, pharyngitis, rhinitis, tinnitus
ENDO: Gynecomastia, hyperglycemia
GI: Anorexia, constipation, diarrhea, elevated liver function test results, indigestion, nausea, thirst, vomiting
GU: Dysuria, nocturia, polyuria, sexual dysfunction, urinary frequency

HEME: Anemia, leukopenia, thrombocytopenia
MS: Joint stiffness, muscle spasms
RESP: Bronchitis, cough, upper respiratory tract infection
SKIN: Dermatitis, diaphoresis, erythema multiforme, flushing, photosensitivity, pruritus, rash, Stevens-Johnson syndrome, urticaria
Other: Hypokalemia, weight gain

Nursing Considerations

- Check blood pressure and pulse rate before nicardipine therapy begins, during dosage changes, and periodically throughout therapy. During prolonged therapy, periodically assess ECG tracings for arrhythmias and other changes.
- Dilute each 25-mg ampule of nicardipine with 240 ml of compatible solution to yield 0.1 mg/ml. Mixture is stable at room temperature for 24 hours when prepared with D_5W, dextrose 5% in normal saline solution, dextrose 5% in half-normal (0.45) saline solution, half-normal saline solution, or normal saline solution.
- Administer continuous infusion by I.V. pump or controller, and adjust according to patient's blood pressure, as prescribed.
- Change peripheral I.V. site every 12 hours, if feasible.
- Give first dose of oral nicardipine 1 hour before stopping I.V. infusion, as prescribed.
- Monitor fluid intake and output and daily weight for signs of fluid retention, which may precipitate heart failure. Also assess for signs of heart failure, such as crackles, dyspnea, jugular vein distention, peripheral edema, and weight gain.
- Monitor patient's liver and renal function test results periodically during long-term therapy. Patients with impaired hepatic or renal function may require dosage adjustment. Expect elevated liver function test results to return to normal after drug is discontinued.
- Monitor serum potassium level during prolonged therapy. Hypokalemia increases the risk of arrhythmias.
- Because of drug's negative inotropic effect on some patients, closely monitor patients who take a beta blocker or have heart failure or significant left ventricular dysfunction.
- **WARNING** Expect to taper dosage gradually before discontinuing drug to prevent angina or dangerously high blood pressure.
- Store drug at 20° to 25° C (68° to 77° F); protect from light and elevated temperatures.

PATIENT TEACHING
- Advise patient to change position slowly during nicardipine therapy to minimize effects of orthostatic hypotension.
- Urge patient to avoid potentially hazardous activities until drug's CNS effects are known.
- Advise patient to immediately report chest pain that is not relieved by rest or nitroglycerin, constipation, irregular heartbeat, nausea, pronounced dizziness, severe or persistent headache, and swelling of hands or feet.
- Urge patient to take oral nicardipine as prescribed, even if she feels well.
- Instruct patient to swallow E.R. capsules whole, not to chew, crush, cut, or open them.
- Advise patient not to take drug within 1 hour of eating a high-fat meal or grapefruit product. Urge her not to alter the amount of grapefruit products in her diet without consulting prescriber.
- **WARNING** Caution against stopping nicardipine abruptly; angina or dangerously high blood pressure could result.
- Teach patient how to take her pulse, and urge her to notify prescriber immediately if it falls below 50 beats/minute.
- Teach patient how to measure her blood pressure, and advise her to do so weekly if nicardipine was prescribed for hypertension. Suggest that she keep a log of blood pressure readings to take to follow-up appointments with her doctor.
- Encourage patient to comply with suggested lifestyle changes, such as alcohol moderation, low-sodium or low-fat diet, regular exercise, smoking cessation, stress management, and weight loss.
- Inform patient that saunas, hot tubs, and prolonged hot showers may cause dizziness or fainting.
- Instruct patient to avoid prolonged sun exposure and to use sunscreen when going outdoors.

nitroglycerin
(glyceryl trinitrate)
Deponit, Minitran, Nitro-Bid, Nitrocot, Nitro-Dur, Nitrogard, Nitroglyn E-R, Nitroject, Nitrol, Nitrolingual, Nitrong SR, Nitropar, Nitrostat, Nitro-time, Transderm-Nitro, Tridil

Class and Category
Chemical: Nitrate
Therapeutic: Antianginal, antihypertensive, vasodilator
Pregnancy category: C

Indications and Dosages

▶ *To prevent or treat angina, to manage hypertension or heart failure*
I.V. INFUSION
Adults. 5 mcg/min, increased by 5 mcg/min every 3 to 5 min to 20 mcg/min, as prescribed, and then by 10 to 20 mcg/min every 3 to 5 min until desired effect occurs.

Route	Onset	Peak	Duration
I.V.	1 to 2 min	Unknown	3 to 5 min

Mechanism of Action

May interact with nitrate receptors in vascular smooth-muscle cell membranes. This interaction reduces nitroglycerin to nitric oxide, as shown, which activates the enzyme guanylate cyclase, increasing intracellular formation of cGMP. The increased cGMP level may relax vascular smooth muscle by forcing calcium out of muscle cells, causing vasodilation. Venous dilation decreases venous return to the heart, reducing left ventricular end-diastolic pressure and pulmonary artery wedge pressure. Arterial dilation decreases systemic vascular resistance, systolic arterial pressure, and mean arterial pressure. Thus, nitroglycerin reduces preload and afterload, decreasing myocardial workload and oxygen demand. It also dilates coronary arteries, increasing blood flow to ischemic myocardial tissue.

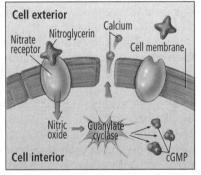

Incompatibilities

Don't administer I.V. nitroglycerin through I.V. bags or tubing made of polyvinyl chloride. Don't mix drug with other solutions.

Contraindications

Acute MI (S.L.), angle-closure glaucoma, cerebral hemorrhage, concurrent use of phosphodiesterase inhibitors, constrictive pericarditis (I.V.), head trauma, hypersensitivity to adhesive in transdermal form, hypersensitivity to nitrates, hypotension (I.V.), hypovolemia (I.V.), inadequate cerebral circulation (I.V.), increased intracranial pressure, orthostatic hypotension, pericardial tamponade, severe anemia

Interactions
DRUGS

acetylcholine, norepinephrine: Possibly decreased therapeutic effects of these drugs

heparin: Possibly decreased anticoagulant effect of heparin (I.V. nitroglycerin)

opioid analgesics, other antihypertensives, vasodilators: Possibly increased orthostatic hypotension

phosphodiesterase inhibitors, such as sildenafil: Possibly severe hypotensive effect of nitroglycerin

sympathomimetics: Possibly decreased antianginal effect of nitroglycerin and increased risk of hypotension

ACTIVITIES

alcohol use: Possibly increased orthostatic hypotension

Adverse Reactions
CNS: Agitation, anxiety, dizziness, headache, insomnia, restlessness, syncope, weakness

CV: Arrhythmias (including tachycardia), edema, hypotension, orthostatic hypotension, palpitations

EENT: Blurred vision, burning or tingling in mouth (buccal, S.L. forms), dry mouth

GI: Abdominal pain, diarrhea, indigestion, nausea, vomiting

GU: Dysuria, impotence, urinary frequency

HEME: Methemoglobinemia

MS: Arthralgia

RESP: Bronchitis, pneumonia

SKIN: Contact dermatitis (transdermal forms), flushing of face and neck, rash

Nursing Considerations
- Use nitroglycerin cautiously in elderly patients, especially those who are volume depleted or taking several medications, because of the increased risk of hypotension and falls. Hypotension may be accompanied by angina and paradoxical slowing of the heart rate. Notify prescriber if these occur, and provide appropriate treatment, as ordered.
- Be aware that I.V. nitroglycerin should be diluted only in D$_5$W or normal saline solution and shouldn't be mixed with other infusions. The pharmacist should add drug to a glass bottle, not a container made of polyvinyl chloride. Don't use a filter be-

cause plastic absorbs drug. Administer drug with infusion pump.
- Check vital signs before every dosage adjustment and frequently during therapy.
- Monitor heart and breath sounds, level of consciousness, fluid intake and output, and pulmonary artery wedge pressure closely.
- Store premixed containers in the dark; don't freeze them.
- **WARNING** Assess for signs of overdose, such as confusion, diaphoresis, dyspnea, flushing, headache, hypotension, nausea, palpitations, tachycardia, vertigo, vision changes, and vomiting. Treat as prescribed by removing nitroglycerin source, if possible; elevating the legs above heart level; and administering an alpha-adrenergic agonist, such as phenylephrine, as prescribed, to treat severe hypotension.

PATIENT TEACHING
- Teach patient to recognize signs and symptoms of angina pectoris, including chest fullness, pain, and pressure, which may be accompanied by sweating and nausea. Pain may radiate down left arm or into neck or jaw. Inform female patients and those with diabetes mellitus or hypertension that they may experience only fatigue and shortness of breath.
- Advise patient to notify prescriber immediately about blurred vision, dizziness, and severe headache.
- Suggest that patient change positions slowly to minimize effects of orthostatic hypotension.
- Advise patient to avoid potentially hazardous activities until drug's CNS effects are known.
- Warn patient to avoid alcohol and erectile dysfunction drugs during therapy.

nitroprusside sodium
Nipride, Nitropress

Class and Category
Chemical: Cyanonitrosylferrate
Therapeutic: Antihypertensive, vasodilator
Pregnancy category: C

Indications and Dosages
▶ *To treat hypertensive crisis and manage severe heart failure*
I.V. INFUSION
Adults and children. *Initial:* 0.25 to 0.3 mcg/kg/min, increased

gradually every few minutes until blood pressure reaches desired level. *Maintenance:* 3 mcg/kg/min (range, 0.25 to 10 mcg/kg/min). *Maximum:* 10 mcg/kg/min for 10 min.

Route	Onset	Peak	Duration
I.V.	1 to 2 min	Immediate	1 to 10 min

Mechanism of Action

May interact with nitrate receptors in vascular smooth-muscle–cell membranes. This interaction reduces nitroprusside to nitric oxide, which activates the enzyme guanylate cyclase, increasing intracellular formation of cGMP. The increased cGMP level may relax vascular smooth muscle by forcing calcium out of muscle cells. Smooth-muscle relaxation causes arteries and veins to dilate, which reduces peripheral vascular resistance and blood pressure.

Incompatibilities

Don't mix nitroprusside with any other drug.

Contraindications

Acute heart failure with decreased peripheral vascular resistance, congenital optic atrophy, decreased cerebral perfusion, hypersensitivity to nitroprusside or its components, hypertension from aortic coarctation or AV shunting, tobacco-induced amblyopia

Interactions

DRUGS

dobutamine: Increased cardiac output, decreased pulmonary artery wedge pressure

ganglionic blockers, general anesthetics, hypotension-producing drugs: Increased hypotensive effect

sympathomimetics: Decreased antihypertensive effect of nitroprusside

Adverse Reactions

CNS: Anxiety, dizziness, headache, increased ICP, nervousness, restlessness

CV: Hypotension, tachycardia

ENDO: Hypothyroidism

GI: Abdominal pain, ileus, nausea, vomiting

HEME: Methemoglobinemia

MS: Muscle twitching

SKIN: Diaphoresis, flushing, rash

Other: Infusion site phlebitis

Nursing Considerations

- Obtain baseline vital signs before administering nitroprusside.
- **WARNING** Don't infuse drug undiluted. Reconstitute with 2 ml of D_5W, and add solution to 250 to 500 ml of D_5W to produce 200 mcg/ml or 100 mcg/ml, respectively.
- Be aware that solution is stable at room temperature for 24 hours when protected from light. Don't use reconstituted solution if it contains particles or is blue, green, red, or darker than faint brown.
- Use an infusion pump. Place opaque covering over infusion container because drug is metabolized by light. I.V. tubing doesn't need to be covered.
- Keep patient supine when starting drug or titrating dose up or down.
- Monitor blood pressure continuously with intra-arterial pressure monitor. Record blood pressure every 5 minutes at start of infusion and every 15 minutes thereafter.
- If patient has severe heart failure, expect to administer an inotropic drug, such as dopamine or dobutamine, as prescribed.
- Monitor level of serum thiocyanate (which forms during nitroprusside metabolism) at least every 72 hours; levels exceeding 100 mcg/ml are associated with toxicity.
- **WARNING** Monitor patients receiving prolonged or high-dose nitroprusside therapy for signs of thiocyanate toxicity (ataxia, blurred vision, delirium, dizziness, dyspnea, headache, hyperreflexia, loss of consciousness, nausea, tinnitus, vomiting). Toxicity can cause arrhythmias, metabolic acidosis, severe hypotension, and death.
- **WARNING** Assess for signs of cyanide toxicity (absence of reflexes, coma, distant heart sounds, hypotension, metabolic acidosis, mydriasis, pink skin, shallow respirations, and weak pulse). If you detect such signs, discontinue nitroprusside, as ordered, and give 4 to 6 mg/kg of sodium nitrite over 2 to 4 minutes to convert hemoglobin to methemoglobin. Follow with 150 to 200 mg/kg of sodium thiosulfate. Repeat this regimen at one-half the original doses after 2 hours, as ordered.
- Monitor infusion site for redness, swelling, and pain.
- Store nitroprusside at 15° to 30° C (59° to 86° F), and protect it from light.

PATIENT TEACHING

- Advise patient to change position slowly during nitroprusside

therapy to minimize dizziness caused by sudden, severe hypotension.
• Instruct patient to report adverse reactions, such as rash, dizziness, headache, and abdominal pain.

norepinephrine bitartrate
(levarterenol bitartrate)
Levophed

Class and Category
Chemical: Catecholamine
Therapeutic: Cardiac stimulant, vasopressor
Pregnancy category: C

Indications and Dosages
▶ *To treat acute hypotension, cardiogenic shock, and septic shock*
I.V. INFUSION
Adults. *Initial:* 0.5 to 1 mcg/min; increased, as ordered, until systolic blood pressure reaches desired level. *Maintenance:* 2 to 12 mcg/min.
Children. 0.1 mcg/kg/min. *Maximum:* 1 mcg/kg/min.
▶ *To treat refractory shock*
I.V. INFUSION
Adults. Up to 30 mcg/min.

Route	Onset	Peak	Duration
I.V.	Rapid	Unknown	1 to 2 min

Mechanism of Action
At high doses (more than 4 mcg/min), directly stimulates alpha-adrenergic receptors and inhibits activity of the intracellular enzyme adenyl cyclase, which then inhibits cAMP production. Inhibition of cAMP causes arterial and venous constriction and increases peripheral vascular resistance and systolic blood pressure. At low doses (less than 2 mcg/min), norepinephrine directly stimulates beta-adrenergic receptors in the myocardium and increases adenyl cyclase activity, producing positive inotropic and chronotropic effects.

Incompatibilities
Don't mix norepinephrine with iron salts, alkalies, or oxidizing solutions. Don't mix with normal saline solution alone.

Contraindications

Concurrent use of hydrocarbon inhalation anesthetics, hypersensitivity to norepinephrine or its components, hypovolemia, mesenteric or peripheral vascular thrombosis

Interactions

DRUGS

alpha blockers: Decreased vasopressor effects of norepinephrine

beta blockers: Decreased cardiac-stimulating effect of norepinephrine, possibly decreased therapeutic effects of both drugs

digoxin: Increased risk of arrhythmias, possibly potentiated inotropic effect

doxapram: Possibly increased vasopressor effects of both drugs

ergonovine, ergotamine, methylergonovine, methysergide, oxytocin: Possibly increased vasoconstriction

general anesthetics: Increased risk of arrhythmias

guanadrel, guanethidine: Increased vasopressor response to norepinephrine, possibly severe hypertension

MAO inhibitors: Possibly life-threatening adverse effects, including arrhythmias, hyperpyrexia, severe headache, severe hypertension, and vomiting

maprotiline, tricyclic antidepressants: Possibly potentiated cardiovascular and pressor effects of norepinephrine, including arrhythmias, severe hypertension, and hyperpyrexia

methylphenidate: Possibly potentiated vasopressor effects

nitrates: Possibly decreased therapeutic effects of both drugs

phenoxybenzamine: Possibly arrhythmias or hypotension

sympathomimetics: Increased risk of adverse cardiovascular effects

thyroid hormones: Increased risk of coronary insufficiency

Adverse Reactions

CNS: Anxiety, dizziness, headache, insomnia, nervousness, tremor, weakness

CV: Angina, bradycardia, ECG changes, edema, hypertension, hypotension, palpitations, peripheral vascular insufficiency (including gangrene), PVCs, sinus tachycardia

GI: Nausea, vomiting

GU: Decreased renal perfusion

RESP: Apnea, dyspnea

SKIN: Pallor

Other: Infusion site sloughing and tissue necrosis, metabolic acidosis

Nursing Considerations

- Dilute norepinephrine concentrate for infusion in D_5W or D_5 in normal saline solution before administering. Concentrations typically range from 16 to 32 mcg/ml. Discard any unused portion of prepared solution.
- Make sure solution contains no particles and isn't discolored before administering.
- Give drug with infusion pump or other flow-control device.
- Check blood pressure every 2 to 3 minutes, preferably by direct intra-arterial monitoring, until stabilized and then every 5 minutes.
- **WARNING** Because extravasation can cause severe tissue damage and necrosis, expect prescriber to give multiple subcutaneous injections of phentolamine (5 to 10 mg diluted in 10 to 15 ml of normal saline solution) around extravasated infusion site.
- If blanching occurs along vein, change infusion site and notify prescriber immediately.
- Monitor ECG tracing continuously during drug administration.
- Store drug in light-resistant container at 15° to 30° C (59° to 86° F); don't freeze.

PATIENT TEACHING
- Urge patient receiving norepinephrine to immediately report burning, leaking, or tingling around I.V. site.

octreotide acetate
Sandostatin

Class and Category
Chemical: Cyclic octapeptide, somatostatin analogue
Therapeutic: Antidiarrheal, hormone suppressant
Pregnancy category: B

Indications and Dosages
▶ *To treat symptoms of acromegaly, to suppress the release of growth hormone from pituitary tumors*
I.V. INJECTION
Adults. *Initial:* 50 mcg t.i.d. *Usual:* 100 mcg t.i.d. *Maximum:* 1,500 mcg daily.

Incompatibilities
Don't mix octreotide in same syringe with fat emulsions or total parenteral nutrition solutions.

Mechanism of Action

Controls many types of secretory diarrhea by inhibiting secretion of serotonin and pituitary and GI hormones (including insulin, glucagon, growth hormone, thyrotropin, and, possibly, thyroid-stimulating hormone) as well as vasoactive intestinal peptides and pancreatic polypeptides (including gastrin, secretin, and motilin). Inhibition of serotonin and peptides increases intestinal absorption of water and electrolytes, decreases pancreatic and gastric acid secretions, and increases intestinal transit time by slowing gastric motility.

By inhibiting hormones involved in vasodilation, octreotide increases splanchnic arterial resistance and decreases GI blood flow, hepatic vein wedge pressure, hepatic blood flow, portal vein pressure, and intravariceal pressure, thus raising seated and standing blood pressures. By inhibiting serotonin secretion, the drug decreases symptoms of acromegaly, including diarrhea, flushing, wheezing, and urinary excretion of 5-hydroxyindoleacetic acid.

Contraindications

Hypersensitivity to octreotide or its components

Interactions

DRUGS

beta blockers, calcium channel blockers: Additive cardiovascular effects of these drugs

bromocriptine: Increased blood bromocriptine level

cisapride: Decreased effectiveness of both drugs

cyclosporine: Decreased blood cyclosporine level

CYP3A4 metabolizers such as quinidine, terfenadine: Decreased metabolic clearance and increased blood levels of these drugs

diuretics: Increased risk of fluid and electrolyte imbalances

insulin, oral antidiabetic drugs: Increased risk of hypoglycemia

vitamin B_{12}: Decreased blood levels of vitamin B_{12}

Adverse Reactions

CNS: Dizziness, drowsiness, fatigue, headache

CV: Arrhythmias (including conduction abnormalities), edema, hypotension, orthostatic hypotension

EENT: Vision changes

ENDO: Hyperglycemia, hypoglycemia

GI: Abdominal distention, guarding, pain, or tenderness; acute cholecystitis; ascending cholangitis; biliary obstruction; cholelithiasis; cholestatic hepatitis; constipation; diarrhea; epigastric pain; flatulence; nausea; pancreatitis; vomiting

GU: Increased urine output
Other: Dehydration, electrolyte imbalances, injection site irritation

Nursing Considerations

- Give octreotide by I.V. injection only in an emergency, as ordered.
- Be aware that octreotide increases risk of acute cholecystitis, ascending cholangitis, biliary obstruction, cholestatic hepatitis, and pancreatitis.
- Monitor vital signs, bowels sounds, and stool consistency. Assess for abdominal pain and signs of gallbladder disease. Although rare, GI side effects such as progressive abdominal distension, severe epigastric pain, and abdominal distension, severe epigastric pain, and abdominal tenderness and guarding may occur together, giving the appearance of acute intestinal obstruction.
- Monitor serum liver enzyme levels, as appropriate.
- Monitor patient for electrolyte imbalances and dehydration.
- Carefully monitor diabetic patient for altered glucose control.
- If patient has periodic flare-ups of symptoms, expect to give additional subcutaneous octreotide temporarily, as prescribed.

PATIENT TEACHING

- Advise patient to change position slowly to minimize effects of orthostatic hypotension.
- Instruct patient to notify prescriber about adverse reactions, especially abdominal pain, which may indicate pancreatitis.
- Urge diabetic patient to monitor blood glucose level often.

ofloxacin

Floxin

Class and Category

Chemical: Fluoroquinolone
Therapeutic: Antibiotic
Pregnancy category: C

Indications and Dosages

▶ *To treat acute, uncomplicated cystitis caused by* Escherichia coli *or* Klebsiella pneumoniae
I.V. INFUSION
Adults. 200 mg every 12 hr for 3 days.

▶ *To treat uncomplicated cystitis from* Citrobacter diversus, Enterobacter aerogenes, Proteus mirabilis, *or* Pseudomonas aeruginosa
I.V. INFUSION
Adults. 200 mg every 12 hr for 7 days.

▶ *To treat complicated UTI caused by* C. diversus, E. coli, K. pneumoniae, P. mirabilis, *or* P. aeruginosa
I.V. INFUSION
Adults. 200 mg every 12 hr for 10 days.
▶ *To treat uncomplicated gonorrhea*
I.V. INFUSION
Adults and adolescents. 400 mg as single dose.
▶ *To treat urethritis or cervicitis caused by* Chlamydia trachomatis *or* Neisseria gonorrhoeae
I.V. INFUSION
Adults and adolescents. 300 mg b.i.d. for 7 days as an alternative to doxycycline or azithromycin.
▶ *To treat pelvic inflammatory disease caused by susceptible organisms*
I.V. INFUSION
Adults and adolescents. 400 mg every 12 hr with metronidazole I.V. and then switched to oral therapy, as prescribed, after 24 hr. Full course of therapy lasts 14 days.
▶ *To treat prostatitis caused by* E. coli
I.V. INFUSION
Adults. 300 mg every 12 hr for 6 wk.
▶ *To treat lower respiratory tract infections caused by* Haemophilus influenzae *or* Streptococcus pneumoniae *and skin and soft-tissue infections caused by* Staphylococcus aureus *or* Streptococcus pyogenes
I.V. INFUSION
Adults. 400 mg every 12 hr for 10 days.
DOSAGE ADJUSTMENT If creatinine clearance is 20 to 50 ml/min/1.73 m^2, dosing interval possibly reduced to every 24 hr; if clearance is less than 10 ml/min/1.73 m^2, dosage possibly reduced by 50% and given every 24 hr.

Incompatibilities
Don't mix ofloxacin with other I.V. drugs or additives.

Contraindications
Hypersensitivity to ofloxacin, other fluoroquinolones, or their components

Interactions
DRUGS
aluminum-, calcium-, or magnesium-containing antacids; didanosine; ferrous sulfate; magnesium-containing laxatives; multivitamins; sevelamer; sucralfate; zinc: Decreased absorption of oral ofloxacin

probenecid: Decreased ofloxacin excretion, increased risk of toxicity
procainamide: Decreased renal clearance of procainamide

Mechanism of Action

Normally, the enzyme DNA gyrase is responsible for unwinding and supercoiling of bacterial DNA before it replicates, as shown top right. Ofloxacin inhibits synthesis of this enzyme, as shown bottom right, by counteracting the excessive supercoiling of DNA during replication and transcription. In this way, ofloxacin causes the death of both rapidly growing and slow-growing bacterial cells.

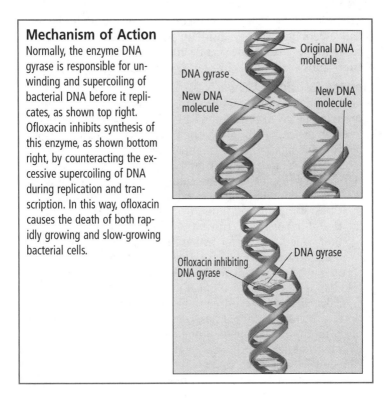

Adverse Reactions

CNS: Dizziness, drowsiness, headache, insomnia, peripheral neuropathy

CV: Arrhythmias, prolonged QT interval, torsades de pointes, vasculitis

GI: Abdominal cramps or pain, acute hepatic necrosis or failure, diarrhea, hepatitis, jaundice, nausea, pseudomembranous colitis, vomiting

GU: Acute renal insufficiency or failure, interstitial nephritis, vaginal candidiasis

HEME: Agranulocytosis, aplastic or hemolytic anemia, leukopenia, pancytopenia, thrombocytopenia

MS: Tendinitis; tendon inflammation, pain, or rupture

HEME: Agranulocytosis, aplastic or hemolytic anemia, leukopenia, pancytopenia, thrombocytopenia
MS: Tendinitis; tendon inflammation, pain, or rupture
RESP: Allergic pneumonitis
SKIN: Blisters, diaphoresis, erythema, erythema multiforme, exfoliative dermatitis, photosensitivity, pruritus, rash, Stevens-Johnson syndrome, toxic epidermal necrolysis, urticaria
Other: Infusion site phlebitis, serum sickness

Nursing Considerations

- Review patient's medical history before giving ofloxacin. Drug shouldn't be given to patients with a history of prolonged QT interval, patients with uncorrected electrolyte disorders, or patients receiving class IA or III antiarrhythmics because of an increased risk of prolonged QT interval. Monitor elderly patients closely; they may be more susceptible to prolonged QT interval.
- For I.V. infusion, dilute drug in normal saline solution or D_5W to at least 4 mg/ml, and infuse over 60 minutes to minimize the risk of hypotension. Discard unused portion.
- Monitor patient closely for hypersensitivity reaction, which can occur as early as the first dose. If evidence of hypersensitivity occurs, such as angioedema, bronchospasm, dyspnea, itching, rash, jaundice, shortness of breath, or urticaria, notify prescriber immediately and expect drug to be discontinued.
- Notify prescriber if patient has symptoms of peripheral neuropathy (pain, burning, tingling, numbness, weakness, or altered sensations of light touch, pain, temperature, position sense, or vibration sense), which could be permanent; tendon rupture (pain and inflammation), which requires immediate rest; or a severe photosensitivity reaction. In each case, expect to stop ofloxacin.
- Maintain adequate hydration to prevent development of highly concentrated urine and crystalluria.
- Expect an increased risk of toxicity in severe hepatic disease, including cirrhosis.
- Be aware that ofloxacin may stimulate the CNS and aggravate seizure disorders.
- If profuse, watery diarrhea develops, notify prescriber and expect to obtain a stool specimen to test for pseudomembranous colitis. If confirmed, withhold ofloxacin and treat diarrhea with fluids, electrolytes, and antibiotics effective against *Clostridium difficile.*
- Be alert for secondary fungal infection.

PATIENT TEACHING
- Advise patient to avoid hazardous activities until CNS effects of drug are known.
- Tell patient to limit exposure to sun and ultraviolet light to prevent phototoxicity.
- Advise patient to notify prescriber immediately about burning skin, hives, itching, rash, rapid heart rate, abnormal motor or sensory function, and tendon pain.
- Encourage patient to seek medical attention immediately for trouble breathing or swallowing, which may signal an allergic reaction.
- Instruct a diabetic patient who takes insulin or an antidiabetic to notify prescriber immediately if he develops a hypoglycemic reaction; ofloxacin will have to be stopped.
- Urge patient to report watery, bloody stools to prescriber immediately, even up to 2 months after drug therapy has ended.

ondansetron hydrochloride
Zofran

Class and Category
Chemical: Carbazole
Therapeutic: Antiemetic
Pregnancy category: B

Indications and Dosages
▶ *To prevent chemotherapy-induced nausea and vomiting*
I.V. INFUSION
Adults. 32 mg infused over 15 min starting 30 min before chemotherapy; or three 0.15-mg/kg doses, each infused over 15 min, starting with the first dose given 30 min before chemotherapy and second and third doses given 4 and 8 hr after first dose.
Children ages 6 months to 18 years. Three 0.15-mg/kg doses, each infused over 15 min, starting with first dose given 30 min before chemotherapy and second and third doses given 4 and 8 hr after first dose.
▶ *To prevent postoperative nausea and vomiting*
I.V. INJECTION
Adults and children age 12 and over. 4 mg as a single dose over 2 to 5 min just before anesthesia induction or if nausea or vomiting develops shortly after surgery.
Children ages 2 to 12 weighing more than 40 kg (88 lb).

4 mg as a single dose over 2 to 5 min just before anesthesia induction or if nausea or vomiting develops shortly after surgery. **Children ages 1 month to 12 years weighing less than 40 kg.** 0.1 mg/kg as a single dose over 2 to 5 min just before or

---

Mechanism of Action

Blocks serotonin receptors centrally in the chemoreceptor trigger zone and peripherally at vagal nerve terminals in the intestine. This action reduces nausea and vomiting by preventing serotonin release in the small intestine (the probable cause of chemotherapy- and radiation-induced nausea and vomiting) and by blocking signals to the CNS. Ondansetron may also bind to other serotonin receptors and to mu-opiate receptors.

---

immediately after anesthesia induction or if nausea or vomiting develops shortly after surgery.

DOSAGE ADJUSTMENT For patients with hepatic impairment, maximum dosage limited to 8 mg daily.

Incompatibilities

Don't give ondansetron in same I.V. line as acyclovir, allopurinol, aminophylline, amphotericin B, ampicillin, ampicillin and sulbactam, amsacrine, cefepime, cefoperazone, furosemide, ganciclovir, lorazepam, methylprednisolone, mezlocillin, piperacillin, or sargramostim. Alkaline solutions and highly concentrated fluorouracil solutions are physically incompatible.

Contraindications

Hypersensitivity to ondansetron or its components

Interactions

DRUGS

cisplatin, cyclophosphamide: Possibly altered blood levels of these drugs

ACTIVITIES

alcohol use: Increased stimulant and sedative effects, including mood and physical sensations

Adverse Reactions

CNS: Agitation, akathisia, anxiety, ataxia, dizziness, drowsiness, fever, headache, hypotension, restlessness, seizures, syncope, somnolence, weakness

CV: Arrythmias, chest pain, hypotension, prolonged QT interval, pulmonary embolism, shock, tachycardia
EENT: Accommodation disturbances, altered taste, blurred vision, dry mouth, laryngeal edema, laryngospasm, transient blindness
GI: Abdominal pain, anorexia, constipation, diarrhea, elevated liver function test results, flatulence, indigestion, intestinal obstruction, thirst
RESP: Bronchospasm, shortness of breath
SKIN: Flushing, hyperpigmentation, maculopapular rash, pruritus
Other: Anaphylaxis, angioedema, injection site burning, pain, and redness

Nursing Considerations

• Give up to 4 mg I.V. diluted in 50 ml of D₅W or normal saline solution.
• **WARNING** Be aware that drug may mask signs and symptoms of adynamic ileus or gastric distention after abdominal surgery.

PATIENT TEACHING

• Advise patient to notify prescriber immediately about signs of hypersensitivity reaction, such as rash.
• Reassure patient who has transient blindness after administration of ondansetron that vision returns within a few minutes to 48 hours.

orphenadrine citrate

Aniflex, Banflex, Flexoject, Miolin, Mio-Rel, Myotrol, Norflex, Orfro, Orphenate

Class and Category

Chemical: Tertiary amine
Therapeutic: Skeletal muscle relaxant
Pregnancy category: C

Indications and Dosages

▶ *To relieve muscle spasms in painful musculoskeletal conditions*

Mechanism of Action

May reduce muscle spasms by acting on the cerebral motor centers or the medulla. Postganglionic anticholinergic effects and some antihistaminic and local anesthetic action contribute to skeletal muscle relaxation.

I.V. INJECTION
Adults and adolescents. 60 mg every 12 hr, p.r.n.

Route	Onset	Peak	Duration
I.V.	Immediate	Unknown	4 to 6 hr

Contraindications

Angle-closure glaucoma; hypersensitivity to orphenadrine or its components; myasthenia gravis; obstruction of bladder neck, duodenum, or pylorus; prostatic hypertrophy; stenosing peptic ulcers

Interactions

DRUGS

amantadine, amitriptyline, amoxapine, antimuscarinics, atropine, bupropion, carbinoxamine, chlorpromazine, clemastine, clomipramine, clozapine, cyclobenzaprine, diphenhydramine, disopyramide, doxepin, imipramine, maprotiline, mesoridazine, methdilazine, nortriptyline, phenothiazines, procainamide, promazine, promethazine, protriptyline, thioridazine, triflupromazine, trimeprazine, trimipramine: Possibly additive anticholinergic effects
CNS depressants: Increased CNS depression
haloperidol: Increased schizophrenic symptoms, possibly tardive dyskinesia
propoxyphene: Increased risk of anxiety, confusion, and tremor
ACTIVITIES
alcohol use: Increased CNS depression

Adverse Reactions

CNS: Agitation, confusion, dizziness, drowsiness, light-headedness, syncope, tremor
CV: Palpitations, tachycardia
EENT: Blurred vision, dry eyes and mouth, increased contact lens awareness
GI: Abdominal distention, constipation, nausea, vomiting
GU: Urine retention

Nursing Considerations

- Be aware that orphenadrine shouldn't be given to patients with tachycardia or cardiac insufficiency.
- Administer drug over 5 minutes with patient in supine position. Have patient remain in this position for 5 to 10 minutes to minimize adverse reactions. Then help him to a sitting position.
- Be aware that drug can aggravate myasthenia gravis and cause tachycardia.

- Anticipate that drug's anticholinergic effects may cause blurred vision, dry eyes, and increased contact lens awareness.
- Be aware that elderly patients may be at increased risk for adverse CNS effects, such as confusion and syncope.
- Monitor blood count and liver and renal function test results periodically for patients receiving orphenadrine long-term.
- Before using drug, store it at 15° to 30° C (59° to 86° F); protect from freezing and light.

PATIENT TEACHING

- Advise patient to avoid potentially hazardous activities until orphenadrine's CNS effects are known.
- Inform patient that dry mouth can be relieved by ice chips, sugarless candy or gum, and increased intake of fluid.
- Suggest that patient use artificial tears during therapy (especially if he wears contact lenses) to reduce discomfort from dry eyes.
- Instruct patient to avoid alcohol and other CNS depressants during orphenadrine therapy.

oxacillin sodium
Bactocill, Prostaphlin

Class and Category
Chemical: Penicillin
Therapeutic class: Antibiotic
Pregnancy category: B

Indications and Dosages
▶ *To treat mild to moderate infections caused by penicillinase-producing strains of* Staphylococcus *or other susceptible organisms*
I.V. INFUSION
Adults and children weighing 40 kg or more. 250 to 500 mg every 4 to 6 hr.
Infants and children weighing less than 40 kg. 50 mg/kg daily in divided doses every 4 to 6 hr.
Neonates over age 7 days weighing more than 2,000 g. 25 to 50 mg/kg every 6 hr.
Neonates over age 7 days weighing less than 2,000 g. 25 to 50 mg/kg every 8 hr.
Neonates age 7 days and younger weighing more than 2,000 g. 25 to 50 mg/kg every 8 hr.
Neonates age 7 days and younger weighing 2,000 g or less. 25 to 50 mg/kg every 12 hr.
▶ *To treat severe infections caused by penicillinase-producing strains of*

Staphylococcus *or other susceptible organisms*
I.V. INFUSION
Adults and children weighing 40 kg or more. 1,000 mg every 4 to 6 hr.
Infants and children weighing less than 40 kg. 100 to 200 mg/kg daily in divided doses every 4 to 6 hr.
Neonates over age 7 days weighing more than 2,000 g. 25 to 50 mg/kg every 6 hr.
Neonates over age 7 days weighing less than 2,000 g. 25 to 50 mg/kg every 8 hr.
Neonates age 7 days and younger weighing more than 2,000 g. 25 to 50 mg/kg every 8 hr.
Neonates age 7 days and younger weighing 2,000 g or less. 25 to 50 mg/kg every 12 hr.
▶ *To treat endocarditis caused by methicillin-susceptible* Staphylococcus aureus *in patients without a prosthetic valve*

Mechanism of Action
Inhibits bacterial cell wall synthesis. In susceptible bacteria, the rigid, cross-linked cell wall is assembled in several steps. Oxacillin exerts its effects in the final stage of the cross-linking process by binding with and inactivating penicillin-binding proteins (enzymes responsible for linking the cell wall strands). This action causes bacterial cell lysis and death.

I.V. INFUSION
Adults. 2 g every 4 hr for 4 to 6 wk.
▶ *To treat endocarditis caused by methicillin-susceptible* S. aureus *in patients with a prosthetic valve*
I.V. INFUSION
Adults. 2 g every 4 hr for at least 6 wk.

Incompatibilities
Don't give oxacillin at same time or in same admixture as aminoglycosides because they are chemically and physically incompatible and will inactivate each other.

Contraindications
Hypersensitivity to oxacillin, penicillins, or their components

Interactions
DRUGS
aminoglycosides: Inactivation of both drugs

chloramphenicol, erythromycins, sulfonamides, tetracyclines: Decreased therapeutic effects of oxacillin
oral contraceptives: Decreased contraceptive efficacy
probenecid: Increased blood oxacillin level
FOODS
all foods: Altered absorption of oxacillin

Adverse Reactions

CNS: Anxiety, depression, fatigue, hallucinations, headache, seizures
EENT: Oral candidiasis
GI: Diarrhea, nausea, pseudomembranous colitis, vomiting
GU: Interstitial nephritis, vaginal candidiasis
HEME: Agranulocytosis, anemia, granulocytopenia, neutropenia
SKIN: Exfoliative dermatitis, pruritus, rash, urticaria
Other: Anaphylaxis

Nursing Considerations

- Administer oxacillin at least 1 hour before other antibiotics.
- Before reconstitution, tap bottle several times to loosen powder. For I.V. infusion, reconstitute only with normal saline solution or D_5W. For I.M. injection, reconstitute with sterile water for injection, 0.45 normal saline solution, or normal saline solution. Shake until solution is clear.
- When giving drug to patient at risk for hypertension or fluid overload, be aware that each gram of oxacillin contains 4.02 mEq of sodium.

PATIENT TEACHING
- Instruct patient to notify prescriber immediately if rash develops.
- Advise female patient who uses an oral contraceptive to use an additional contraceptive method during oxacillin therapy.

oxymorphone hydrochloride

Numorphan

Class, Category, and Schedule

Chemical: Phenanthrene derivative
Therapeutic: Analgesic
Pregnancy category: Not rated
Controlled substance schedule: II

Indications and Dosages

▶ *To relieve moderate to severe pain; to relieve anxiety in patients with dyspnea from pulmonary edema caused by acute left ventricular dysfunction*

Mechanism of Action

Alters the perception of and emotional response to pain at the spinal cord and higher levels of the CNS by blocking the release of inhibitory neurotransmitters, such as gamma-aminobutyric acid and acetylcholine.

I.V. INJECTION

Adults. *Initial:* 0.5 mg, repeated every 3 to 6 hr, p.r.n.

DOSAGE ADJUSTMENT For patients with creatinine clearance less than 50 ml/min, dosage reduced; for patients taking other CNS depressants, dosage reduced to ⅓ to ½ usual dosage.

Route	Onset	Peak	Duration
I.V.	5 to 10 min	15 to 30 min	3 to 4 hr

Contraindications

Acute or severe asthma; hypercarbia; hypersensitivity to oxymorphone, other morphine analogues, or their components; ileus; moderate to severe hepatic impairment; pulmonary edema from a chemical respiratory irritant; severe respiratory depression; upper airway obstruction

Interactions

DRUGS

agonist and antagonist analgesics such as butorphanol, buprenorphine, nalbuphine, or pentazocine: Possibly reduced analgesic effect of oxymorphone and increased risk of withdrawal symptoms

anticholingerics: Increased risk of urine retention, severe constipation

antidiarrheals, antiperistaltics: Increased risk of severe constipation, CNS depression

antihypertensives, diuretics, hypotension-producing drugs: Increased hypotensive effects

cimetidine: Increased risk of CNS and respiratory adverse reactions

CNS depressants: Additive CNS depressant effects, increased risk of habituation

hydroxyzine, other opioid analgesics: Increased analgesia, CNS depression, and hypotensive effects

MAO inhibitors: Increased risk of unpredictable, severe, sometimes fatal adverse reactions *metoclopramide:* Antagonized effects of metoclopramide on GI motility

naloxone: Antagonized analgesic, CNS, and respiratory depressant effects of oxymorphone

naltrexone: Withdrawal symptoms in oxymorphone-dependent patients

neuromuscular blockers: Additive respiratory depression

propofol: Increased incidence of bradycardia

ACTIVITIES

alcohol use: Additive CNS depressant effects, increased risk of habituation

Adverse Reactions

CNS: Asthenia, confusion, delusions, depersonalization, dizziness, drowsiness, euphoria, fatigue, headache, insomnia, light-headedness, nervousness, nightmares, restlessness, seizures, somnolence, tiredness, tremor, weakness

CV: Bradycardia, hypertension, hypotension, palpitations, tachycardia

EENT: Blurred vision, diplopia, dry mouth, laryngeal edema, laryngospasm, miosis, tinnitus

GI: Abdominal cramps or pain, anorexia, biliary colic, constipation, hepatotoxicity, nausea, paralytic ileus, vomiting

GU: Decreased urine output; dysuria; urinary frequency, hesitation or retention

MS: Muscle rigidity (with large doses), uncontrolled muscle movements

RESP: Apnea, atelectasis, bradypnea, bronchospasm, dyspnea, irregular breathing, respiratory depression, wheezing

SKIN: Allergic dermatitis, diaphoresis, erythema, flushing or swelling of face, pruritus, urticaria

Other: Angioedema, injection site burning, pain, redness, and swelling

Nursing Considerations

- Use with extreme caution in patients with conditions accompanied by hypoxia, hypercapnia, or decreased respiratory reserve such as asthma, chronic obstructive pulmonary disease or cor pulmonale, severe obesity, sleep apnea syndrome, myxedema, kyphoscoliosis, CNS depression or coma.
- Use with extreme caution in patients with increased intracranial pressure or a head injury because oxymorphone may obscure neurologic signs of increasing severity.

- Use cautiously in patients with circulatory shock because vaso-dilation produced by oxymorphone may further reduce cardiac output and blood pressure.
- Use oxymorphone cautiously in patients with mild hepatic function because plasma oxymophone level may increase, in-creaing the patient's risk of serious adverse reactions such as hypotension and respiratory depression.
- Use oxymorphone cautiously in elderly or debilitated patients and in patients with underlying medical conditions such as acute alcoholism, adrenocortical insufficiency, biliary tract dis-ease, CNS depression or coma, delirium tremens, kyphoscoliosis associated with respiratory depression, myxedema or hypothy-roidism, prostatic hypertrophy or urethral stricture, severe pul-monary or renal function, or toxic pyschosis.
- Monitor vital signs during oxymorphone therapy to detect res-piratory depression and hypotension, especially in elderly patents, debilitated patients, and patients with conditions ac-companied by hypoxia. In these patients, even moderate dosage may severely decrease pulmonary ventilation.
- **WARNING** Be aware that oxymophone may obscure neuro-logic signs of increased intracranial pressure or in the pres-ence of head injury, intracranial lesions or a preexisting in-crease in intracranial pressure, cause an exaggerated response to respiratory depression and elevated cerebrospinal fluid pressure. Monitor the patient closely and notify prescriber immediately if significant alterations occur in the patient's vi-tal signs or neurologic status.
- **WARNING** Know that oxymorphone therapy may obscure the clinical presentation of acute abdominal conditions or ag-gravate seizures in patients with seizure disorders. Provide protective measures such as seizure precautions and assess patients GI function regularly throughout the course of oxy-morphone therapy.
- Monitor patient closely for withdrawal symptoms following abrupt discontinuation of oxymorphone such as irritability, ab-dominal cramps, vomiting, diarrhea, restlessness, rhinorrhea, yawning, perspiration, chills, myalgia and mydriasis, and changes in vital signs. If present, alert prescriber.
- Monitor urinary and bowel status; constipation may become so severe that it causes ileus.
- Offer fluids to relieve dry mouth.

PATIENT TEACHING
- Warn patient that drug can cause physical dependence.

P

paclitaxel
Taxol

Class and Category
Chemical: Diterpenoid taxane
Therapeutic: Antimicrotubule antineoplastic
Pregnancy category: D

Indications and Dosages
▶ *To treat ovarian cancer*
I.V. INFUSION
Previously untreated adults. 135 mg/m^2 infused over 24 hr, followed by 75 mg/m^2 of cisplatin; repeated every 21 days. Alternatively, 175 mg/m^2 over 3 hr, followed by 75 mg/m^2 of cisplatin; repeated every 21 days.
Previously treated adults. 135 mg/m^2 or 175 mg/m^2 over 3 hr every 21 days.
▶ *To treat metastatic breast cancer, as a single agent or in combination with other drugs, as first-line treatment; to treat metastatic breast cancer if initial chemotherapy regimen fails or if relapse occurs within 6 months of adjuvant chemotherapy that included an anthracycline antineoplastic*
I.V. INFUSION
Adults. 175 mg/m^2 over 3 hr every 21 days.
▶ *To treat node-positive breast cancer sequentially with doxorubicin-containing combination therapy*
I.V. INFUSION
Adults. 175 mg/m^2 over 3 hr every 21 days for four courses, administered sequentially with doxorubicin-containing combination chemotherapy
▶ *To treat non–small-cell lung cancer*
I.V. INFUSION
Adults. 135 mg/m^2 over 24 hr, followed by 75 mg/m^2 of cisplatin.
▶ *To treat AIDS-related Kaposi's sarcoma*
I.V. INFUSION
Adults. 135 mg/m^2 over 3 hr every 21 days. Or, 100 mg/m^2 over 3 hr every 14 days.

DOSAGE ADJUSTMENT Subsequent dosage reduced by 20% if peripheral neuropathy occurs or if patient's neutrophil count falls below 500/mm^3 for 1 week or longer during paclitaxel therapy.

Mechanism of Action

Stabilizes microtubules, which normally contribute to cell structure and movement, and promotes microtubule assembly. In this way, paclitaxel inhibits the normal reorganization of the microtubule network, which is active during interphase and mitotic cellular functions. Paclitaxel also causes abnormal groups of microtubules to form throughout the cell cycle and multiple asters of microtubules to form during mitosis, when cell division normally occurs.

Incompatibilities

Don't let paclitaxel come in contact with plasticized polyvinyl chloride (PVC) equipment or devices, such as infusion bags or sets, to avoid exposing patient to plasticizer DEHP, which can be leached from these materials.

Contraindications

Hypersensitivity to paclitaxel or its components; hypersensitivity to other drugs formulated in polyoxyethylated castor oil, such as cyclosporine or teniposide; patients with solid tumors whose baseline neutrophil count is less than 1,500/mm^3; patients with AIDS-related Kaposi's sarcoma whose baseline neutrophil count is less than 1,000/mm^3

Interactions
DRUGS

blood-dyscrasia–causing drugs (such as cephalosporins and sulfasalazine): Increased risk of leukopenia and thrombocytopenia
bone marrow depressants (such as carboplatin and lomustine): Possibly additive bone marrow depression
vaccines, killed virus: Possibly decreased antibody response to vaccine
vaccines, live virus: Possibly decreased antibody response to vaccine, increased adverse effects of vaccine, and severe infection

Adverse Reactions

CNS: Motor dysfunction, paresthesia, peripheral neuropathy, seizures
CV: Arrhythmias (including bradycardia and ventricular tachycardia), AV block, chest pain, ECG changes, hypotension, MI
EENT: Mucositis

GI: Anorexia, diarrhea, elevated liver function test results, esophageal necrosis and ulceration, nausea, vomiting
GU: Nephrotoxicity
HEME: Anemia, leukopenia, neutropenia, thrombocytopenia
MS: Arthralgia, myalgia
RESP: Dyspnea
SKIN: Alopecia, extravasation with phlebitis or cellulitis, rash, urticaria
Other: Anaphylaxis, angioedema, hypersensitivity reaction, infection

Nursing Considerations

- Follow facility protocols for preparation and handling of antineoplastic drugs and for appropriate disposal of used equipment.
- Monitor CBC, including hematocrit, platelet count, and WBC with differential, before and frequently during paclitaxel therapy, as ordered.
- **WARNING** Don't administer paclitaxel to patients with AIDS-related Kaposi's sarcoma whose neutrophil count is below 1,000/mm^3. For all other indications, don't administer paclitaxel if neutrophil count falls below 1,500/mm^3.
- If paclitaxel solution comes in contact with your skin or mucosa, wash it off thoroughly with warm water. If drug comes in contact with your eye, irrigate it thoroughly with water or normal saline solution.
- Dilute and store drug in glass or polypropylene bottles or in plastic bags made of polypropylene or polyolefin, and administer it through polyethylene-line administration sets to avoid exposing patient to plasticizer DEHP, which can be leached from PVC supplies.
- Dilute paclitaxel with normal saline solution, D$_5$W, dextrose 5% in normal saline solution, or dextrose 5% in lactated Ringer's solution to a final concentration of 0.3 to 1.2 mg/ml. Use solution within 27 hours if stored at controlled room temperature and in ambient lighting.
- Use an in-line filter no greater than 0.22 micron when administering paclitaxel. Be aware that filter may need to be changed periodically if clogging occurs during infusion.
- To prevent a hypersensitivity reaction, expect to premedicate patient, as ordered, with 20 mg P.O. of dexamethasone (10 mg P.O. for treatment of AIDS-associated Kaposi's sarcoma) about 12 and 6 hours before paclitaxel administration; 50 mg of

diphenhydramine I.V. 30 to 60 minutes before paclitaxel administration; and 300 mg of cimetidine or 50 mg of ranitidine 30 to 60 minutes before paclitaxel administration.

- Observe patient continuously for first 30 minutes of each paclitaxel infusion and frequently thereafter. If anaphylaxis occurs, administer epinephrine, antihistamines, corticosteroids, or oxygen, as prescribed.
- Monitor vital signs during paclitaxel therapy, especially during the first hour of administration, assessing for signs of bradycardia or hypotension. Patients with a history of angina, cardiac conduction abnormalities, MI within past 6 months, or heart failure may be at increased risk for adverse cardiac effects.
- Maintain continuous cardiac monitoring, as prescribed, of patients with a history of cardiac conduction abnormalities.
- Be aware that adverse reactions can vary when paclitaxel is administered in combination therapy. Review information for all drugs administered as part of a specific regimen, including drug interactions and adverse effects.
- If extravasation occurs, stop the infusion immediately and notify prescriber. Then resume the infusion in another vein.
- Monitor patients who have, or have recently been exposed to, chicken pox and those who have herpes zoster for signs and symptoms of severe generalized disease.
- Be aware that patients who have previously received cytotoxic therapy and those who are receiving concurrent or consecutive radiation therapy are at risk for additive bone marrow depression.
- If patient develops thrombocytopenia, implement protective precautions according to facility policy.
- Assess for signs of infection, such as fever, if patient develops leukopenia. Expect to obtain appropriate specimens for culture and sensitivity testing.
- Before diluting paclitaxel, store it at controlled room temperature of 20° to 25° C (68° to 77° F). Protect from light.

PATIENT TEACHING

- Advise patient to have dental work completed before beginning paclitaxel treatment, if possible, or to defer such work until blood counts return to normal because drug can delay healing and cause gingival bleeding. Teach patient proper oral hygiene, and advise her to use a soft-bristled toothbrush.
- Advise patient to immediately report burning at injection site or other signs of extravasation.
- Also instruct patient to immediately report unusual bleeding or

bruising, black or tarry stools, blood in urine or stools, or red pinpoint spots on skin.

- Stress the importance of avoiding accidental cuts from sharp objects, such as razor blades and fingernail clippers, because excessive bleeding or infection may occur.
- Caution patient to avoid contact sports and other activities that put her at risk for bruising or injury.
- Suggest that patient with mucositis eat bland, soft foods served cold or at room temperature to decrease irritation.
- Instruct patient who develops bone marrow depression to avoid people with infections and to report fever, chills, cough, hoarseness, lower back or side pain, and painful or difficult urination because these signs and symptoms may signal an infection.
- Instruct patient to wash her hands immediately before touching her eyes or inside of her nose.
- Caution patient to avoid receiving immunizations unless approved by prescriber. Instruct her to avoid people who have recently received vaccines or to wear a protective mask that covers her nose and mouth when in their presence.
- Stress the importance of complying with the dosage regimen and of keeping follow-up medical appointments and appointments for laboratory tests.
- Inform patient that her hair should grow back after paclitaxel therapy has been completed.
- Advise patient to use contraception because of the risk of fetal harm from paclitaxel therapy. Instruct her to notify prescriber immediately if she becomes pregnant.

palonosetron hydrochloride
Aloxi

Class and Category
Chemical: Selective serotonin subtype 3 (5-HT$_3$) receptor antagonist
Therapeutic: Antiemetic
Pregnancy category: B

Indications and Dosages
▶ *To prevent acute and delayed nausea and vomiting from chemotherapy*
I.V. INJECTION
Adults. 0.25 mg over 30 sec approximately 30 min before start of chemotherapy.

▶ *To prevent postoperative nausea and vomiting for up to 24 hours following surgery*

I.V. INJECTION

Adults. 0.075 mg over 10 sec immediately before induction of anesthesia.

Mechanism of Action

Chemotherapy-induced nausea and vomiting may occur when a chemotherapeutic drug irritates the small intestine's mucosa, causing enterochromaffin cells within the mucosa to release serotonin (5-HT$_3$). Then, 5-HT$_3$ stimulates sympathetic receptors on afferent vagal nerve endings and the vagus nerve initiates the vomiting reflex.

Palonosetron selectively blocks 5-HT$_3$ receptors in afferent vagal nerve endings, preventing the vagus nerve from inducing the vomiting reflex and thereby averting or reducing the nausea and vomiting associated with chemotherapy. Palonosetron may also block 5-HT$_3$ receptors centrally, in the chemoreceptor trigger zone of the brain's area postrema.

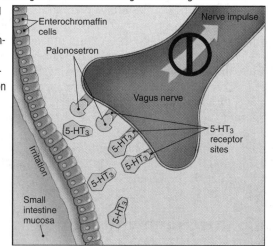

Incompatibilities

Palonosetron should not be mixed with any other drug.

Contraindications

Hypersensitivity to palonosetron or its components

Interactions

DRUGS
None reported.

Adverse Reactions

CNS: Anxiety, dizziness, drowsiness, fatigue, headache, insomnia, weakness
CV: Bradycardia, hypotension, prolonged QT interval, tachycardia
GI: Abdominal pain, constipation, diarrhea
SKIN: Dermatitis, pruritus, rash
Other: Hyperkalemia, hypersensitivity reactions, injection site reactions (burning, induration, pain)

Nursing Considerations

- Use palonosetron cautiously in patients who have or may develop prolonged cardiac conduction intervals—especially QT interval—such as those with congenital QT syndrome, hypokalemia, or hypomagnesemia; those taking a diuretic known to induce electrolyte abnormalities, an antiarrhythmic, or another drug that may prolong QT interval; and those who have received cumulative high-dose anthracycline therapy. With these patients, obtain a baseline ECG before giving palonosetron; repeat the ECG 15 minutes or 24 hours after giving drug, as ordered. Notify prescriber of any delayed conduction.
- Flush I.V. line before and after palonosetron administration with normal saline solution.
- Closely monitor any patient hypersensitive to other selective serotonin receptor antagonists for a similar reaction. If a reaction occurs, notify prescriber immediately.

PATIENT TEACHING

- Advise patient to avoid hazardous activities until drug's CNS effects are known.
- Instruct patient to notify prescriber of any hypersensitivity reaction, such as rash or allergic dermatitis.

pamidronate disodium

Aredia

Class and Category

Chemical: Bisphosphonate
Therapeutic: Antihypercalcemic, bone resorption inhibitor
Pregnancy category: D

Indications and Dosages

▶ *To treat cancer-induced hypercalcemia that's inadequately managed by oral hydration alone*

I.V. INFUSION

Adults. 60 to 90 mg over 2 to 24 hr as a single dose when corrected serum calcium level is 12 to 13.5 mg/dl; 90 mg over 2 to 24 hr when corrected serum calcium level is greater than 13.5 mg/dl. May be repeated as prescribed after 7 days if hypercalcemia recurs.

DOSAGE ADJUSTMENT For patients with renal failure, dosage is limited to 30 mg over 4 to 24 hr, as prescribed. For patients with cardiac or renal failure, drug is given in a smaller volume of fluid or at a slower rate, as prescribed.

▶ *To treat moderate to severe Paget's disease of bone*
I.V. INFUSION

Adults. 30 mg daily over 4 hr on 3 consecutive days for a total dose of 90 mg. Repeated as needed and tolerated.

▶ *To treat osteolytic bone metastases of breast cancer*
I.V. INFUSION

Adults. 90 mg over 2 hr every 3 to 4 wk.

▶ *To treat osteolytic bone metastases of multiple myeloma*
I.V. INFUSION

Adults. 90 mg over 4 hr every mo.

Mechanism of Action

Inhibits bone resorption, possibly by impairing attachment of osteoclast precursors to mineralized bone matrix, thus reducing the rate of bone turnover in Paget's disease and osteolytic metastases. Pamidronate also reduces the flow of calcium from resorbing bone into the bloodstream.

Incompatibilities

Don't mix pamidronate with calcium-containing infusion solutions, such as Ringer's solution.

Contraindications

Hypersensitivity to pamidronate, other bisphosphonates, or their components

Interactions

DRUGS

calcium-containing preparations; vitamin D preparations, such as calcifediol and calcitriol: Antagonized pamidronate effects when used to treat hypercalcemia

thalidomide: Possibly increased risk of renal dysfunction in patients with multiple myeloma

Adverse Reactions

CNS: Confusion, fever, psychosis
CV: Hypotension
GI: Abdominal cramps, anorexia, GI bleeding, indigestion, nausea, vomiting
GU: Azotemia, glomerulosclerosis, renal failure, renal toxicity
HEME: Leukopenia, lymphopenia
MS: Bone pain, muscle spasms or stiffness, osteonecrosis (mainly of jaw)
RESP: Dyspnea
Other: Anaphylaxis, angioedema, hyperkalemia, hypernatremia, hypocalcemia, hypokalemia, hypomagnesemia, hypophosphatemia, injection site pain and swelling

Nursing Considerations

- Make sure that patient has had a dental checkup before invasive dental procedures during pamidronate therapy, especially if the patient has cancer; is receiving chemotherapy, head or neck radiation, or corticosteroid therapy; or has poor oral hygiene because the risk of osteonecrosis is increased in these patients.
- Stay alert for fever during the first 3 days of pamidronate therapy, especially in patients receiving high doses. If fever develops, obtain the patient's CBC with differential, as ordered.
- Obtain serum creatinine level before each treatment. Notify prescriber of abnormal results because drug may need to be held or dosage adjusted until the creatinine level returns to normal.
- Be aware that patients have developed renal failure requiring dialysis with just one dose of pamidronate.
- Monitor patient with a history of thyroid surgery closely because he may be predisposed to hypocalcemia during pamidronate therapy.
- Assess patient with anemia, leukopenia, or thrombocytopenia for worsening of the condition during first 2 weeks of pamidronate therapy.

PATIENT TEACHING

- Stress the importance of complying with prescribed administration schedule for pamidronate.
- Advise patient to avoid calcium and vitamin D supplements during pamidronate therapy.
- Instruct patient on proper oral hygiene and on need to notify prescriber about invasive dental procedures.

pantoprazole sodium

Pantoloc (CAN), Protonix I.V.

Class and Category

Chemical: Substituted benzimidazole
Therapeutic: Antiulcer, gastric acid proton pump inhibitor
Pregnancy category: B

Indications and Dosages

▶ *To treat gastroesophageal reflux disease (GERD)*

I.V. INFUSION

Adults. 40 mg daily infused over 2 min or 15 min for 7 to 10 days, followed by oral doses.

▶ *To treat pathological hypersecretion associated with Zollinger-Ellison syndrome or other neoplastic conditions*

I.V. INFUSION

Adults. 80 mg every 12 hr infused over 2 min or 15 min; adjusted based on patient's acid output measurements up to 80 mg every 8 hr.

Route	Onset	Peak	Duration
I.V.	1 day	Unknown	1 wk

Mechanism of Action

Interferes with gastric acid secretion by inhibiting the hydrogen-potassium-adenosine triphosphatase (H^+-K^+-ATPase) enzyme system, or proton pump, in gastric parietal cells. Normally, the proton pump uses energy from the hydrolysis of ATPase to drive H^+ and chloride (Cl^-) out of parietal cells and into the stomach lumen in exchange for potassium (K^+), which leaves the stomach lumen and enters parietal cells. After this exchange, H^+ and Cl^- combine in the stomach to form hydrochloric acid (HCl). Pantoprazole irreversibly inhibits the final step in gastric acid production by blocking the exchange of intracellular H^+ and extracellular K^+, thus preventing H^+ from entering the stomach and additional HCl from forming.

Incompatibilities

Midazolam and products containing zinc may cause precipitation or discoloration.

Contraindications

Hypersensitivity to pantoprazole, substituted benzimidazoles (omeprazole, lansoprazole, rabeprazole sodium), or their components

Interactions
DRUGS
ampicillin, cyanocobalamin, digoxin, iron salts, ketoconazole: Possibly impaired absorption of these drugs
atazanavir: Substantially decreased plasma atazanavir level and reduced therapeutic effect
warfarin: Increased INR, PT, and bleeding risk

Adverse Reactions
CNS: Anxiety, asthenia, confusion, dizziness, headache, hypertonia, hypokinesia, insomnia, malaise, migraine, speech disorder vertigo
CV: Chest pain, hypercholesterolemia, hyperlipidemia
EENT: Anterior ischemic optic neuropathy, blurred vision, increased salivation, pharyngitis, rhinitis, sinusitis, tinnitus
ENDO: Hyperglycemia
GI: Abdominal pain, constipation, diarrhea, elevated liver function tests results, flatulence, gastroenteritis, hepatotoxicity, indigestion, nausea, pancreatitis, vomiting
GU: Elevated serum creatinine level, interstitial nephritis
HEME: Pancytopenia
MS: Arthralgia, back or neck pain, rhabdomyolysis
RESP: Bronchitis, dyspnea, increased cough, upper respiratory tract infection
SKIN: Erythema multiforme, rash, Stevens-Johnson syndrome, toxic epidermal necrolysis
Other: Anaphylaxis, angioedema, elevated creatine kinase and phosphokinase levels, flulike symptoms, generalized pain, hyperuricemia, infection, injection site reaction

Nursing Considerations
- Ensure the continuity of gastric acid suppression during transition from oral to I.V. pantoprazole (or vice versa); even a brief interruption of suppression can lead to serious complications.
- Don't give pantoprazole within 4 weeks of testing for *Helicobacter pylori* because antibiotics, proton pump inhibitors, and bismuth preparations suppress *H. pylori* and may lead to false-negative results. Be aware that drug may cause false-positive results in urine screening tests for tetrahydrocannabinol. Obtain guidelines for pantoprazole use from prescriber before testing.
- Flush I.V. line with D_5W, normal saline solution, or lactated Ringer's injection before and after giving drug.
- When giving I.V. over 2 minutes, reconstitute with 10 ml of normal saline solution injection. Solution may be stored up to

2 hours at room temperature.

- When giving I.V. over 15 minutes, reconstitute with 10 ml normal saline solution injection. Then, further reconstitute with 100 ml (for GERD) or 80 ml (for pathological hypersecretion in Zollinger-Ellison syndrome) of D_5W, normal saline injection, or lactated Ringer's injection. Solution may be stored up to 2 hours before further dilution and up to 22 hours before use.
- Monitor PT or INR, as ordered, if patient takes an oral anticoagulant.
- Be aware that, if drug is given for more than 3 years, patient may not be able to absorb vitamin B_{12} because of hypochlorhydria or achlorhydria. Treatment for cyanocobalamin deficiency may be needed.

PATIENT TEACHING
- Advise patient to expect relief of symptoms within 2 weeks of starting therapy.
- Advise patient who takes warfarin to follow bleeding precautions and to notify prescriber immediately if bleeding occurs.

paricalcitol

Zemplar

Class and Category

Chemical: Sterol derivative, vitamin D analogue
Therapeutic: Antihyperparathyroid
Pregnancy category: Not rated

Indications and Dosages

▶ *To prevent and treat secondary hyperparathyroidism in patients with chronic renal failure stage 3 or 4*

I.V. INJECTION

Adults. *Initial:* 0.04 to 0.1 mcg/kg (2.8 to 7 mcg) no more than every other day at any time during dialysis. *Maintenance:* If initial dosage doesn't produce a satisfactory response, 2 to 4 mcg given every 2 to 4 wk. *Maximum:* 0.24 mcg/kg/dose or up to 16.8 mcg/dose.

Children age 5 and older. *Initial:* 0.04 mcg/kg three times weekly if baseline intact parathyroid hormone (iPTH) level is less than 500 pg/ml. Give 0.08 mcg/kg three times weekly if baseline iPTH level is 500 pg/ml or more. *Maintenance:* If initial dosage isn't adequate, adjust it in 0.04-mcg/kg increments as needed and ordered.

DOSAGE ADJUSTMENT If serum PTH level remains the same

or increases, dosage is increased. If serum PTH level decreases by less than 30%, dosage is increased. If serum PTH level decreases by 30% to 60%, dosage is maintained. If serum PTH level decreases by more than 60%, dosage is decreased. If serum PTH level is 1.5 to 3 times the upper limit of normal, dosage is maintained.

DOSAGE ADJUSTMENT Dosage is immediately reduced or stopped if serum calcium level is elevated or serum calcium-phosphorus product exceeds 75. Dosage restarted at a lower dose when these levels return to normal.

Route	Onset	Peak	Duration
I.V.	Unknown	Unknown	15 hr

Mechanism of Action

Reduces serum PTH level by an unknown mechanism. In chronic renal failure, decreased renal synthesis of vitamin D leads to chronic hypocalcemia. In response, parathyroid glands secrete PTH to stimulate vitamin D synthesis, but serum calcium levels can't normalize because of renal failure.

Contraindications

Evidence of vitamin D toxicity, hypercalcemia, hypersensitivity to paricalcitol or components

Interactions

DRUGS

atazanavir, clarithromycin, indinavir, itraconazole, ketoconazole, nefazodone, nelfinavir, ritonavir, saquinavir, telithromycin, voriconazole: Increased effects of oral paricalcitol

digoxin: Possibly increased risk of digitalis toxicity

drugs, such as cholestyramine, that impair absorption of fat-soluble vitamins: Possibly impaired absorption of oral paricalcitol

Adverse Reactions

CNS: Arthritis, asthenia, chills, depression, dizziness, fever, headache, insomnia, light-headedness, malaise, neuropathy, syncope, vertigo

CV: Cardiomyopathy, chest pain, congestive heart failure, edema, hypertension, hypotension, MI, orthostatic hypotension, palpitations

EENT: Amblopia, dry mouth, epistaxis, pharyngitis, retinal abnormality, rhinitis, sinusitis, taste perversion

ENDO: Hypoglycemia
GI: Abdominal pain, constipation, diarrhea, dyspepsia, gastritis, gastroenteritis, GI bleeding, nausea, vomiting
GU: Abnormal kidney function, uremia, UTI
MS: Back pain, leg cramps, myalgia
RESP: Bronchitis, increased cough, pneumonia
SKIN: Ecchymosis, hypertrophy, pruritus, rash (including vesiculobullous), ulceration, urticaria
Other: Acidosis; allergic reaction; dehydration; facial, oral or generalized edema; gout; hyperkalemia; hyperphosphatemia; hypervolemia; hypokalemia; infections; influenza; sepsis

Nursing Considerations

- Before giving paricalcitol, look for particles and discoloration; if present, discard drug.
- Give as I.V. bolus; discard unused portion.
- Monitor serum calcium and phosphorus levels, as ordered, twice weekly to guide dosage adjustments and then monthly.
- **WARNING** Drug may lead to vitamin D toxicity and hypercalcemia. Look for early evidence, including arthralgia, constipation, dry mouth, headache, metallic taste, myalgia, nausea, somnolence, vomiting, and weakness. Also look for late evidence, including albuminuria, anorexia, arrhythmias, azotemia, conjunctivitis (calcific), decreased libido, elevated BUN and serum ALT and AST levels, vascular calcification, hypercholesterolemia, hypertension, hyperthermia, irritability, mild acidosis, nephrocalcinosis, nocturia, pancreatitis, photophobia, polydipsia, polyuria, pruritus, rhinorrhea, and weight loss.
- If toxicity occurs, notify prescriber immediately and expect to decrease or stop drug. Place patient on bed rest and give fluids, low-calcium diet, and laxative, as prescribed. For hypercalcemic crisis and dehydration, expect to infuse normal saline solution and a loop diuretic to prompt renal calcium excretion.
- Expect to check patient's serum PTH level every 3 months.
- If patient also takes digoxin, monitor her for evidence of digitalis glycoside toxicity, which is potentiated by hypercalcemia.
- Store drug at 25° C (77° F).

PATIENT TEACHING

- Advise patient to follow high-calcium, low-phosphorus diet.
- Explain that patient may need phosphate binders to control serum phosphorus level.
- Review early evidence of hypercalcemia and vitamin D toxicity. Tell patient to contact prescriber immediately if it develops.

- Urge patient to avoid hazardous activities until drug's adverse CNS effects are known.
- If patient takes digoxin, explain evidence of toxicity and the need to contact prescriber immediately if it develops.

penicillin G potassium
Megacillin (CAN), Pentids, Pfizerpen
penicillin G sodium
Class and Category
Chemical: Penicillin
Therapeutic: Antibiotic
Pregnancy category: B

Indications and Dosages
▶ *To treat systemic infections caused by gram-positive organisms (including* Bacillus anthracis, Corynebacterium diphtheriae, *enterococci,* Listeria monocytogenes, Staphylococcus aureus, *and* Staphylococcus epidermidis*), gram-negative organisms (including* Neisseria gonorrhoeae, Neisseria meningitidis, Pasteurella multocida, *and* Streptobacillus moniliformis *[rat-bite fever]), and gram-positive anaerobes (including* Actinomyces israelii *[actinomycosis],* Clostridium perfringens, Clostridium tetani, Peptococcus *species,* Peptostreptococcus *species, and spirochetes, especially* Treponema cara-teum *[pinta],* Treponema pallidum, *and* Treponema pertenue *[yaws])*
I.V. INFUSION
Adults and adolescents. 1 to 5 million units every 4 to 6 hr. *Maximum:* 80 million units daily.
Children. 8,333 to 16,667 units/kg every 4 hr or 12,500 to 25,000 units/kg every 6 hr.
▶ *To treat bacterial meningitis*
I.V. INFUSION
Adults. 50,000 units/kg every 4 hr or 24 million units daily in divided doses every 2 to 4 hr.

Mechanism of Action
Inhibits the final stage of bacterial cell wall synthesis by competitively binding to penicillin-binding proteins inside the cell wall. Penicillin-binding proteins are responsible for various steps in bacterial cell wall synthesis. By binding to these proteins, penicillin leads to cell wall lysis.

Contraindications
Hypersensitivity to penicillin or its components

Incompatibilities
Don't mix any penicillin in the same syringe or container with aminoglycosides because aminoglycosides will be inactivated. Don't mix penicillin G with drugs that may result in a pH below 5.5 or above 8.

Interactions
DRUGS

ACE inhibitors, potassium-containing drugs, potassium-sparing diuretics: Increased risk of hyperkalemia (penicillin G potassium)

chloramphenicol, erythromycin, sulfonamides, tetracycline, thrombolytics: Possibly interference with penicillin's bactericidal effect

cholestyramine, colestipol: Possibly impaired absorption of oral penicillin G

methotrexate: Decreased methotrexate clearance, increased risk of toxicity

oral contraceptives: Decreased contraceptive effectiveness (with penicillin V)

probenecid: Increased blood penicillin level

FOODS

acidic beverages, such as fruit juices: Possibly altered effects of oral penicillin G

Adverse Reactions
CNS: Confusion, dizziness, dysphasia, hallucinations, headache, lethargy, sciatic nerve irritation, seizures

CV: Labile blood pressure, palpitations

EENT: Black "hairy" tongue, oral candidiasis, stomatitis, taste perversion

GI: Abdominal pain, diarrhea, elevated liver function test results (transient), indigestion, nausea, pseudomembranous colitis

GU: Interstitial nephritis (acute), vaginal candidiasis

MS: Muscle twitching

SKIN: Rash

Other: Electrolyte imbalances; injection site necrosis, pain, or redness

Nursing Considerations
- Obtain body tissue and fluid samples for culture and sensitivity tests as ordered before giving first dose. Expect to begin drug therapy before test results are known.

- Reconstitute vials of penicillin for injection with sterile water for injection, D_5W, or sodium chloride for injection.
- Give penicillin at least 1 hour before giving other antibiotics.
- Assess patient for signs of secondary infection, such as profuse, watery diarrhea.
- Monitor serum sodium level and assess patiebt for early signs of heart failure in patients receiving high doses of penicillin G sodium.
- When giving penicillin G potassium to patient at risk for hypertension or fluid overload, be aware that each gram of pencillin G potassium also contains 1.02 mEq of sodium.
- Monitor patients with renal impairment closely throughout therapy because they're at increased risk for toxic reactions as penicillin G is primarily excreted primarily by the kidneys.

PATIENT TEACHING
- Instruct patient to report previous allergies to penicillins and to immediately report adverse reactions, including fever.

pentamidine isethionate

Pentacarinat (CAN), Pentam 300

Class and Category

Chemical: Diamidine derivative
Therapeutic: Antiprotozoal
Pregnancy category: C

Indications and Dosages

▶ *To treat* Pneumocystis jiroveci (carinii) *pneumonia*

I.V. INFUSION

Adults and children. 4 mg/kg daily infused over 1 to 2 hr for 14 to 21 days.

DOSAGE ADJUSTMENT Dosage possibly reduced or I.V. infusion time or dosing interval extended in renal failure.

Mechanism of Action

May bind to DNA and inhibit DNA replication in *Pneumocystis jiroveci* (formerly *carinii*). Pentamidine also may inhibit dihydrofolate reductase, an enzyme needed to convert dihydrofolic acid to tetrahydrofolic acid in this organism. This action inhibits the formation of coenzymes that are essential to the growth and replication of *P. jiroveci.*

Incompatibilities

Don't mix pentamidine with other drugs or with saline solutions because precipitation may occur.

Contraindications

History of anaphylactic reaction to pentamidine or its components, hypersensitivity to pentamidine or its components

Interactions

DRUGS

blood-dyscrasia–causing drugs, bone marrow depressants: Increased risk of adverse hematologic effects

didanosine: Increased risk of pancreatitis

erythromycin: Increased risk of torsades de pointes

foscarnet: Increased risk of severe but reversible hypocalcemia, hypomagnesemia, and nephrotoxicity

nephrotoxic drugs: Increased risk of nephrotoxicity

Adverse Reactions

CNS: Chills, confusion, dizziness, fatigue, fever, hallucinations, headache

CV: Arrhythmias, edema, hypotension, prolonged QT interval, torsades de pointes, ventricular tachycardia

EENT: Bitter or metallic taste

ENDO: Diabetes mellitus, hyperglycemia, hypoglycemia

GI: Abdominal pain, anorexia, diarrhea, elevated liver function test results, nausea, vomiting, pancreatitis

GU: Elevated serum creatinine level

HEME: Anemia, leukopenia, thrombocytopenia, unusual bleeding or bruising

MS: Myalgia

SKIN: Night sweats, rash

Other: Hyperchloremic acidosis, hyperkalemia, hypocalcemia, hypomagnesemia, infusion site phlebitis

Nursing Considerations

- To prepare initial dilution, add 3 to 5 ml of sterile water for injection or D_5W to 300-mg vial of pentamidine. Use drug prepared with D_5W within 24 hours of reconstitution, and protect from light until ready to use. Further dilute in 50 to 250 ml of D_5W, and infuse over 1 to 2 hours.
- Keep patient supine during infusion, and monitor blood pressure frequently during and after administration. Keep emergency resuscitation equipment readily available.

- Assess for hypoglycemia and arrhythmias. Although uncommon, these adverse reactions can be severe.
- Monitor CBC; platelet count; liver function test results; BUN, serum creatinine and calcium, and blood glucose levels; and ECG tracing throughout therapy, as ordered.
- Monitor blood glucose level because pentamidine use can induce insulin release from pancreas, causing severe hypoglycemia that can last from 1 day to several weeks.
- Be aware that hyperglycemia and diabetes mellitus can occur up to several months after parenteral pentamidine therapy stops.
- Before reconstituting pentamidine, store it at 2° to 8° C (36° to 46° F) and protect from light.

PATIENT TEACHING
- Advise patient to avoid potentially hazardous activities until pentamidine's CNS effects are known.
- Instruct patient to report unusual bleeding or bruising and to take precautions to avoid bleeding, such as using a soft-bristled toothbrush and an electric shaver.
- Caution patient about possible hypoglycemic effects of pentamidine therapy.
- Advise patient to undergo follow-up testing for diabetes mellitus, which can occur up to several months after pentamidine therapy is completed.

pentazocine lactate
Talwin

Class, Category, and Schedule
Chemical: Synthetic opioid
Therapeutic: Analgesic
Pregnancy category: C
Controlled substance schedule: IV

Indications and Dosages
▶ *To relieve moderate to severe pain*
I.V. INJECTION
Adults. *Initial:* 30 mg every 3 to 4 hr, p.r.n. *Maximum:* 30 mg/single dose I.V., 360 mg/24 hr
▶ *To relieve obstetric pain*
I.V. INJECTION
Adults. 20 mg when contractions become regular; repeated 2 or 3 times every 2 to 3 hr, as prescribed.

Route	Onset	Peak	Duration
I.V.	2 to 3 min	15 to 30 min	2 to 3 hr

Mechanism of Action
Binds with opiate receptors, primarily kappa and sigma receptors, at many CNS sites to alter the perception of and emotional response to pain.

Incompatibilities
Don't mix pentazocine in same syringe with a soluble barbiturate because precipitation will occur.

Contraindications
Hypersensitivity to pentazocine or its components

Interactions
DRUGS

anticholinergics: Increased risk of urine retention and severe constipation

antidiarrheals, antiperistaltics: Increased risk of severe constipation and CNS depression

antihypertensives, diuretics, other hypotension-producing drugs: Additive hypotensive effects

buprenorphine: Decreased pentazocine effectiveness, increased respiratory depression

CNS depressants: Increased CNS depression, increased risk of habituation

hydroxyzine, other opioid analgesics: Increased analgesia, CNS depression, and hypotensive effects

MAO inhibitors: Increased risk of unpredictable, severe, and sometimes fatal adverse reactions

metoclopramide: Antagonized metoclopramide effects on GI motility

naloxone: Antagonized analgesic, CNS, and respiratory depressant effects of pentazocine

naltrexone: Withdrawal symptoms in patients physically dependent on pentazocine

neuromuscular blockers: Increased respiratory depression

ACTIVITIES

alcohol use: Additive CNS depression and increased risk of habituation

Adverse Reactions
CNS: Chills, dizziness, drowsiness, euphoria, fatigue, headache, insomnia, light-headedness, nervousness, nightmares, paresthesia,

restlessness, weakness
CV: Hypotension, tachycardia
EENT: Blurred vision, diplopia, dry mouth, laryngeal edema, laryngospasm
GI: Constipation, hepatotoxicity, nausea, vomiting
GU: Decreased urine output, dysuria, urinary frequency, urine retention
MS: Muscle rigidity (with large doses)
RESP: Atelectasis, bronchospasm, dyspnea, hypoventilation, wheezing
SKIN: Diaphoresis, erythema multiforme, facial flushing, pruritus, rash, Stevens-Johnson syndrome, toxic epidermal necrolysis, urticaria
Other: Facial edema; injection site burning, pain, redness, or swelling; physical and psychological dependence

Nursing Considerations

- Use pentazocine with extreme caution in patients who have head injury, intracranial lesion, or increased intracranial pressure because drug may mask neurologic signs and symptoms.
- Use drug cautiously in patients who are physically dependent on opioid agonists because drug may prompt withdrawal symptoms; in patients with acute MI because drug's cardiovascular effects can increase cardiac workload; in patients with renal or hepatic dysfunction because drug is metabolized in the liver and excreted in urine; and in patients with respiratory conditions because drug depresses the respiratory system.
- After giving parenteral form, expect to taper dosage gradually, as prescribed, to reduce the risk of withdrawal symptoms.

PATIENT TEACHING
- Caution that prolonged use of pentazocine cause dependence.
- Advise patient to avoid potentially hazardous activities until drug's CNS effects are known.
- Caution patient not to use alcohol or OTC drugs without consulting prescriber.
- Advise patient to notify prescriber if she notices signs of an allergic reaction, such as a rash or itching.

pentobarbital sodium
Nembutal

Class, Category, and Schedule
Chemical: Barbiturate

Therapeutic: Anticonvulsant, sedative-hypnotic
Pregnancy category: D
Controlled substance schedule: II

Indications and Dosages

▶ *To provide short-term treatment of insomnia*

I.V. INJECTION

Adults. *Initial:* 100 mg, with additional small doses at 1-min intervals, as prescribed. *Maximum:* 500 mg.

▶ *To provide emergency treatment of seizures associated with eclampsia, meningitis, status epilepticus, tetanus, or toxic reactions to local anesthetics or strychnine*

I.V. INJECTION

Adults. 100 mg, with additional small doses at 1-min intervals, as prescribed. *Maximum:* 500 mg.

Children. 50 mg, with additional small doses at 1-min intervals, as prescribed, until desired effect occurs.

DOSAGE ADJUSTMENT Dosage possibly reduced for elderly or debilitated patients and those with hepatic dysfunction.

Route	Onset	Peak	Duration
I.V.	In 1 min	Unknown	15 min

Mechanism of Action

Inhibits ascending conduction of impulses in the reticular formation, which controls CNS arousal to produce drowsiness, hypnosis, and sedation. Pentobarbital also decreases the spread of seizure activity in the cortex, thalamus, and limbic system. It promotes an increased threshold for electrical stimulation in the motor cortex, which may contribute to its anticonvulsant properties.

Contraindications

Hepatic disease; history of addiction to hypnotics or sedatives; hypersensitivity to pentobarbital, other barbiturates, or their components; nephritis; porphyria; severe respiratory disease with airway obstruction or dyspnea

Interactions

DRUGS

acetaminophen: Possibly decreased effects of acetaminophen (with long-term pentobarbital use)

carbamazepine, chloramphenicol, corticosteroids, cyclosporine, dacar-

bazine, digoxin, disopyramide, doxycycline, griseofulvin, metronidazole, oral contraceptives, phenylbutazone, quinidine, theophyllines, vitamin D: Decreased effectiveness of these drugs

CNS depressants: Increased CNS depression and risk of habituation

divalproex sodium, valproic acid: Increased risk of CNS toxicity and neurotoxicity

guanadrel, guanethidine: Possibly increased risk of orthostatic hypotension

halogenated hydrocarbon anesthetics: Increased risk of hepatotoxicity (with long-term pentobarbital use)

haloperidol: Possibly decreased blood haloperidol level, possibly altered seizure pattern or frequency

hydantoins: Possibly interference with hydantoin metabolism

leucovorin: Possibly decreased anticonvulsant effect of pentobarbital

maprotiline: Possibly enhanced CNS depression and decreased therapeutic effects of pentobarbital

mexiletine: Possibly decreased blood mexiletine level

oral anticoagulants: Possibly decreased therapeutic effects of these drugs, possibly increased risk of bleeding when pentobarbital is discontinued

tricyclic antidepressants: Possibly decreased therapeutic effects of these drugs

ACTIVITIES
alcohol use: Increased CNS depression

Adverse Reactions

CNS: Agitation, anxiety, ataxia, confusion, delusions, depression, dizziness, drowsiness, fever, hallucinations, headache, insomnia, irritability, nervousness, nightmares, paradoxical stimulation, seizures, syncope, tremor
CV: Orthostatic hypotension
EENT: Vision changes
GI: Anorexia, constipation, hepatic dysfunction, nausea, vomiting
HEME: Agranulocytosis
MS: Arthralgia, bone pain, muscle twitching or weakness
RESP: Respiratory depression
SKIN: Exfoliative dermatitis, rash, Stevens-Johnson syndrome
Other: Physical and psychological dependence, weight loss

Nursing Considerations

- Inject pentobarbital at 50 mg or less/minute to prevent adverse respiratory and circulatory reactions.
- Be aware that pentobarbital shouldn't be given during third

trimester of pregnancy because repeated use can cause dependence in neonate. It also shouldn't be given to breast-feeding women because it may cause CNS depression in infants.

- Closely monitor blood pressure, pulse, and respirations during administration. Keep emergency equipment and drugs nearby in case respiratory depression or adverse hemodynamic effects occur. Be aware that patients with cardiovascular disease are at increased risk for adverse circulatory reactions, particularly if drug is administered too fast, and that those with pulmonary diseases associated with obstruction or dyspnea are at increased risk for ventilatory depression. Anticipate the risk of hypotension, even when giving drug at recommended rate.
- Monitor patients for hypersensitivity reactions, such as bronchospasm, trouble breathing, facial edema, and urticaria, especially those with a history of asthma, angioedema, or urticaria.
- Anticipate that pentobarbital's CNS effects may exacerbate major depression, suicidal tendencies, or other mental disorders.
- Be aware that pentobarbital may cause paradoxical stimulation (excitement, euphoria, restlessness) in patients with acute pain, children, and elderly or debilitated patients. Elderly or debilitated patients are also more likely to experience such adverse CNS reactions as confusion and depression; monitor these patients closely and take safety precautions.
- Assess hyperthyroid patients for worsened symptoms, such as increased nervousness and palpitations.
- Be aware that barbiturate-induced respiratory depression may cause complications in patients with severe anemia.
- Be aware that drug may trigger signs and symptoms in patients with acute intermittent porphyria.
- If patient shows premonitory signs of hepatic coma, withhold drug and notify prescriber immediately.
- Monitor I.V. site closely and be careful to avoid extravasation. Drug is highly alkaline and may cause local tissue damage and necrosis.
- Store drug at 2° to 15° (36° to 59° F) in a tightly closed container.

PATIENT TEACHING
- Inform patient that pentobarbital is habit-forming.
- Advise patient to avoid potentially hazardous activities until pentobarbital's CNS effects are known.
- Urge patient to avoid alcohol and other CNS depressants because they may increase drug's adverse CNS effects.

perphenazine

Apo-Perphenazine (CAN), PMS Perphenazine (CAN), Trilafon, Trilafon Concentrate

Class and Category

Chemical: Piperazine phenothiazine
Therapeutic: Antiemetic
Pregnancy category: Not rated

Indications and Dosages

▶ *To treat severe nausea and vomiting*

I.V. INFUSION, I.V. INJECTION

Adults and adolescents. 1 mg every 1 to 2 min, up to total of 5 mg.

DOSAGE ADJUSTMENT Initial dose possibly reduced and gradually increased for elderly, emaciated, or debilitated patients. Lower end of adult dosage range possibly needed for adolescents.

Mechanism of Action

Prevents nausea and vomiting by inhibiting or blocking dopamine receptors in the medullary chemoreceptor trigger zone and peripherally by blocking the vagus nerve in the GI tract.

Contraindications

Blood dyscrasias; bone marrow depression; cerebral arteriosclerosis; coma; concurrent use of CNS depressants (large doses); coronary artery disease; hepatic impairment; hypersensitivity to perphenazine, other phenothiazines, or their components; myeloproliferative disorders; severe CNS depression; severe hypertension or hypotension; subcortical brain damage

Interactions

DRUGS

amantadine, anticholinergics, antidyskinetics, antihistamines: Increased adverse anticholinergic effects
amphetamines: Decreased therapeutic effects of both drugs
anticonvulsants: Decreased seizure threshold, inhibited metabolism and toxicity of anticonvulsant
antithyroid drugs: Increased risk of agranulocytosis
apomorphine: Additive CNS depression, decreased emetic response to apomorphine if perphenazine is given first

appetite suppressants (except phenmetrazine): Antagonized anorectic effect of appetite suppressants

beta blockers: Increased blood levels of both drugs and risk of arrhythmias, hypotension, irreversible retinopathy, and tardive dyskinesia

bromocriptine: Possibly interference with bromocriptine's effects

CNS depressants: Increased CNS and respiratory depression, increased hypotensive effects

dopamine: Antagonized peripheral vasoconstriction with high doses of dopamine

ephedrine: Decreased vasopressor response to ephedrine

epinephrine: Blocked alpha-adrenergic effects of epinephrine, possibly causing severe hypotension and tachycardia

hepatotoxic drugs: Increased risk of hepatotoxicity

hypotension-causing drugs: Increased risk of severe orthostatic hypotension

levodopa: Inhibited antidyskinetic effects of levodopa

lithium: Possibly neurotoxicity (disorientation, extrapyramidal symptoms, unconsciousness)

maprotiline, tricyclic antidepressants: Prolonged and intensified sedative and anticholinergic effects of these drugs or perphenazine

metrizamide: Decreased seizure threshold

opioid analgesics: Increased CNS and respiratory depression, increased risk of orthostatic hypotension and severe constipation

ototoxic drugs (especially antibiotics): Possibly masking of some symptoms of ototoxicity, such as dizziness, tinnitus, and vertigo

probucol, other drugs that prolong QT interval: Prolonged QT interval, which may increase risk of ventricular tachycardia

thiazide diuretics: Possibly hyponatremia and water intoxication

ACTIVITIES

alcohol use: Increased CNS and respiratory depression, hypotensive effects, and risk of heatstroke

Adverse Reactions

CNS: Behavioral changes, cerebral edema, dizziness, drowsiness, extrapyramidal reactions (such as akathisia, dystonia, pseudoparkinsonism), fever, headache, neuroleptic malignant syndrome, seizures, syncope, tardive dyskinesia (persistent)

CV: Bradycardia, cardiac arrest, hypertension, hypotension, orthostatic hypotension, tachycardia

EENT: Blurred vision, dry mouth, glaucoma, laryngeal edema, miosis, mydriasis, nasal congestion, ocular changes (corneal opacification, retinopathy)

ENDO: Decreased libido, galactorrhea, gynecomastia, syndrome of inappropriate ADH secretion
GI: Anorexia, constipation, diarrhea, fecal impaction, nausea, vomiting
GU: Bladder paralysis, ejaculation failure, menstrual irregularities, polyuria, urinary frequency, urinary incontinence, urine retention
HEME: Agranulocytosis, eosinophilia, hemolytic anemia, leukopenia, pancytopenia, thrombocytopenic purpura
RESP: Asthma
SKIN: Diaphoresis, eczema, erythema, exfoliative dermatitis, hyperpigmentation, jaundice, pallor, photosensitivity, pruritus, urticaria
Other: Anaphylaxis, angioedema

Nursing Considerations

- Wear gloves when working with perphenazine because the parenteral solution may cause contact dermatitis.
- Dilute drug to 0.5 mg/ml with sodium chloride for injection. Protect solution from light. Slight yellowing is acceptable, but discard solution if it is markedly discolored or contains precipitate.
- Be aware that some perphenazine solutions contain sulfites. Patients with a history of sulfite sensitivity may be at increased risk for a hypersensitivity reaction.
- Obtain blood samples for CBC and liver and renal function tests, as ordered, to detect adverse reactions.
- Monitor temperature frequently, and notify prescriber if it rises; a significant increase suggests drug intolerance.
- Monitor blood pressure of patient who takes large doses of perphenazine, especially if surgery is indicated, because of the increased risk of hypotension.
- **WARNING** Be alert for possible suppressed cough reflex, which increases patient's risk of aspirating vomitus.
- Monitor patients (especially children) with chronic respiratory disorders (such as severe asthma or emphysema) or acute respiratory tract infections for exacerbations of these conditions caused by perphenazine's CNS depressant effects. Be aware that patients with cardiovascular or renal disease are at increased risk for developing hypotension, heart failure, and arrhythmias.
- **WARNING** If patient develops neuroleptic malignant syndrome (hyperpyrexia, muscle rigidity, altered mental status, autonomic instability), notify prescriber immediately and expect to stop drug and start intensive medical treatment. Watch carefully for recurrence if perphenazine therapy resumes.

- Be aware that patient with impaired hepatic function is at risk for decreased perphenazine metabolism or further hepatic dysfunction. If patient has history of hepatic encephalopathy from cirrhosis, watch for increased sensitivity to drug's CNS effects.
- Because of perphenazine's anticholinergic effects, monitor patients with a history of, or predisposition to, glaucoma for signs and symptoms of this disorder, such as eye pain, vision changes, or nausea and vomiting from increased intraocular pressure.
- Be aware that drug should be used cautiously in those who are exposed to organophosphorus insecticides.
- Monitor patients who have been exposed to extreme heat for heatstroke due to drug-induced suppression of temperature regulation. Symptoms include tachycardia, fever, and confusion.
- Be aware that children and elderly patients are at increased risk for developing hypotension amd extrapyramidal reactions, especially if they're acutely ill or debilitated.
- Store drug at 15° to 30° C (59 to 86° F); protect from freezing and light.

PATIENT TEACHING
- Stress the importance of reporting persistent or severe adverse reactions resulting from perphenazine therapy.
- Urge patient to avoid alcohol and other CNS depressants during perphenazine therapy and to avoid potentially hazardous activities until drug's CNS effects are known.
- Advise patient to avoid excessive sun exposure and to protect skin when outdoors.
- Advise patient, especially if elderly, to rise slowly from a supine or seated position to avoid feeling dizzy or faint.
- Inform patient that drug may reduce body's response to heat and cold; advise her to avoid temperature extremes, as in very cold or hot showers.
- Suggest sugarless chewing gum, hard candy, and fluids to relieve dry mouth.
- Urge patient to report sore throat or other signs of infection.

phenobarbital sodium
Luminal

Class, Category, and Schedule
Chemical: Barbiturate
Therapeutic: Anticonvulsant, sedative-hypnotic
Pregnancy category: D

Controlled substance schedule: IV

Indications and Dosages

▶ *To treat seizures*
I.V. INJECTION
Adults. 100 to 320 mg, repeated as needed and as prescribed. *Maximum:* 600 mg daily.
Children. *Initial:* 10 to 20 mg/kg as a single dose. *Maintenance:* 1 to 6 mg/kg daily.

▶ *To treat status epilepticus*
I.V. INFUSION, I.V. INJECTION
Adults. 10 to 20 mg/kg given slowly and repeated as needed and as prescribed.
Children. 15 to 20 mg/kg over 10 to 15 min.

▶ *To provide short-term treatment of insomnia*
I.V. INJECTION
Adults. 100 to 325 mg at bedtime.

▶ *To provide daytime sedation*
I.V. INJECTION
Adults. 30 to 120 mg daily in divided doses b.i.d. or t.i.d.

▶ *To provide preoperative sedation*
I.V. INJECTION
Children. 1 to 3 mg/kg 60 to 90 min before surgery.

DOSAGE ADJUSTMENT Possibly reduced for elderly or debilitated patients to reduce confusion, depression, and excitement.

Route	Onset	Peak	Duration
I.V.	5 min	30 min	4 to 6 hr

Mechanism of Action

Inhibits ascending conduction of impulses in the reticular formation, which controls CNS arousal to produce drowsiness, hypnosis, and sedation. Phenobarbital also decreases the spread of seizure activity in the cortex, thalamus, and limbic system. It promotes an increased threshold for electrical stimulation in the motor cortex, which may contribute to its anticonvulsant properties.

Contraindications

Hepatic disease; history of addiction to hypnotics or sedatives; hypersensitivity to phenobarbital, other barbiturates, or their components; nephritis; porphyria; severe respiratory disease with airway obstruction or dyspnea

Interactions

DRUGS

acetaminophen: Decreased acetaminophen effectiveness with long-term phenobarbital therapy

anticonvulsants (hydantoin): Unpredictable effects on metabolism of anticonvulsant

anticonvulsants (succinimide, including carbamazepine): Decreased blood levels and elimination half-lives of these drugs

calcium channel blockers: Possibly excessive hypotension

carbonic anhydrase inhibitors: Enhanced osteopenia induced by phenobarbital

chloramphenicol, corticosteroids, cyclosporine, dacarbazine, digoxin, metronidazole, quinidine: Decreased effectiveness of these drugs from enhanced metabolism

CNS depressants: Additive CNS depression

cyclophosphamide: Possibly reduced half-life and increased leukopenic activity of cyclophosphamide

disopyramide: Possibly ineffectiveness of disopyramide

doxycycline, fenoprofen: Shortened half-life of these drugs

griseofulvin: Possibly decreased absorption and effectiveness of griseofulvin

guanadrel, guanethidine: Possibly increased orthostatic hypotension

halogenated hydrocarbon anesthetics: Possibly hepatotoxicity

haloperidol: Decreased seizure threshold, decreased blood haloperidol level

ketamine (high doses): Increased risk of hypotension and respiratory depression

leucovorin: Interference with phenobarbital's anticonvulsant effect

levothyroxine, oral contraceptives, phenylbutazone, tricyclic antidepressants: Decreased effectiveness of these drugs

loxapine, phenothiazines, thioxanthenes: Decreased seizure threshold

MAO inhibitors: Prolonged phenobarbital effects, possibly altered pattern of seizure activity

maprotiline: Increased CNS depression, decreased seizure threshold at high doses, decreased phenobarbital effectiveness

methoxyflurane: Possibly hepatotoxicity and nephrotoxicity

methylphenidate: Increased risk of phenobarbital toxicity

mexiletine: Decreased blood mexiletine level

oral anticoagulants: Decreased anticoagulant activity, increased risk of bleeding when phenobarbital is discontinued

pituitary hormones (posterior): Increased risk of arrhythmias and coronary insufficiency *primidone:* Altered pattern of seizures, increased CNS effects of both drugs

valproate, valproic acid: Decreased phenobarbital metabolism, increased risk of barbiturate toxicity

vitamin D: Decreased phenobarbital effectiveness

xanthines: Increased xanthine metabolism, antagonized hypnotic effect of phenobarbital

ACTIVITIES

alcohol use: Additive CNS depression

Adverse Reactions

CNS: Anxiety, depression, dizziness, drowsiness, headache, irritability, lethargy, mood changes, paradoxical stimulation, sedation, vertigo

CV: Hypotension, sinus bradycardia

EENT: Miosis, ptosis

GI: Constipation, diarrhea, nausea, vomiting

GU: Decreased libido, impotence, sexual dysfunction

MS: Arthralgia, bone tenderness

RESP: Bronchospasm, respiratory depression

SKIN: Dermatitis, photosensitivity, rash, urticaria

Other: Injection site phlebitis, physical and psychological dependence

Nursing Considerations

- Be aware that phenobarbital shouldn't be given during third trimester of pregnancy because repeated use can cause dependence in neonate. The drug also shouldn't be given to breast-feeding women because it may cause CNS depression in infants.
- Because drug can cause respiratory depression, assess respiratory rate and depth before use, especially in patient with bronchopneumonia, pulmonary disease, respiratory tract infection, or status asthmaticus.
- Be aware that phenobarbital is available as a solution and as a powder that can be reconstituted. Reconstitute sterile powder with the recommended amount of sterile water for injection. Don't use reconstituted solution if it fails to clear within 5 minutes. Use within 30 minutes. Further dilute prescribed dose with normal saline solution or D_5W, and infuse over 30 to 60 minutes.
- Don't give I.V. injection at more than 60 mg/minute to prevent respiratory depression.
- Monitor blood pressure, respiratory rate, and heart rate and

rhythm during drug administration. Anticipate an increased risk of hypotension, even when giving drug at recommended rate. Keep resuscitation equipment readily available. Patients with cardiovascular disease are at increased risk for adverse circulatory reactions, particularly if drug is administered too rapidly. Patients with pulmonary diseases associated with obstruction or dyspnea are at increased risk for ventilatory depression.

- Watch for hypersensitivity reactions, such as bronchospasm, difficulty breathing, facial edema, and urticaria, especially in patients with a history of asthma, angioedema, or urticaria.
- Be aware that I.V. phenobarbital may not reach peak effects for up to 30 minutes. Expect to wait for drug to take effect before a second dose is ordered.
- Be aware that drug may cause physical and psychological dependence.
- Anticipate that phenobarbital's CNS effects may worsen major depression, suicidal tendencies, and other mental disorders.
- Take safety precautions for elderly patients, as appropriate, because they're more likely to experience confusion, depression, and excitement as adverse CNS reactions.
- Be aware that phenobarbital may cause paradoxical stimulation (excitement, euphoria, restlessness) in patients with acute pain, children, and elderly or debilitated patients. Elderly or debilitated patients are also more likely to experience such adverse CNS reactions as confusion and depression; monitor these patients closely and take safety precautions.
- Be aware that drug may trigger signs and symptoms in patients with acute intermittent porphyria.
- Assess hyperthyroid patients for exacerbated symptoms resulting from phenobarbital use, such as increased nervousness and palpitations.
- Be aware that barbiturate-induced respiratory depression may cause complications in patients with severe anemia.
- Store phenobarbital at 15° to 30° C (59° to 86° F), and don't freeze it.

PATIENT TEACHING

- Caution patient about possible drowsiness and reduced alertness. Advise her to avoid potentially hazardous activities until phenobarbital's CNS effects are known.
- Urge patient to avoid alcohol during therapy.
- Inform parents that child may react to phenobarbital with paradoxical excitement. Tell them to notify prescriber if it occurs.

- Instruct female patient to report suspected, known, or intended pregnancy. Advise against breast-feeding during therapy.

phentolamine mesylate

Regitine, Rogitine (CAN)

Class and Category

Chemical: Imidazoline
Therapeutic: Antihypertensive, diagnostic aid, vasodilator
Pregnancy category: Not rated

Indications and Dosages

▶ *To diagnose pheochromocytoma*

I.V. INJECTION

Adults. 2.5 mg as a single dose. After negative result, repeat test with 5-mg dose, as prescribed.

Children. 1 mg as a single dose. After negative result, repeat test with 0.1-mg/kg dose, as prescribed.

▶ *To manage hypertension before or during pheochromocytomectomy*

I.V. INJECTION

Adults. 5 mg 1 to 2 hr before surgery, repeated as needed and as prescribed. During surgery, 5 mg, as ordered.

Children. 1 mg 1 to 2 hr before surgery, repeated as needed and as prescribed. During surgery, 1 mg, as ordered.

▶ *To prevent dermal necrosis or sloughing after extravasation of I.V. norepinephrine*

I.V. INJECTION

Adults, children, and infants. 10 mg/L of I.V. fluid that contains norepinephrine at rate determined by patient response.

Mechanism of Action

Blocks the actions of circulating epinephrine and norepinephrine by antagonizing alpha$_1$ and alpha$_2$ receptors. Phentolamine causes peripheral vasodilation through direct relaxation of vascular smooth muscle and alpha blockade. Positive inotropic and chronotropic effects increase cardiac output. A positive inotropic effect primarily raises blood pressure, but in larger doses, phentolamine causes peripheral vasodilation and can reduce blood pressure.

In patients with pheochromocytoma, phentolamine causes systolic and diastolic blood pressures to fall dramatically. In those without pheochromocytoma, it causes blood pressure to fall or rise slightly or remain the same.

Contraindications

Angina, hypersensitivity to phentolamine or its components, MI

Interactions

DRUGS

antihypertensives: Additive hypotensive effect
dopamine: Antagonized vasopressor activity of dopamine
epinephrine, methoxamine, norepinephrine, phenylephrine: Inhibited alpha-adrenergic effects of these drugs
metaraminol: Possibly decreased vasopressor effect of metaraminol

ACTIVITIES

alcohol use: Additive vasodilation, increased risk of hypotension and tachycardia

Adverse Reactions

CNS: Dizziness
CV: Angina; arrhythmias, including tachycardia; hypotension
EENT: Nasal congestion
GI: Diarrhea, nausea, vomiting
GU: Ejaculation disorders, priapism
MS: Muscle weakness
SKIN: Flushing

Nursing Considerations

- Reconstitute each 5-mg vial of phentolamine with 1 ml of sterile water for injection.
- Use reconstituted solution immediately; don't store unused portion.
- Dilute 5 to 10 mg of reconstituted solution in 500 ml of D_5W.
- Inspect drug for particles and discoloration before giving it.
- When using drug to diagnose pheochromocytoma, withhold all nonessential drugs, as ordered, for at least 24 hours (preferably 48 to 72 hours) before test.
- Before giving an I.V. test dose for pheochromocytoma, place patient in supine position and determine baseline blood pressure by taking readings every 10 minutes for at least 30 minutes.
- Expect patient with pheochromocytoma to have excessive hypotension after receiving drug.
- Take safety precautions according to facility policy if patient experiences dizziness.
- Store drug at 15° to 30° C (59° to 86° F).

PATIENT TEACHING

- Instruct patient to move slowly after phentolamine administration to minimize dizziness and avoid falls.

phenylephrine hydrochloride
Neo-Synephrine

Class and Category
Chemical: Sympathomimetic amine
Therapeutic: Antiarrhythmic, vasoconstrictor, vasopressor
Pregnancy category: C

Indications and Dosages
▶ *To manage mild to moderate hypotension*
I.V. INJECTION
Adults. *Initial:* 0.1 to 0.5 mg. *Usual:* 0.2 mg, repeated no more often than every 10 to 15 min, as prescribed.
▶ *To treat severe hypotension or shock*
I.V. INFUSION
Adults. *Initial:* 100 to 180 mcg/min (0.1 to 0.18 mg/min) until blood pressure is stable. *Maintenance:* 40 to 60 mcg/min (0.04 to 0.06 mg/min). Infusion concentration and flow rate, adjusted as prescribed, based on patient response.
▶ *To treat hypotension during spinal anesthesia*
I.V. INJECTION
Adults. *Initial:* 0.2 mg, increased by no more than 0.2 mg, as prescribed. *Maximum:* 0.5 mg/dose.
Children. 0.5 to 1 mg for each 11.3 kg (25 lb).
▶ *To treat paroxysmal supraventricular tachycardia*
I.V. INJECTION
Adults. *Initial:* Up to 0.5 mg by rapid injection; later doses increased to 0.1 to 0.2 mg above preceding dose, as prescribed. *Maximum:* 1 mg/dose.

Route	Onset	Peak	Duration
I.V.	Immediately	Unknown	15 to 20 min

Mechanism of Action
Directly stimulates alpha-adrenergic receptors and inhibits activity of the intracellular enzyme adenyl cyclase, which then inhibits production of cAMP. The inhibition of cAMP causes arterial and venous constriction and increases peripheral vascular resistance and systolic blood pressure. With greater-than-therapeutic doses, phenylephrine directly stimulates beta-adrenergic receptors in the myocardium, which increases the activity of adenyl cyclase and produces positive inotropic and chronotropic effects.

Contraindications

Hypersensitivity to bisulfites, phenylephrine, or their components; severe coronary artery disease or hypertension; use within 14 days of MAO inhibitor therapy; ventricular tachycardia

Interactions

DRUGS

alpha blockers, haloperidol, loxapine, phenothiazines, thioxanthenes: Possibly decreased vasoconstrictor effect of phenylephrine

antihypertensives, diuretics: Possibly decreased antihypertensive effects

atropine, methylphenidate: Possibly enhanced vasopressor effect of phenylephrine

beta blockers: Decreased therapeutic effects of both drugs

bretylium: Possibly potentiated vasopressor effect and arrhythmias

doxapram: Increased vasopressor effect of both drugs

ergot alkaloids: Possibly cerebral blood vessel rupture, increased vasopressor effect, peripheral vascular ischemia, and gangrene (with ergotamine)

guanadrel, guanethidine: Increased vasopressor effect of phenylephrine, increased risk of severe hypertension and arrhythmias

hydrocarbon anesthetics (inhaled): Increased risk of serious arrhythmias

MAO inhibitors: Increased and prolonged cardiac stimulation, increased vasopressor effect, increased risk of severe cardiovascular and cerebrovascular effects, hyperpyrexia, vomiting

maprotiline, tricyclic antidepressants: Increased risk of severe cardiovascular effects (including arrhythmias, hyperpyrexia, severe hypertension); possibly increased or decreased sensitivity to phenylephrine

mecamylamine, methyldopa: Decreased hypotensive effects of these drugs, increased vasopressor effect of phenylephrine

nitrates: Possibly decreased vasopressor effect of phenylephrine and decreased antianginal effect of nitrates

other sympathomimetics (such as dopamine and isoproterenol): Possibly increased cardiovascular effects or adverse reactions

oxytocin: Possibly severe, persistent hypertension

phenoxybenzamine: Decreased vasoconstrictor effect of phenylephrine, possibly hypotension and tachycardia

thyroid hormones: Increased cardiovascular effects of both drugs

Adverse Reactions

CNS: Dizziness, headache, insomnia, nervousness, paresthesia, restlessness, tremor, weakness

CV: Angina, bradycardia, hypertension, hypotension, palpitations, peripheral vasoconstriction that may lead to necrosis or gangrene, tachycardia, ventricular arrhythmias
GI: Nausea, vomiting
RESP: Dyspnea
SKIN: Extravasation with tissue necrosis and sloughing, pallor
Other: Allergic reaction

Nursing Considerations

- Be aware that phenylephrine may not be prescribed for patients with occlusive vascular disease, such as atherosclerosis, Buerger's disease, diabetic endarteritis, or Raynaud's disease, because of the risk of decreased peripheral circulation.
- For I.V. use, dilute with D_5W or sodium chloride for injection and prepare as prescribed—usually 10 mg/500 ml. Administer infusions using an infusion pump to ensure appropriate administration rate.
- Assess patient for signs and symptoms of angina, arrhythmias, and hypertension because phenylephrine may increase myocardial oxygen demand and the risk of proarrhythmias and blood pressure changes.
- **WARNING** Monitor patient with thyroid disease for increased sensitivity to catecholamines and, possibly, thyrotoxicity or cardiotoxicity.
- **WARNING** Be aware that extravasation may cause tissue necrosis, gangrene, and other reactions around injection site. If extravasation occurs, expect to use phentolamine to antagonize vasoconstriction and minimize sloughing and tissue necrosis.
- Store drug at 15° to 30° C (59° to 86° F); protect from freezing and light.

PATIENT TEACHING

- Advise patient to avoid potentially hazardous activities until phenylephrine's CNS effects are known.

phenytoin sodium
Dilantin

Class and Category
Chemical: Hydantoin derivative
Therapeutic: Anticonvulsant
Pregnancy category: C

Indications and Dosages

▶ *To treat status epilepticus*

I.V. INJECTION

Adults and adolescents. *Initial:* 15 to 20 mg/kg by slow push in 50 ml of sodium chloride for injection at a rate not to exceed 50 mg/min. *Maintenance:* Beginning within 12 to 24 hr of initial dose, 100 mg every 6 to 8 hr or 5 mg/kg daily P.O. in divided doses b.i.d. to q.i.d.

Children. 15 to 20 mg/kg at no more than 1 mg/kg/min. *Maximum:* 50 mg/min.

DOSAGE ADJUSTMENT For elderly or very ill patients and those with cardiovascular or hepatic disease, dosage reduced to 25 mg/min, as prescribed, or possibly to as low as 5 to 10 mg/min to reduce the risk of adverse reactions.

▶ *To prevent or treat seizures during neurosurgery*

I.V. INJECTION

Adults. 100 to 200 mg every 4 hr at no more than 50 mg/min during or immediately after neurosurgery.

Mechanism of Action

Limits the spread of seizure activity and the start of new seizures by regulating voltage-dependent sodium and calcium channels in neurons, inhibiting calcium movement across neuronal membranes, and enhancing sodium–potassium–adenosine triphosphatase activity in neurons and glial cells. These actions all help stabilize the neurons.

Incompatibilities

Don't mix phenytoin in same syringe with any other drugs or with any I.V. solutions other than sodium chloride for injection because a precipitate will form.

Contraindications

Adams-Stokes syndrome, hypersensitivity to phenytoin or its components, SA block, second- or third-degree heart block, sinus bradycardia

Interactions

DRUGS

acetaminophen: Possibly hepatoxicity, decreased acetaminophen effects

activated charcoal, antacids, calcium salts, enteral feedings, sucralfate:

Decreased absorption of oral phenytoin

allopurinol, benzodiazepines, chloramphenicol, cimetidine, disulfiram, fluconazole, isoniazid, itraconazole, methylphenidate, metronidazole, miconazole, omeprazole, phenacemide, ranitidine, sulfonamides, trazodone, trimethoprim: Decreased metabolism and increased effects of phenytoin

amiodarone, ticlopidine: Possibly increased blood phenytoin level

antifungals (azole): Increased blood phenytoin level, decreased blood antifungal level

antineoplastics, nitrofurantoin, pyridoxine: Decreased phenytoin effects

barbiturates: Variable effects on blood phenytoin level

bupropion, clozapine, loxapine, MAO inhibitors, maprotiline, molindone, phenothiazines, pimozide, thioxanthenes, tricyclic antidepressants: Decreased seizure threshold, decreased anticonvulsant effect of phenytoin

calcium channel blockers: Increased metabolism and decreased effects of these drugs, possibly increased blood phenytoin level

carbamazepine: Decreased blood level and effects of carbamazepine, possibly phenytoin toxicity

carbonic anhydrase inhibitors: Increased risk of osteopenia from phenytoin

chlordiazepoxide, diazepam: Possibly increased blood phenytoin level, decreased effects of these drugs

clonazepam: Possibly decreased blood level and effects of clonazepam, possibly phenytoin toxicity

corticosteroids, cyclosporine, dicumarol, digoxin, disopyramide, doxycycline, estrogens, furosemide, lamotrigine, levodopa, methadone, metyrapone, mexiletine, oral contraceptives, quinidine, sirolimus, tacrolimus, theophylline: Increased metabolism and decreased effects of these drugs

dopamine: Increased risk of severe hypotension and bradycardia

fluoxetine: Increased blood phenytoin level and risk of phenytoin toxicity

folic acid, leucovorin: Decreased blood phenytoin level, increased risk of seizures

haloperidol: Decreased effects of haloperidol, decreased anticonvulsant effect of phenytoin

halothane anesthetics: Increased risk of hepatotoxicity and phenytoin toxicity

ifosfamide: Decreased phenytoin effects, possibly increased toxicity

influenza virus vaccine: Possibly decreased phenytoin effects

insulin, oral antidiabetic drugs: Possibly hyperglycemia, increased blood phenytoin level (with tolbutamide)

levonorgestrel, mebendazole, streptozocin, sulfonylureas: Decreased effects of these drugs

lidocaine, propranolol (possibly other beta blockers): Increased cardiac depressant effects, possibly decreased blood level and increased adverse effects of phenytoin

lithium: Increased risk of lithium toxicity, increased risk of neurologic symptoms with normal blood lithium level

meperidine: Increased metabolism and decreased effects of meperidine, possibly meperidine toxicity

methadone: Possibly increased metabolism of methadone and withdrawal symptoms

neuromuscular blockers: Shorter duration of action and decreased effects of neuromuscular blockers

oral anticoagulants: Decreased metabolism and increased effects of phenytoin; early increase in anticoagulant effect followed by decrease

paroxetine: Decreased bioavailability of both drugs

phenylbutazone, salicylates: Increased phenytoin effects, possibly phenytoin toxicity

primidone: Increased primidone effects, possibly primidone toxicity

rifampin: Increased hepatic metabolism of phenytoin

valproic acid: Possibly decreased phenytoin metabolism, resulting in increased phenytoin effects; possibly decreased blood valproic acid level

vitamin D: Possibly decreased vitamin D effects, resulting in rickets or osteomalacia (with long-term use of phenytoin)

ACTIVITIES

alcohol use: Additive CNS depression, increased phenytoin clearance

Adverse Reactions

CNS: Ataxia, confusion, depression, dizziness, drowsiness, excitement, fever, headache, involuntary motor activity, lethargy, nervousness, peripheral neuropathy, restlessness, slurred speech, tremor, weakness

CV: Cardiac arrest, hypotension, vasculitis

EENT: Amblyopia, conjunctivitis, diplopia, earache, epistaxis, eye pain, gingival hyperplasia, hearing loss, loss of taste, nystagmus, pharyngitis, photophobia, rhinitis, sinusitis, taste perversion, tinnitus

ENDO: Gynecomastia, hyperglycemia

GI: Abdominal pain, anorexia, constipation, diarrhea, epigastric pain, hepatic dysfunction, hepatic necrosis, hepatitis, nausea, vomiting

GU: Glycosuria, priapism, renal failure

HEME: Acute intermittent porphyria (exacerbation), agranulocytosis, anemia, eosinophilia, leukopenia, pancytopenia, thrombocytopenia

MS: Arthralgia, arthropathy, bone fractures, muscle twitching, osteomalacia, polymyositis

RESP: Apnea, asthma, bronchitis, cough, dyspnea, hypoxia, increased sputum production, pneumonia, pneumothorax, pulmonary fibrosis

SKIN: Exfoliative dermatitis, jaundice, maculopapular or morbilliform rash, purpuric dermatitis, Stevens-Johnson syndrome, toxic epidermal necrolysis, unusual hair growth, urticaria

Other: Facial feature enlargement, injection site pain, lupuslike symptoms, lymphadenopathy, polyarteritis, weight gain or loss

Nursing Considerations

- Be aware that preferred administration routes for phenytoin are I.V. injection and oral. Phenytoin has a variable absorption rate when administered by I.M. route.
- Inspect I.V. form for particles and discoloration before administering.
- Administer I.V. injection through a large vein, using a large-gauge needle or an I.V. catheter.
- **WARNING** Avoid rapid I.V. injection because it may cause cardiac arrest, CNS depression, or severe hypotension. Administer at a rate not to exceed 50 mg/minute.
- To decrease vein irritation, follow I.V. injection with flush of sodium chloride for injection through same I.V. catheter.
- Continuously monitor ECG tracings and blood pressure when administering I.V. phenytoin.
- Frequently assess I.V. site for signs of extravasation because drug can cause tissue necrosis.
- Administer oral phenytoin at least 2 hours before or after antacids and calcium salts.
- If patient has difficulty swallowing, open prompt (rapid-release) capsules and mix contents with food or fluid.
- Shake oral suspension before measuring dose, and use a calibrated measuring device.
- To minimize GI distress, give phenytoin with or just after meals.
- If patient has an NG tube in place, minimize drug absorption by polyvinyl chloride tubing by diluting suspension threefold with

sodium chloride for injection, D_5W, or sterile water. After administering drug, flush tube with at least 20 ml of diluent.

- Expect continuous enteral feedings to disrupt phenytoin absorption and, possibly, reduce blood phenytoin level. Discontinue tube feedings 1 to 2 hours before and after phenytoin administration, as prescribed. Anticipate increasing phenytoin dosage, as prescribed, to compensate for reduced bioavailability during continuous tube feedings.
- Monitor blood phenytoin level. Therapeutic level ranges from 10 to 20 mg/L.
- **WARNING** Monitor hematologic status during therapy because phenytoin can cause blood dyscrasias. Patients with a history of agranulocytosis, leukopenia, or pancytopenia may have an increased risk of infection because phenytoin can cause myelosuppression.
- Anticipate that drug may worsen intermittent porphyria.
- Frequently monitor blood glucose level of patient with diabetes mellitus because drug can stimulate glucagon and impair insulin secretion, either of which can raise blood glucose level.
- Monitor blood thyroid hormone levels of patients receiving thyroid replacement therapy, as appropriate, because phenytoin may decrease circulating thyroid hormone levels and increase thyroid-stimulating hormone level.
- Be aware that long-term phenytoin therapy may increase patient's requirements for folic acid or vitamin D supplements. However, keep in mind that a diet high in folic acid may decrease seizure control.
- Store drug at 15° to 30° C (59° to 86° F); don't freeze.

PATIENT TEACHING

- Caution patient to avoid potentially hazardous activities until phenytoin's CNS effects are known.
- Explain to patient with diabetes mellitus that she may be at increased risk for hyperglycemia and may need an increased dosage of antidiabetic drug during phenytoin therapy. Inform her that her blood glucose level will be monitored frequently.
- Instruct patient to crush or thoroughly chew phenytoin chewable tablets or to shake oral solution well before swallowing.
- Advise patient to take drug exactly as prescribed and not to change brands or dosage or stop taking drug unless instructed by prescriber.
- Instruct patient to avoid taking antacids or calcium products within 2 hours of oral phenytoin.

- Urge patient to avoid alcohol during phenytoin therapy.
- Stress the importance of good oral hygiene, and encourage patient to inform her dentist that she's taking phenytoin.
- Encourage patient to carry medical identification indicating her diagnosis and drug therapy.

physostigmine salicylate
Antilirium

Class and Category
Chemical: Salicylic acid derivative
Therapeutic: Anticholinergic antidote, cholinesterase inhibitor
Pregnancy category: Not rated

Indications and Dosages
▶ *To counteract toxic anticholinergic effects (anticholinergic syndrome)*
I.V. INJECTION
Adults and adolescents. 0.5 to 2 mg at no more than 1 mg/min; then 1 to 4 mg, repeated every 20 to 30 min as needed and as prescribed.
Children. 0.02 mg/kg at a rate not to exceed 0.5 mg/min, repeated every 5 to 10 min as needed and as prescribed. *Maximum:* 2 mg/dose.

Route	Onset	Peak	Duration
I.V.	3 to 8 min	5 min	30 to 60 min

Mechanism of Action
Inhibits the destruction of acetylcholine by acetylcholinesterase. This action increases the concentration of acetylcholine at cholinergic transmission sites and prolongs and exaggerates the effects of acetylcholine that are blocked by toxic doses of anticholinergics.

Contraindications
Asthma; cardiovascular disease; diabetes mellitus; gangrene; GI or GU obstruction; hypersensitivity to physostigmine, sulfites, or their components

Interactions
DRUGS
choline esters: Enhanced effects of carbachol and bethanechol with

concurrent use of physostigmine, enhanced effects of acetylcholine and methacholine with prior use of physostigmine
succinylcholine: Prolonged neuromuscular paralysis

Adverse Reactions

CNS: CNS stimulation, fatigue, hallucinations, restlessness, seizures (with too-rapid administration), weakness
CV: Bradycardia (with too-rapid administration), irregular heartbeat, palpitations
EENT: Increased salivation, lacrimation, miosis
GI: Abdominal pain, diarrhea, nausea, vomiting
GU: Urinary urgency
MS: Muscle twitching
RESP: Bronchospasm, chest tightness, dyspnea (with too-rapid administration), increased bronchial secretions, wheezing
SKIN: Diaphoresis

Nursing Considerations

- Avoid rapid administration of physostigmine because it may lead to bradycardia, respiratory distress, or seizures.
- Frequently monitor pulse and respiratory rates, blood pressure, and neurologic status during therapy.
- Monitor ECG tracing during drug administration. Patients with a history of bradycardia may be at increased risk for drug-induced bradycardia.
- Closely monitor patients with asthma for an asthma attack; drug may precipitate an attack by causing bronchoconstriction.
- Monitor for drug-induced seizures due to drug's CNS-stimulating effects in patients with a history of seizures.
- Assess patients with Parkinson's disease for increased tremors, akinesia, or rigidity.
- **WARNING** Be alert for evidence of a life-threatening cholinergic crisis, which may indicate a physostigmine overdose: confusion, diaphoresis, hypotension, miosis, muscle weakness, nausea, paralysis (including respiratory paralysis), salivation, seizures, sinus bradycardia, and vomiting. If you detect such signs, prepare to give atropine (the antidote) and use resuscitation equipment. Keep in mind that atropine counteracts only muscarinic cholinergic effects; paralytic effects may continue.
- Store drug at 15° to 30° C (59° to 86° F); protect from freezing and light.

PATIENT TEACHING
- Reassure patient that her vital signs will be monitored frequently during physostigmine administration to help prevent or detect adverse reactions.
- Instruct patient to notify prescriber immediately about signs of cholinergic crisis.

piperacillin sodium
Pipracil

Class and Category
Chemical: Piperazine derivative of ampicillin, acylureidopenicillin
Therapeutic: Antibiotic
Pregnancy category: B

Indications and Dosages
▶ *To treat moderate to severe bacterial infections, including bone and joint infections, gynecologic infections, intra-abdominal infections, lower respiratory tract infections, septicemia, and skin and soft-tissue infections, caused by susceptible strains of* Acinetobacter *species, anaerobic cocci,* Bacteroides *species,* Enterobacter *species,* Escherichia coli, Haemophilus influenzae, Klebsiella *species,* Proteus *species,* Pseudomonas aeruginosa, *and* Serratia *species*

I.V. INFUSION
Adults and adolescents. 12 to 18 g daily or 200 to 300 mg/kg daily in divided doses every 4 to 6 hr. *Maximum:* 24 g daily.
▶ *To treat bacterial meningitis*
I.V. INFUSION
Adults and adolescents. 4 g every 4 hr or 75 mg/ kg every 6 hr. *Maximum:* 24 g daily.
▶ *To treat uncomplicated UTI and community-acquired pneumonia caused by susceptible organisms, including* E. coli, Klebsiella *species, and* Serratia *species*
I.V. INFUSION
Adults. 6 to 8 g daily or 100 to 125 mg/kg daily in divided doses every 6 to 12 hr.
▶ *To treat complicated UTI caused by susceptible organisms, including* Acinetobacter *species,* Klebsiella *species, and* Serratia *species*
I.V. INFUSION
Adults. 8 to 16 g daily or 125 to 200 mg/kg daily in divided doses every 6 to 8 hr.

I.V. INFUSION

Adults. 2 g 20 to 30 min before anesthesia, 2 g during surgery, and 2 g every 6 hr for 24 hr after surgery.

▶ *To provide surgical prophylaxis in abdominal hysterectomy*

I.V. INFUSION

Adults. 2 g 20 to 30 min before anesthesia, 2 g just after surgery, and 2 g 6 hr later.

▶ *To provide surgical prophylaxis in vaginal hysterectomy*

I.V. INFUSION

Adults. 2 g 20 to 30 min before anesthesia, then 2 g 6 and 12 hr after initial dose.

▶ *To provide surgical prophylaxis in cesarean section*

I.V. INFUSION

Adults. 2 g after cord is clamped, then 2 g 4 and 8 hr after initial dose.

Mechanism of Action

Binds to specific penicillin-binding proteins and inhibits the third and final stage of bacterial cell wall synthesis by interfering with an autolysin inhibitor. Uninhibited autolytic enzymes destroy the cell wall and result in cell lysis.

Incompatibilities

Don't mix piperacillin sodium in same container with aminoglycosides because of chemical incompatibility (depending on concentrations, diluents, pH, and temperature). Don't mix with solutions that contain only sodium bicarbonate because of chemical instability.

Contraindications

Hypersensitivity to cephalosporins, penicillins, or their components

Interactions

DRUGS

aminoglycosides: Additive or synergistic effects against some bacteria, possibly mutual inactivation

anti-inflammatory drugs (including aspirin and NSAIDs), heparin, oral anticoagulants, platelet aggregation inhibitors, sulfinpyrazone, thrombolytics: Increased risk of bleeding

hepatotoxic drugs (including labetalol and rifampin): Increased risk of hepatotoxicity

methotrexate: Increased blood methotrexate level and risk of toxicity
probenecid: Increased blood piperacillin level and risk of toxicity
vecuronium: Possibly prolonged perioperative neuromuscular
blockade of vecuronium

Adverse Reactions

CNS: CVA, dizziness, fever, hallucinations, headache, lethargy,
seizures
CV: Cardiac arrest, hypotension, palpitations, tachycardia, vasodi-
lation, vasovagal reactions
EENT: Oral candidiasis, pharyngitis
GI: Diarrhea, epigastric distress, intestinal necrosis, nausea,
pseudomembranous colitis, vomiting
GU: Hematuria, impotence, nephritis, neurogenic bladder, pri-
apism, proteinuria, renal failure, vaginal candidiasis
HEME: Agranulocytosis, eosinophilia, hemolytic anemia,
leukopenia, neutropenia, pancytopenia, prolonged bleeding time,
thrombocytopenia
MS: Arthralgia
RESP: Dyspnea, pulmonary embolism, pulmonary hypertension
SKIN: Exfoliative dermatitis, mottling, rash, toxic epidermal
necrolysis, urticaria
Other: Anaphylaxis; facial edema; hypokalemia; hyponatremia;
injection site pain, phlebitis, and skin ulcer; superinfection

Nursing Considerations

- Obtain blood, sputum, or other samples for culture and sensitivity testing, as ordered, before giving piperacillin. Expect to
  begin piperacillin therapy before results are available.
- Be aware that sunlight may darken powder for dilution but
  won't alter drug potency.
- For initial dilution for I.V. infusion, reconstitute each gram of
  drug with at least 5 ml of sterile water for injection, sodium
  chloride for injection, D_5W, dextrose 5% in normal saline solution, or bacteriostatic water that contains parabens or benzyl alcohol. Shake solution vigorously after adding diluent to help
  drug dissolve, and inspect for particles and discoloration before
  giving.
- For further dilution, use sodium chloride for injection, D_5W,
  dextrose 5% in normal saline solution, lactated Ringer's solution, or dextran 6% in normal saline solution. Solutions diluted
  with lactated Ringer's solution should be given within 2 hours.
- For intermittent infusion, infuse dose over 20 to 30 minutes.

- Give aminoglycosides 1 hour before or after piperacillin; use a separate site, I.V. bag, and tubing.
- Watch for bleeding or excessive bruising because drug can decrease platelet aggregation. If bleeding occurs, notify prescriber and expect to stop piperacillin.
- Monitor CBC regularly, as ordered, to detect hematologic abnormalities, such as leukopenia and neutropenia.
- Monitor serum potassium level to detect hypokalemia from urinary potassium loss.
- Check for diarrhea (possible pseudomembranous colitis) during and after therapy.
- Watch closely for hypersensitivity reactions, especially if patient has cystic fibrosis. Notify prescriber, and expect to stop drug.

PATIENT TEACHING

- Advise patient to consult prescriber before using OTC drugs during piperacillin therapy because of the risk of interactions.
- Inform patient that increased bruising may occur if she takes anti-inflammatory drugs during piperacillin therapy.
- Advise patient to report signs of superinfection, such as severe diarrhea or white patches on tongue or in mouth.
- Instruct patient to complete full course of therapy, even if symptoms subside.

piperacillin sodium and tazobactam sodium

Tazocin (CAN), Zosyn

Class and Category

Chemical: Piperazine derivative of ampicillin, acylureidopenicillin (piperacillin); penicillinate sulfone (tazobactam)
Therapeutic: Antibiotic
Pregnancy category: B

Indications and Dosages

▶ *To treat moderate to severe gram-negative or anaerobic infections, such as appendicitis, community-acquired pneumonia, diabetic foot ulcers, intra-abdominal infections, pelvic inflammatory disease, peritonitis, postpartum endometritis, and uncomplicated or complicated skin or soft-tissue infections caused by susceptible organisms, such as* Bacteroides species (including many strains of Bacteroides fragilis), Clostridium species, Enterobacter *species,* Enterococcus faecalis, Escherichia coli, Haemophilus influenzae, Klebsiella pneumoniae, Morganella

morganii, Neisseria gonorrhoeae, Proteus mirabilis, Proteus vulgaris, Pseudomonas aeruginosa, *and* Serratia *species*
I.V. INFUSION
Adults and adolescents. 3.375 g every 6 hr. *Maximum:* 4.5 g every 6 to 8 hr.
▶ *To treat nosocomial pneumonia caused by susceptible organisms*
I.V. INFUSION
Adults and adolescents. 4.5 g every 6 hr in addition to aminoglycoside therapy for 7 to 14 days.
DOSAGE ADJUSTMENT Dosage possibly decreased to 2.25 g every 6 hr for patients with creatinine clearance of 20 to 40 ml/min/1.73 m^2; to 2.25 g every 8 hr for those with creatinine clearance of less than 20 ml/min/1.73 m^2.

Mechanism of Action

Binds to specific penicillin-binding proteins and inhibits the third and final stage of bacterial cell wall synthesis. Piperacillin does this by interfering with an autolysin inhibitor. Uninhibited autolytic enzymes destroy the cell wall and result in cell lysis.

Tazobactam doesn't change piperacillin's action, but it protects piperacillin against Richmond and Sykes types II, III, IV, and V beta-lactamases; staphylococcal beta-lactamases; and extended-spectrum beta-lactamases.

Incompatibilities

Don't mix piperacillin and tazobactam in same container with aminoglycosides because of chemical incompatibility (depending on concentrations, diluents, pH, and temperature), except when using reformulated piperacillin and tazobactam containing EDTA with amikacin and gentamicin.

Contraindications

Hypersensitivity to beta-lactamase inhibitors, cephalosporins, penicillins, piperacillin, tazobactam, or their components

Interactions

DRUGS
aminoglycosides: Additive or synergistic effects against some bacteria, possibly mutual inactivation
anti-inflammatory drugs (including aspirin and NSAIDs), heparin, oral anticoagulants, platelet aggregation inhibitors, sulfinpyrazone, thrombolytics: Increased risk of bleeding

hepatotoxic drugs (including labetalol and rifampin): Increased risk of hepatotoxicity
methotrexate: Increased blood methotrexate level and risk of toxicity
probenecid: Increased blood piperacillin level and risk of toxicity
vecuronium: Possibly prolonged neuromuscular blockade in perioperative period

Adverse Reactions

CNS: Chills, CVA, dizziness, fever, hallucinations, headache, lethargy, seizures
CV: Cardiac arrest, hypotension, palpitations, tachycardia, vasodilation, vasovagal reactions
EENT: Epistaxis, oral candidiasis, pharyngitis
GI: Cholestatic jaundice, diarrhea, elevated liver function test results, epigastric distress, hepatitis, intestinal necrosis, nausea, pseudomembranous colitis, vomiting
GU: Hematuria, impotence, nephritis, neurogenic bladder, priapism, proteinuria, renal failure, vaginal candidiasis
HEME: Agranulocytosis, anemia, eosinophilia, hemolytic anemia, leukopenia, neutropenia, pancytopenia, thrombocytopenia, thrombocytosis
MS: Arthralgia, prolonged muscle relaxation
RESP: Dyspnea, pulmonary embolism, pulmonary hypertension
SKIN: Erythema multiforme, exfoliative dermatitis, mottling, rash, Stevens-Johnson syndrome, toxic epidermal necrolysis
Other: Anaphylaxis, facial edema, hypokalemia, hyponatremia

Nursing Considerations

- Expect to obtain blood, sputum, or other samples for culture and sensitivity testing before giving piperacillin and tazobactam. Therapy may start before tests are complete.
- Be aware that sunlight may darken powder for dilution but won't alter drug potency.
- Reconstitute with sterile water for injection, sodium chloride for injection, D_5W, or bacteriostatic water or normal saline solution that contains parabens or benzyl alcohol.
- For additional dilution (50 to 150 ml except as noted), use appropriate solution, such as sodium chloride for injection, sterile water for injection (no more than 50 ml), D_5W, or dextran 6% in normal saline solution.
- Shake solution vigorously after adding diluent to help drug dissolve, and inspect for particles and discoloration before giving.
- Administer over at least 30 minutes.

- Assess for bleeding or excessive bruising because drug can decrease platelet aggregation, especially in patients with renal failure. If bleeding occurs, notify prescriber and expect to discontinue piperacillin.
- Monitor serum potassium level; hypokalemia may result from urinary potassium loss.
- Monitor patients who need to limit salt intake for fluid retention and unexplained sudden weight gain because piperacillin and tazobactam contains 64 mg of sodium/gram of the drug; at the usual dose, a patient would receive between 768 and 1024 mg of sodium daily. Also monitor elderly patients closely because they may exhibit a blunted natriuresis to excessive salt intake.
- Monitor patient for diarrhea during or shortly after drug therapy; diarrhea may signal pseudomembranous colitis.
- Give aminoglycosides 1 hour before or after piperacillin and tazobactam; use a separate site, I.V. bag, and tubing.

PATIENT TEACHING
- Instruct patient to take drug for as long as prescribed, even after feeling better.
- Inform diabetic patients who test urine glucose level that drug may alter results of copper reduction tests, such as Clinitest. Advise using a test based on enzymatic glucose oxidase reaction, such as Diastix or TesTape.
- Advise patient to consult prescriber before using OTC drugs during treatment with piperacillin and tazobactam because of the risk of interactions.
- Inform patient that increased bruising may occur if she takes anti-inflammatory drugs, such as aspirin and NSAIDs, during piperacillin and tazobactam therapy.
- Advise patient to notify prescriber about signs of superinfection, such as severe diarrhea or white patches on tongue or in mouth.

polymyxin B sulfate
Aerosporin

Class and Category
Chemical: Bacillus polymyxa derivative
Therapeutic: Antibiotic
Pregnancy category: Not rated

Indications and Dosages

▶ *To treat infections that are resistant to less toxic drugs, such as bacteremia, septicemia, and UTI caused by susceptible organisms, including* Enterobacter aerogenes, Escherichia coli, Haemophilus influenzae, *and* Klebsiella pneumoniae

I.V. INFUSION

Adults and children age 2 and over. 15,000 to 25,000 units/kg daily in divided doses every 12 hr or as a continuous infusion. *Maximum:* 2 million units daily.

Infants and children under age 2. Up to 40,000 units/kg daily in divided doses every 12 hr or as a continuous infusion.

DOSAGE ADJUSTMENT Dosage reduced by 50% for patients with creatinine clearance of 5 to 20 ml/min/1.73 m² and by 85% for patients with creatinine clearance of less than 5 ml/min/1.73 m².

▶ *To treat meningitis caused by susceptible strains of* Pseudomonas aeruginosa *or* H. influenzae

INTRATHECAL INJECTION

Adults and children age 2 and over. 50,000 units daily for 3 to 4 days; then 50,000 units every other day for at least 2 wk after CSF cultures are negative and glucose content is normal.

Infants and children under age 2. 20,000 units daily for 3 to 4 days, then 25,000 units every other day for at least 2 wk after CSF cultures are negative and glucose content is normal.

Mechanism of Action

Binds to cell membrane phospholipids in gram-negative bacteria, increasing the permeability of the bacterial cell membrane. Polymyxin B also acts as a cationic detergent, altering the osmotic barrier of the cell membrane and causing essential intracellular metabolites to leak out. Both actions lead to cell death.

Incompatibilities

Don't mix polymyxin B sulfate with amphotericin B, calcium salts, chloramphenicol, chlorothiazide, heparin sodium, magnesium salts, nitrofurantoin, penicillins, prednisolone, or tetracyclines because these drugs are incompatible.

Contraindications

Hypersensitivity to polymyxin B or its components

Interactions
DRUGS

general anesthetics, neuromuscular blockers, skeletal muscle relaxants: Increased or prolonged skeletal muscle relaxation, possibly respiratory paralysis

nephrotoxic and neurotoxic drugs (such as aminoglycosides, amphotericin B, colistin, sodium citrate, streptomycin, tobramycin, and vancomycin): Increased risk of nephrotoxicity and neurotoxicity

Adverse Reactions

CNS: Ataxia, confusion, dizziness, drowsiness, fever, giddiness, headache, increased leukocyte and protein levels in CSF, neurotoxicity, paresthesia (circumoral or peripheral), slurred speech
CV: Thrombophlebitis
EENT: Blurred vision, nystagmus
GU: Albuminuria, azotemia, cylindruria, decreased urine output, hematuria, nephrotoxicity
HEME: Eosinophilia
RESP: Respiratory muscle paralysis
SKIN: Rash, urticaria
Other: Anaphylaxis, drug-induced fever, facial flushing, injection site pain, stiff neck (with intrathecal injection), superinfection

Nursing Considerations

- Be aware that patients receiving polymyxin B sulfate are hospitalized to allow appropriate supervision.
- Obtain blood, urine, or other specimens for culture and sensitivity tests, as ordered, before giving drug. Expect to begin polymyxin B therapy before results are known. Keep in mind that baseline renal function tests should have been performed before administration. Check these test results, if available, and notify prescriber of abnormalities.
- For I.V. infusion, dissolve polymyxin B in 300 to 500 ml of D$_5$W and infuse over 60 to 90 minutes.
- For intrathecal administration, add 10 ml of sodium chloride for injection to vial of polymyxin B.
- Inspect for particles and discoloration before giving drug.
- Monitor renal function, including BUN and serum creatinine levels, during therapy, especially in patients with a history of renal insufficiency.
- **WARNING** Be aware that declining urine output and rising BUN level suggest nephrotoxicity, which also is characterized by albuminuria, azotemia, cylindruria, excessive excretion of

electrolytes, hematuria, leukocyturia, and rising blood drug level. Notify prescriber immediately if you detect such signs.

• **WARNING** Notify prescriber immediately if patient experiences blurred vision, circumoral or peripheral paresthesia, confusion, dizziness, drowsiness, facial flushing, giddiness, myasthenia, nystagmus, or slurred speech. These may be signs of neurotoxicity, a serious adverse reaction that may lead to respiratory arrest or paralysis if untreated.

• Assess for signs of superinfection, such as mouth sores, severe diarrhea, and white patches on tongue or in mouth, especially in debilitated or elderly patients.

• Monitor fluid intake and output, and provide adequate fluids to reduce the risk of nephrotoxicity.

PATIENT TEACHING

• Encourage patient to maintain adequate fluid intake during polymyxin B therapy.

• Instruct patient to immediately report diarrhea, mouth sores, or vaginitis, which may be early signs of superinfection.

potassium acetate
(contains 2 or 4 mEq of elemental potassium per 1 ml of injection)
potassium chloride
(contains 0.1, 0.2, 0.3, 0.4, 1.5, 2, 3, or 10 mEq of elemental potassium per 1 ml of injection)

Class and Category
Chemical: Electrolyte cation
Therapeutic: Electrolyte replacement
Pregnancy category: C

Indications and Dosages
▶ *To prevent or treat hypokalemia in patients who can't ingest sufficient dietary potassium or who are losing potassium because of certain conditions (such as hepatic cirrhosis and prolonged vomiting) or drugs (such as potassium-wasting diuretics and certain antibiotics)*
I.V. INFUSION (POTASSIUM ACETATE AND POTASSIUM CHLORIDE)
Adults and adolescents with serum potassium level above 2.5 mEq/L. Up to 10 mEq/hr. *Maximum:* 200 mEq daily.
Adults and adolescents with serum potassium level below 2 mEq/L, ECG changes, or paralysis. Up to 20 mEq/hr. *Maximum:* 400 mEq daily.
Children. 3 mEq/kg daily.

DOSAGE ADJUSTMENT Dosage adjusted as prescribed based on patient's ECG patterns and serum potassium level.

Mechanism of Action

Acts as the major cation in intracellular fluid, activating many enzymatic reactions that are essential for physiologic processes, including nerve impulse transmission and cardiac and skeletal muscle contraction. Potassium also helps maintain electroneutrality in cells by controlling the exchange of intracellular and extracellular ions. It also helps maintain normal renal function and acid-base balance.

Incompatibilities

Don't mix potassium chloride for injection in same syringe with amino acid solutions, lipid solutions, or mannitol because these drugs may precipitate from solution. Administration with blood or blood products can cause lysis of infused RBCs.

Contraindications

Acute dehydration, Addison's disease (untreated), concurrent use of potassium-sparing diuretics, crush syndrome, heat cramps, hyperkalemia, hypersensitivity to potassium salts or their components, renal impairment with azotemia or oliguria, severe hemolytic anemia

Interactions

DRUGS

ACE inhibitors, beta blockers, blood products, cyclosporine, heparin, NSAIDs, potassium-containing drugs, potassium-sparing diuretics: Increased risk of hyperkalemia

amphotericin B, corticosteroids (glucocorticoids or mineralocorticoids), gentamicin, penicillins, polymyxin B: Possibly hypokalemia

anticholinergics, drugs with anticholinergic activity: Increased risk of GI ulceration, stricture, and perforation

calcium salts (parenteral): Possibly arrhythmias

digoxin: Increased risk of digitalis toxicity

insulin, laxatives, sodium bicarbonate: Decreased serum potassium level

sodium polystyrene sulfonate: Possibly decreased serum potassium level and fluid retention

thiazide diuretics: Possibly hyperkalemia when diuretic is discontinued

FOODS

low-salt milk, salt substitutes: Increased risk of hyperkalemia

Adverse Reactions

CNS: Confusion, paralysis, paresthesia, weakness

CV: Arrhythmias, ECG changes

EENT: Throat pain when swallowing

GI: Abdominal pain; bloody stools; diarrhea; flatulence; GI bleeding, perforation, or ulceration; intestinal obstruction; nausea; vomiting

RESP: Dyspnea

SKIN: Rash

Other: Hyperkalemia

Nursing Considerations

- **WARNING** Be aware that direct injection of potassium concentrate may be immediately fatal. Dilute potassium for injection with an adequate volume of solution before I.V. use. Maximum recommended concentration is 40 mEq/L, although concentrations up to 80 mEq/L may be used for severe hypokalemia. Inappropriate solutions or improper technique may cause extravasation, fever, hyperkalemia, hypervolemia, I.V. site infection, phlebitis, venospasm, and venous thrombosis.
- Infuse potassium slowly to avoid phlebitis and decrease the risk of adverse cardiac reactions. Keep in mind that different forms of potassium salts contain different amounts of elemental potassium per gram and that not all forms are dosage equivalent.
- Monitor serum potassium level before and during administration of I.V. potassium.
- **WARNING** Be aware that some forms of potassium contain tartrazine, which may cause an allergic reaction, such as asthma. Some forms may also contain aluminum, which may become toxic in a patient with impaired renal function.
- Regularly assess patient for evidence of hypokalemia (such as arrhythmias, fatigue, and weakness) or hyperkalemia (such as arrhythmias, confusion, dyspnea, and paresthesia).
- Because adequate renal function is needed for potassium supplementation, monitor serum creatinine level and urine output during administration. Notify prescriber about signs of decreased renal function.

PATIENT TEACHING

- Teach patient how to take her radial pulse, and advise her to notify prescriber about significant changes in heart rate or rhythm.

- Advise patient to watch stools for changes in color and consistency and to notify prescriber if they become black or tarry or bright red from blood.
- Tell patient that her serum potassium level will be checked regularly.

potassium phosphates
sodium phosphates
Class and Category
Chemical: Anion, soluble salts
Therapeutic: Electrolyte replenisher
Pregnancy category: C

Indications and Dosages
▶ *To prevent or treat hypophosphatemia*
I.V. INFUSION (POTASSIUM PHOSPHATES)
Adults and adolescents. 10 mmol (310 mg) daily.
Children. 1.5 to 2 mmol (46.5 to 62 mg) daily.
I.V. INFUSION (SODIUM PHOSPHATES)
Adults and adolescents. 10 to 15 mmol (310 to 465 mg) daily.
Children. 1.5 to 2 mmol (46.5 to 62 mg) daily.

Mechanism of Action
Reverses symptoms of hypophosphatemia by replenishing the body's supply of phosphate.

Incompatibilities
Don't add potassium or sodium phosphates to calcium- or magnesium-containing solutions because a precipitate may form.

Contraindications
Hyperkalemia (potassium formulations only), hypernatremia (sodium formulations only), hyperphosphatemia, magnesium ammonium phosphate urolithiasis accompanied by infection, severe renal insufficiency, UTIs caused by urea-splitting organisms

Interactions
DRUGS
ACE inhibitors, cyclosporine, heparin (long-term use), NSAIDs, potassium-containing drugs, potassium-sparing diuretics: Increased risk of hyperkalemia (potassium formulations only)

anabolic steroids, androgens, corticosteroids, estrogens: Increased risk of edema (sodium formulations only)

calcium-containing drugs: Increased risk of calcium deposition in soft tissues

phosphate-containing drugs, vitamin D: Increased risk of hyperphosphatemia

salicylates: Increased blood salicylate level

zinc supplements: Reduced zinc absorption

FOODS

low-salt milk, salt substitutes: Increased risk of hyperkalemia

Adverse Reactions

CNS: Anxiety, confusion, dizziness, fatigue, headache, paresthesia, seizures, tremor, weakness

CV: Arrhythmias, edema of legs, tachycardia

GI: Thirst

GU: Decreased urine output

MS: Muscle cramps or weakness

RESP: Dyspnea

Other: Hyperkalemia, hypernatremia, hyperphosphatemia, hypocalcemia, weight gain

Nursing Considerations

- Avoid mixing potassium or sodium phosphates with solutions containing calcium or magnesium to prevent the formation of precipitates. Dilute phosphates, as prescribed, before administration.
- Monitor serum phosphorus level, as appropriate, of patients with a condition that may be associated with an elevated phosphorus level, such as chronic renal disease, hypoparathyroidism, and rhabdomyolysis; phosphates may further increase serum phosphorus level.
- Monitor serum calcium level, as appropriate, of patients with a condition that may be associated with a low calcium level, such as acute pancreatitis, chronic renal disease, hypoparathyroidism, osteomalacia, rhabdomyolysis, and rickets; phosphates may further decrease serum calcium level.
- Monitor serum potassium level, as appropriate, of patients who receive potassium phosphates and have a condition that may be associated with an elevated potassium level, such as acute dehydration, adrenal insufficiency, extensive tissue breakdown (as in severe burns), myotonia congenita, pancreatitis, rhabdomyolysis, and severe renal insufficiency; they may be at increased risk for hyperkalemia.

- Monitor serum sodium level of patients who receive sodium phosphates and have a condition that may be exacerbated by sodium excess, such as heart failure, hypernatremia, hypertension, peripheral or pulmonary edema, preeclampsia, renal impairment, and severe hepatic disease.
- Monitor ECG tracing frequently during I.V. infusion of sodium phosphates to detect arrhythmias.
- Store drug at 15° to 30° C (59° to 86° F); don't freeze.

PATIENT TEACHING
- Urge patient receiving potassium or sodium phosphates to immediately report muscle weakness or cramps, unexplained weight gain, or shortness of breath.
- Encourage increased intake of fluids (8 oz/hour, if not contraindicated) to prevent kidney stones.

pralidoxime chloride
(2-PAM chloride, 2-pyridine aldoxime methochloride)
Protopam Chloride

Class and Category
Chemical: Quaternary ammonium oxime
Therapeutic: Anticholinesterase antidote
Pregnancy category: C

Indications and Dosages
▶ *As adjunct to reverse organophosphate pesticide toxicity*
I.V. INFUSION, I.M. OR SUBCUTANEOUS INJECTION
Adults. *Initial:* 1 to 2 g in 100 ml of normal saline solution infused over 15 to 30 min, given with atropine 2 to 6 mg every 5 to 60 min until muscarinic signs and symptoms disappear; may be repeated in 1 hr and then every 3 to 8 hr if muscle weakness persists. If I.V. route isn't feasible, give I.M. or subcutaneously.
Children. *Initial:* 20 mg/kg in 100 ml of normal saline solution infused over 15 to 30 min, given with atropine (dosage individualized); may be repeated in 1 hr and then every 3 to 8 hr if muscle weakness persists. If I.V. route isn't feasible, give I.M. or subcutaneously.
▶ *To treat anticholinesterase overdose secondary to myasthenic drugs (including ambenonium, neostigmine, and pyridostigmine)*
I.V. INJECTION
Adults. *Initial:* 1 to 2 g, followed by 250 mg every 5 min.

▶ *To treat exposure to nerve agents*
I.V. INJECTION
Adults. *Initial:* 1 atropine-containing autoinjector followed by 1 pralidoxime-containing autoinjector as soon as atropine's effects are evident; both injections repeated every 15 min for 2 additional doses if nerve agent symptoms persist.
DOSAGE ADJUSTMENT Dosage reduced for patients with renal insufficiency.

Mechanism of Action
Reverses muscle paralysis by removing the phosphoryl group from inhibited cholinesterase molecules at the neuromuscular junction of skeletal and respiratory muscles. Reactivation of cholinesterase restores the body's ability to metabolize acetylcholine, which is inhibited by the effects of organophosphate pesticides, anticholinesterase overdose, or nerve agent poisoning.

Contraindications
Hypersensitivity to pralidoxime chloride or its components

Interactions
DRUGS
aminophylline, morphine, phenothiazines, reserpine, succinylcholine, theophylline: Increased symptoms of organophosphate poisoning
barbiturates: Potentiated barbiturate effects

Adverse Reactions
CNS: Dizziness, drowsiness, headache
CV: Increased systolic and diastolic blood pressure, tachycardia
EENT: Accommodation disturbances, blurred vision, diplopia
GI: Nausea, vomiting
MS: Muscle weakness
RESP: Hyperventilation
Other: Injection site pain

Nursing Considerations
• Be aware that pralidoxime must be administered within 36 hours of toxicity to be effective.
• Use drug with extreme caution in patients with myasthenia gravis who are being treated for organophosphate poisoning because pralidoxime may precipitate myasthenic crisis.

- Reconstitute drug according to manufacturer's guidelines and administration route.
- For intermittent infusion, further dilute with normal saline solution to a volume of 100 ml and infuse over 15 to 30 minutes.
- Avoid too-rapid administration, which may cause hypertension, laryngospasm, muscle spasms, neuromuscular blockade, and tachycardia. Also be sure to avoid intradermal injection.
- Closely monitor neuromuscular status during therapy.
- Monitor BUN and serum creatinine levels, as appropriate, in patients with renal insufficiency because pralidoxime is excreted in urine.
- When pralidoxime is given with atropine, expect signs of atropinization (dry mouth and nose, flushing, mydriasis, tachycardia), to occur earlier than when atropine is given alone.
- Store drug at room temperature.

PATIENT TEACHING
- Inform patient receiving I.M. pralidoxime that she'll experience pain at the injection site for 40 to 60 minutes afterward.
- Reassure patient that she'll be closely monitored during therapy.

procainamide hydrochloride
Pronestyl

Class and Category
Chemical: Ethyl benzamide monohydrochloride
Therapeutic: Antiarrhythmic
Pregnancy category: C

Indications and Dosages
▶ *To treat life-threatening ventricular arrhythmias, to treat ventricular extrasystoles and arrhythmias associated with anesthesia and surgery*
I.V. INFUSION, I.V. INJECTION
Adults. *Initial:* 100 mg diluted in D_5W and administered at no more than 50 mg/min. Dosage repeated every 5 min until arrhythmia is controlled or maximum total dose of 1 g is reached. Alternatively, 10 to 15 mg/kg I.V. bolus administered at 25 to 50 mg/min. *Maintenance:* 1 to 4 mg/min by continuous infusion.
DOSAGE ADJUSTMENT For elderly patients or patients with cardiac or hepatic insufficiency, dosage possibly reduced or dosing intervals increased. For patients with creatinine clearance less than 50 ml/min/1.73 m², initial dosage reduced to 1 to 2 mg/min.

Route	Onset	Peak	Duration
I.V.	Unknown	Immediate	Unknown

Mechanism of Action

Prolongs the recovery period after myocardial repolarization by inhibiting sodium influx through myocardial cell membranes. This action prolongs the refractory period, causing myocardial automaticity, excitability, and conduction velocity to decline.

Contraindications

Complete heart block, hypersensitivity to procainamide or its components, systemic lupus erythematosus, torsades de pointes

Interactions

DRUGS

antiarrhythmics: Additive cardiac effects

anticholinergics, antidyskinetics, antihistamines: Possibly intensified atropine-like adverse effects, increased risk of ileus

antihypertensives: Additive hypotensive effects

antimyasthenics: Possibly antagonized effect of antimyasthenic on skeletal muscle

bethanechol: Possibly antagonized cholinergic effect of bethanechol

bone marrow depressants: Possibly increased leukopenic or thrombocytopenic effects

bretylium: Possibly decreased inotropic effect of bretylium and enhanced hypotension

neuromuscular blockers: Possibly increased or prolonged neuromuscular blockade

pimozide: Possibly prolonged QT interval, leading to life-threatening arrhythmias

Adverse Reactions

CNS: Chills, disorientation, dizziness, light-headedness

CV: Heart block (second-degree), hypotension, pericarditis, prolonged QT interval, tachycardia

EENT: Bitter taste

GI: Abdominal distress, anorexia, diarrhea, nausea, vomiting

HEME: Agranulocytosis, neutropenia, thrombocytopenia

MS: Arthralgia, myalgia

RESP: Pleural effusion

SKIN: Pruritus, rash

Other: Drug-induced fever, lupuslike symptoms

Nursing Considerations
- Place patient in a supine position before administering procainamide to minimize hypotensive effects. Monitor blood pressure frequently and ECG tracings continuously during administration and for 30 minutes afterward.
- Inspect parenteral solution for particles and discoloration before administering; discard if particles are present or solution is darker than light amber.
- Dilute procainamide with D$_5$W according to manufacturer's instructions.
- For I.V. infusion, dilute 200 to 1,000 mg of procainamide with 50 to 500 ml of D$_5$W, respectively, to yield a concentration of 2 or 4 mg/ml.
- Administer I.V. infusion with an infusion pump or other controlled-delivery device.
- Don't administer more than 500 mg in 30 minutes by I.V. infusion or 50 mg/minute by I.V. injection because heart block or cardiac arrest may occur.
- Anticipate that patient has reached maximum clinical response when ventricular tachycardia resolves, hypotension develops, or QRS complex is 50% wider than it was originally.
- If patient is switching to oral form, expect to administer first oral dose 3 or 4 hours after last I.V. dose.
- Before diluting procainamide, store it at 15° to 30° C (59° to 86° F).

PATIENT TEACHING
- Advise patient receiving procainamide to immediately report bruising, chills, diarrhea, fever, or rash.
- Urge patient to obtain needed dental work before therapy starts or after blood count returns to normal, if possible, because drug can cause myelosuppression and increase the risk of bleeding and infection. Stress the need for good oral hygiene during therapy, and urge patient to consult prescriber before scheduling dental procedures.

prochlorperazine edisylate
Compazine

Class and Category
Chemical: Phenothiazine, piperazine
Therapeutic: Antianxiety agent, antiemetic
Pregnancy category: Not rated

Indications and Dosages

▶ *To control nausea and vomiting related to surgery*

I.V. INFUSION, I.V. INJECTION

Adults and adolescents. 5 to 10 mg at no more than 5 mg/ml 15 to 30 min before anesthesia or during or after surgery, as needed. Dosage repeated once, if necessary. *Maximum:* 10 mg/ dose, 40 mg daily.

▶ *To control severe nausea and vomiting*

I.V. INFUSION, I.V. INJECTION

Adults and adolescents. 2.5 to 10 mg at no more than 5 mg/ min. *Maximum:* 40 mg daily.

▶ *To provide short-term treatment of anxiety*

I.V. INFUSION, I.V. INJECTION

Adults and adolescents. 2.5 to 10 mg at no more than 5 mg/ min. *Maximum:* 40 mg daily.

DOSAGE ADJUSTMENT Initial dose usually reduced and subsequent dosage increased more gradually for elderly, emaciated, and debilitated patients.

Route	Onset	Peak	Duration
I.V.	Unknown	Up to 6 mo	Unknown

Mechanism of Action

Alleviates nausea and vomiting by centrally blocking dopamine receptors in the medullary chemoreceptor trigger zone and by peripherally blocking the vagus nerve in the GI tract. In addition, prochlorperazine's anticholinergic effects and alpha-adrenergic blockade reduce anxiety by decreasing arousal and filtering internal stimuli to the reticular activating system.

Incompatibilities

Don't mix prochlorperazine in same syringe with other drugs. A precipitate may form when prochlorperazine edisylate is mixed in same syringe with morphine sulfate.

Contraindications

Age younger than 2 years, blood dyscrasias, bone marrow depression, cerebral arteriosclerosis, coma, coronary artery disease, hepatic dysfunction, hypersensitivity to phenothiazines, myeloproliferative disorders, pediatric surgery, severe CNS depression, severe hypertension or hypotension, subcortical brain damage, use of large quantities of CNS depressants, weight less than 9 kg (20 lb)

Interactions
DRUGS

amantadine, anticholinergics, antidyskinetics, antihistamines: Possibly intensified anticholinergic adverse effects, increased risk of prochlorperazine-induced hyperpyretic effect

amphetamines: Decreased stimulant effect of amphetamines, decreased antipsychotic effect of prochlorperazine

anticonvulsants: Lowered seizure threshold

antithyroid drugs: Increased risk of agranulocytosis

apomorphine: Possibly decreased emetic response to apomorphine, additive CNS depression

appetite suppressants: Possibly antagonized anorectic effect of appetite suppressants (except for phenmetrazine)

astemizole, cisapride, disopyramide, erythromycin, pimozide, probucol, procainamide: Additive QT interval prolongation, increased risk of ventricular tachycardia

beta blockers: Increased risk of additive hypotensive effects, irreversible retinopathy, arrhythmias, and tardive dyskinesia

bromocriptine: Decreased effectiveness of bromocriptine

CNS depressants: Additive CNS depression

dopamine: Possibly antagonized peripheral vasoconstriction (with high doses of dopamine)

ephedrine, epinephrine: Decreased vasopressor effects of these drugs

hepatotoxic drugs: Increased incidence of hepatotoxicity

hypotension-producing drugs: Possibly severe hypotension and syncope

levodopa: Inhibited antidyskinetic effect of levodopa

lithium: Reduced absorption of oral prochlorperazine, increased excretion of lithium, increased extrapyramidal effects, possibly masking of early symptoms of lithium toxicity

MAO inhibitors, maprotiline, tricyclic antidepressants: Possibly prolonged and intensified anticholinergic and sedative effects, increased blood antidepressant levels, inhibited prochlorperazine metabolism, and increased risk of neuroleptic malignant syndrome

mephentermine: Possibly antagonized antipsychotic effect of prochlorperazine and vasopressor effect of mephentermine

metrizamide: Increased risk of seizures

opioid analgesics: Increased risk of CNS and respiratory depression, orthostatic hypotension, severe constipation, and urine retention

ototoxic drugs: Possibly masking of some symptoms of ototoxicity, such as dizziness, tinnitus, and vertigo

phenytoin: Possibly inhibited phenytoin metabolism and increased risk of phenytoin toxicity

thiazide diuretics: Possibly potentiated hyponatremia and water intoxication

ACTIVITIES

alcohol use: Additive CNS depression

Adverse Reactions

CNS: Akathisia, altered temperature regulation, dizziness, drowsiness, extrapyramidal reactions (such as dystonia, pseudoparkinsonism, tardive dyskinesia)

CV: Hypotension, orthostatic hypotension, tachycardia

EENT: Blurred vision, dry mouth, nasal congestion, ocular changes, pigmentary retinopathy

ENDO: Galactorrhea, gynecomastia

GI: Constipation, epigastric pain, nausea, vomiting

GU: Dysuria, ejaculation disorders, menstrual irregularities, urine retention

SKIN: Decreased sweating, photosensitivity, pruritus, rash

Other: Weight gain

Nursing Considerations

- Wear gloves when working with prochlorperazine because the parenteral solution may cause contact dermatitis.
- Be aware that I.V. form may be administered undiluted as an injection or diluted in isotonic solution as an infusion. Don't administer more than 10 mg as a single dose or exceed a rate of 5 mg/minute.
- Be aware that parenteral solution may develop a slight yellowing that won't affect potency. Don't use if discoloration is pronounced or precipitate is present.
- **WARNING** Monitor closely for numerous adverse reactions that may be serious.
- **WARNING** Monitor patients with chronic respiratory disorders (such as severe asthma or emphysema) or acute respiratory tract infections for exacerbations of these conditions caused by prochlorperazine's CNS depressant effects. Be alert for possible suppressed cough reflex, which increases patient's risk of aspirating vomitus.
- Be aware that patients with cardiovascular or renal disease are at increased risk for developing hypotension, heart failure, and arrhythmias.
- **WARNING** If patient develops neuroleptic malignant syndrome (hyperpyrexia, muscle rigidity, altered mental status, autonomic instability), notify prescriber immediately and ex-

pect to discontinue drug and begin intensive medical treatment.

- Be aware that patients with impaired hepatic function are at risk for decreased prochlorperazine metabolism or further hepatic dysfunction. Monitor patients with a history of hepatic encephalopathy from cirrhosis for increased sensitivity to drug's CNS effects.
- Because prochlorperazine may have anticholinergic effects, monitor patients with a history of, or predisposition to, glaucoma for signs and symptoms of this disorder, such as eye pain, vision changes, or nausea and vomiting from increased intraocular pressure.
- Be aware that drug should be used cautiously in those who are exposed to organophosphorus insecticides.
- Monitor patients who have been exposed to extreme heat for heatstroke caused by drug-induced suppression of temperature regulation. Signs and symptoms include tachycardia, fever, and confusion.
- Be aware that pediatric and elderly patients are at increased risk for developing hypotension and extrapyramidal reactions, especially if they're acutely ill or debilitated.
- Store drug at less than 30° C (86° F); protect from freezing and light.

PATIENT TEACHING

- Advise patient to rise slowly from a lying or sitting position during prochlorperazine therapy to minimize effects of orthostatic hypotension.
- Instruct patient to avoid potentially hazardous activities because of the risk of drowsiness and impaired judgment and coordination.
- Urge patient to report involuntary movements and restlessness.
- Advise patient to report sudden sore throat or other signs of infection.
- Inform patient that drug may reduce body's response to heat and cold; advise her to avoid temperature extremes, such as very cold or hot showers.
- Suggest sugarless chewing gum, hard candy, and fluids to relieve dry mouth.
- Urge patient to avoid alcohol and OTC drugs that may contain CNS depressants.
- Instruct patient to avoid excessive sun exposure and to wear sunscreen when outdoors.

promethazine hydrochloride

Anergan 25, Anergan 50, Antinaus 50, Histantil (CAN), Pentazine, Phenazine 25, Phenazine 50, Phencen-50, Phenergan, Phenerzine, Phenoject-50, Pro-50, Promacot, Pro-Med 50, Promet, Prorex-25, Prorex-50, Prothazine, Shogan, V-Gan-25, V-Gan-50

Class and Category

Chemical: Phenothiazine derivative
Therapeutic: Antiemetic, antihistamine, antivertigo, sedative-hypnotic
Pregnancy category: C

Indications and Dosages

▶ *To prevent or treat nausea and vomiting in certain types of anesthesia and surgery*

I.V. INJECTION

Adults and adolescents. 12.5 to 25 mg every 4 hr, p.r.n. *Maximum:* 150 mg daily.

▶ *To treat signs and symptoms of allergic response*

I.V. INJECTION

Adults and adolescents. 25 mg, repeated within 2 hr, if needed.

▶ *To provide nighttime, preoperative, or postoperative sedation*

I.V. INJECTION

Adults and adolescents. 25 to 50 mg as a single dose. Alternatively, for preoperative and postoperative sedation, 25 to 50 mg combined with appropriately reduced dosages of analgesics and anticholinergics.

DOSAGE ADJUSTMENT Dosage usually decreased for elderly patients.

▶ *To provide obstetric sedation*

I.V. INJECTION

Adults and adolescents. 50 mg for early stages of labor, followed by 1 or 2 doses of 25 to 75 mg after labor is definitely established, repeated every 4 hr during normal labor.

Route	Onset	Peak	Duration
I.V.	3 to 5 min	Unknown	4 to 6 hr

Contraindications

Age younger than 2; angle-closure glaucoma; benign prostatic hyperplasia; bladder neck obstruction; bone marrow depression;

breast-feeding; coma; hypersensitivity or history of idiosyncratic reaction to promethazine, other phenothiazines, or their components; hypertensive crisis; lower respiratory tract disorders (including asthma) when used as an antihistamine; pyloroduodenal obstruction; stenosing peptic ulcer; use of large quantities of CNS depressants

---

Mechanism of Action

Competes with histamine for H_1-receptor sites, thereby antagonizing many histamine effects and reducing allergy signs and symptoms. Promethazine also prevents motion sickness, nausea, and vertigo by acting centrally on the medullary chemoreceptive trigger zone and by decreasing vestibular stimulation and labyrinthine function in the inner ear. In addition, it promotes sedation and relieves anxiety by blocking receptor sites within the CNS, directly reducing stimuli to the brain.

Interactions

DRUGS

amphetamines: Decreased stimulant effect of amphetamines
anticholinergics: Possibly intensified anticholinergic adverse effects
anticonvulsants: Lowered seizure threshold
appetite suppressants: Possibly antagonized anorectic effect of appetite suppressants
beta blockers: Increased risk of additive hypotensive effects, irreversible retinopathy, arrhythmias, and tardive dyskinesia
bromocriptine: Decreased effectiveness of bromocriptine
CNS depressants: Additive CNS depression
dopamine: Possibly antagonized peripheral vasoconstriction (with high doses of dopamine)
ephedrine, metaraminol, methoxamine: Decreased vasopressor response to these drugs
epinephrine: Blocked alpha-adrenergic effects of epinephrine, increased risk of hypotension
guanadrel, guanethidine: Decreased antihypertensive effects of these drugs
hepatotoxic drugs: Increased risk of hepatotoxicity
hypotension-producing drugs: Possibly severe hypotension with syncope
levodopa: Inhibited antidyskinetic effects of levodopa

MAO inhibitors: Possibly prolonged and intensified anticholinergic and CNS depressant effects of promethazine
metrizamide: Increased risk of seizures
ototoxic drugs: Possibly masking of some symptoms of ototoxicity, such as dizziness, tinnitus, and vertigo
quinidine: Additive cardiac effects
riboflavin: Increased riboflavin requirements
ACTIVITIES
alcohol use: Additive CNS depression

Adverse Reactions

CNS: Akathisia, CNS stimulation, confusion, dizziness, drowsiness, dystonia, euphoria, excitation, fatigue, hallucinations, hysteria, incoordination, insomnia, irritability, nervousness, neuroleptic malignant syndrome, paradoxical stimulation, pseudoparkinsonism, restlessness, sedation, seizures, syncope, tardive dyskinesia, tremor
CV: Bradycardia, hypertension, hypotension, tachycardia
EENT: Blurred vision; diplopia; dry mouth, nose, and throat; nasal congestion; tinnitus; vision changes
ENDO: Hyperglycemia
GI: Anorexia, cholestatic jaundice, ileus, nausea, vomiting
GU: Dysuria
HEME: Agranulocytosis, leukopenia, thrombocytopenia, thrombocytopenic purpura
RESP: Apnea, respiratory depression, tenacious bronchial secretions
SKIN: Dermatitis, diaphoresis, jaundice, photosensitivity, rash, urticaria
Other: Angioedema, paradoxical reactions

Nursing Considerations

- Use promethazine cautiously in children because they may be more sensitive to drug effects, especially respiratory effects, which may include life-threatening respiratory depression and apnea despite weight-calculated dosage. Also use cautiously in elderly patients and patients with cardiovascular disease or hepatic dysfunction.
- Use drug cautiously in patients with asthma because of its anticholinergic effects and in patients with seizure disorders or those who use medication that may affect seizure threshold because drug may lower patient's seizure threshold.
- **WARNING** Avoid inadvertent intra-arterial injection of promethazine because it can cause arteriospasm; gangrene

may develop from impaired circulation.
- Give I.V. injection at a rate not to exceed 25 mg/min; rapid I.V. administration may produce a transient fall in blood pressure.
- **WARNING** Monitor respiratory function because drug may suppress cough reflex and cause thickening of bronchial secretions, aggravating such conditions as asthma and COPD, and, in rare cases, may depress respirations and induce apnea.
- Monitor patient's hematologic status as ordered because promethazine may cause bone marrow depression, especially when used with other marrow-toxic agents. Assess patient for evidence of infection or bleeding.
- **WARNING** Monitor patient for evidence of neuroleptic malignant syndrome, such as fever, hypertension or hypotension, involuntary motor activity, mental changes, muscle rigidity, tachycardia, and tachypnea. Be prepared to provide supportive treatment and additional drug therapy, as prescribed.
- Be aware that patient shouldn't have intradermal allergen tests within 72 hours of receiving promethazine because drug may significantly alter flare response.

PATIENT TEACHING
- Advise patient to avoid OTC drugs unless approved by prescriber.
- Instruct patient to notify prescriber immediately if she experiences involuntary movements and restlessness.
- Urge patient to avoid alcohol and other CNS depressants while taking promethazine.
- Instruct patient to avoid hazardous activities until drug's CNS effects are known.
- Suggest frequent rinsing and use of sugarless gum or hard candy to relieve dry mouth.
- Advise patient to avoid excessive sun exposure and to use sunscreen when outdoors.

propofol
(disoprofol)
Diprivan

Class and Category
Chemical: 2,6-Diisopropylphenol derivative
Therapeutic: Sedative-hypnotic
Pregnancy category: B

Indications and Dosages

▶ *To provide sedation for critically ill patients in intensive care*
I.V. INFUSION
Adults. 2.8 to 130 mcg/kg/min. *Usual:* 27 mcg/kg/min.
DOSAGE ADJUSTMENT For elderly, debilitated or ASA-PS
III or IV patients, induction dose decreased and a slower maintenance rate of administration is required.

Route	Onset	Peak	Duration
I.V.	Within 40 sec	Unknown	3 to 5 min

Mechanism of Action

Decreases cerebral blood flow, cerebral metabolic oxygen consumption, and ICP and increases cerebrovascular resistance, which may play a role in propofol's hypnotic effects.

Incompatibilities

Don't mix propofol with other drugs before administration. Don't administer propofol through same I.V. line as blood or plasma products because globular component of emulsion will aggregate.

Contraindications

Hypersensitivity to propofol or its components, to eggs or egg products, or to soy or soy products

Interactions

DRUGS
CNS depressants: Additive CNS depressant, respiratory depressant, and hypotensive effects; possibly decreased emetic effects of opioids
droperidol: Possibly decreased control of nausea and vomiting
ACTIVITIES
alcohol use: Additive CNS depressant, respiratory depressant, and hypotensive effects

Adverse Reactions

CV: Bradycardia, hypotension
GI: Nausea, vomiting
MS: Involuntary muscle movements (transient)
RESP: Apnea
Other: Anaphylaxis, injection site burning, pain, or stinging

Nursing Considerations

• If ordered to dilute propofol before administration, use only

D₅W to yield a final concentration of 2 mg/ml or more.

- Consult prescriber about pretreating injection site with 1 ml of 1% lidocaine to minimize pain, burning, or stinging that may occur with propofol administration. Administering drug through a larger vein in the forearm or antecubital fossa may also minimize injection site discomfort.
- Shake container well before using, and administer drug promptly after opening. Use vial for only one patient. Use prefilled syringes within 6 hours of opening.
- Use a drop counter, syringe pump, or volumetric pump to safely control infusion rate. Don't infuse drug through filter with a pore size of less than 5 microns because doing so could cause emulsion to break down.
- Discard all unused portions of propofol solution as well as reservoirs, I.V. tubing, and solutions immediately after or within 12 hours of administration (6 hours if propofol was transferred from original container) to prevent bacterial growth in stagnant solution. Also, protect solution from light.
- Be aware that dosage may be reduced for debilitated or hypovolemic patients and in those older than age 55. Propofol is not approved to treat sedation in children.
- Taper dosage before discontinuing drug, as ordered. Abrupt discontinuation will cause rapid awakening with anxiety, agitation, and resistance to mechanical ventilation.
- **WARNING** Monitor patient for propofol infusion syndrome, which includes severe metabolic acidosis, hyperkalemia, lipemia, rhabdomyolysis, hepatomegaly, and cardiac and renal failure, especially in patients receiving prolonged high-dose infusions. Alert prescriber immediately, and be prepared to provide emergency supportive care as ordered.
- Expect patient to recover from sedation within 8 minutes.
- Monitor patients with cardiac disease, peripheral vascular disease, impaired cerebral circulation, or increased ICP for signs or symptoms of exacerbation because drug may aggravate these disorders.
- Store drug at 4° to 22° C (40° to 72° F); don't refrigerate. Protect from light.

PATIENT TEACHING

- Encourage patient and family to voice concerns and ask questions before propofol administration.
- Reassure patient that she'll be closely monitored throughout drug administration and that her vital functions, including breathing, will be supported as needed.

propranolol hydrochloride
Inderal

Class and Category
Chemical: Beta-adrenergic blocker
Therapeutic: Antiarrhythmic,
Pregnancy category: C

Indications and Dosages
▶ *To treat supraventricular arrhythmias and ventricular tachycardia*
I.V. INJECTION
Adults. 1 to 3 mg at a rate not to exceed 1 mg/min; repeated after 2 min and again after 4 hr, if needed.
Children. 0.01 to 0.1 mg/kg at no more than 1 mg/min; repeated every 6 to 8 hr, as needed. *Maximum:* 1 mg/dose.
DOSAGE ADJUSTMENT Dosage decreased for patients with hepatic insufficiency

---

Mechanism of Action
Exerts the following effects through its beta-blocking actions:
- prevents arterial dilation and inhibits renin secretion, resulting in decreased blood pressure (in hypertension and pheochromocytoma) and relief of migraine headaches
- decreases the heart rate, which helps resolve tachyarrhythmias
- improves myocardial contractility, which helps ease the symptoms of hypertrophic cardiomyopathy
- decreases myocardial oxygen demand, which helps prevent angina pain and death of myocardial tissue.

In addition, peripheral beta-adrenergic blockade may play a role in propranolol's ability to alleviate tremor.

Contraindications
Asthma, cardiogenic shock, greater than first-degree AV block, heart failure (unless secondary to tachyarrhythmia that's responsive to propranolol), hypersensitivity to propranolol or its components, sinus bradycardia

Interactions
DRUGS
ACE inhibitors, calcium channel blockers, clonidine, diazoxide, guanabenz, resperpine, other hypotension-producing drugs: Additive hypotensive effect and possibly other beta blockade effects

allergen immunotherapy, allergenic extracts for skin testing: Increased risk of serious systemic adverse reactions or anaphylaxis

amiodarone: Additive depressant effects on conduction, negative inotropic effects

anesthetics (hydrocarbon inhalation): Increased risk of myocardial depression and hypotension

antidepressants such as tricyclic agents: Increased risk of hypotension

beta blockers: Additive beta blockade effects

cimetidine: Possibly interference with propranolol clearance

digoxin: Increased risk of bradycardia

dobutamine, isoproterenol: Inhibited effect of propranolol

epinephrine: Possibly uncontrolled hypertension

estrogens: Decreased antihypertensive effect of propranolol

fentanyl, fentanyl derivatives: Possibly increased risk of initial bradycardia after induction doses of fentanyl or a derivative (with long-term propranolol use)

glucagon: Possibly blunted hyperglycemic response

haloperidol: Possibly increased risk of hypotension and cardiac arrest

indomethacin: Possibly reduced effect of propranolol to reduce blood pressure and heart rate

insulin, oral antidiabetic drugs: Possibly impaired glucose control, masking of tachycardia in response to hypoglycemia

lidocaine: Decreased lidocaine clearance, increased risk of lidocaine toxicity

MAO inhibitors: Increased risk of significant hypertension

neuromuscular blockers: Possibly potentiated and prolonged action of these drugs

NSAIDs: Possibly decreased hypotensive effects

phenothiazines: Increased blood levels of both drugs

phenytoin: Additive cardiac depressant effects (with parenteral phenytoin)

propafenone: Increased blood level and half-life of propranolol

quinidine: Possibly increased serum propranolol levels with greater degree of beta blockade and increased risk of postural hypotension

sympathomimetics, xanthines: Possibly mutual inhibition of therapeutic effects

thyroxine: Decreased T_3 concentration

warfarin: Increased concentration of warfarin increasing risk of bleeding

ACTIVITIES

nicotine chewing gum, smoking cessation, smoking deterrents: Increased therapeutic effects of propranolol

Adverse Reactions

CNS: Anxiety, depression, disorientation, dizziness, drowsiness, emotional lability, fatigue, fever, hallucinations, insomnia, lethargy, light headedness, nervousness, paresthesia of hands, short term memory loss, weakness

CV: Arterial insufficiency, AV conduction disorders, bradycardia, cardiac arrest, cold extremities, heart failure, hypotension, sinus bradycardia

EENT: Laryngospasm, nasal congestion, pharyngitis, sore throat, visual disturbances

ENDO: Hyperglycemia or hypoglycemia in diabetic patients

GI: Abdominal pain, constipation, diarrhea, epigastric distress, ischemic colitis, mesenteric arterial thrombosis, nausea, vomiting

GU: Sexual dysfunction

HEME: Agranulocytosis, thrommbocytopenia

MS: Muscle weakness

RESP: Bronchospasm, dyspnea, respiratory distress, wheezing

SKIN: Cutaneous ulcers, erythema multiforme, erythematous rash, exfoliative dermatitis, Stevens-Johnson syndrome, toxic epidermal necrolysis, urticaria

Other: Anaphylaxis, flulike symptoms, systemic lupus erythematosus

Nursing Considerations

- Use with extreme caution in patients with bronchospastic lung disease (because of risk of inducing a bronchial asthmatic attack) and in patients with Wolff-Parkinson-White syndrome and tachycardia (because drug may cause severe bradycardia requiring emergency treatment).
- Monitor blood pressure, apical and radial pulses, fluid intake and output, daily weight, respiration, and circulation in extremities before and during propranolol therapy.
- Give I.V. injection at no more than 1 mg/ minute.
- **WARNING** Monitor ECG continuously, as ordered, when giving I.V. injection. Have emergency drugs and equipment available in case of hypotension or cardiac arrest.
- Protect injection solution from light.
- Because drug's negative inotropic effect can depress cardiac output, monitor it in patients with heart failure, particularly those with severely compromised left ventricular dysfunction.
- Be aware that propranolol can mask tachycardia in hyperthyroidism and that abrupt withdrawal of drug in patients with hyperthyroidism or thyrotoxicosis can precipitate thyroid storm.

- Monitor diabetic patient who is receiving antidiabetic drugs because propranolol can prolong hypoglycemia or promote hyperglycemia. Propranolol also can mask signs of hypoglycemia, especially tachycardia, palpitations, and tremor, but it doesn't suppress diaphoresis or hypertensive response to hypoglycemia.
- **WARNING** Be aware that abruptly stopping drug may cause myocardial ischemia, MI, ventricular arrhythmias, or severe hypertension, especially in patients with cardiac disease.

PATIENT TEACHING
- Advise patient to notify prescriber immediately if she experiences shortness of breath.
- Instruct diabetic patient to regularly monitor blood glucose level and urine for ketones.
- Advise patient to consult prescriber before taking OTC drugs, especially cold remedies.
- Urge patient to avoid potentially hazardous activities until drug's CNS effects are known.
- Advise smoker to notify prescriber immediately if she stops smoking because smoking cessation may decrease drug metabolism, calling for dosage adjustments.

protamine sulfate

Class and Category

Chemical: Simple low–molecular-weight protein
Therapeutic: Heparin antagonist
Pregnancy category: C

Indications and Dosages

▶ *To treat heparin toxicity or hemorrhage associated with heparin therapy*

I.V. INJECTION

Adults and children. 1 mg for each 100 units of heparin to be neutralized, or as indicated by coagulation test results. *Maximum:* 100 mg (within 2-hr period).

Route	Onset	Peak	Duration
I.V.	5 min	Unknown	2 hr

Mechanism of Action

Combines with strongly acidic heparin complex to form an inactive stable salt, thereby neutralizing the anticoagulant activity of both drugs.

Incompatibilities

Don't mix protamine sulfate in same syringe with other drugs unless they're known to be compatible. Several cephalosporins, penicillins, and other antibiotics are incompatible with protamine.

Contraindications

Allergy to fish, hypersensitivity to protamine or its components

Interactions

DRUGS

heparin: Neutralized anticoagulant effect of both drugs

Adverse Reactions

CNS: Weakness
CV: Bradycardia, hypertension, hypotension, shock
GI: Nausea, vomiting
HEME: Unusual bleeding or bruising
RESP: Dyspnea, pulmonary edema (noncardiogenic), pulmonary hypertension
SKIN: Flushing, sensation of warmth
Other: Anaphylaxis

Nursing Considerations

- Expect to administer protamine undiluted. However, dilute drug if needed (for patients other than neonates) with 5 ml of bacteriostatic water for injection containing 0.9% benzyl alcohol.
- **WARNING** When administering drug to neonates or premature infants, reconstitute with preservative-free sterile water for injection. Avoid using solutions that contain benzyl alcohol because they can cause a fatal toxic syndrome in infants, characterized by CNS, respiratory, circulatory, and renal impairment and metabolic acidosis.
- Inject drug slowly at a rate of 5 mg/minute; administer no more than 50 mg in 10 minutes or 100 mg in 2 hours.
- Discard any unused portion because protamine contains no preservatives.
- **WARNING** Be aware that rapid administration may cause severe hypotension and anaphylaxis.
- Be prepared to obtain coagulation studies (APTT, activated clotting time) 5 to 15 minutes after administering drug and to repeat studies in 2 to 8 hours to assess for heparin-rebound hypotension, shock, and bleeding.
- Monitor vital signs, hemodynamic parameters, and fluid intake and output, and assess for flushing sensation.
- Have fluids—epinephrine 1:1,000, dobutamine, or dopamine—

available for allergic or hypotensive reactions.
- Be aware that vasectomized males have an increased risk of hypersensitivity reaction because of possible accumulation of antiprotamine antibodies.
- Store drug at 2° to 8° C (36° to 46° F); don't freeze.

PATIENT TEACHING
- Instruct patient receiving protamine to report adverse reactions immediately.

pyridostigmine bromide
Mestinon, Mestinon-SR (CAN), Mestinon Timespans, Regonol (CAN)

Class and Category
Chemical: Bromide dimethylcarbamate
Therapeutic: Antimyasthenic
Pregnancy category: Not rated

Indications and Dosages
▶ *To treat symptoms of myasthenia gravis*
I.V. INJECTION
Adults and adolescents. 2 mg every 2 to 3 hr.
▶ *To reverse the effects of neuromuscular blockers*
I.V. INJECTION
Adults and adolescents. 10 to 20 mg after 0.6 to 1.2 mg of I.V. atropine has been given.
DOSAGE ADJUSTMENT Dosage possibly reduced for patients with renal impairment.

Route	Onset	Peak	Duration
I.V.	2 to 5 min	Unknown	2 to 4 hr

Mechanism of Action
Improves muscle strength compromised by myasthenia gravis or neuromuscular blockade by competing with acetylcholine for its binding site on acetylcholinesterase. This action potentiates the effects of acetylcholine on skeletal muscle and the GI tract. Inhibited destruction of acetylcholine allows freer transmission of nerve impulses across the neuromuscular junction.

Contraindications
Hypersensitivity to pyridostigmine or its components, mechanical obstruction of GI or urinary tract

Interactions
DRUGS

aminoglycosides (systemic), capreomycin, hydrocarbon inhalation anesthetics, lidocaine (I.V.), lincomycins, polymyxins, quinine: Possibly antagonized effect of pyridostigmine on skeletal muscle; possibly decreased neuromuscular blocking activity of these drugs (with large doses of pyridostigmine)

anticholinergics: Possibly masking of signs of pyridostigmine overdose and reduced intestinal motility

cholinesterase inhibitors: Increased risk of additive toxicity

edrophonium: Possibly worsening of patient's condition

guanadrel, guanethidine, mecamylamine, neuromuscular blockers, procainamide: Possibly prolonged phase I blocking effect or reversal of nondepolarization blockade

local anesthetics: Inhibited neuronal transmission, increased anesthesia effects

quinidine, trimethaphan: Possibly antagonized pyridostigmine effects

Adverse Reactions
CV: Thrombophlebitis
EENT: Increased salivation, lacrimation, miosis
GI: Abdominal cramps, diarrhea, increased peristalsis, nausea, vomiting
GU: Urinary frequency, incontinence, or urgency
MS: Fasciculations, muscle spasms or weakness
RESP: Increased tracheobronchial secretions
SKIN: Diaphoresis, rash

Nursing Considerations
- **WARNING** Maintain a rigid dosing schedule because a missed or late dose of pyridostigmine can precipitate myasthenic crisis.
- Observe for cholinergic reactions, such as muscle weakness, during drug administration.
- Monitor BUN and serum creatinine levels, as ordered, in patients with renal disease because pyridostigmine is mainly excreted unchanged by the kidneys.
- **WARNING** Be aware that pyridostigmine overdose may obscure the diagnosis of myasthenic crisis because the primary symptom in both is muscle weakness. Respiratory muscle involvement can lead to death. Be prepared to treat cholinergic crisis by immediately stopping pyridostigmine therapy, administering atropine as prescribed, and assisting with endotracheal intubation and mechanical ventilation, if needed.

- Be aware that reversal of neuromuscular blockade usually occurs in 15 to 30 minutes. Be prepared to maintain patent airway and ventilation until normal voluntary respiration returns completely. Assess respiratory measurements and muscle tone with peripheral nerve stimulator device, as indicated.
- Store drug at 15° to 30° C (59° to 86° F); protect from freezing and light.

PATIENT TEACHING
- Instruct patient receiving pyridostigmine to report muscle weakness, difficulty breathing, diarrhea, nausea, or vomiting.
- Ask patient to record pyridostigmine dosage, times taken, and effects to help determine optimal dosage and schedule for her needs.
- Urge patient to carry medical identification describing her condition and drug regimen.

pyridoxine hydrochloride
(vitamin B₆)
Beesix, Doxine, Nestrex, Pyri, Rodex, Vitabee 6

Class and Category
Chemical: Water-soluble B complex vitamin
Therapeutic: Nutritional supplement
Pregnancy category: A

Indications and Dosages
▶ *To prevent vitamin B₆ deficiency based on U.S. and Canadian recommended daily allowances (RDAs)*
I.V. INFUSION
Adults and children. Dosage individualized as part of total parenteral nutrition.
▶ *To treat pyridoxine dependency syndrome*
I.V. INJECTION
Adults and children age 11 and over. 30 to 600 mg daily.
Infants with seizures. *Initial:* 10 to 100 mg; then individualized based on severity of deficiency, as prescribed.
▶ *To treat drug-induced pyridoxine deficiency*
I.V. INJECTION
Adults and children age 11 and over. 50 to 200 mg daily for 3 wk; then 25 to 100 mg daily as needed.

Contraindications
Hypersensitivity to pyridoxine or its components

Mechanism of Action

Replaces vitamin in pyridoxine deficiency. In erythrocytes, pyridoxine breaks down to pyridoxal and pyridoxamine, which act as coenzymes in fat, protein, and carbohydrate metabolism. Pyridoxine is used to help convert tryptophan to niacin or serotonin, to break down glycogen to glucose-1-phosphate, and to convert oxalate to glycine. It's also essential in the synthesis of both gamma-aminobutyric acid (within the CNS) and heme.

Interactions

DRUGS

azathioprine, chlorambucil, corticosteroids, cyclophosphamide, cycloserine, cyclosporine, ethionamide, hydralazine, isoniazid, mercaptopurine, penicillamine: Possibly anemia or peripheral neuritis
estrogens, oral contraceptives: Possibly increased RDA of pyridoxine
levodopa: Reversal of levodopa's antiparkinsonian effects

Adverse Reactions

CNS: Sensory neuropathy

Nursing Considerations

- Assess patient's daily intake of pyridoxine, including any OTC sources. If patient has been ingesting high doses (2 to 6 g daily) for several months, assess for sensory neuropathy, characterized by unstable gait and numbness in feet and hands. If symptoms occur, notify prescriber and expect to discontinue drug.
- Evaluate drug's effectiveness in reversing deficiency by assessing for resolution of signs and symptoms, including xanthurenic aciduria, sideroblastic anemia, neurologic problems, seborrheic dermatitis, and cheilosis.
- Store drug at 15° to 30° C (59° to 86° F); protect from freezing and light.

PATIENT TEACHING

- Instruct patient to report unsteadiness while walking or numbness of hands or feet during pyridoxine therapy.
- Inform patient that vitamin is not a substitute for proper diet. Inform her that best sources of dietary pyridoxine include bananas, egg yolks, lima beans, meat, peanuts, and whole grain cereals.

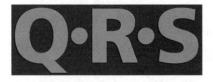

quinidine gluconate

Class and Category

Chemical: Dextrorotatory isomer of quinine
Therapeutic: Class IA antiarrhythmic
Pregnancy category: C

Indications and Dosages

▶ *To prevent or treat cardiac arrhythmias, including established atrial fibrillation, atrial flutter, paroxysmal atrial fibrillation, paroxysmal atrial tachycardia, paroxysmal AV junctional rhythm, paroxysmal ventricular tachycardia not associated with complete heart block, and premature atrial and ventricular contractions*

I.V. INFUSION

Adults. 800 mg in 40 ml of D_5W at up to 0.25 mg/kg/min.

Mechanism of Action

Depresses excitability, conduction velocity, and contractility of the myocardium and increases the effective refractory period to suppress arrhythmic activity in the atria, ventricles, and His-Purkinje system.

Contraindications

Digitalis toxicity; history of quinidine-induced thrombocytopenic purpura or torsades de pointes; hypersensitivity to quinidine, other cinchona derivatives, or their components; long QT syndrome; myasthenia gravis; pacemaker-dependent conduction disturbances

Interactions

DRUGS

antiarrhythmics, phenothiazines, rauwolfia alkaloids, and other drugs that prolong QT interval: Additive cardiac effects
anticholinergics: Possibly intensified atropine-like adverse effects
antimyasthenics: Antagonized antimyasthenic effects on skeletal muscle

barbiturates, rifampin: Possibly accelerated elimination and decreased effectiveness of quinidine

cimetidine: Increased elimination half-life, possibly leading to quinidine toxicity

digoxin: Possibly digitalis toxicity

hepatic enzyme inducers: Possibly decreased blood quinidine level

hepatic enzyme inhibitors: Possibly increased blood quinidine level

neuromuscular blockers: Possibly potentiated neuromuscular blockade

oral anticoagulants: Additive hypoprothrombinemia, increased risk of bleeding

pimozide: Risk of arrhythmias

quinine: Increased risk of quinidine toxicity

urinary alkalizers (such as antacids, carbonic anhydrase inhibitors, citrates, sodium bicarbonate, and thiazide diuretics): Increased renal tubular reabsorption of quinidine, possibly leading to quinidine toxicity

verapamil: Possibly AV block, bradycardia, pulmonary edema, significant hypotension, and ventricular tachycardia

Adverse Reactions

CNS: Anxiety, asthenia, ataxia, confusion, delirium, difficulty speaking, dizziness, drowsiness, extrapyramidal reactions, fever, headache, hypertonia, syncope, vertigo

CV: Complete heart block, orthostatic hypotension, palpitations, peripheral edema, prolonged QT interval, torsades de pointes, vasculitis, ventricular arrhythmias, widening QRS complex

EENT: Blurred vision, change in color perception, diplopia, dry mouth, hearing loss (high-frequency), pharyngitis, photophobia, rhinitis, tinnitus

GI: Abdominal pain, anorexia, constipation, diarrhea, indigestion, nausea, vomiting

HEME: Agranulocytosis, hemolytic anemia, leukopenia, neutropenia, thrombocytopenia, thrombocytopenic purpura

MS: Arthralgia, myalgia

RESP: Dyspnea

SKIN: Diaphoresis, eczema, exfoliative dermatitis, flushing, hyperpigmentation, photosensitivity, pruritus, psoriasis, purpura, rash, urticaria

Other: Angioedema, flulike symptoms, weight gain

Nursing Considerations

- For intermittent I.V. infusion, dilute quinidine in 40 ml of D_5W and administer using an infusion pump at a rate of 0.25 mg/kg/

minute or less. Rapid administration may cause hypotension. Use diluted solutions within 24 hours if stored at room temperature or within 48 hours if refrigerated. Monitor ECG tracings and blood pressure throughout administration.

• Monitor therapeutic blood level of quinidine, as ordered, in all patients receiving drug.

• Monitor heart rate and rhythm closely because quinidine may cause serious adverse reactions and can be cardiotoxic, especially at dosages exceeding 2.4 g daily. Implement continuous cardiac monitoring, as ordered.

• Monitor serum electrolyte levels, especially potassium, as prescribed to identify electrolyte imbalances, which increase patient's risk of developing adverse cardiac reactions such as torsades de pointes.

• Assess for early signs and symptoms of cinchonism, including blurred vision, change in color perception, confusion, diplopia, headache, and tinnitus, which may indicate quinidine toxicity.

• Before diluting quinidine, store it at 15° to 30° C (59° to 86° F).

PATIENT TEACHING
• Urge patient receiving quinidine to immediately report blurred or double vision, change in color perception, confusion, diarrhea, fever, headache, loss of hearing, or tinnitus.

quinupristin and dalfopristin
Synercid

Class and Category
Chemical: Pristinamycin I and IIa derivative, streptogramin
Therapeutic: Antibiotic
Pregnancy category: B

Indications and Dosages
▶ *To treat serious or life-threatening infections, such as bacteremia, caused by vancomycin-resistant* Enterococcus faecium
I.V. INFUSION
Adults and adolescents age 16 and over. 7.5 mg/kg every 8 hr.

▶ *To treat complicated skin and soft-tissue infections caused by methicillin-susceptible strains of* Staphylococcus aureus *or* Streptococcus pyogenes
I.V. INFUSION
Adults and adolescents age 16 and over. 7.5 mg/kg every 12 hr for at least 7 days.

Mechanism of Action

Inhibits bacterial protein synthesis by irreversibly blocking ribosome functioning. Quinupristin inhibits the late phase of protein synthesis by binding to the 50S ribosomal subunit. Dalfopristin inhibits the early phase of protein synthesis by binding to the 70S or 50S ribosomal subunit. This combined activity also inhibits transfer RNA (tRNA) synthetase activity, which decreases the amount of free tRNA within the cell. Without tRNA, the bacterial cell cannot incorporate amino acids into peptide chains and eventually dies.

Incompatibilities

Don't mix quinupristin and dalfopristin in saline solutions, including normal saline solution, 0.45 normal saline solution, 3% sodium chloride, and 5% sodium chloride, because drug is physically incompatible with these solutions.

Contraindications

Hypersensitivity to quinupristin or dalfopristin, other streptogramin antibiotics, or their components

Interactions

DRUGS

alfentanil, alprazolam, carbamazepine, delavirdine, diazepam, diltiazem, disopyramide, dofetilide, donepezil, erythromycin, ethinyl estradiol, felodipine, fexofenadine, indinavir, lidocaine, lovastatin, methylprednisolone, nevirapine, norethindrone, quinidine, ritonavir, saquinavir, simvastatin, tacrolimus, triazolam, trimetrexate, verapamil, vinblastine: Decreased elimination of these drugs, possibly resulting in toxicity
astemizole, cisapride: Decreased elimination of these drugs, possibly prolonged QT interval
cyclosporine, midazolam, nifedipine: Possibly increased blood levels of these drugs
terfenadine: Decreased elimination and increased blood level of terfenadine, possibly prolonged QT interval

Adverse Reactions

CNS: Anxiety, confusion, dizziness, fever, headache, hypertonia, insomnia, paresthesia
CV: Chest pain, palpitations, peripheral edema, thrombophlebitis, vasodilation
EENT: Oral candidiasis, stomatitis
GI: Abdominal pain, constipation, diarrhea, elevated liver function test results, indigestion, nausea, pancreatitis, pseudomembra-

nous colitis, vomiting
GU: Hematuria, vaginitis
MS: Arthralgia, gout, muscle spasms, myalgia, myasthenia
RESP: Dyspnea, pleural effusion
SKIN: Diaphoresis, pruritus, rash, urticaria
Other: Injection site edema, inflammation, pain, or thrombophlebitis

Nursing Considerations

- **WARNING** Reconstitute and further dilute quinupristin and dalfopristin only with dextrose in water or sterile water for injection. Don't use saline solutions because drug is physically incompatible with them.
- Reconstitute 500-mg vial (150 mg quinupristin and 350 mg dalfopristin) only with 5 ml of 5% dextrose for injection or sterile water for injection to yield a concentration of 100 mg/ml.
- Swirl gently to mix; don't shake. Let foam dissipate until solution is clear.
- Further dilute reconstituted solution within 30 minutes. Vials are for single use only. Discard any unused portion.
- Dilute prescribed dose in 250 ml of D₅W. Use diluted solution as soon as possible to avoid possible microbial contamination—within 5 hours if stored at room temperature or within 54 hours if refrigerated; don't freeze. Infuse drug over 1 hour through a peripheral I.V. line. If administered by central venous catheter, dilute prescribed dose in 100 ml of D₅W. Central venous administration may decrease incidence of infusion site reaction. Use an infusion pump or device to control rate of infusion.
- Don't flush I.V. catheter with saline or heparin flush solution because of possible incompatibility. Flush I.V. catheter only with D₅W before and after drug administration.
- Monitor patient for diarrhea, a possible indication of overgrowth of normal intestinal flora, such as *Clostridium difficile*. Be aware that pseudomembranous colitis may result from a toxin produced by *C. difficile*.
- If you suspect that patient has pseudomembranous colitis, notify prescriber and expect to stop drug immediately.
- If patient develops pseudomembranous colitis, be aware that drugs that inhibit peristalsis are contraindicated because of the risk of toxic megacolon.
- Assess infusion area for redness or swelling, and ask patient if he feels discomfort. If irritation occurs, expect to change infusion site, increase amount of diluent to 500 or 750 ml, or administer

drug by peripherally inserted central catheter, if ordered.
• Store unopened vials in refrigerator.
PATIENT TEACHING
• Advise patient receiving quinupristin and dalfopristin to immediately report diarrhea or abdominal pains.
• Emphasize the importance of completing the full course of quinupristin and dalfopristin therapy, as prescribed.
• Inform patient that if he requires long-term therapy, drug will be administered either in the hospital or clinic or by a home health care nurse.

ranitidine hydrochloride
Zantac

Class and Category
Chemical: Aminoalkyl-substituted puran derivative
Therapeutic: Antiulcer agent, gastric acid secretion inhibitor
Pregnancy category: B

Indications and Dosages
▶ *To provide short-term treatment of active duodenal and benign gastric ulcers*
CONTINUOUS I.V. INFUSION
Adults and adolescents. 6.25 mg/hr. *Maximum:* 400 mg daily.
INTERMITTENT I.V. INFUSION
Adults and adolescents. 50 mg diluted to total volume of 100 ml and infused over 15 to 20 min every 6 to 8 hr. *Maximum:* 400 mg daily.
Children. 2 to 4 mg/kg daily diluted to a suitable volume and infused over 15 to 20 min.
I.V. INJECTION
Adults and adolescents. 50 mg diluted to total volume of 20 ml and injected slowly, over no less than 5 min, every 6 to 8 hr. *Maximum:* 400 mg daily.
▶ *To treat acute gastroesophageal reflux disease*
INTERMITTENT I.V. INFUSION
Children. 2 to 8 mg/kg diluted to suitable volume and infused over 15 to 20 min t.i.d.
▶ *To treat hypersecretory GI conditions, such as Zollinger-Ellison syndrome, systemic mastocytosis, and multiple endocrine adenoma syndrome*
CONTINUOUS I.V. INFUSION
Adults and adolescents. *Initial:* 1 mg/kg/hr, increased by

0.5 mg/kg/hr up to 2.5 mg/kg/hr. *Maximum:* 400 mg daily.
INTERMITTENT I.V. INFUSION
Adults. 50 mg diluted to total volume of 100 ml and infused over 15 to 20 min every 6 to 8 hr. *Maximum:* 400 mg daily.
I.V. INJECTION
Adults and adolescents. 50 mg diluted to total volume of 20 ml and injected slowly, over no less than 5 min, every 6 to 8 hr. *Maximum:* 400 mg daily.
DOSAGE ADJUSTMENT For adults with creatinine clearance less than 50 ml/min/1.73 m^2, 50 mg every 18 to 24 hr; dosage interval increased to every 12 hr as needed. Dosage reduction may also be needed for patients with hepatic dysfunction.

Route	Onset	Peak	Duration
I.V.	Unknown	1 to 3 hr	13 hr

Mechanism of Action
Inhibits basal and nocturnal secretion of gastric acid and pepsin by competitively inhibiting the action of histamine at H$_2$ receptors on gastric parietal cells. This action reduces total volume of gastric juices and, thus, irritation of GI mucosa.

Contraindications
Acute porphyria, hypersensitivity to ranitidine or its components

Interactions
DRUGS
bone marrow depressants: Increased risk of neutropenia or other blood dyscrasias
diazepam, itraconazole, ketoconazole, sucralfate: Decreased absorption of these drugs
glipizide, glyburide, metoprolol, midazolam, nifedipine, phenytoin, theophylline, warfarin: Increased effects of these drugs, possibly leading to toxic reactions

Adverse Reactions
CNS: Dizziness, drowsiness, headache, insomnia
GI: Abdominal distress, constipation, diarrhea, nausea, vomiting
GU: Impotence
MS: Arthralgia, myalgia
RESP: Bronchospasm
Other: Anaphylaxis, angioedema

Nursing Considerations

- Be aware that ranitidine must be diluted for I.V. administration if premixed solution is not being used. For I.V. injection, dilute to total volume of 20 ml with normal saline solution, D_5W, $D_{10}W$, lactated Ringer's solution, or 5% sodium bicarbonate. For I.V. infusion, dilute to total volume of 100 ml with any of the above solutions. Use diluted solution within 48 hours if stored at room temperature.
- Administer I.V. injection at no more than 4 ml/minute, intermittent I.V. infusion at 5 to 7 ml/minute, and continuous I.V. infusion at 6.25 mg/hour (except in patients with hypersecretory conditions, for whom initial infusion rate is 1 mg/kg/hour and then gradually increased after 4 hours, as needed, in increments of 0.5 mg/kg/hour).
- Don't introduce additives into premixed solution.
- Stop primary I.V. solution infusion during piggyback administration.
- Store undiluted ranitidine below 30° C (86° F); store premixed form at 2° to 25° C (36° to 77° F). Protect drug from freezing and light.

PATIENT TEACHING

- Instruct patient to report discomfort at ranitidine infusion site.
- Inform patient about potential adverse reactions, such as dizziness, headache, and myalgia, and advise her to report them.
- Inform patient that ulcer may take 4 to 8 weeks to heal.

remifentanil hydrochloride
Ultiva

Class, Category, and Schedule
Chemical: Fentanyl analogue
Therapeutic: Anesthesia adjunct
Pregnancy category: C
Controlled substance schedule: II

Indications and Dosages
▶ *As adjunct to induce general anesthesia*
INTERMITTENT I.V. INFUSION
Adults and children age 2 and over. 0.5 to 1 mcg/kg in addition to inhalation or I.V. anesthetic.
▶ *To maintain general anesthesia*
INTERMITTENT I.V. INFUSION
Adults and children age 2 and over. 0.05 to 0.2 mcg/kg, fol-

lowed by 0.5 to 1 mcg/kg every 2 to 5 min, as needed.

▶ *To continue analgesic effect in immediate postoperative period*

CONTINUOUS I.V. INFUSION

Adults and children age 2 and over. *Initial:* 0.1 mcg/kg/min, adjusted by 0.025 mcg/kg/min every 5 min, as prescribed, to balance the level of analgesia and the respiratory rate. *Maximum:* 0.2 mcg/kg/min.

▶ *To supplement local or regional anesthesia in a monitored anesthetic setting*

I.V. INFUSION

Adults and children age 2 and over. With a benzodiazepine: 0.05 mcg/kg/min, beginning 5 min before placement of local or regional block; after placement of block, decreased to 0.025 mcg/kg/min and then further adjusted every 5 min in increments of 0.025 mcg/kg/min, as needed. Without a benzodiazepine: 0.1 mcg/kg/min, beginning 5 min before placement of local or regional block; after placement of block, decreased to 0.05 mcg/kg/min and then further adjusted every 5 min in increments of 0.025 mcg/kg/min, as needed.

I.V. INJECTION

Adults and children age 2 and over. With a benzodiazepine: 0.5 mcg/kg administered over 30 to 60 sec as a single dose 60 to 90 sec before local anesthetic is administered. Without a benzodiazepine: 1 mcg/kg administered over 30 to 60 sec as a single dose 60 to 90 sec before local anesthetic is administered.

DOSAGE ADJUSTMENT For elderly patients, starting dose possibly reduced by half. If patient is more than 30% over ideal body weight, starting dose should be based on ideal body weight.

Route	Onset	Peak	Duration
I.V.	1 min	1 to 2 min	5 to 10 min

Incompatibilities

Don't administer remifentanil through same I.V. line as blood because nonspecific esterases in blood products may inactivate drug.

Contraindications

Epidural or intrathecal administration, hypersensitivity to fentanyl analogues

Interactions

DRUGS

anesthetics (barbiturate, inhalation), benzodiazepines, propofol: Possibly synergistic effects, increasing risk of hypotension and respiratory depression

atropine, glycopyrrolate: Possibly reversal of remifentanil-induced bradycardia

ephedrine, epinephrine, norepinephrine: Possibly reversal of remifentanil-induced hypotension

neuromuscular blockers: Prolonged remifentanil-induced skeletal muscle rigidity

opioid antagonists: Possibly reversal of remifentanil's effects

Mechanism of Action

Remifentanil decreases the transmission and perception of pain by stimulating mu-opiate receptors in neurons. This action decreases the activity of adenyl cyclase in neurons, which in turn decreases cAMP production. With less cAMP available, potassium (K+) is forced out of neurons, and calcium (Ca++) is prevented from entering neurons. As a result, neuron excitability declines, and fewer neurotransmitters (such as substance P) leave the neurons, thereby decreasing pain transmission.

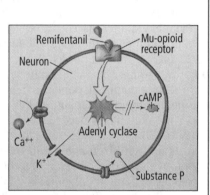

Adverse Reactions

CNS: Headache, shivering
CV: Asystole, bradycardia, hypotension
GI: Nausea, vomiting
MS: Skeletal muscle rigidity
RESP: Apnea, cough, dyspnea, respiratory depression, stridor, wheezing
Other: Anaphylaxis

Nursing Considerations

- Inject remifentanil into I.V. tubing at or as close as possible to venous cannula.
- Use infusion device for continuous infusion.
- Monitor vital signs and oxygenation continuously during administration.
- Expect analgesic effects to dissipate rapidly when drug is discon-

tinued. Expect to start adequate postoperative analgesia, as prescribed, before stopping drug.

• **WARNING** After stopping drug, clear I.V. tubing to prevent
inadvertent later administration.

• Monitor respiratory status continuously because of risk of respiratory depression from residual effects of other anesthetics for
up to 30 minutes after infusion stops.

PATIENT TEACHING

• Explain expected drug effects to patient, and reassure her that
she'll be monitored continuously during drug administration.

reteplase
Retavase

Class and Category
Chemical: Recombinant plasminogen activator (r-PA)
Therapeutic: Thrombolytic
Pregnancy category: C

Indications and Dosages
▶ *To improve ventricular function, prevent heart failure, and reduce
mortality after acute MI*
I.V. INJECTION
Adults. 10 units over 2 min; repeated after 30 min.

Mechanism of Action
Converts plasminogen to plasmin, which works to break up fibrin clots that
have formed in the coronary arteries. Elimination of the clots improves cardiac blood and oxygen flow to the area, thus improving ventricular function.

Incompatibilities
Don't add other drugs to, or administer them through same I.V.
line as, reteplase injection solution.

Contraindications
Active internal bleeding, aneurysm, arteriovenous malformation,
bleeding diathesis, brain tumor, history of CVA or other cerebrovascular disease, hypersensitivity to reteplase or its components,
intracranial or intraspinal surgery or trauma during previous
2 months, severe uncontrolled hypertension (systolic blood pressure 200 mm Hg or higher, diastolic blood pressure 110 mm Hg
or higher)

Interactions
DRUGS

antifibrinolytics (including aminocaproic acid, aprotinin, and tranexamic acid): Decreased effectiveness of reteplase

antineoplastics, antithymocyte globulin, certain cephalosporins (such as cefamandole, cefoperazone, and cefotetan), heparin, oral anticoagulants, platelet aggregation inhibitors (such as abciximab, aspirin, and dipyridamole), strontium-89 chloride, sulfinpyrazone, valproic acid: Increased risk of bleeding

Adverse Reactions
CNS: Intracranial hemorrhage
GI: GI bleeding, nausea, vomiting
HEME: Thrombocytopenia
RESP: Hemoptysis
SKIN: Bleeding from wounds, ecchymosis, hematoma, purpura
Other: Anaphylaxis, injection site bleeding

Nursing Considerations
- Expect to begin reteplase therapy, as prescribed, as soon as possible after MI symptoms begin.
- Closely monitor patient with atrial fibrillation, severe hypertension, or other cardiac disease for signs and symptoms of cerebral embolism.
- Reconstitute drug using diluent, syringe, needle, and dispensing pin provided. Withdraw 10 ml of preservative-free sterile water for injection. Remove and discard needle from syringe, and connect dispensing pin to syringe. Remove protective cap from spike end of dispensing pin, and insert spike into reteplase vial. Inject 10 ml of sterile water into the vial. With the spike still in the vial, swirl gently—don't shake—to dissolve the powder. Expect to see slight foaming. Let vial stand for several minutes. When bubbles dissipate, withdraw 10 ml of reconstituted solution into syringe (about 0.7 ml may remain in vial). Now detach syringe from dispensing pin and attach 20G needle.
- Use solution within 4 hours. Discard if it appears discolored or contains particles.
- Don't administer heparin and reteplase in same solution. Instead, flush heparin line with normal saline solutin or D$_5$W before and after reteplase injection.
- Because fibrin is lysed during therapy, closely monitor all possible bleeding sites (catheter insertions, arterial and venous punctures, cutdowns, and needle punctures).

- Avoid I.M. injections, venipunctures, and nonessential handling of patient during therapy.
- If arterial puncture is necessary, use an arm vessel that can be compressed, if possible. After sample is obtained, apply pressure for at least 30 minutes, and then apply a pressure dressing. Check site frequently for bleeding.
- If bleeding occurs and can't be controlled by local pressure, notify prescriber immediately. Be prepared to stop concurrent anticoagulant therapy immediately and to discontinue second reteplase bolus, as prescribed.
- Anticipate that reperfusion arrhythmias—premature ventricular contractions, ventricular tachycardia—may follow coronary thrombolysis.
- Store drug at 2° to 25° C (36° to 77° F), and protect from light.

PATIENT TEACHING
- Advise patient to immediately report adverse reactions to reteplase, including bleeding or bruising, headache, rash, or difficulty breathing.
- Instruct patient to maintain strict bed rest while receiving reteplase to prevent or minimize bleeding.

rifampin
(rifampicin)
Rifadin, Rifadin IV, Rimactane, Rofact (CAN)

Class and Category
Chemical: Semisynthetic antibiotic derivative of rifamycin
Therapeutic: Antimycobacterial antitubercular
Pregnancy category: C

Indications and Dosages
▶ *As adjunct to treat tuberculosis caused by all strains of* Mycobacterium tuberculosis
I.V. INFUSION
Adults. 10 mg/kg daily in combination with other antitubercular drugs for 2 mo. *Maximum:* 600 mg daily.
Infants and children. 10 to 20 mg/kg daily in combination with other antitubercular drugs for 2 mo. *Maximum:* 600 mg daily.
▶ *To eliminate meningococci from nasopharynx of asymptomatic carriers of* Neisseria meningitidis
I.V. INFUSION
Adults. 600 mg every 12 hr for 2 days (total of 4 doses).

Infants age 1 month and over and children. 10 mg/kg every 12 hr for 2 days (total of 4 doses). *Maximum:* 600 mg daily.
Infants under age 1 month. 5 mg/kg every 12 hr for 2 days (total of 4 doses). *Maximum:* 600 mg daily.
DOSAGE ADJUSTMENT For patients with hepatic impairment, maximum dosage of 8 mg/kg daily. For patients with creatinine clearance of 10 ml/min/1.73 m^2 or less, recommended dosage usually decreased by 50%.

Mechanism of Action

Inhibits bacterial and mycobacterial RNA synthesis by binding to DNA-dependent RNA polymerase, thereby blocking RNA transcription. Exhibits dose-dependent bactericidal or bacteriostatic action. Rifampin is highly effective against rapidly dividing bacilli in extracellular cavitary lesions, such as those found in the nasopharynx.

Incompatibilities

Don't administer rifampin in the same I.V. line as diltiazem.

Contraindications

Concurrent use of nonnucleoside reverse transcriptase inhibitors or protease inhibitors by patients with HIV, hypersensitivity to rifamycins

Interactions

DRUGS

aminophylline, oxtriphylline, theophylline: Increased metabolism and clearance of these theophylline preparations
anesthetics (hydrocarbon inhalation, except isoflurane), hepatotoxic drugs, isoniazid: Increased risk of hepatotoxicity
beta blockers, chloramphenicol, clofibrate, corticosteroids, cyclosporine, dapsone, digitalis glycosides, disopyramide, hexobarbital, itraconazole, ketoconazole, mexiletine, oral anticoagulants, oral antidiabetic drugs, phenytoin, propafenone, quinidine, tocainide, verapamil (oral): Increased metabolism, resulting in lower blood levels of these drugs
bone marrow depressants: Increased leukopenic or thrombocytopenic effects
clofazimine: Reduced absorption of rifampin, delaying its peak concentration and increasing its half-life
diazepam: Enhanced elimination of diazepam, resulting in decreased drug effectiveness
estramustine, estrogens, oral contraceptives: Decreased estrogen effects

methadone: Possibly impaired absorption of methadone, leading to withdrawal symptoms

probenecid: Increased blood level or prolonged duration of rifampin, increasing risk of toxicity

nonnucleoside reverse transcriptase inhibitors, protease inhibitors (indinavir, nelfinavir, ritonavir, saquinavir): Accelerated metabolism of these drugs (by patients with HIV), resulting in subtherapeutic levels; delayed metabolism of rifampin, increasing risk of toxicity

trimethoprim: Increased elimination and shortened elimination half-life of trimethoprim

vitamin D: Increased metabolism and decreased efficacy of vitamin D, leading to decreased serum calcium and phosphate levels and increased parathyroid hormone levels

ACTIVITIES

alcohol use: Increased risk of hepatotoxicity

Adverse Reactions

CNS: Chills, dizziness, drowsiness, fatigue, headache, paresthesia
EENT: Discolored saliva, tears, and sputum; mouth or tongue soreness; periorbital edema
GI: Abdominal cramps, anorexia, diarrhea, discolored feces, elevated liver function test results, epigastric discomfort, flatulence, heartburn, hepatitis, nausea, pseudomembranous colitis, vomiting
GU: Discolored urine
MS: Arthralgia, myalgia
SKIN: Discolored skin and sweat
Other: Facial edema, flulike symptoms

Nursing Considerations

- Obtain blood samples or other specimens for culture and sensitivity testing, as ordered, before giving rifampin and throughout therapy to monitor response to drug.
- Expect to monitor liver function test results before and every 2 to 4 weeks during therapy. Immediately report abnormalities.
- For I.V. infusion, reconstitute by adding 10 ml of sterile water for injection to 600-mg vial of rifampin. Swirl gently to dissolve. Withdraw appropriate dose and add to 500 ml of D_5W (preferred solution) or normal saline solution and infuse over 3 hours. Alternatively, withdraw appropriate dose and add to 100 ml of D_5W (preferred solution) or normal saline solution and infuse over 30 minutes. Use reconstituted drug promptly because rifampin may precipitate out of D_5W solution after 4 hours. Normal saline solution solution is stable for up to 24 hours at room temperature.

- Be aware that patient receiving intermittent therapy (once or twice weekly) is at increased risk for adverse reactions.
- Expect drug to discolor skin and body fluids reddish orange to reddish brown.
- Be aware that rifampin can cause myelosuppression and increase risk of infection. Notify prescriber immediately if signs of infection, such as fever, develop.

PATIENT TEACHING

- Explain that drug may turn urine, feces, saliva, sputum, sweat, tears, and skin reddish orange to reddish brown.
- Caution patient against wearing soft contact lenses during therapy because drug may permanently stain them.
- Advise patient who takes an oral contraceptive to use an additional form of birth control during rifampin therapy.
- Urge patient to report flulike symptoms, anorexia, darkened urine, fever, joint pain or swelling, malaise, nausea, vomiting, and yellowish skin or eyes, which may indicate hepatitis.
- Advise patient to avoid alcohol during rifampin therapy.
- Instruct patient to notify prescriber if no improvement occurs within 2 to 3 weeks.

rituximab

Rituxan

Class and Category

Chemical: Chimeric murine-human monoclonal antibody
Therapeutic: Antirheumatic
Pregnancy category: C

Indications and Dosages

▶ *To reduce signs and symptoms in patients with moderate to severe active rheumatoid arthritis who take methotrexate and had an inadequate response to one or more tumor necrosis factor antagonists*

I.V. INFUSION

Adults. 1,000 mg at an initial rate of 50 mg/hr. If no hypersensitivity or infusion reaction occurs, increased in increments of 50 mg/hr every 30 minutes to a maximum of 400 mg/hr. Dosage repeated in 2 wk at an initial rate of 100 mg/hr if no reaction occurred with first infusion given 2 wk prior. Increased in increments of 100 mg/hr every 30 minutes to a maximum of 400 mg/hr.

▶ *To treat relapsed or refractory, low-grade or follicular, CD20-positive, B-cell non-Hodgkin's lymphoma*

I.V. INFUSION

Adults. 375 mg/m^2 once/wk for 4 to 8 doses.

▶ *To treat previously untreated follicular, CD20-positive, B-cell non-Hodgkin's lymphoma or diffuse large B-cell, CD20-positive non-Hodgkin's lymphoma*

I.V. INFUSION

Adults. 375 mg/m^2 on day 1 of each cycle of chemotherapy for up to 8 infusions.

▶ *To treat nonprogressive, low-grade, CD20-positive, B-cell non-Hodgkin's lymphoma after first-line treatment with CVP chemotherapy regimen*

I.V. INFUSION

Adults. 375 mg/m^2 once/wk for 4 doses every 6 months for maximum of 16 doses.

DOSAGE ADJUSTMENT For patients who have a hypersensitivity or infusion reaction with first dose, infusion temporarily slowed or stopped until symptoms resolve. Infusion restarted at half the previous rate. For patients who have a hypersensitivity or infusion reaction to first dose, second dose given in the same manner as first dose.

Mechanism of Action

Binds to the CD20 antigen on pre-B and mature B lymphocytes. B lymphocytes may play a role in autoimmune and inflammatory processes, including the pathogenesis of rheumatoid arthritis. Processes may include production of rheumatoid factor and other autoantibodies, antigen presentation, T-cell activation, and production of pro-inflammatory cytokines. Interference with these activities hinders the autoimmune and inflammatory processes, reducing signs and symptoms of rheumatoid arthritis.

Contraindications

Hepatitis, history of anaphylaxis or IgE-mediated hypersensitivity to murine proteins, hypersensitivity to rituximab or its components, renal impairment

Interactions

DRUGS

anticoagulants: Additive risk of bleeding in thrombocytopenic patients

antihypertensives: Inreased risk of hypotension

cisplatin: Possibly increased risk of renal toxicity

fludarabine: Additive cytotoxic effects

vaccines: Suboptimal antibody response, particularly to live-virus vaccines

Adverse Reactions

CNS: Anxiety, asthenia, chills, fever, insomnia, migraine head-aches, paresthesia, progressive multifocal leukoencephalopathy, rigors, vertigo

CV: Angina, cardiogenic shock, hypercholesterolemia, hyperten-sion, hypotension, MI, supraventricular tachycardia, ventricular tachycardia or fibrillation

EENT: Nasopharyngitis, rhinitis, sneezing, sinusitis, throat irrita-tion

GI: Anorexia, dyspepsia, nauseaupper abdominal pain

GU: Acute renal failure, UTI

MS: Arthralgia

RESP: Acute respiratory distress syndrome, bronchitis, bron-chospasm, cough, hypoxia, pneumonitis, pulmonary infiltrates, upper respiratory tract infection

SKIN: Flushing, paraneoplastic pemphigus, Stevens-Johnson syn-drome, lichenoid or vesiculobullous dermatitis, toxic epidermal necrolysis, pruritus, urticaria

Other: Anaphylaxis, angioedema, fatal infusion reaction, injec-tion site reaction, tumor lysis syndrome, weight loss

Nursing Considerations

- **WARNING** Severe infusion reactions are common during the first infusion, starting within 30 to 120 minutes, especially in patients with cardiac or pulmonary conditions, those with previous adverse cardiopulmonary reactions, and those with large numbers (more than 25,000/mm³) of circulating malig-nant cells. Monitor patient for urticaria, hypotension, an-gioedema, hypoxia, bronchospasm, pulmonary infiltrates, acute respiratory distress syndrome, myocardial infarction, ventricular fibrillation, cardiogenic shock, and anaphylaxis. If a reaction occurs, stop drug and provide emergency treatment immediately, as needed.
- Expect to give methylprednisolone 100 mg IV or its equilvalent 30 minutes before each rituximab dose to reduce the risk and severity of infusion reactions.
- Expect to give methotrexate with rituximab.
- Dilute rituximab before giving it by transferring prescribed amount from vial to an infusion bag containing normal saline solution or D₅W to make a final concentration of 1 to 4 mg/ml. Gently invert bag to mix the contents. If solution won't be

given immediately, refrigerate and use within 48 hours.
- Administer drug only as an I.V. infusion and not as an I.V. push or bolus.
- Monitor patient's blood pressure and cardiac function during and after rituximab therapy to detect abnormalities. Drug-induced infusion reaction may also cause adverse cardiac effects. If a serious event occurs, such as a life-threatening arrhythmia or angina, stop infusion, notify prescriber, and provide supportive care.
- Inspect patient's skin regularly because rituximab therapy may cause serious to life-threatening adverse dermatological effects.

PATIENT TEACHING
- Inform patient that rituxmab may cause infusion reactions. Review signs and symptoms that should be reported immediately. Reassure patient that he will receive a steroid 30 minutes before the rituxmab infusion to reduce the risk and severity of infusion reactions.
- Tell patient that drug will be given twice, 2 weeks apart.
- Alert patient that adverse effects may appear after infusion is finished and patient is at home. Emphasize the need to report unusual or serious adverse effects immediately to prescriber.

scopolamine hydrobromide

Class and Category
Chemical: Belladonna alkaloid, tertiary amine
Therapeutic: Anesthesia adjunct, anticholinergic, antiemetic, antispasmodic, antivertigo agent
Pregnancy category: C

Indications and Dosages
▶ *To treat biliary tract disorders, enuresis, nausea and vomiting, and nocturia*
I.V. INJECTION
Adults and adolescents. 300 to 600 mcg (0.3 to 0.6 mg) as a single dose.
Children. 6 mcg (0.006 mg)/kg as a single dose.
▶ *As adjunct to anesthesia to induce sleep and calmness*
I.V. INJECTION
Adults and adolescents. 0.6 mg t.i.d. or q.i.d.
▶ *As adjunct to anesthesia to induce amnesia*
I.V. INJECTION
Adults and adolescents. 0.32 to 0.65 mg.

DOSAGE ADJUSTMENT Dosage reduction possible for elderly patients because of their increased sensitivity to scopolamine.

Route	Onset	Peak	Duration
I.V.*	10 min	50 to 80 min	2 hr

Mechanism of Action

Competitively inhibits acetylcholine at autonomic postganglionic cholinergic receptors. Because the most sensitive receptors are in the salivary, bronchial, and sweat glands, this action reduces secretions from these glands. Scopolamine also decreases nasal and oropharyngeal secretions, GI smooth-muscle tone and bladder detrusor muscle tone, and gastric secretions and GI motility. It also relaxes smooth muscles in the bronchi and bronchioles, resulting in decreased airway resistance.

In addition, scopolamine blocks neural pathways in the inner ear. This action relieves motion sickness and depresses the cerebral cortex to produce sedation and hypnotic effects.

Contraindications

Angle-closure glaucoma; hemorrhage with hemodynamic instability; hepatic dysfunction; hypersensitivity to barbiturates, scopolamine, other belladonna alkaloids, or their components; ileus; intestinal atony; myasthenia gravis; myocardial ischemia; obstructive GI disease, such as pyloric stenosis; obstructive uropathy, as in prostatic hyperplasia; renal impairment; tachycardia; toxic megacolon; ulcerative colitis

Interactions

DRUGS

antimyasthenics: Possibly reduced intestinal motility

CNS depressants: Possibly potentiated effects of either drug, resulting in additive sedation

cyclopropane: Increased risk of ventricular arrhythmias

haloperidol: Decreased antipsychotic effect of haloperidol

ketoconazole: Decreased absorption of ketoconazole

lorazepam (parenteral): Possibly hallucinations, irrational behavior, and sedation

metoclopramide: Possibly antagonized effect of metoclopramide on GI motility

* For amnesia.

opioid analgesics: Increased risk of severe constipation and ileus
other anticholinergics: Possibly intensified anticholinergic effects
potassium chloride: Possibly increased severity of potassium
chloride–induced GI lesions
urinary alkalizers (antacids, carbonic anhydrase inhibitors, citrates, sodium bicarbonate): Delayed excretion of scopolamine, possibly leading to increased therapeutic and adverse effects
ACTIVITIES
alcohol use: Additive CNS effects

Adverse Reactions

CNS: Dizziness, drowsiness, euphoria, insomnia, memory loss,
paradoxical stimulation
CV: Palpitations, tachycardia
EENT: Blurred vision; dry eyes, mouth, nose, and throat; mydriasis
GI: Constipation, dysphagia
GU: Urinary hesitancy, urine retention
SKIN: Decreased sweating, dry skin, flushing
Other: Injection site irritation or redness

Nursing Considerations

• Dilute scopolamine with sterile water for injection.
• Assess patient for bladder distention, and monitor urine output. Drug's antimuscarinic effects can cause urine retention.
• Know that, if patient has pain, drug may act as a stimulant and produce delirium if given without morphine or meperidine.
• Monitor heart rate for transient tachycardia, which may occur with high doses of scopolamine. Expect normal rate to return within 30 minutes.
• Store scopolamine at 15° to 30° C (59° to 86° F) in a light-resistant container; don't freeze.
PATIENT TEACHING
• Advise patient to avoid potentially hazardous activities until scopolamine's CNS effects are known.
• Instruct patient to avoid alcohol while receiving scopolamine.
• Suggest lubricating drops to relieve dry eyes.

sodium bicarbonate

Class and Category

Chemical: Electrolyte
Therapeutic: Electrolyte replenisher, systemic and urinary alkalizer
Pregnancy category: C

Indications and Dosages

▶ *To provide urinary alkalization*

I.V. INFUSION

Adults and children. 2 to 5 mEq/kg over 4 to 8 hr.

▶ *To treat metabolic acidosis during cardiac arrest*

I.V. INJECTION

Adults and children. *Initial:* 1 mEq/kg, followed by 0.5 mEq/kg every 10 min while arrest continues.

▶ *To treat less urgent forms of metabolic acidosis*

I.V. INFUSION

Adults and children. 2 to 5 mEq/kg over 4 to 8 hr.

DOSAGE ADJUSTMENT Dosage reduction possible for elderly patients because of age-related renal impairment.

Mechanism of Action

Increases plasma bicarbonate level, buffers excess hydrogen ions, and raises blood pH, thereby reversing metabolic acidosis. Sodium bicarbonate also increases the excretion of free bicarbonate ions in urine, raising urine pH; increased alkalinity of urine may help to dissolve uric acid calculi.

Incompatibilities

Don't mix sodium bicarbonate in same solution or give through same I.V. line as other drugs because a precipitate may form.

Contraindications

Hypocalcemia in which alkalosis may lead to tetany; hypochloremic alkalosis secondary to vomiting, diuretics, or nasogastric suction; preexisting metabolic or respiratory alkalosis

Interactions

DRUGS

amphetamines, quinidine: Decreased urinary excretion of these drugs, possibly resulting in toxicity

anticholinergics: Decreased anticholinergic absorption and effectiveness

chlorpropamide, lithium, salicylates, tetracyclines: Increased renal excretion of these drugs

ciprofloxacin, norfloxacin, ofloxacin: Decreased solubility of these drugs, leading to crystalluria and nephrotoxicity

citrates: Increased risk of systemic alkalosis; increased risk of calcium calculus formation and hypernatremia in patients with history of uric acid calculi

digoxin: Possibly elevated blood digoxin level
ephedrine: Increased ephedrine half-life and duration of action
mecamylamine: Decreased excretion and prolonged effect of mecamylamine
methenamine: Decreased methenamine effectiveness
mexiletine: Possibly mexiletine toxicity
potassium supplements: Decreased serum potassium level
urinary acidifiers (ammonium chloride, ascorbic acid, potassium and sodium phosphates): Counteracted effects of urinary acidifiers

Adverse Reactions

CNS: Mental or mood changes
CV: Irregular heartbeat, peripheral edema (with large doses), weak pulse
EENT: Dry mouth
GI: Abdominal cramps, thirst
MS: Muscle spasms, myalgia
SKIN: Extravasation with necrosis, tissue sloughing, or ulceration

Nursing Considerations

- Dilute sodium bicarbonate with normal saline solution, D_5W, or other standard electrolyte solution before administration.
- **WARNING** Avoid rapid I.V. infusion, which can cause severe alkalosis. However, be aware that during cardiac arrest, the risk of death from acidosis may outweigh the risks associated with rapid infusion. In addition, rapid administration in children under age 2 poses a risk of hypernatremia with decreased CSF pressure and, possibly, intracranial hemorrhage.
- Monitor urine pH, as ordered, to determine drug's effectiveness as urinary alkalizer.
- Be aware that parenteral formulations are hypertonic and that increased sodium intake can produce edema and weight gain. Patients with impaired renal function, heart failure, or other conditions that predispose them to sodium retention or edema are at increased risk.
- Assess I.V. site often for evidence of extravasation. If it occurs, notify prescriber immediately and remove I.V. catheter. Elevate the extremity, apply warm compresses, and expect prescriber to administer a local injection of hyaluronidase or lidocaine.
- When calculating sodium intake for patients on a sodium-restricted diet, keep in mind that sodium bicarbonate contains varying amounts of sodium, depending on concentration of solution used; check label to calculate amount of sodium that patient is receiving.

- Store drug at 15° to 30° C (59° to 86° F); don't freeze.

PATIENT TEACHING

- Advise patient receiving sodium bicarbonate to report pain, swelling, or redness at I.V. insertion site.
- Instruct patient to avoid taking OTC drugs without prescriber's approval because many drugs interact with sodium bicarbonate.

sodium ferric gluconate
(contains 62.5 mg of elemental iron per 5 ml)
Ferrlecit

Class and Category
Chemical: Iron salt, mineral
Therapeutic: Antianemic
Pregnancy category: B

Indications and Dosages
▶ *To treat iron deficiency anemia in patients receiving long-term hemodialysis and erythropoietin*

I.V. INFUSION, I.V. INJECTION

Adults. 125 mg of elemental iron. *Usual:* Minimum cumulative dose of 1 g of elemental iron given over eight sequential dialysis treatment. Dosage repeated at lowest dosage needed to maintain target levels of hemoglobin and hematocrit and acceptable limits of blood iron levels.

Mechanism of Action
Acts to replenish iron stores lost during hemodialysis because of increased blood loss or increased iron utilization from epoetin therapy. Iron is an essential component of hemoglobin, myoglobin, and several enzymes, including cytochromes, catalase, and peroxidase, and is needed for catecholamine metabolism and normal neutrophil function. Sodium ferric gluconate also normalizes RBC production by binding with hemoglobin or being stored as ferritin in the reticuloendothelial cells of the liver, spleen, and bone marrow.

Incompatibilities
Don't mix sodium ferric gluconate with other drugs or parenteral nutrition solutions for I.V. infusion.

Contraindications
Anemia other than iron deficiency, hypersensitivity to iron salts or their components, iron overload

Interactions
DRUGS
oral iron preparations: Possibly reduced absorption of oral iron

Adverse Reactions
CNS: Asthenia, dizziness, fatigue, fever, headache, hypertonia, hypoesthesia, loss of consciousness, nervousness, paresthesia, seizures, syncope
CV: Chest pain, generalized edema, hypertension, hypotension, phlebitis, shock, tachycardia
EENT: Dry mouth
GI: Abdominal pain, diarrhea, nausea, vomiting
HEME: Hemorrhage
MS: Back pain, leg cramps
RESP: Cough, dyspnea, upper respiratory tract infection, wheezing
SKIN: Discoloration, diaphoresis, pallor, pruritus
Other: Anaphylaxis, generalized pain, hyperkalemia, hypersensitivity, infusion or injection site reaction

Nursing Considerations
- To reconstitute sodium ferric gluconate for I.V. infusion, dilute prescribed dose in 100 ml of normal saline solution immediately before infusion. Infuse over 1 hour. Discard any unused diluted solution.
- Inspect drug for particles and discoloration before administration, and discard if present.
- Administer undiluted drug by slow I.V. injection at up to 12.5 mg/min, not to exceed 125 mg per injection.
- Be aware that most patients need a minimum cumulative dose of 1 gram of elemental iron administered over eight sequential dialysis treatments.
- **WARNING** Assess patient for signs and symptoms of an allergic reaction, including chills, facial flushing, pruritus, and rash, and of a hypersensitivity reaction, including diaphoresis, dyspnea, nausea, severe lower back pain, vomiting, and wheezing. Discontinue drug and notify prescriber immediately if patient develops an allergic or hypersensitivity reaction, and be prepared to provide emergency interventions.
- **WARNING** Assess blood pressure often after drug administration because hypotension may occur and may be related to infusion rate or total cumulative dose. Avoid rapid infusion, and be prepared to provide I.V. fluids for volume expansion.
- Expect to monitor blood hemoglobin level, hematocrit, serum ferritin level, and transferrin saturation, as ordered, before, dur-

ing, and after sodium ferric gluconate therapy. Make sure that serum iron level is tested 48 hours after last dose. To prevent iron toxicity, notify prescriber and expect to discontinue therapy if blood iron level is normal or elevated.

• Assess patient for possible iron overload (bleeding in GI tract and lungs, decreased activity, pale conjunctivae, and sedation).

PATIENT TEACHING

• Warn patient not to take oral iron preparations during sodium ferric gluconate therapy without first consulting prescriber.

• Inform patient that iron deficiency may cause decreased stamina, learning problems, shortness of breath, and fatigue.

sodium thiosalicylate

Rexolate, Tusal

Class and Category

Chemical: Salicylic acid derivative
Therapeutic: Analgesic, anti-inflammatory
Pregnancy category: Not rated

Indications and Dosages

▶ *To relieve symptoms of acute gout*

I.V. INJECTION

Adults. *Initial:* 100 mg every 3 to 4 hr for 2 days, followed by 100 mg daily.

▶ *To relieve pain from musculoskeletal conditions*

I.V. INJECTION

Adults. 50 to 100 mg daily or every other day.

▶ *To relieve symptoms of osteoarthritis*

I.V. INJECTION

Adults. 100 mg 3 times/wk for several wk, followed by 100 mg once/wk, usually up to a total dose of 2.5 g. After 1 to 2 wk, another course of treatment may be given.

▶ *To treat rheumatic fever*

I.V. INJECTION

Adults. *Initial:* 100 to 150 mg every 4 to 8 hr for 3 days, followed by 100 mg b.i.d.

Mechanism of Action

Exerts peripherally induced analgesic and anti-inflammatory effects by blocking pain impulses and inhibiting prostaglandin synthesis.

Contraindications

GI bleeding; hemophilia; hemorrhage; hypersensitivity to sodium thiosalicylate, NSAIDs, or their components; Reye's syndrome

Interactions

DRUGS

ACE inhibitors, beta blockers: Decreased antihypertensive effect
activated charcoal: Decreased sodium thiosalicylate absorption
antacids, urinary alkalizers: Increased sodium thiosalicylate excretion, leading to reduced effectiveness and shortened half-life
carbonic anhydrase inhibitors (such as acetazolamide): Increased risk of salicylate toxicity; possibly displacement of acetazolamide from protein-binding sites, resulting in toxicity
corticosteroids: Possibly increased sodium thiosalicylate excretion
insulin, oral antidiabetic drugs: Altered glucose control (with large doses of sodium thiosalicylate)
loop diuretics: Possibly decreased effectiveness of loop diuretics in patients with renal or hepatic impairment
methotrexate: Increased risk of methotrexate toxicity
nizatidine: Increased blood sodium thiosalicylate level
probenecid, sulfinpyrazone: Decreased uricosuric effects
spironolactone: Possibly inhibited diuretic effect of spironolactone
urinary acidifiers (including ammonium chloride, ascorbic acid, and methionine): Decreased sodium thiosalicylate excretion, possibly leading to salicylate toxicity

ACTIVITIES

alcohol use: Increased risk of GI ulceration

Adverse Reactions

GI: Anorexia, diarrhea, GI bleeding, heartburn, hepatotoxicity, indigestion, nausea, thirst, vomiting
HEME: Leukopenia, platelet dysfunction, prolonged bleeding time, thrombocytopenia
RESP: Bronchospasm
SKIN: Rash, urticaria
Other: Angioedema

Nursing Considerations

- Inspect vial before administration. If drug contains slight precipitate from oxidation, shake well. Discard if precipitate persists.
- Administer sodium thiosalicylate by slow injection.
- Watch for evidence of a hypersensitivity reaction, such as angioedema, bronchospasm, and rash. Patients with asthma, chronic urticaria, or nasal polyps are more prone to drug hypersensitivity.

- Expect to monitor hepatic and renal function during long-term drug therapy.
- After repeated administration or large doses, assess patient for evidence of salicylate toxicity: CNS depression, confusion, diaphoresis, diarrhea, difficulty hearing, dizziness, headache, hyperventilation, lassitude, tinnitus, and vomiting.
- Be aware that tinnitus usually means blood sodium thiosalicylate has reached or exceeded upper limit of therapeutic effects.
- Store drug at 15° to 30° C (59° to 86° F).

PATIENT TEACHING
- Instruct patient to report bleeding or symptoms of salicylate toxicity immediately.

streptokinase
Kabikinase, Streptase

Class and Category
Chemical: Purified beta-hemolytic *Streptococcus* filtrate
Therapeutic: Thrombolytic
Pregnancy category: C

Indications and Dosages
▶ *To lyse coronary artery thrombi*
I.V. INFUSION
Adults. 1,500,000 international units within 60 min of event.
INTRACORONARY INFUSION
Adults. 20,000–international unit bolus, followed by 2,000 international units/min for 60 min for total dose of 140,000 international units.
▶ *To lyse acute arterial thromboembolism or thrombosis, acute pulmonary embolism, or deep vein thrombosis*
I.V. INFUSION
Adults. 250,000–international unit bolus over 30 min, followed by 100,000 international units/hr for 24 to 72 hr.
▶ *To clear occluded arteriovenous cannula*
I.V. INJECTION
Adults. 100,000 to 250,000 international units instilled slowly into each occluded lumen.

Route	Onset	Peak	Duration
I.V.	Immediate	20 to 120 min	4 hr

Mechanism of Action

Binds to fibrin in a thrombus and converts trapped plasminogen to plasmin. Plasmin breaks down fibrin, fibrinogen, and other clotting factors, thereby dissolving the thrombus.

Incompatibilities

Don't mix streptokinase in same syringe or administer through same I.V. line as other drugs.

Contraindications

Active internal bleeding, arteriovenous malformation or aneurysm, bleeding diathesis, CVA or intracranial or intraspinal surgery within the past 2 months, hypersensitivity to streptokinase or its components, intracranial cancer, severe uncontrolled hypertension

Interactions

DRUGS

anticoagulants, enoxaparin, heparin, NSAIDs, platelet aggregation inhibitors: Increased risk of bleeding
antifibrinolytics: Antagonized effects of both drugs
antihypertensives: Increased risk of severe hypotension, especially when streptokinase is give rapidly for coronary artery occlusion
cefamandole, cefoperazone, cefotetan, plicamycin, valproic acid: Possibly hypoprothrombinemia and increased risk of severe hemorrhage
corticosteroids, ethacrynic acid, salicylates: Possibly GI ulceration or bleeding

Adverse Reactions

CNS: Chills, fever
CV: Arrhythmias, hypotension
HEME: Unusual bleeding or bruising
Other: Allergic reaction

Nursing Considerations

• Obtain hematocrit, platelet count, APTT, PT, and INR, as ordered, before, during, and after streptokinase therapy.
• Consult manufacturer's instructions for reconstituting and diluting drug for I.V. and intracoronary infusions. If drug will be used to clear occluded arteriovenous cannula, slowly reconstitute 250,000-international unit vial with 2 ml of sodium chloride injection or 5% dextrose injection.
• To prevent foaming, don't shake drug during reconstitution.

- Watch for bleeding at I.V. site and for blood in urine and stools. Perform neurologic assessment to detect intracranial bleeding.
- Monitor the following patients for signs and symptoms of bleeding or hemorrhage because they're at increased risk during streptokinase therapy: pregnant women and patients with acute pericarditis (risk of hemopericardium, possibly leading to cardiac tamponade); cerebrovascular disease; hemorrhagic ophthalmic conditions; history of major surgery, GI or GU bleeding, or trauma within past 10 days; hypertension; mitral stenosis with atrial fibrillation (risk of embolism); septic thrombophlebitis; severe hepatic or renal disease; or subacute bacterial endocarditis.
- Closely monitor all puncture sites, such as catheter insertion and needle puncture sites, for bleeding.
- If serious spontaneous bleeding occurs and can't be controlled by local pressure, stop streptokinase infusion immediately and notify prescriber.
- Monitor patient for evidence of a hypersensitivity reaction, such as nausea, pruritus, rash, or wheezing. Keep equipment and drugs used to treat anaphylaxis, such as epinephrine, glucocorticoids, and antihistamines, nearby.
- Monitor heart rate and rhythm by continuous ECG, as ordered.
- Avoid giving I.M. injections and handling patient unnecessarily during streptokinase therapy. Perform venipuncture only when necessary, using a 23G or smaller needle.
- If an arterial puncture is needed after streptokinase administration, use an arm vessel that allows easy manual compression. Apply manual pressure for 30 minutes. Then apply a pressure dressing and check puncture site frequently for bleeding.
- Treat fever with acetaminophen, as prescribed, rather than aspirin to reduce the risk of bleeding.
- Store drug at 15° to 30° C (59° to 86° F).

PATIENT TEACHING
- Explain to patient that he'll be on bed rest during therapy.
- Inform patient that minor bleeding may occur at arterial puncture or surgical sites. Reassure him that appropriate care measures will be taken if bleeding occurs.
- Advise patient to obtain medical alert identification stating that he's receiving streptokinase.
- If patient experiences chest pain within 12 months of receiving streptokinase, instruct him to inform health care providers about his streptokinase therapy because repeated administration within 12 months may be ineffective.

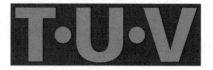

tenecteplase
TNKase

Class and Category
Chemical: Purified glycoprotein
Therapeutic: Thrombolytic
Pregnancy category: C

Indications and Dosages
▶ *To reduce mortality in acute MI*
I.V. INJECTION
Adults. Single bolus given over 5 sec in individualized dosage based on patient's weight, as follows: 30 mg (6 ml) for patients weighing less than 60 kg; 35 mg (7 ml) for patients weighing 60 to 69 kg; 40 mg (8 ml) for patients weighing 70 to 79 kg; 45 mg (9 ml) for patients weighing 80 to 89 kg; 50 mg (10 ml) for patients weighing 90 kg or more. *Maximum:* 50 mg total dose.

Mechanism of Action
Activates plasminogen, a naturally occurring substance secreted by endothelial cells in response to arterial wall injury that contributes to clot formation. Plasminogen is converted into plasmin, which breaks down the fibrin mesh that binds the clot together, resulting in dissolution of the clot.

Incompatibilities
Don't administer tenecteplase through an I.V. line containing dextrose because precipitation may occur.

Contraindications
Active internal bleeding, aneurysm, arteriovenous malformation, bleeding diathesis, brain tumor, history of CVA, hypersensitivity to tenecteplase or its components, intracranial or intraspinal surgery or trauma within past 2 months, severe uncontrolled hypertension

Interactions

DRUGS

abciximab, aspirin, clopidogrel, dipyridamole, heparin, oral anticoagulants, ticlopidine: Possibly increased risk of bleeding

Adverse Reactions

CNS: Intracranial hemorrhage
EENT: Epistaxis, gingival bleeding, pharyngeal bleeding
GI: GI and retroperitoneal bleeding
GU: Genitourinary bleeding, prolonged or heavy menstrual bleeding
HEME: Hematoma
RESP: Hemoptysis
SKIN: Bleeding at puncture sites, surgical incision sites, or venous cutdown sites

Nursing Considerations

- **WARNING** Reconstitute tenecteplase for injection immediately before use because drug contains no antibacterial preservatives. If reconstituted drug isn't used immediately, refrigerate vial at 2° to 8° C (36° to 46° F). Discard solution if not used within 8 hours.
- To reconstitute and administer drug, use supplied 10-ml syringe with dual cannula device. Withdraw 10 ml of supplied (preservative-free) sterile water for injection into syringe, and inject entire contents into vial containing tenecteplase dry powder, directing stream of diluent into powder. Gently swirl—don't shake—vial until contents are completely dissolved. If slight foaming occurs during reconstitution, allow drug to stand undisturbed for a few minutes to allow large bubbles to dissipate. Then, using supplied syringe, withdraw prescribed dose of tenecteplase from reconstituted drug in vial. Make sure that reconstituted preparation is a colorless to pale yellow transparent solution. Discard any unused portion.
- Administer drug as a single I.V. bolus over 5 seconds. Although supplied syringe is intended for use with needleless I.V. systems, be aware that it is also compatible with a conventional needle. Follow manufacturer's directions for use with each system. Flush any dextrose-containing I.V. lines with saline solution before and after administering tenecteplase.
- **WARNING** Monitor patient for signs and symptoms of GI bleeding, including bloody or black, tarry stools; bloody or coffee-ground vomitus; and severe stomach pain. Notify prescriber at once if patient develops such signs or symptoms.

- Assess tenecteplase injection site for signs and symptoms of hematoma, including deep, dark purple bruises under skin and itching, pain, redness, or swelling. Also monitor for superficial bleeding, delayed bleeding at puncture sites, and bleeding from surgical incisions.
- Assess for signs and symptoms of intracranial bleeding (such as decreased LOC), retroperitoneal bleeding (such as abdominal pain or swelling and back pain), genitourinary bleeding (such as hematuria), or respiratory tract bleeding (such as hemoptysis). Notify prescriber immediately if patient develops any of these signs or symptoms.
- If serious bleeding (not controllable by local pressure) occurs, expect to discontinue concomitant heparin or oral antiplatelet therapy immediately.
- If possible, avoid I.M. injections and nonessential handling of patient for first few hours after drug administration.
- If arterial puncture becomes necessary during first few hours after tenecteplase administration, expect to use an upper extremity that is accessible to manual compression. Apply pressure for at least 30 minutes after procedure, use a pressure dressing, and frequently monitor puncture site for signs of bleeding.
- Before reconstituting tenecteplase, store it at controlled room temperature or refrigerate it.

PATIENT TEACHING
- Instruct patient to limit physical activity during tenecteplase administration to reduce the risk of injury or bleeding.
- Advise patient to immediately report any bleeding, including from nose or gums.

theophylline in dextrose injection

Class and Category
Chemical: Xanthine derivative
Therapeutic: Bronchodilator
Pregnancy category: C

Indications and Dosages
▶ *As loading dose to treat reversible airway obstruction in patients not currently receiving theophylline*
I.V. INFUSION
Adults and children. 5 mg/kg infused over 20 to 30 min.
▶ *As partial loading dose to treat reversible airway obstruction in patients currently receiving theophylline*

I.V. INFUSION
Adults and children. Dosage individualized based on blood theophylline level, as prescribed. Loading dose based on principle that 0.5 mg/kg of theophylline will produce a 1-mcg/ml increase in blood theophylline level.

▶ *To provide maintenance treatment of reversible airway obstruction associated with asthma or COPD*
I.V. INFUSION
Adults and adolescents age 16 and over. 0.4 mg/kg/hr for nonsmokers, 0.7 mg/kg/hr for smokers.
Children ages 9 to 16. 0.7 mg/kg/hr.
Children ages 1 to 9. 0.8 mg/kg/hr.
Full-term infants up to age 1. Dosage highly individualized.
DOSAGE ADJUSTMENT For elderly patients and adults with cardiac decompensation, cor pulmonale, or hepatic impairment, dosage reduced to 0.2 mg/kg/hr.

Mechanism of Action
Inhibits phosphodiesterase enzymes, causing bronchodilation. Normally, these enzymes inactivate cAMP and cGMP, which are responsible for bronchial smooth-muscle relaxation. Theophylline also may cause calcium translocation, antagonize prostaglandins and adenosine receptors, stimulate catecholamines, and inhibit cGMP metabolism.

Incompatibilities
Don't mix parenteral theophylline solution with any additives. Don't infuse theophylline through same I.V. line as Hetastarch (Hespan), a colloidal plasma volume expander, which is incompatible with theophylline.

Contraindications
Hypersensitivity to theophylline or its components, peptic ulcer disease, uncontrolled seizure disorder

Interactions
DRUGS
adenosine: Decreased adenosine effectiveness
allopurinol, cimetidine, ciprofloxacin, clarithromycin, disulfiram, enoxacin, erythromycin, fluvoxamine, interferon alfa (human recombinant), methotrexate, mexiletine, pentoxifylline, propafenone, propranolol, tacrine, thiabendazole, ticlopidine, troleandomycin, verapamil: Increased blood theophylline level and risk of toxicity

aminoglutethimide, carbamazepine, isoproterenol (I.V.), moricizine, oral contraceptives (containing estrogen), phenobarbital, phenytoin, rifampin: Decreased blood level and possibly effectiveness of theophylline
benzodiazepines: Possibly reversal of benzodiazepine sedation
beta blockers: Possibly decreased bronchodilator effect of theophylline
ephedrine: Increased adverse effects, including insomnia, nausea, and nervousness
halothane anesthetics: Increased risk of ventricular arrhythmias
ketamine: Lowered seizure threshold
lithium: Decreased lithium effectiveness
neuromuscular blockers: Possibly antagonized neuromuscular blockade
FOODS
caffeine: Possibly increased risk of adverse CNS effects
high-carbohydrate, low-protein diet: Possibly decreased theophylline elimination
low-carbohydrate, high-protein diet; daily intake of charbroiled beef: Possibly increased theophylline elimination
ACTIVITIES
alcohol use: Increased blood theophylline level and risk of toxicity
smoking: Increased drug clearance, decreased drug effectiveness
smoking cessation: Possibly decreased drug clearance

Adverse Reactions
CNS: Agitation, anxiety, behavioral changes, confusion, disorientation, headache, insomnia, nervousness, seizures, tremor
CV: Hypotension, tachycardia, ventricular arrhythmias
ENDO: Hyperglycemia
GI: Abdominal pain, diarrhea, heartburn, nausea, vomiting
GU: Increased urine output

Nursing Considerations
• Be aware that ideal body weight is used to calculate theophylline dosages because drug doesn't bind well in body fat.
• Discard unused portions of theophylline and dextrose solutions because they contain no preservatives.
• Infuse theophylline loading dose, bolus, or intermittent infusion at a rate not exceeding 25 mg/minute.
• Administer continuous infusion with a rate-controlled device.
• Frequently assess heart rate and rhythm because theophylline can exacerbate existing arrhythmias.
• Monitor blood theophylline level, as ordered, to gauge therapeutic level and detect toxicity.
• Be especially alert for signs of toxicity in patients with acute pulmonary edema, hypothyroidism, prolonged fever, sepsis with

multiple organ failure, shock, or viral pulmonary infection and those who have recently received an influenza vaccine because drug clearance is decreased in these patients. Patients with uncorrected acidemia also have an increased risk of toxicity.

- Suspect toxicity if patient experiences vomiting; be prepared to obtain blood theophylline level.
- Expect patients with cystic fibrosis or hyperthyroidism to experience increased theophylline clearance and decreased drug effectiveness. Monitor blood theophylline level, as ordered.
- Store drug at 15° to 30° C (59° to 86° F); don't freeze.

PATIENT TEACHING

- Advise patient to report if she develops a fever, makes a significant dietary change, or starts or stops smoking or taking other drugs because these factors may alter blood theophylline level.
- Urge patient to avoid excessive intake of caffeine because it can increase the risk of adverse CNS reactions, such as agitation and nervousness.

thiamine hydrochloride
(vitamin B$_1$)
Betaxin (CAN), Biamine

Class and Category
Chemical: Water-soluble B-complex vitamin
Therapeutic: Nutritional supplement
Pregnancy category: A (parenteral)

Indications and Dosages
▶ *To provide nutritional supplementation based on U.S. and Canadian recommended daily allowances (RDAs), to prevent thiamine deficiency*
I.V. INFUSION
Adults and children. Dosage individualized and added to total parenteral nutrition solution.
▶ *To treat beriberi*
I.V. INJECTION
Adults. *Initial:* 5 to 100 mg every 8 hr, then switched to P.O. therapy as soon as possible and continued for 1 mo.
Children and infants. 10 to 25 mg daily.
▶ *To treat Wernicke's encephalopathy*
I.V. INJECTION
Adults. *Initial:* 100 mg. *Maintenance:* 50 to 100 mg daily until normal RDA is achieved.

Mechanism of Action

Replaces vitamin in thiamine deficiency, which can lead to beriberi or Wernicke's encephalopathy. Thiamine combines with ATP to produce thiamine pyrophosphate, a coenzyme needed for carbohydrate metabolism. Thiamine is necessary for the conversion of pyruvic acid to acetyl-CoA so that it can enter the Krebs cycle; in patients without adequate thiamine, pyruvic acid accumulates in the blood, where it's converted to lactic acid.

Incompatibilities

Don't add thiamine to alkaline or neutral solutions or mix it with oxidizing and reducing agents, including barbiturates, carbonates, citrates, and copper ions.

Contraindications

Hypersensitivity to thiamine preparations or their components

Interactions

None known.

Adverse Reactions

CNS: Restlessness, weakness
EENT: Sneezing, throat tightness
GI: Nausea, vomiting
SKIN: Diaphoresis, pruritus, sensation of warmth, urticaria

Nursing Considerations

- Be aware that symptoms of thiamine deficiency may appear as a syndrome of nonspecific symptoms that include headache, malaise, myalgia, and nausea.
- **WARNING** Severe thiamine deficiency causes beriberi, which can affect the CNS and cardiovascular system. Monitor patient for neurologic effects, such as ataxia, confabulation, impaired ability to learn, neuropathy, and retrograde amnesia, as well as cardiovascular effects, such as biventricular failure, edema, and peripheral vasodilation.
- Expect an intradermal test dose to be prescribed before I.V. administration of thiamine.
- Use thiamine immediately if mixed in solutions containing sodium bisulfite as an antioxidant or preservative because drug stability is poor in such solutions.
- Be aware that a high-carbohydrate diet and dextrose-containing I.V. solutions may increase thiamine requirements and worsen symptoms of thiamine deficiency.

- Be aware that thiamine absorption is decreased in patients with alcoholism, cirrhosis, or GI disease.
- Assess patient and laboratory test results for signs of lactic acidosis. In patients with a thiamine deficiency, pyruvic acid accumulates in the blood and is converted to lactic acid.
- Keep in mind that thiamine is a water-soluble vitamin that won't accumulate in the body.
- Store drug at 15° to 30° C (59° to 86° F); protect from freezing and light.

PATIENT TEACHING

- Inform breast-feeding patient that she and her infant must be treated with thiamine if infant has beriberi.
- Encourage patient to improve dietary intake of thiamine to prevent disease recurrence.

ticarcillin disodium
Ticar

Class and Category
Chemical: Penicillin
Therapeutic: Antibiotic
Pregnancy category: B

Indications and Dosages
▶ *To treat moderate to severe infections, such as bacteremia, diabetic foot ulcers, empyema, intra-abdominal infections, lower respiratory tract infections (including pneumonia), lung abscess, peritonitis, pulmonary infections due to complications of cystic fibrosis (including bronchiectasis and pneumonia), septicemia, and skin and soft-tissue infections (including cellulitis) caused by susceptible organisms*

I.V. INFUSION

Adults and children. 200 to 300 mg/kg daily in divided doses every 4 to 6 hr. *Usual:* 3 g every 4 hr or 4 g every 6 hr.

▶ *To treat severe infections (including sepsis) caused by susceptible strains of* Pseudomonas *species,* Proteus *species, and* Escherichia coli

Neonates within 7 days after birth weighing less than 2 g. 75 mg/kg every 12 hr.

Neonates within first 7 days after birth weighing more than 2 g. 75 mg/kg every 8 hr.

Neonates more than 7 days after birth weighing less than 2 g. 75 mg/kg every 8 hr.

Neonates more than 7 days after birth weighing more than 2 g. 100 mg/kg every 8 hr or 75 mg/kg every 6 hr.

▶ *To treat uncomplicated UTI*
I.V. INFUSION
Adults and children weighing 40 kg (88 lb) or more. 1 g every 6 hr.
Children over age 1 month weighing less than 40 kg. 50 to 100 mg/kg daily in divided doses every 6 to 8 hr.
▶ *To treat complicated UTI*
I.V. INFUSION
Adults and children. 150 to 200 mg/kg in equally divided doses every 4 to 6 hr. *Usual:* 3 g every 6 hr.
DOSAGE ADJUSTMENT Adult patients with renal impairment given a loading dose of 3 g, then dosage adjusted as follows: for creatinine clearance of 30 to 60 ml/min/1.73 m², 2 g every 4 hr; for creatinine clearance of 10 to 30 ml/min/1.73 m², 2 g every 8 hr; for creatinine clearance of less than 10 ml/min/1.73 m², 2 g every 12 hr; for creatinine clearance of less than 10 ml/min/1.73 m² *and* impaired hepatic function, 2 g every 24 hr; for patients who undergo hemodialysis, 2 g every 12 hr and 3 g after each dialysis session; for patients who undergo peritoneal dialysis, 3 g every 12 hr.

Mechanism of Action
Inhibits bacterial cell wall synthesis by binding to specific penicillin-binding proteins located inside the bacterial cell wall. Ultimately, this leads to cell wall lysis and death.

Incompatibilities
Don't administer ticarcillin through same I.V. line as amikacin, gentamicin, or tobramycin or within 1 hour of aminoglycosides.

Contraindications
Hypersensitivity to ticarcillin, other penicillins, or their components

Interactions
DRUGS
aminoglycosides: Additive or synergistic activity against some bacteria, possibly mutual inactivation
anticoagulants: Possibly interference with platelet aggregation, prolonged PT
methotrexate: Prolonged blood methotrexate level, increased risk of methotrexate toxicity
probenecid: Prolonged blood ticarcillin level

Adverse Reactions

CV: Thrombophlebitis, vasculitis
GI: Elevated liver function test results, nausea, pseudomembranous colitis, vomiting
GU: Proteinuria
HEME: Anemia, eosinophilia, hemorrhage, leukopenia, neutropenia, prolonged bleeding time, thrombocytopenia
SKIN: Erythema nodosum, exfoliative dermatitis, pruritus, rash, toxic epidermal necrolysis, urticaria
Other: Anaphylaxis, hypernatremia, hypokalemia, superinfection

Nursing Considerations

- Obtain body fluid or tissue specimens for culture and sensitivity testing, as ordered. Review test results, if possible, before giving first dose of ticarcillin.
- Before starting ticarcillin therapy, make sure patient has had no previous hypersensitivity reactions to ticarcillin or other penicillins.
- Reconstitute each gram of ticarcillin with 4 ml of a compatible diluent, such as 5% dextrose injection or 0.9% sodium chloride injection. Further dilute reconstituted I.V. solution to 10 to 100 mg/ml with a compatible I.V. solution. To minimize vein irritation, don't exceed concentration of 100 mg/ml (concentrations of 50 mg/ml or greater are preferred). Infuse appropriate adult or children's dose over 30 to 120 minutes; infuse neonatal dose over 10 to 20 minutes.
- Assess for local injection site reaction, including thrombophlebitis, during therapy.
- **WARNING** Monitor patient's platelet count, PT, and APTT because ticarcillin may increase bleeding time and, in rare cases, may induce thrombocytopenia.
- Be aware that ticarcillin may exacerbate symptoms in patients with a history of GI disease or colitis.
- Implement seizure precautions according to facility policy for patients with renal impairment because they're at increased risk for seizures.
- Assess patient for signs of pseudomembranous colitis, such as abdominal cramps and severe watery diarrhea. Also assess for other signs of superinfection, such as oral candidiasis and rash in breast-feeding infant.
- Monitor serum electrolyte levels for hypernatremia due to drug's high sodium content and for hypokalemia due to increased urinary potassium loss.

• When calculating sodium intake for patients on a sodium-restricted diet, keep in mind that each gram of ticarcillin contains approximately 5.2 to 6.5 mEq of sodium.
• Before reconstituting drug, store it at 15° to 30° C (59° to 86° F).

PATIENT TEACHING

• Instruct patient receiving ticarcillin to immediately report adverse reactions, including rash, difficulty breathing, or fever.
• Advise patient to decrease sodium intake to reduce the risk of electrolyte imbalance.
• Advise patient to report diarrhea and to check with prescriber before taking an antidiarrheal because it may mask symptoms of pseudomembranous colitis.

ticarcillin disodium and clavulanate potassium

Timentin

Class and Category

Chemical: Penicillin
Therapeutic: Antibiotic combination
Pregnancy category: B

Indications and Dosages

▶ *To treat moderate to severe infections, such as appendicitis, bacteremia, bone and joint infections (including osteomyelitis), diabetic foot ulcers, diverticulitis, gynecologic infections (including endometritis), infectious arthritis, intra-abdominal infections, lower respiratory tract infections (including pneumonia), peritonitis, septicemia, skin and soft-tissue infections (including cellulitis), and UTI caused by susceptible organisms; to manage febrile neutropenia*

I.V. INFUSION

Adults and children age 12 and over weighing 60 kg (132 lb) or more. 3.1 g (3 g of ticarcillin and 100 mg of clavulanic acid) infused over 30 min every 4 to 6 hr.

Adults and children age 12 and over weighing less than 60 kg. 200 to 300 mg/kg daily (based on ticarcillin content) in divided doses every 4 to 6 hr.

Children and infants over age 3 months. For mild to moderate infections, 200 mg/kg daily (based on ticarcillin content) in divided doses every 6 hr; for severe infections, 300 mg/kg daily (based on ticarcillin content) in divided doses every 4 to 6 hr.

DOSAGE ADJUSTMENT Adults with renal impairment given

loading dose of 3.1 g (3 g of ticarcillin and 100 mg of clavulanic acid). Then dosage adjusted as follows: for creatinine clearance of 30 to 60 ml/min/1.73 m², 2 g every 4 hr; for clearance of 10 to 30 ml/min/1.73 m², 2 g every 8 hr; for clearance of less than 10 ml/min/1.73 m², 2 g every 12 hr; for clearance of less than 10 ml/min/1.73 m² *and* impaired hepatic function, 2 g every 24 hr; in hemodialysis, 2 g every 12 hr and 3.1 g after each dialysis; in peritoneal dialysis, 3.1 g every 12 hr.

▶ *To treat pulmonary infections caused by complications of cystic fibrosis, such as bronchiectasis or pneumonia*

I.V. INFUSION

Children. 350 to 450 mg/kg daily (based on ticarcillin content) in divided doses.

Mechanism of Action

Inhibits bacterial cell wall synthesis by binding to specific penicillin-binding proteins located inside bacterial cell walls. In this way, ticarcillin ultimately leads to cell wall lysis and death. Clavulanic acid, which doesn't alter the action of ticarcillin, binds with bound and extracellular beta-lactamase, preventing beta-lactamase from inactivating ticarcillin.

Incompatibilities

Don't give ticarcillin and clavulanate through same I.V. line as amikacin, gentamicin, or tobramycin. Don't combine with sodium bicarbonate or give within 1 hour of aminoglycosides.

Contraindications

Hypersensitivity to ticarcillin or other penicillins, clavulanic acid, or their components

Interactions

DRUGS

aminoglycosides: Additive or synergistic activity against some bacteria, possibly mutual inactivation

anticoagulants: Possibly interference with platelet aggregation

methotrexate: Prolonged blood methotrexate level, increased risk of methotrexate toxicity

probenecid: Prolonged blood ticarcillin level

Adverse Reactions

CV: Thrombophlebitis, vasculitis

GI: Elevated liver function test results, nausea, pseudomembranous colitis, vomiting

GU: Proteinuria
HEME: Anemia, eosinophilia, hemorrhage, leukopenia, neutropenia, prolonged bleeding time, thrombocytopenia
SKIN: Erythema nodosum, exfoliative dermatitis, pruritus, rash, toxic epidermal necrolysis, urticaria
Other: Anaphylaxis, hypernatremia, hypokalemia, infusion site pain

Nursing Considerations

- Obtain body fluid or tissue specimens for culture and sensitivity testing, as ordered. Review test results, if possible, before giving first dose of ticarcillin and clavulanate.
- Before starting drug, make sure patient has had no previous hypersensitivity reactions to ticarcillin, other penicillins, or clavulanic acid.
- Keep in mind that 3.1 g of combination drug ticarcillin and clavulanate corresponds to 3 g of ticarcillin and 100 mg of clavulanic acid.
- Dilute reconstituted I.V. solution to concentration of 10 to 100 mg/ml with compatible I.V. solution. To minimize vein irritation, don't exceed concentration of 100 mg/ml. Concentrations of 50 mg/ml or greater are preferred. Infuse appropriate I.V. dose over 30 to 120 min.
- Be aware that premixed minibags are available for use in concentration of 3.1 g (3 g of ticarcillin and 100 mg of clavulanic acid) in 100 ml. Before using minibags, store them below −10° C (14° F). Allow them to thaw at room temperature. Examine contents closely before administration to make sure that ice crystals have melted. When administering minibags, don't use I.V. lines with series connections because they may cause air embolism.
- Know that ticarcillin and clavulanate may exacerbate symptoms in patients with a history of GI disease, especially colitis.
- Assess patient for signs of pseudomembranous colitis, such as abdominal cramps and severe watery diarrhea. Also assess for other signs of superinfection, such as oral candidiasis and rash in breast-feeding infant.
- Implement seizure precautions, according to facility policy, for patients with renal impairment because they're at increased risk for seizures.
- Monitor serum electrolyte levels for hypernatremia due to drug's high sodium content and for hypokalemia due to increased urinary potassium loss.

- **WARNING** Monitor patient's platelet count, PT, and APTT because drug may increase bleeding time and, in rare cases, may induce thrombocytopenia.
- Be aware that patient receiving high doses of ticarcillin may develop pseudoproteinuria.
- When calculating sodium intake for patients on a sodium-restricted diet, keep in mind that each gram of ticarcillin contains approximately 4.75 mEq of sodium.
- Before reconstituting drug, store it at 15° to 30° C (59° to 86° F). Store premixed minibags below −10° C (14° F) before thawing.

PATIENT TEACHING
- Instruct patient receiving ticarcillin and clavulanate to immediately report adverse reactions, including fever, rash, and difficulty breathing.
- Advise patient to decrease sodium intake to reduce the risk of electrolyte imbalance.
- Advise patient to report diarrhea and to check with prescriber before taking an antidiarrheal because it may mask symptoms of pseudomembranous colitis.

tigecycline
Tygacil

Class and Category
Chemical: Glycylcycline
Therapeutic: Antibiotic
Pregnancy category: D

Indications and Dosages
▶ *To treat complicated skin and skin structure infections caused by* Escherichia coli, Enterococcus faecalis *(vancomycin-susceptible isolates only)*, Staphylococcus aureus *(methicillin-susceptible and -resistant isolates)*, Streptococcus agalactiae, Streptococcus anginosus *group (includes* S. anginosus, S. intermedius, *and* S. constellatus*)*, Streptococcus pyogenes, *and* Bacteroides fragilis; *to treat complicated intra-abdominal infections caused by* Citrobacter freundii, Enterobacter cloacae, Escherichia coli, Klebsiella oxytoca, Klebsiella pneumoniae, Enterococcus faecalis *(vancomycin-suseptible isolates only)*, Staphylococcus aureus *(methicillin-susceptible isolates only)*, Streptococcus anginosus *group*, Bacteroides fragilis, Bacteroides thetaiotaomicron, Bacteroides uniformis, Bacteroides vulgatus, Clostridium perfringens, *and* Peptostreptococcus micros

I.V. INFUSION

Adults. *Initial:* 100 mg infused over 30 to 60 min followed by 50 mg infused over 30 to 60 min every 12 hr for 5 to 14 days.

DOSAGE ADJUSTMENT For patients with severe hepatic impairment, initial dosage of 100 mg should be followed by a reduced maintenance dosage of 25 mg every 12 hr.

Mechanism of Action

Inhibits protein translation in bacteria by binding to the 30S ribosomal subunit, which prevents binding of amino-acyl tRNA molecules to the ribosome complex, thus interfering with protein synthesis. Through this bacteriostatic action, bacteria are weakened.

Incompatibilities

Don't give amphotericin B, chlorpromazine, methylprednisolone, or voriconazole simultaneously through the same Y-site.

Contraindications

Hypersensitivity to tigecycline or its components

Interactions

None known.

Adverse Reactions

CNS: Asthenia, chills, dizziness, fever, headache, insomnia, somnolence

CV: Bradycardia, hypertension, hypotension, peripheral edema, phlebitis, septic shock, tachycardia, thrombophlebitis, vasodilation

EENT: Dry mouth, taste perversion

ENDO: Hyperglycemia, hypoglycemia

GI: Abdominal pain, acute pancreatitis, anorexia, constipation, diarrhea, dyspepsia, elevated liver enzyme levels, jaundice, nausea, pseudomembranous colitis, vomiting

GU: Acute pancreatitis, elevated BUN and creatinine levels, vaginal candidiasis

HEME: Anemia, leukocytosis, thrombocythemia

MS: Back pain

RESP: Increased cough, dyspnea

SKIN: Diaphoresis, photosensitivity, pruritus, rash

Other: Hypersensitivity reaction, hypocalcemia; hypokalemia; hyponatremia; hypoproteinemia; injection site reaction, such as edema, phlebitis, inflammation, and pain

Nursing Considerations

• Obtain body tissue and fluid samples for culture and sensitivity tests as ordered before giving first dose. Expect to begin drug therapy before test results are known.

• Avoid giving tigecycline to children younger than age 8 because drug may cause permanent brown or yellow tooth discoloration and enamel hypoplasia.

• Use tigecycline cautiously in patients hypersensitive to tetracycline class antibiotics because glycylcycline class antibiotics are structurally similar to tetracycline class antibiotics.

• Also use cautiously in patients with complicated intra-abdominal infections secondary to intestinal perforation because of the risk of septic shock.

• Determine whether female patient could be pregnant before starting tigecycline therapy because drug may harm fetus.

• Reconstitute each vial of tigecycline with 5.3 ml normal saline injection or 5% dextrose injection to yield 10 mg/ml. The color should be yellow to orange. If not, discard the solution. Immediately withdraw reconstituted solution from the vial and add to a 100-ml I.V. bag for infusion. Drug may be stored in the I.V. bag at room temperature for up to 6 hours or refrigerated up to 24 hours before use.

• If I.V. line is used to infuse other drugs, flush the line with either normal saline injection or 5% dextrose injection before and after tigecycline infusion.

• Infuse tigecycline over 30 to 60 minutes.

• Monitor patient closely for diarrhea, which may indicate pseudomembranous colitis, which is known to occur with many antibiotics. If diarrhea occurs during therapy, notify prescriber and expect to withhold drug. Expect to treat psuedomembranous colitis, if confirmed, with fluids, electrolytes, protein, and an antibiotic effective against *Clostridium difficile.*

• Monitor patient for adverse reactions, keeping in mind the similarity between tigecycline and tetracycline.

• Assess patient for superinfection, such as vaginal candiasis, that may result from overgrowth of nonsusceptible organisms, including fungi. If signs of infection are present, notify prescriber and provide supportive care, as prescribed.

PATIENT TEACHING

• Instruct patient to report adverse reactions to prescriber, especially hypersensitivity reactions, such as a rash or itching, as well as diarrhea.

• Tell patient to report discomfort at infusion site because site may need to be changed.

tirofiban hydrochloride
Aggrastat

Class and Category
Chemical: Tyrosine derivative
Therapeutic: Platelet aggregation inhibitor
Pregnancy category: B

Indications and Dosages
▶ *To treat acute coronary syndrome*
I.V. INFUSION
Adults. 0.4 mcg/kg/min for 30 min, followed by 0.1 mcg/kg/min.
DOSAGE ADJUSTMENT For patients with creatinine clearance of less than 30 ml/min/1.73 m^2, infusion rate reduced by one-half.

Route	Onset	Peak	◌ Duration
I.V.	Immediate	30 min	4 to 8 hr

Mechanism of Action
Binds to glycoprotein IIb/IIIa receptor sites on the surface of activated platelets. Circulating fibrinogen can bind to these receptor sites and link platelets together, forming a clot that eventually blocks a coronary artery. By binding to receptor sites, tirofiban prevents the normal binding of fibrinogen and other factors and inhibits platelet aggregation.

Incompatibilities
Don't infuse tirofiban in same I.V. line with any drug other than atropine sulfate, dobutamine, dopamine, epinephrine hydrochloride, furosemide, heparin, lidocaine, midazolam hydrochloride, morphine sulfate, nitroglycerin, potassium chloride, propranolol hydrochloride, or famotidine (Pepcid injection).

Contraindications
Acute pericarditis; arteriovenous malformation; coagulopathy; CVA that occurred within previous 30 days or a history of hemorrhagic CVA; GI or GU bleeding; hemophilia; history of thrombocytopenia after tirofiban use; hypersensitivity to tirofiban or its

components; intracranial aneurysm or mass, intracranial bleeding, retinal bleeding, aortic dissection, or any evidence of active abnormal bleeding within previous 30 days; major surgery or trauma within previous 6 weeks; severe uncontrolled hypertension (systolic blood pressure above 180 mm Hg, diastolic blood pressure above 110 mm Hg)

Interactions
DRUGS

antineoplastics, antithymocyte globulin, NSAIDs, oral anticoagulants, platelet aggregation inhibitors, strontium-89 chloride, thrombolytics: Increased risk of bleeding
levothyroxine, omeprazole: Increased rate of tirofiban clearance
porfimer: Decreased effects of porfimer photodynamic therapy
salicylates: Increased risk of bleeding, possibly hypoprothrombinemia

Adverse Reactions

CNS: Chills, dizziness, fever, headache, intracranial hemorrhage
CV: Edema, hemopericardium, peripheral edema, sinus bradycardia
GI: Hematemesis, nausea, retroperitoneal bleeding, vomiting
GU: Hematuria, pelvic pain
HEME: Severe thrombocytopenia with chills, fever, and possibly fatal bleeding complications
RESP: Pulmonary hemorrhage
SKIN: Diaphoresis, rash, urticaria
Other: Allergic reaction, anaphylaxis, infusion site bleeding

Nursing Considerations

- **WARNING** Dilute 50-ml vial of tirofiban before use; don't dilute 500-ml container because it holds premixed solution ready for I.V. infusion. Don't use solution unless it's clear and the seal is intact.
- If prescribed, administer tirofiban with heparin for 48 to 108 hours. Expect to continue infusion throughout angiography and for 12 to 24 hours after angioplasty or ather-ectomy.
- **WARNING** If patient is also receiving a heparin infusion, expect to monitor APTT before treatment, 6 hours after heparin infusion starts, and regularly thereafter. Expect to adjust heparin dosage to maintain APTT at about two times the control. Notify prescriber immediately if patient develops an abnormally high APTT. Also, assess patient for signs and symptoms of abnormal bleeding and report them to prescriber immedi-

ately because potentially life-threatening bleeding may occur.
- After cardiac catheterization or percutaneous transluminal coronary angioplasty, maintain patient on bed rest and keep head of bed elevated. Ensure percutaneous site hemostasis at least 4 hours before discharge. Minimize invasive procedures, including epidural procedures, to reduce the risk of bleeding.
- Monitor patient's platelet count, hemoglobin level, and hematocrit, as ordered. Expect to discontinue tirofiban if patient's platelet count is less than 90,000/mm^3. Expect to administer a platelet transfusion, as prescribed, if patient's platelet count falls below 50,000/mm^3.

PATIENT TEACHING
- Advise patient to immediately report any bleeding, bruising, headache, pain, or swelling during I.V. infusion of tirofiban.

tobramycin sulfate
Tobi

Class and Category
Chemical: Aminoglycoside
Therapeutic: Antibiotic
Pregnancy category: D

Indications and Dosages
▶ *To treat bacteremia; bone and joint, gynecologic, intra-abdominal, lower respiratory tract, skin and soft-tissue, and urinary tract infections; endocarditis; meningitis; neonatal sepsis; pyelonephritis; and septicemia caused by susceptible strains of* Acinetobacter *species,* Aeromonas *species,* Citrobacter *species,* Enterobacter *species,* Escherichia coli, Haemophilus influenzae *(beta-lactamase–negative and –positive),* Klebsiella *species,* Morganella morganii, Proteus mirabilis, Proteus vulgaris, Providencia rettgeri, Pseudomonas aeruginosa, Salmonella *species,* Serratia *species,* Shigella *species,* Staphylococcus aureus, *and* Staphylococcus epidermidis; *to treat febrile neutropenia*
I.V. INFUSION
Adults. 3 to 6 mg/kg daily in divided doses every 8 to 12 hr.
Children over age 5. 2 to 2.5 mg/kg every 8 hr.
Children under age 5. 2.5 mg/kg every 8 to 16 hr.
Neonates over age 7 days weighing more than 2 kg (4.4 lb). 2.5 mg/kg every 8 hr.
Neonates over age 7 days weighing 1.2 to 2 kg (2.6 to 4.4 lb). 2.5 mg/kg every 8 to 12 hr.

Neonates age 7 days and under weighing 2 kg or more.
2.5 mg/kg every 12 hr.
Neonates age 7 days and under weighing 1.2 to 2 kg.
2.5 mg/kg every 12 to 18 hr.
Preterm neonates weighing 1 to 1.2 kg (2.2 to 2.6 lb).
2.5 mg/kg every 18 to 24 hr.
Preterm neonates weighing less than 1 kg. 3.5 mg/kg every
24 hr.

▶ *To treat pulmonary infection caused by* P. aeruginosa *in patients with cystic fibrosis*
I.V. INFUSION
Adults and children. 2.5 to 3.3 mg/kg every 8 hr; dosage adjusted to achieve peak blood drug level of 8 to 12 mcg/ml and trough blood drug level below 2 mcg/ml.
DOSAGE ADJUSTMENT For patients with renal impairment, dosage possibly reduced.

Mechanism of Action

Inhibits bacterial protein synthesis by binding irreversibly to one of two aminoglycoside-binding sites on the 30S ribosomal subunit, resulting in bacteriostatic effects. Bactericidal effects may stem tobramycin accumulation in cells, so the intracellular drug level exceeds the extracellular level.

Incompatibilities

Don't mix tobramycin in same solution with parenteral aminoglycosides or beta-lactam antibiotics because mutual inactivation may result. Don't dilute or mix inhalation solution in nebulizer with dornase alfa.

Contraindications

Concurrent cidofovir therapy; hypersensitivity to tobramycin, aminoglycosides, sodium bisulfite, or their components

Interactions

DRUGS

acyclovir, aminoglycosides, amphotericin B, carboplatin, cisplatin, NSAIDs, vancomycin: Additive nephrotoxicity
carbenicillin, ticarcillin: Possibly inactivation of tobramycin
dimenhydrinate: Possibly masking of symptoms of ototoxicity
ethacrynic acid, furosemide: Additive ototoxicity
general anesthetics, neuromuscular blockers: Possibly exaggerated neuromuscular blockade

Adverse Reactions

CNS: Confusion, dizziness, headache, lethargy, neurotoxicity, vertigo
EENT: Hearing loss, tinnitus
GI: Diarrhea, elevated liver function test results, nausea, vomiting
GU: Elevated BUN and serum creatinine levels, nephrotoxicity, oliguria, proteinuria, renal failure
HEME: Anemia, leukocytosis, leukopenia, neutropenia, thrombocytopenia
SKIN: Exfoliative dermatitis, pruritus, rash, urticaria
Other: Hypocalcemia, hypokalemia, hypomagnesemia, hyponatremia, injection site pain

Nursing Considerations

- Obtain body fluid and tissue samples for culture and sensitivity testing before and during tobramycin treatment, as ordered. Review test results, if available, before therapy begins.
- After reconstituting drug with 30 ml of sterile or bacteriostatic water for injection, dilute further with normal saline solution or D_5W.
- Give each I.V. dose over 20 to 60 minutes.
- **WARNING** Don't infuse tobramycin over less than 20 minutes because doing so may result in neuromuscular blockade and excessive peak blood drug level.
- Because drug can cause bilateral and irreversible hearing loss, assess for early signs of cochlear and vestibular ototoxicity, including high-frequency hearing loss and vertigo.
- Monitor serum calcium, magnesium, potassium, and sodium levels to detect electrolyte imbalances.
- **WARNING** Be alert for allergic reactions, including anaphylaxis, because some forms of tobramycin contain sodium bisulfite.
- Discontinue tobramycin therapy 7 days before starting cidofovir therapy, as prescribed.
- Assess for signs of nephrotoxicity, such as elevated BUN and serum creatinine levels.
- Expect dehydration to increase the risk of nephrotoxicity.
- **WARNING** Monitor patient with myasthenia gravis or parkinsonism for increased muscle weakness because of tobramycin's potential curare-like effect.

PATIENT TEACHING
- Urge patient to immediately report high-frequency hearing loss and vertigo.

• Instruct female patients to notify prescriber immediately about known or suspected pregnancy because drug poses danger to fetus.

torsemide
Demadex

Class and Category
Chemical: Anilinopyridine sulfonylurea derivative
Therapeutic: Antihypertensive, diuretic
Pregnancy category: B

Indications and Dosages
▶ *To treat edema in heart failure*
I.V. INJECTION
Adults. *Initial:* 10 to 20 mg daily, adjusted by doubling, as prescribed, to achieve desired effect. *Maximum:* 200 mg daily.
▶ *To treat edema in chronic renal failure*
I.V. INJECTION
Adults. *Initial:* 20 mg daily, adjusted by doubling, as prescribed, to achieve desired effect. *Maximum:* 200 mg daily.
▶ *To treat ascites, alone or with amiloride or spironolactone*
I.V. INJECTION
Adults. *Initial:* 5 to 10 mg daily. *Maximum:* 40 mg daily.

Route	Onset	Peak	Duration
I.V.	10 min	1 hr	6 to 8 hr

Mechanism of Action
Blocks active sodium and chloride reabsorption in the ascending loop of Henle by promoting rapid excretion of water, sodium, and chloride. Torsemide also increases the production of renal prostaglandins, increasing the plasma renin level and renal vasodilation. As a result, systolic and diastolic blood pressures fall, reducing preload and afterload.

Contraindications
Hypersensitivity to torsemide, sulfonamides, or their components

Interactions
DRUGS
ACE inhibitors, other antihypertensives: Additive hypotension
amiloride, spironolactone, triamterene: Possibly counteraction of

torsemide-induced hypokalemia

amphotericin B: Increased risk of nephrotoxicity and severe, prolonged hypokalemia or hypomagnesemia

cisplatin: Increased risk of significant hypokalemia or hypomagnesemia, possibly permanent ototoxicity

cortisone, hydrocortisone: Increased risk of sodium retention and hypokalemia

digoxin: Increased risk of arrhythmias and digitalis toxicity due to hypokalemia or hypomagnesemia

indomethacin: Possibly decreased diuretic and antihypertensive effects of torsemide and increased risk of renal failure

lithium: Possibly lithium toxicity

metolazone, thiazide diuretics: Increased risk of severe fluid and electrolyte loss

neuromuscular blockers: Possibly increased neuromuscular blockade due to hypokalemia

probenecid: Possibly decreased diuretic effect of torsemide

quinidine and other ototoxic drugs: Increased risk of ototoxicity

salicylates: Increased risk of salicylate toxicity

ACTIVITIES

alcohol use: Additive diuresis and, possibly, dehydration

Adverse Reactions

CNS: Dizziness, drowsiness, fatigue, headache, insomnia, lethargy, nervousness, restlessness, weakness

CV: Chest pain, ECG abnormalities, edema, hypotension, tachycardia

EENT: Dry mouth, hearing loss, ototoxicity, pharyngitis, rhinitis, tinnitus

GI: Constipation, diarrhea, indigestion, nausea, thirst, vomiting

GU: Azotemia (prerenal), oliguria, urinary frequency

MS: Muscle spasms, myalgia

RESP: Cough

Other: Hypochloremia, hypokalemia, hypomagnesemia, hyponatremia, hypovolemia

Nursing Considerations

- Examine torsemide before administering it; discard if it contains particles or is discolored.
- Inject drug slowly over 2 minutes. Flush I.V. line with normal saline solution before and after administration.
- Don't exceed 200 mg in a single dose.
- Monitor serum electrolyte levels, as ordered, and fluid intake and output to detect hypovolemia.

- **WARNING** Expect drug-induced electrolyte imbalances, such as hypokalemia and hypomagnesemia, to increase the risk of toxicity and fatal arrhythmias in a patient who takes a digitalis glycoside. Hypokalemia also potentiates neuromuscular blockade effects of nondepolarizing neuromuscular blockers.
- Store drug at 15° to 30° C (59° to 86° F); don't freeze.

PATIENT TEACHING

- Advise patient to change position slowly during torsemide therapy to minimize effects of orthostatic hypotension.
- Instruct patient to immediately report drowsiness, dry mouth, hearing changes, lethargy, muscle cramps or pain, nausea, restlessness, thirst, vomiting, and weakness.
- Inform diabetic patient that her blood glucose level will be monitored frequently because torsemide may increase it.

trastuzumab
Herceptin

Class and Category
Chemical: Recombinant DNA-derived humanized monoclonal antibody
Therapeutic: Antineoplastic
Pregnancy category: D

Indications and Dosages
▶ *To treat metastatic breast cancer in patients whose tumors overexpress the protein human epidermal growth factor receptor 2 (HER2), either as a single agent (for those who have previously received at least one chemotherapy regimen for metastatic disease) or in combination with paclitaxel (for those who have not previously received chemotherapy for metastatic disease)*

I.V. INFUSION

Adults. *Initial:* 4 mg/kg infused over 90 min. *Maintenance:* 2 mg/kg infused over 30 min if initial dose was well tolerated.

Route	Onset	Peak	Duration
I.V.	Unknown	16 to 32 wk	Unknown

Incompatibilities
Don't mix trastuzumab with dextrose solutions or any other drug.

Contraindications
None known.

Mechanism of Action

Preferentially binds to the HER2 protein, which is associated with more aggressive forms of breast cancer. In this way, trastuzumab inhibits the proliferation of tumor cells and mediates antibody-dependent cellular toxicity in cancer cells that overexpress HER2.

Interactions

DRUGS

cyclophosphamide, doxorubicin, epirubicin: Increased risk of cardiac dysfunction

paclitaxel: Possibly increased blood level and effects of trastuzumab

Adverse Reactions

CNS: Asthenia, headache, insomnia, paresthesia

CV: Cardiomyopathy, cardiotoxicity (including heart failure), hypotension, ventricular dysfunction

EENT: Rhinitis

GI: Anorexia, diarrhea, nausea, vomiting

HEME: Anemia, leukopenia

RESP: Adult respiratory distress syndrome, bronchospasm, cough, dyspnea, hypoxia, pleural effusion, pulmonary edema (noncardiogenic), pulmonary infiltrates, pulmonary insufficiency, sinusitis, wheezing

SKIN: Rash, urticaria

Other: Allergic reaction, anaphylaxis, angioedema, infection, infusion reaction

Nursing Considerations

- Perform baseline cardiac assessment before trastuzumab therapy. Expect patient to have an echocardiogram, an ECG, or a multigated acquisition (MUGA) scan. Be aware that elderly patients and patients with a history of cardiac disease or dysfunction are at increased risk for cardiomyopathy. Also, patients who have received a cardiotoxic drug or radiation therapy to the chest wall are at increased risk for cardiotoxicity.
- Be aware that adverse reactions can vary when trastuzumab is administered in combination therapy. Review information for all drugs administered as part of a specific regimen, including drug interactions and adverse effects.
- **WARNING** Reconstitute trastuzumab with 20 ml of the 30 ml of bacteriostatic water for injection (containing benzyl alco-

hol) provided by manufacturer to produce a multidose vial of 21 mg/ml. Discard the remaining 10 ml of diluent; using all of it would result in a lower-than-intended dose. Label vial with "DO NOT USE AFTER" and insert date that is 28 days after date of reconstitution. Use contents within 28 days if stored at 2° to 8° C (36° to 46° F).

- If patient is hypersensitive to benzyl alcohol, prepare initial dilution using 20 ml of sterile water for injection *without* preservative. Use immediately.

- When reconstituting drug, slowly inject the stream of diluent directly into lyophilized cake of trastuzumab. Swirl gently; don't shake. Let vial stand for about 5 minutes to allow slight foaming that may have formed to dissipate. Expect solution to be clear to slightly opalescent and colorless to pale yellow. Discard if solution contains particles.

- Dilute reconstituted drug with a 250-ml infusion bag of normal saline solution; use within 24 hours if stored at 2° to 8° C.

- Administer trastuzumab by I.V. infusion, *not* by I.V. push or bolus.

- **WARNING** Monitor patient for possibly life-threatening infusion reaction, pulmonary complications, or allergic reaction. Assess for such signs as dizziness, fever or chills, headache, nausea, rash, shortness of breath, vomiting, or weakness, particularly during and for at least 24 hours after administration. Infusion reaction typically occurs with the first dose but may occur with subsequent doses. Patients with pulmonary compromise from lung disease or pulmonary malignancy are at increased risk for pulmonary complications.

- Continue to assess cardiac function, including left ventricular function, in all patients during trastuzumab treatment. Prescriber may discontinue drug if patient develops a clinically significant decrease in left ventricular function. Patients who receive trastuzumab in combination with anthracyclines and cyclophosphamide are at increased risk.

- Expect to discontinue infusion if patient has dyspnea or clinically significant hypotension. Assess patient until signs and symptoms completely resolve. Prescriber may discontinue drug if patient develops anaphylaxis, angioedema, or acute respiratory distress syndrome.

- Before reconstituting trastuzumab, store it at 2° to 8° C.

PATIENT TEACHING

- Advise patient to immediately report signs of an infusion or allergic reaction or pulmonary complications, including difficulty breathing, rash, and facial swelling. Inform her that such reactions may occur 24 hours or longer after infusion.

- Instruct female patients not to breast-feed during trastuzumab therapy and for 6 months afterward.
- Stress the importance of complying with the dosage regimen and of keeping follow-up medical appointments and appointments for laboratory tests.
- **WARNING** Instruct women of childbearing age to use effective contraception throughout trastuzumab therapy and to notify prescriber immediately if they become pregnant. Urge them to enroll in the Cancer and Childbirth Registry (1-800-690-6720) if they continue receiving trastuzumab during pregnancy.

treprostinil sodium
Remodulin

Class and Category
Chemical: Prostaglandin, tricyclic benzidene analogue
Therapeutic: Vasodilator
Pregnancy category: B

Indications and Dosages
▶ *To treat pulmonary artery hypertension in patients who have New York Heart Association Class II to IV symptoms in order to diminish exercise-induced symptoms*
I.V. INFUSION
Adults. *Initial:* 1.25 nanograms/kg/min. *Maintenance:* Infusion rate increased in increments of no more than 1.25 nanograms/kg/min each wk for first 4 wk, and in increments of no more than 2.5 nanograms/kg/min each wk thereafter, as needed. *Maximum:* 40 nanograms/kg/min.
DOSAGE ADJUSTMENT If initial dosage isn't tolerated or if patient has mild to moderate hepatic insufficiency, decrease initial dose to 0.625 nanogram/kg/min (using ideal body weight).

Contraindications
Hypersensitivity to treprostinil, its components, or structurally related compounds

Interactions
DRUGS
anticoagulants: Increased risk of bleeding

antihypertensives, diuretics, other vasodilators: Increased risk of hypotension

---

Mechanism of Action

Acts directly on pulmonary and systemic arterial vascular beds to produce vasodilation. The vasodilatory effects reduce right and left ventricular afterload and increase cardiac output and stroke volume. These effects improve symptoms of pulmonary hypertension, such as dyspnea, and enable patients with pulmonary hypertension to walk greater distances with less discomfort.

Adverse Reactions

CNS: Anxiety, dizziness, headache, restlessness
CV: Edema, hypotension, right ventricular heart failure, vasodilation
EENT: Jaw pain
GI: Diarrhea, nausea, vomiting
SKIN: Cellulitis, pruritus, rash
Other: Infusion site pain or reaction (erythema, induration, rash)

Nursing Considerations

- Use treprostinil cautiously in patients with hepatic or renal impairment.
- Assess patient's ability to care for an I.V. catheter and to use an infusion pump. Discuss findings with prescriber before starting treprostinil therapy.
- For I.V. use, dilute with sterile water for injection or normal saline solution according to manufacturer's instructions.
- Calculate infusion rate using the formula provided in the package insert, or refer to charts in package insert to find infusion delivery rate for prescribed dosage and administration route.
- **WARNING** Don't abruptly stop treprostinil infusion or make sudden large reductions in dose because symptoms of pulmonary hypertension may worsen.
- Assess patient frequently for drug effectiveness and for adverse reactions. Know that the goal of chronic dosage adjustments is to find a dose that will improve symptoms of pulmonary hypertension, such as dyspnea and fatigue, while minimizing the drug's adverse effects, such as headache, nausea, vomiting, restlessness, anxiety, and infusion site pain or reaction.
- Monitor patients with mild to moderate hepatic insufficiency closely for adverse reactions, especially after dosage increases,

because treprostinil is metabolized primarily by the liver.
- Be aware that patient must be discharged with a backup infusion pump. It should be one that's adjustable to about 0.002 ml/hr and has alarms that indicate occlusion/no delivery, low battery, programming error, and motor malfunction. Also, the pump should have a delivery accuracy of 66% or better, be positive-pressure driven, and have a reservoir made of polyvinyl chloride, polypropylene, or glass. Make sure patient has additional I.V. or subcutaneous infusion sets to prevent interruptions in drug delivery.

PATIENT TEACHING
- Explain to patient that treprostinil is infused continuously through an I.V. catheter via an infusion pump.
- Teach patient to operate and maintain the I.V. infusion pump and to recognize the drug's adverse effects.
- To reduce the risk of infection, caution patient to always use aseptic technique when preparing and giving drug.
- Tell patient that a single vial of the drug shouldn't be used beyond 14 days after opening and that once the drug is placed in the pump's reservoir, it shouldn't be used after 72 hours.
- Instruct patient to store treprostinil vials at room temperature (about 25° C [77° F]).
- Inform patient that drug will be needed for prolonged periods, possibly years. Stress the importance of not stopping drug abruptly or making sudden large reductions in dosage without consulting prescriber because symptoms could worsen.
- Make sure patient understands that treprostinil use doesn't preclude the subsequent use of an alternative I.V. prostacyclin therapy such as epoprostenol.
- Make sure patient has emergency contact information for problems or questions about giving treprostinil at home.

triflupromazine hydrochloride
Vesprin

Class and Category
Chemical: Phenothiazine
Therapeutic: Antiemetic, antipsychotic
Pregnancy category: Not rated

Indications and Dosages
▶ *To treat nausea and vomiting*

I.V. INJECTION
Adults. 1 mg p.r.n. *Maximum:* 3 mg daily.

Mechanism of Action

Prevents nausea and vomiting by inhibiting or blocking dopamine receptors in the medullary chemoreceptor trigger zone and, peripherally, by blocking the vagus nerve in the GI tract. Triflupromazine also blocks postsynaptic dopamine receptors, increasing dopamine turnover and decreasing dopamine neurotransmission. This action may depress the areas of the brain that control activity and aggression, including the cerebral cortex, hypothalamus, and limbic system.

Contraindications

Blood dyscrasias, bone marrow depression, cerebral arteriosclerosis, coma or severe CNS depression, concurrent use of large quantity of CNS depressants, coronary artery disease, hepatic dysfunction, hypersensitivity to phenothiazines, severe hypertension or hypotension, subcortical brain damage

Interactions

DRUGS

amantadine, anticholinergics, antidyskinetics, antihistamines: Possibly intensified adverse anticholinergic effects, increased risk of triflupromazine-induced hyperpyrexia

amphetamines: Decreased stimulant effect of amphetamines, decreased antipsychotic effect of triflupromazine

anticonvulsants: Lowered seizure threshold

antithyroid drugs: Increased risk of agranulocytosis

apomorphine: Possibly decreased emetic response to apomorphine, additive CNS depression

appetite suppressants: Decreased anorectic effect of appetite suppressants

astemizole, cisapride, disopyramide, erythromycin, pimozide, probucol, procainamide, quinidine: Prolonged QT interval, increased risk of ventricular tachycardia

beta blockers: Increased blood levels of both drugs, possibly leading to additive hypotensive effect, arrhythmias, irreversible retinopathy, and tardive dyskinesia

bromocriptine: Impaired therapeutic effects of bromocriptine

CNS depressants: Additive CNS depression

ephedrine: Decreased vasopressor response to ephedrine

epinephrine: Blocked alpha-adrenergic effects of epinephrine
extrapyramidal reaction–causing drugs (droperidol, haloperidol, metoclopramide, metyrosine, risperidone): Increased severity and frequency of extrapyramidal reactions
hepatotoxic drugs: Increased risk of hepatotoxicity
hypotension-producing drugs: Possibly severe hypotension with syncope
levodopa: Decreased antidyskinetic effect of levodopa
lithium: Possibly encephalopathy and additive extrapyramidal effects
MAO inhibitors, maprotiline, tricyclic antidepressants: Increased CNS depression, impaired triflupromazine metabolism, increased risk of neuroleptic malignant syndrome
mephentermine: Possibly antagonized antipsychotic effect of triflupromazine and vasopressor effect of mephentermine
metaraminol: Decreased vasopressor effect of metaraminol
methoxamine, phenylephrine: Decreased vasopressor effect and shortened duration of action of these drugs
metrizamide: Increased risk of seizures
opioid analgesics: Increased risk of CNS and respiratory depression, orthostatic hypotension, severe constipation, and urine retention
ototoxic drugs: Possibly masking of symptoms of ototoxicity, such as dizziness, tinnitus, and vertigo
phenytoin: Lowered seizure threshold; inhibited phenytoin metabolism, possibly leading to phenytoin toxicity
photosensitizing drugs: Possibly additive photosensitivity and intraocular photochemical damage to choroid, lens, or retina
thiazide diuretics: Possibly hyponatremia and water intoxication
ACTIVITIES
alcohol use: Increased CNS and respiratory depression, increased hypotensive effect

Adverse Reactions

CNS: Akathisia, altered temperature regulation, dizziness, drowsiness, extrapyramidal reactions (dystonia, pseudoparkinsonism, tardive dyskinesia), neuroleptic malignant syndrome
CV: Hypotension, orthostatic hypotension, tachycardia
EENT: Blurred vision, dry mouth, nasal congestion, ocular changes (deposits of fine particles in cornea and lens), pigmentary retinopathy
ENDO: Galactorrhea, gynecomastia
GI: Constipation, epigastric pain, nausea, vomiting
GU: Ejaculation disorders, menstrual irregularities, urine retention

SKIN: Decreased sweating, photosensitivity, pruritus, rash
Other: Injection site irritation and sterile abscess, weight gain

Nursing Considerations

- Be aware that I.V. triflupromazine is not recommended for use in children because of its hypotensive and severe, rapid-onset extrapyramidal effects.
- Before giving triflupromazine, observe parenteral solution; it may turn slightly yellow without altering potency. Don't use solution if discoloration is pronounced or precipitate is present.
- Don't let solution come in contact with your skin because contact dermatitis may result.
- **WARNING** Monitor patient closely for tardive dyskinesia, which may continue after treatment stops. Notify prescriber if patient exhibits such signs as uncontrolled movements of arms, body, cheeks, jaw, legs, mouth, or tongue.
- Closely monitor elderly patients and severely ill or dehydrated children because they're at increased risk for certain adverse CNS reactions. Elderly patients are also at increased risk for developing hypotension amd extrapyramidal reactions, especially if they're acutely ill or debilitated.
- Monitor patients with glaucoma for signs and symptoms of this disorder, such as eye pain, vision changes, and nausea or vomiting from increased intraocular pressure, because of drug's anticholinergic effects.
- Monitor patients with chronic respiratory disorders (such as asthma and emphysema) or acute respiratory tract infections for exacerbations due to drug's CNS depressant effects.
- Monitor patients with cardiovascular, hepatic, or renal disease because they're at increased risk for developing hypotension, heart failure, and arrhythmias.
- Be aware that triflupromazine should be used cautiously in patients who will be exposed to organophosphate insecticides.
- **WARNING** If patient develops neuroleptic malignant syndrome (hyperpyrexia, muscle rigidity, altered mental status, autonomic instability), notify prescriber immediately and expect to stop therapy and start intensive medical treatment.
- **WARNING** Be alert for suppressed cough reflex, which increases patient's risk of aspirating vomitus.
- Monitor patients with a history of hepatic encephalopathy due to cirrhosis for increased sensitivity to drug's CNS effects.
- Monitor patients who have been exposed to extreme heat for heatstroke due to drug-induced suppression of temperature reg-

ulation. Symptoms include tachycardia, fever, and confusion.
• Before using triflupromazine, store it at 15° to 30° C (59° to 86° F); protect from freezing and light.

PATIENT TEACHING
• Instruct patient to change position slowly during triflupromazine therapy to minimize effects of orthostatic hypotension.
• Urge patient to avoid potentially hazardous activities until drug's CNS effects are known.
• Instruct patient to immediately report difficulty swallowing or speaking and tongue protrusion.
• Caution patient to avoid alcohol during therapy.
• Urge patient to avoid exposure to the sun and extreme heat because drug may cause photosensitivity and interfere with thermoregulation. Encourage her to wear sunscreen when outdoors.

tromethamine
Tham

Class and Category
Chemical: Organic amine
Therapeutic: Alkalinizer
Pregnancy category: C

Indications and Dosages
▶ *To treat metabolic acidosis associated with cardiac arrest*
I.V. INFUSION
Adults and children. 3.6 to 10.8 g (111 to 333 ml) of 0.3 M solution.
▶ *To treat metabolic acidosis during cardiac bypass surgery*
I.V. INFUSION
Adults and children. 9 ml (2.7 mEq or 0.32 g) of 0.3 M solution/kg as a single dose. *Usual:* 500 ml (150 mEq or 18 g) infused over 1 hr. *Maximum:* 500 mg/kg over 1 hr.

Mechanism of Action
Combines with hydrogen ions and their associated acid anions, including lactic, pyruvic, and carbonic acid, to form salts that are excreted in urine. Tromethamine exerts additional alkalinizing effects by acting as an osmotic diuretic, promoting the excretion of alkaline urine that contains increased amounts of carbon dioxide and electrolytes.

Contraindications

Anuria, chronic respiratory acidosis, hypersensitivity to tromethamine or its components, uremia

Interactions

DRUGS

amphetamines, quinidine, other pH-dependent drugs: Altered excretion of these drugs

Adverse Reactions

CNS: Fever
CV: Vasospasm
ENDO: Hypoglycemia
GI: Hepatic necrosis (hemorrhagic)
RESP: Respiratory depression
Other: Hypervolemia; infusion site infection, phlebitis, or venous thrombosis; metabolic alkalosis

Nursing Considerations

- Evaluate blood pH, blood glucose, and serum bicarbonate and electrolyte levels, and partial pressure of arterial carbon dioxide before, during, and after tromethamine therapy, as ordered.
- Administer infusion by an indwelling catheter inserted into a large vein, such as one in the antecubital area.
- **WARNING** Be aware that exceeding the recommended dosage can cause alkalosis, respiratory depression, and reduced carbon dioxide level. Because of the risk of alkalosis, tromethamine therapy is limited to 1 day, except in life-threatening situations.
- Be aware that I.V. administration of tromethamine increases the risk of hypervolemia and subsequent pulmonary edema.
- Assess infusion site frequently for signs of infiltration, which may cause inflammation, necrosis, thrombosis, tissue sloughing, and vasospasm.
- Be aware that patients with renal failure have an increased risk of hyperkalemia. For such patients, be prepared to monitor ECG continuously and assess serum potassium level often.
- Monitor blood glucose level often during and after therapy because rapid administration can cause hypoglycemia for several hours.
- Protect drug from freezing and extreme heat.

PATIENT TEACHING

- Inform family members that patient's vital signs and laboratory test results will be evaluated frequently to monitor her progress.

urea
(carbamide)
Ureaphil

Class and Category
Chemical: Carbonic acid diamide salt
Therapeutic: Antiglaucoma agent, diuretic
Pregnancy category: C

Indications and Dosages
▶ *To reduce cerebral edema and intracranial pressure (ICP)*
I.V. INFUSION
Adults and children age 2 and over. 500 mg to 1.5 g/kg as
30% solution in D_5W, $D_{10}W$, or 10% invert sugar solution infused
over 30 min to 2 hr at 4 ml/min or as ordered, according to
manufacturer's instructions. *Maximum:* 2 g/kg daily.
Children under age 2. 100 mg to 1.5 g/kg as 30% solution in
D_5W, $D_{10}W$, or 10% invert sugar solution infused over 30 min to
2 hr at 4 ml/min or as ordered, according to manufacturer's instructions.
▶ *To treat malignant or secondary glaucoma*
I.V. INFUSION
Adults. 500 mg to 1.5 g/kg as 30% solution in D_5W, $D_{10}W$, or
10% invert sugar solution infused over 30 min to 2 hr at 4 ml/
min or as ordered, according to manufacturer's instructions. *Maximum:* 2 g/kg daily.
DOSAGE ADJUSTMENT Dosage reduced or drug withheld
for patients with renal impairment if BUN level rises to 75 mg/
dl or more or if diuresis fails to occur within 2 hr after administration.

Route	Onset	Peak	Duration
I.V.	10 min	1 to 2 hr	3 to 10 hr*

Incompatibilities
If patient is receiving blood simultaneously, don't administer urea
through same administration set.

Contraindications
Active intracranial bleeding, hepatic failure, hypersensitivity to
urea or its components, renal impairment, severe dehydration

---

* For diuresis; 5 to 6 hr for reduction of intraocular pressure in malignant or secondary glaucoma.

Mechanism of Action

Elevates blood plasma osmolality, creating an osmotic effect that increases the movement of water from the brain, CSF, and anterior portion of the eyes into interstitial fluid and plasma. This action reduces cerebral edema, ICP, CSF volume, and intraocular pressure. Large doses of urea inhibit the reabsorption of water and solutes in the renal tubules and induce diuresis by affecting the osmotic pressure gradient of the glomerular filtrate.

Interactions

DRUGS

carbonic anhydrase inhibitors, other diuretics: Additive diuretic and intraocular pressure–reducing effects

lithium: Increased renal excretion of lithium

Adverse Reactions

CNS: Agitation, confusion, fever, headache, hyperthermia, nervousness, subarachnoid hemorrhage, subdural hematoma, syncope

CV: Tachycardia

EENT: Dry mouth, intraocular hemorrhage

GI: Nausea, thirst, vomiting

GU: Elevated BUN level

HEME: Hemolysis

SKIN: Blemishes, extravasation with tissue necrosis and sloughing

Other: Dehydration, hypokalemia, hyponatremia, infusion site phlebitis or thrombosis

Nursing Considerations

- Expect to give urea 1 hour before intracranial or ocular surgery to obtain maximum reduction of ICP or intraocular pressure.
- Don't mix urea with invert sugar solution if patient has fructose intolerance from aldolase deficiency.
- Avoid infusing drug into leg veins to reduce the risk of phlebitis and thrombosis.
- Discard unused portion of drug after 24 hours.
- Be aware that rapid administration may cause hemolysis, increased capillary bleeding, and, in patients with glaucoma, intraocular hemorrhage.
- Maintain adequate hydration to minimize adverse reactions. Assess patient for signs of dehydration, including dry mucous membranes or tenting.
- Monitor BUN and serum electrolyte levels and fluid intake and

output during urea therapy; prolonged use can cause diuresis.
• Store drug at 15° to 30° C (59° to 86° F); don't freeze.

PATIENT TEACHING

• Instruct patient to immediately report difficulty breathing or shortness of breath because urea can cause transient increases in circulatory volume, leading to circulatory overload, exacerbations of heart failure, or pulmonary edema.
• Advise patient to expect increased urine output.
• Encourage patient to remain on bed rest during urea therapy.

urokinase
Abbokinase, Abbokinase Open-Cath

Class and Category
Chemical: Renal enzymatic protein
Therapeutic: Thrombolytic
Pregnancy category: B

Indications and Dosages
▶ *To treat acute coronary artery thrombosis*

INTRACORONARY INFUSION

Adults. 6,000 international units/min until artery is maximally opened (up to 2 hr may be required). *Usual:* 500,000 international units.

▶ *To treat acute pulmonary thromboembolism including massive events*

I.V. INFUSION

Adults. *Initial:* 4,400 international units/kg over 10 min, followed by 4,400 international units/kg/hr for 12 hr.

▶ *To clear I.V. catheter occlusion*

INSTILLATION

Adults and children. 5,000 international units/ml instilled into occluded line.

Route	Onset	Peak	Duration
I.V.	Unknown	20 min to 2 hr	4 hr
Intracoronary	Unknown	Unknown	4 hr

Mechanism of Action
Indirectly promotes conversion of plasminogen to plasmin, an enzyme that breaks down fibrin clots, fibrinogen, and other plasma proteins, including procoagulant factors V and VIII.

Incompatibilities
Don't administer I.V. urokinase through the same I.V. line as other drugs or add other drugs to urokinase solution.

Contraindications
Arteriovenous malformation, bleeding disorder, CVA during previous 2 months, hypersensitivity to urokinase or its components, internal bleeding, intracranial aneurysm, intracranial or intraspinal surgery during previous 2 months, intracranial tumor, recent cardiopulmonary resuscitation, recent trauma, severe uncontrolled hypertension (systolic blood pressure of 200 mm Hg or higher, or diastolic blood pressure of 110 mm Hg or higher)

Interactions
DRUGS
antifibrinolytics (aminocaproic acid, aprotinin): Mutual antagonism
antihypertensives: Increased risk of severe hypotension
cefamandole, cefoperazone, cefotetan, plicamycin, valproic acid: Increased risk of hypoprothrombinemia and severe hemorrhage
corticosteroids, ethacrynic acid, salicylates (nonacetylated): Increased risk of GI ulceration and bleeding
enoxaparin, heparin, NSAIDs, oral anticoagulants, platelet-aggregation inhibitors: Increased risk of hemorrhage
thiotepa: Increased therapeutic effects of thiotepa

Adverse Reactions
CNS: Chills, CVA, fever, headache
CV: Arrhythmias, including tachycardia; chest pain; cholesterol embolization, hypertension; hypotension
EENT: Orolingual edema
GI: Nausea, vomiting
HEME: Unusual bleeding
MS: Back pain, myalgia
RESP: Bronchospasm, dyspnea, hypoxemia, wheezing
SKIN: Cyanosis, ecchymosis, flushing, pruritus, rash, urticaria
Other: Anaphylaxis, infusion site reactions, metabolic acidosis

Nursing Considerations
• To prevent foaming, don't shake urokinase when reconstituting. Consult with pharmacist about giving drug through 0.45-micron or smaller cellulose membrane filter.
• Assess baseline hematocrit, platelet count, thrombin time, APTT, PT, and INR as ordered.
• Monitor heart rate and rhythm by continuous ECG during therapy, especially during rapid lysis of coronary thrombi, because

arrhythmias can occur with reperfusion.
• Monitor blood pressure for hypotension. If hypotension occurs, notify prescriber and expect to reduce infusion rate.
• Check for bleeding at puncture sites and in urine and stool. Check for intracranial bleeding by performing frequent neurologic assessments.
• After arterial puncture is performed, apply pressure for at least 30 minutes and then apply pressure dressing. Check often for bleeding during therapy.
• To prevent bleeding and associated complications, avoid venipunctures; use an external blood pressure cuff to measure blood pressure; give acetaminophen (not aspirin), as prescribed, for fever; and handle patient as little as possible.
• **WARNING** If serious bleeding begins and can't be controlled with local pressure, stop infusion immediately and notify prescriber.

PATIENT TEACHING
• Instruct patient to remain on bed rest during urokinase therapy.
• Inform patient that minor bleeding may occur at wounds or puncture sites.

valproic acid
Alti-Valproic (CAN), Depakene, Deproic (CAN), Dom-Proic (CAN), Med-Valproic (CAN), Novo-Valproic (CAN), Nu-Valproic (CAN), PMS-Valproic Acid (CAN)

valproate sodium
Depacon

divalproex sodium
Depakote, Epival (CAN)

Class and Category
Chemical: Carboxylic acid derivative
Therapeutic: Anticonvulsant
Pregnancy category: D

Indications and Dosages
▶ *To treat simple or complex absence seizures, complex partial seizures, myoclonic seizures, and generalized tonic-clonic seizures as monotherapy*
I.V. INFUSION
Adults and adolescents. *Initial:* 10 to 15 mg/kg daily in divided doses b.i.d. or t.i.d., increased by 5 to 10 mg/kg daily every wk, as needed and as prescribed. *Maximum:* 60 mg/kg daily.

Children. *Initial:* 15 to 45 mg/kg daily in divided doses b.i.d. or t.i.d., increased by 5 to 10 mg/kg daily every wk, as needed and as prescribed.

▶ *As adjunct to treat simple or complex absence seizures, complex partial seizures, myoclonic seizures, and generalized tonic-clonic seizures*

I.V. INFUSION

Adults and adolescents. 10 to 30 mg/kg daily in divided doses, increased by 5 to 10 mg/kg daily every wk, as needed and as prescribed.

Children. 30 to 100 mg/kg daily in divided doses, as prescribed.

DOSAGE ADJUSTMENT For adults being converted from immediate-release divalproex tablets to delayed-release tablets, dosage increased to 8% to 20% more than total daily dose of immediate-release tablets and given once daily.

Mechanism of Action

May decrease seizure activity by blocking the reuptake of gamma-aminobutyric acid (GABA), the most common inhibitory neurotransmitter in the brain. GABA is known to suppress the rapid firing of neurons by inhibiting voltage-sensitive sodium channels.

Contraindications

Hepatic dysfunction; hypersensitivity to valproic acid, valproate sodium, divalproex sodium, or their components; urea cycle disorders

Interactions

DRUGS

aspirin, heparin, NSAIDs, oral anticoagulants, thrombolytics: Increased inhibition of platelet aggregation and risk of bleeding

barbiturates, primidone: Increased blood levels of both drugs, additive CNS effects

carbamazepine: Possibly decreased valproic acid effectiveness

cholestyramine: Decreased bioavailability of valproic acid

clonazepam: Increased risk of absence seizures

CNS depressants: Increased CNS depression

diazepam: Inhibited diazepam metabolism

ethosuximide: Unpredictable blood ethosuximide level

felbamate: Impaired valproic acid metabolism and increased blood drug level

haloperidol, loxapine, MAO inhibitors, maprotiline, phenothiazines, thioxanthenes, tricyclic antidepressants: Increased CNS depression, lowered seizure threshold

lamotrigine: Decreased lamotrigine clearance

mefloquine: Decreased blood levels of valproic acid, divalproex, and valproate sodium; increased risk of seizures

phenytoin: Increased risk of phenytoin toxicity, loss of seizure control

topiramate: Increased risk of hyperammonemia and encephalopathy

ACTIVITIES

alcohol use: Additive CNS depression

Adverse Reactions

CNS: Agitation, ataxia, confusion, depression, dizziness, drowsiness, euphoria, hallucinations, headache, hyperesthesia, lack of coordination, lethargy, loss of seizure control, paresthesia, psychosis, sedation, tremor, vertigo, weakness

EENT: Diplopia, nystagmus, pharyngitis, spots before eyes

ENDO: Galactorrhea, hyperglycemia

GI: Abdominal pain, anorexia, constipation, diarrhea, elevated liver function test results, hepato-renal syndrome, hepatotoxicity, increased appetite, indigestion, nausea, pancreatitis, vomiting

GU: Menstrual irregularities, nephritis, oliguria

HEME: Eosinophilia, hematoma, leukopenia, neutropenia, prolonged bleeding time, thrombocytopenia

MS: Arthralgia, dysarthria

SKIN: Alopecia, diaphoresis, erythema multiforme, jaundice, petechiae, photosensitivity, pruritus, rash, Stevens-Johnson syndrome

Other: Facial edema, hyperammonemia, injection site pain, lymphadenopathy, multi-organ hypersensitivity reaction, weight gain or loss

Nursing Considerations

• For I.V. administration, dilute prescribed dose with at least 50 ml of compatible diluent and infuse over 60 minutes.

• Be aware that patient should be switched from I.V. to P.O. form of valproic acid as soon as possible.

• **WARNING** Although rare, life-threatening multi-organ hypersensitivity reaction have occurred, during initiation of valproic acid therapy. Monitor patient closely for fever and rash accompanied by organ involvement such as lymphadenopathy, hepatitis, liver function test abnormalities, eosinophilia, thrombocytopenia, neutropenia, nephritis, pruritis, oliguria, hepato-renal syndrome, arthralgia, and asthenia. Notify prescriber immediately if present, discontinue drug, as ordered, and be prepared to provide supportive care.

- Be aware that hypoalbuminemia or other protein-binding deficiency increases the risk of valproic acid toxicity.
- Assess patient for signs and symptoms of decreased hepatic function, including anorexia, facial edema, jaundice, lethargy, loss of seizure control, malaise, vomiting, and weakness.
- Monitor liver function test results, as or dered. Assess for signs and symptoms of hepatotoxicity during first 6 months of treatment, especially in children under age 2. Notify prescriber immediately if you suspect hepatotoxicity.
- Monitor platelet count, as ordered, for signs of thrombocytopenia, and notify prescriber if they appear.
- **WARNING** Be aware that hyperammonemia may occur even if patient's liver function test results are normal. Monitor ammonia levels, as ordered. If patient develops unexplained lethargy, vomiting, or changes in mental status with an increase in ammonia level or if asymptomatic ammonia elevations are detected and persist, expect valproic acid to be discontinued.

PATIENT TEACHING

- Instruct patient to report any unusual, persistent or severe signs and symptoms to prescriber, especially unexplained fever and rash accompanied by other complaints.
- Advise patient to avoid hazardous activities during therapy because drug may affect mental and motor performance.
- Urge patient to avoid alcohol during therapy.
- Urge female patient to notify prescriber immediately about suspected or known pregnancy.
- Advise patient to notify prescriber if tremor develops during therapy; occurrence of tremor may be dose-related.

vancomycin hydrochloride

Vancocin

Class and Category

Chemical: Tricyclic glycopeptide derivative
Therapeutic: Antibiotic
Pregnancy category: C (parenteral)

Indications and Dosages

▶ *To treat bacterial endocarditis caused by methicillin-resistant* Staphylococcus aureus

I.V. INFUSION

Adults. 30 mg/kg daily in equally divided doses b.i.d. for 4 to 6 wk. *Maximum:* 2 g daily.

▶ *As adjunct to treat bacterial endocarditis caused by methicillin-resistant* S. aureus *in patients with prosthetic heart valve*

I.V. INFUSION

Adults. 30 mg/kg daily in equally divided doses b.i.d. to q.i.d. for 6 wk or longer in conjunction with rifampin and gentamicin. *Maximum:* 2 g daily.

▶ *To treat bacterial endocarditis caused by* Streptococcus bovis *or* Streptococcus viridans

I.V. INFUSION

Adults. 30 mg/kg daily in equally divided doses b.i.d. for 4 wk. *Maximum:* 2 g daily.

▶ *As adjunct to treat bacterial endocarditis caused by enterococci*

I.V. INFUSION

Adults. 30 mg/kg daily in equally divided doses b.i.d. for 4 to 6 wk in conjunction with gentamicin. *Maximum:* 2 g daily.

▶ *To treat bacterial septicemia, bone and joint infections, pneumonia, and skin and soft-tissue infections caused by* Staphylococcus, *including methicillin-resistant strains, and life-threatening infections*

I.V. INFUSION

Adults and children age 12 and over. 500 mg every 6 hr or 1 g every 12 hr infused over at least 60 min. *Maximum:* 4 g daily.

Children ages 1 month to 12 years. 10 mg/kg every 6 hr or 20 mg/kg every 12 hr infused over at least 60 min.

Neonates ages 1 week to 1 month. *Initial:* 15 mg/kg followed by 10 mg/kg every 8 hr infused over at least 60 min.

Neonates under age 1 week. *Initial:* 15 mg/kg followed by 10 mg/kg every 12 hr infused over at least 60 min.

Mechanism of Action

Inhibits bacterial RNA and cell wall synthesis; alters permeability of bacterial membranes, causing cell wall lysis and cell death.

Incompatibilities

Don't give I.V. vancomycin through the same I.V. line as other drugs. Don't add vancomycin to albumin-containing solutions, alkaline solutions, aminophylline, amobarbital sodium, aztreonam, cefepime, ceftazidime, chloramphenicol sodium succinate, chlorothiazide sodium, dexamethasone sodium phosphate, foscarnet sodium, heparin sodium, methicillin sodium, penicillin G, pentobarbital sodium, phenobarbital sodium, piperacillin sodium and tazobactam sodium, secobarbital sodium, and sodium bicarbonate. Drug may precipitate with heavy metals.

Contraindications

Hypersensitivity to vancomycin or its components, hypersensitivity to corn or corn products when vancomycin is given with dextrose solutions

Interactions

DRUGS

aminoglycosides (amikacin, gentamicin, tobramycin), amphotericin B, bacitracin (parenteral), bumetanide, capreomycin, carmustine, cidofovir, cisplatin, cyclosporine, ethacrynic acid, furosemide, paromomycin, pentamidine (parenteral), polymyxins, salicylates (parenteral), streptozocin: Additive nephrotoxicity or ototoxicity

antihistamines, buclizine, cyclizine, meclizine, phenothiazines, thioxanthenes, trimethobenzamide: Masked symptoms of ototoxicity

cholestyramine, colestipol: Decreased antibacterial activity of oral vancomycin

dexamethasone: Decreased penetration of vancomycin into CSF

nephrotoxic drugs: Increased risk of nephrotoxicity

Adverse Reactions

CNS: Chills, dizziness, vertigo
CV: Hypotension
EENT: Ototoxicity
GI: Nausea, pseudomembranous colitis
GU: Nephrotoxicity
HEME: Eosinophilia, neutropenia
RESP: Dyspnea, wheezing
SKIN: Exfoliative dermatitis; extravasation with pain, tenderness, thrombophlebitis, and tissue necrosis; pruritus; rash; toxic epidermal necrolysis; urticaria
Other: Anaphylaxis, drug-induced fever, injection site inflammation, superinfection

Nursing Considerations

• To reconstitute 500-mg vial of vancomycin for I.V. use, add 10 ml of sterile water for injection; further dilute with at least 100 ml of compatible I.V. solution. For 1-g vial of dry, sterile powder, add 20 ml of sterile water for injection; further dilute with at least 200 ml of compatible I.V. solution.

- **WARNING** Infuse vancomycin over at least 1 hour. Rapid delivery may cause hypotension or transient "red man syndrome," with chills; fainting; fever; flushing of face, neck, upper arms, and torso; hypotension; nausea; tachycardia; and vomiting.
- Monitor blood vancomycin level, as ordered; be aware that therapeutic levels are 10 to 15 mcg/ml trough and 30 to 40 mcg/ml peak.
- If patient has an inflammatory intestinal disorder, assess him often for adverse reactions because vancomycin absorption may be increased in these conditions.
- Monitor CBC results and serum creatinine and BUN levels during therapy, especially if patient has renal impairment or takes an aminoglycoside.
- Monitor I.V. infusion site for signs and symptoms of extravasation, including necrosis, pain, tenderness, and thrombophlebitis. If extravasation occurs, discontinue infusion immediately and notify prescriber.
- Monitor hearing during therapy. Transient or permanent ototoxicity may occur if patient receives excessive vancomycin, has a hearing loss, or receives concurrent aminoglycosides.
- Monitor patient closely for diarrhea, which may indicate pseudomembranous colitis. If diarrhea occurs, notify prescriber. Expect to obtain a stool specimen to test for *Clostridium difficile*, to discontinue vancomycin, and to treat confirmed pseudomembranous colitis with fluids, electrolytes, protein, and an antibiotic effective against *C. difficile*.

PATIENT TEACHING
- Advise patient to notify prescriber if no improvement occurs after a few days.
- Urge patient to report watery, bloody stools to prescriber immediately, even up to 2 months after drug therapy has ended.
- Instruct patient to keep follow-up appointments during and after treatment.

verapamil hydrochloride
Isoptin

Class and Category
Chemical: Phenylalkylamine derivative
Therapeutic: Antianginal, antiarrhythmic, antihypertensive
Pregnancy category: C

Indications and Dosages

▶ *To prevent or treat supraventricular tachycardia*
I.V. INJECTION
Adults and adolescents age 15 and over. *Initial:* 5 to 10 mg slowly over 2 min; then 10 mg, as prescribed, if response isn't adequate after 30 min.
Children ages 1 to 15. *Initial:* 100 to 300 mcg/kg slowly over 2 min, up to maximum of 5 mg; then 10 mg, as prescribed, if response isn't adequate after 30 min.
Infants up to age 1. *Initial:* 100 to 200 mcg/kg slowly over 2 min.
DOSAGE ADJUSTMENT I.V. drug administered over 3 minutes in elderly patients.

Route	Onset	Peak	Duration
I.V.	1 to 5 min	3 to 5 min	10 min to 6 hr

Mechanism of Action

Inhibits calcium movement into coronary and vascular smooth-muscle cells by blocking slow calcium channels in cell membranes. The resulting decrease in the intracellular calcium level has the following effects:

- inhibits smooth-muscle cell contractions
- decreases myocardial oxygen demand by relaxing coronary and vascular smooth muscle, reducing peripheral vascular resistance, and decreasing systolic and diastolic pressures
- slows AV conduction time and prolongs AV nodal refractoriness
- interrupts reentry circuit in AV nodal reentrant tachycardias.

Incompatibilities

Don't mix I.V. verapamil with albumin, amphotericin B injection, hydralazine hydrochloride injection, nafcillin, or sulfamethoxazole and trimethoprim injection. Solutions with pH above 6.0 cause precipitation.

Contraindications

Cardiogenic shock, concomitant use of beta blockers (with I.V. verapamil), hypersensitivity to verapamil or its components, hypotension, severe heart failure unless secondary to supraventricular tachycardia that responds to verapamil, severe left ventricular dysfunction, sick sinus syndrome or second- or third-degree heart block unless artificial pacemaker is in place, ventricular tachycardia (with I.V. verapamil)

Interactions
DRUGS
alpha blockers, antihypertensives, general anesthetics (hydrocarbon), prazosin: Hypotensive effects
aspirin: Increased bleeding time
beta blockers: Increased risk of heart failure, hypotension, and severe bradycardia
calcium supplements: Decreased response to verapamil
carbamazepine, cyclosporine, theophylline, valproate: Increased risk of toxicity from these drugs
cimetidine: Decreased metabolism and increased blood level of verapamil
dantrolene: Increased risk of hyperkalemia and myocardial depression
digoxin: Increased blood digoxin level and risk of digitalis toxicity
disopyramide, flecainide: Additive negative inotropic effects
erythromycin, ritonavir: Increased blood verapamil level
lithium: Increased risk of neurotoxicity
neuromuscular blockers: Prolonged recovery from neuromuscular blockade
NSAIDs, sympathomimetics: Decreased antihypertensive effect of verapamil
phenobarbital: Increased verapamil clearance
procainamide: Increased QT interval, additive negative inotropic effects
protein-bound drugs (hydantoins, salicylates, sulfonamides, sulfonylureas, and warfarin and other oral anticoagulants): Altered blood levels of these drugs
quinidine: Increased risk of quinidine toxicity, increased QT interval, additive negative inotropic effects
rifampin: Decreased bioavailability of oral verapamil
telithromycin: Increased risk of bradyarrhythmias, hypotension, lactic acidosis
FOODS
grapefruit juice: Increased concentrations of verapamil
ACTIVITIES
alcohol use: Increased blood alcohol level and prolonged CNS effects

Adverse Reactions
CNS: Confusion, CVA, disequilibrium, dizziness, extrapyramidal reactions, fatigue, headache, insomnia, paresthesia, psychosis, shakiness, somnolence

CV: Angina, AV conduction disorders, bradycardia, claudication, heart failure, hypotension, peripheral edema, tachycardia
GI: Constipation, elevated liver function test results, nausea
GU: Galactorrhea, menstrual irregularities
MS: Muscle spasms
RESP: Dyspnea, pulmonary edema, wheezing
SKIN: Flushing, rash

Nursing Considerations

- Administer I.V. verapamil with compatible solutions, including Ringer's injection, D_5W, or normal saline solution.
- Maintain continuous ECG monitoring and keep emergency resuscitation equipment readily available during I.V. therapy.
- Assess patient with hypertrophic cardiomyopathy for early development of hypotension and pulmonary edema because second-degree AV block and sinus arrest can result.
- Assess for bradycardia and hypotension, and notify prescriber if heart rate or blood pressure declines significantly.
- Be aware that disopyramide or flecainide shouldn't be given within 48 hours before or 24 hours after verapamil because additive negative inotropic effects can result.
- Institute measures to prevent constipation, including a high-fiber diet and a stool softener, as prescribed.

PATIENT TEACHING

- Direct patient to check her pulse rate before taking verapamil and to notify prescriber if it's below 50 beats/minute or as instructed by prescriber.
- Caution patient about possible dizziness and the need to avoid hazardous activities until drug's CNS effects are known.
- Explain that adverse skin reactions may subside with continued use. Advise her to notify prescriber about persistent rash.
- Encourage patient to increase dietary fiber intake to help prevent constipation. Advise her to notify prescriber if problem becomes persistent or severe.

vinblastine sulfate

Velban, Velbe (CAN)

Class and Category

Chemical: Vinca alkaloid
Therapeutic: Antimicrotubule antineoplastic
Pregnancy category: D

Indications and Dosages

▶ *To treat breast or testicular cancer, gestational trophoblastic tumors, histiocytosis X, Hodgkin's disease or non-Hodgkin's lymphoma, Kaposi's sarcoma, or mycosis fungoides*

I.V. INJECTION

Adults. *Initial:* 100 mcg (0.1mg)/kg or 3.7 mg/m^2 over 1 min every 7 days, increased in weekly increments of 50 mcg (0.05 mg)/kg or 1.8 to 1.9 mg/m^2 until leukocyte count falls to 3,000/mm^3. *Maintenance:* 50 mcg (0.05 mg/kg) or 1.8 to 1.9 mg/m^2 less than final initial dose. *Maximum:* 500 mcg (0.5 mg)/kg or 18.5 mg/m^2.

Adolescents and children. *Initial:* 2.5 mg/m^2 over 1 min every 7 days, increased in weekly increments of 1.25 mg/m^2 until leukocyte count falls to 3,000/mm^3. *Maintenance:* 1.25 mg/m^2 less than final initial dose. *Maximum:* 7.5 mg/m^2.

DOSAGE ADJUSTMENT Dosage decreased by 50% for patients with direct serum bilirubin concentration above 3 mg/dl.

Mechanism of Action

Binds to tubulin, a protein component of microtubules, which normally contribute to cell structure and movement, thereby inhibiting microtubule assembly and arresting cells in metaphase. Vinblastine may also interfere with amino acid metabolism. This drug is cell-cycle–phase specific for the M phase of cell division.

Incompatibilities

Prepare vinblastine solution using normal saline solution. Don't mix solution with any other drug.

Contraindications

Bacterial infection; granulocytopenia resulting from condition other than disease being treated

Interactions

DRUGS

blood-dyscrasia–causing drugs (such as cephalosporins and sulfasalazine): Increased risk of leukopenia and thrombocytopenia

bone marrow depressants (such as carboplatin and lomustine): Possibly additive bone marrow depression

hepatic enzyme inhibitors (such as allopurinol and cimetidine): Possibly earlier onset or increased severity of vinblastine adverse effects *itraconazole:* Possibly earlier onset or increased severity of neuromuscular adverse effects

phenytoin: Possibly decreased blood phenytoin level and increased risk of seizures

vaccines, killed virus: Possibly decreased antibody response to vaccine

vaccines, live virus: Possibly decreased antibody response to vaccine, increased adverse effects of vaccine, and severe infection

Adverse Reactions

CNS: Malaise, neurotoxicity, weakness
CV: Hypertension
EENT: Jaw pain, stomatitis
GI: Anorexia, constipation, nausea, vomiting
GU: Uric acid nephropathy
HEME: Anemia, leukopenia, thrombocytopenia (transient)
MS: Bone pain, tissue pain at tumor site
SKIN: Alopecia
Other: Hyperuricemia, injection site pain or redness

Nursing Considerations

- Follow facility protocols for preparation and handling of antineoplastic drugs and for appropriate disposal of used equipment.
- Be aware that vinblastine dosage may vary, depending on dosage schedule and regimen being used.
- Be aware that adverse reactions can vary when vinblastine is administered in combination therapy. Review information for all drugs administered as part of a specific regimen, including drug interactions and adverse effects.
- Monitor liver function test results; hematocrit, hemoglobin, and platelet count; and leukocyte count (total and differential) before and periodically during treatment, as ordered.
- Monitor blood uric acid level of patients with a history of gout or renal calculi before and periodically during vinblastine therapy to detect hyperuricemia. Expect to give allopurinol to patients with elevated blood uric acid levels to prevent uric acid nephropathy. Be aware that patients already receiving antigout drugs, such as allopurinol, colchicine, probenecid, or sufinpyrazone, may require an adjustment in antigout drug dosage.
- Be aware that vinblastine is available in a 1-mg/ml preparation or as a powder for reconstitution. To reconstitute vinblastine, add 10 ml of 0.9% sodium chloride injection to a vial containing 10 mg/ml to yield a final concentration of 1 mg/ml. If the diluent contains a preservative, such as benzyl alcohol, use di-

luted solution within 28 days if stored at 2° to 8° C (36° to 46° F). If the diluent doesn't contain a preservative, use solution immediately and discard unused portion.

- **WARNING** When preparing vinblastine for neonates or premature infants, don't use a diluent that contains benzyl alcohol because this preservative has been linked to a fatal toxic syndrome characterized by CNS, respiratory, circulatory, and renal impairment and metabolic acidosis.
- If vinblastine solution comes in contact with your skin or mucosa, wash if off thoroughly with warm water. If drug comes in contact with your eye, irrigate eye thoroughly with water to prevent irritation or corneal ulceration.
- **WARNING** Clearly label syringe containing prepared dose "FATAL IF GIVEN INTRATHECALLY. FOR I.V. USE ONLY" and place in overwrap. Label overwrap with the same warning and the additional statement "DO NOT REMOVE COVERING UNTIL THE MOMENT OF INJECTION." Don't administer drug intrathecally because potentially fatal paralysis may occur.
- Inspect I.V. site for signs of infiltration and leakage into surrounding tissues. If extravasation occurs, stop injection immediately and notify prescriber. Then resume injection in another vein. Apply warm heat to affected area, and expect to administer a local injection of hyaluronidase, if ordered, to help decrease discomfort and reduce the risk of cellulitis.
- Be aware that subsequent doses of vinblastine shouldn't be administered until leukocyte count after previous dose has returned to at least 4,000/mm^3, even if 7 days has passed.
- Monitor patients who have, or have recently been exposed to, chicken pox or who have herpes zoster for signs and symptoms of severe generalized disease.
- Be aware that patients who have received cytotoxic therapy and those who are receiving concurrent or consecutive radiation therapy are at risk for additive bone marrow depression.
- If patient develops thrombocytopenia, implement protective precautions according to facility policy.
- Assess for signs of infection, such as fever, if patient develops leukopenia. Expect to obtain appropriate specimens for culture and sensitivity testing and implement protective precautions according to facility policy.
- Before reconstituting powder form or using diluted form, store vinblastine at 2° to 8° C (36° to 46° F).

PATIENT TEACHING
- Advise patient to have any needed dental work completed be-

fore beginning vinblastine treatment, if possible, or to defer such work until blood counts return to normal; vinblastine can delay healing and cause gingival bleeding. Teach patient proper oral hygiene, and advise her to use a soft-bristled toothbrush.

- Advise patient to immediately report burning at injection site or other signs of extravasation.
- Instruct patient who develops bone marrow depression to avoid people with infections and to report fever, chills, cough, hoarseness, lower back or side pain, or painful or difficult urination because these signs and symptoms may indicate an infection.
- Instruct patient to avoid touching her eyes or inside of her nose unless she washes her hands immediately beforehand.
- Caution patient to avoid receiving immunizations unless approved by prescriber. Instruct her to avoid people who have recently received vaccines or to wear a protective mask over her nose and mouth if she must be around them.
- Instruct patient to immediately report unusual bleeding or bruising, black or tarry stools, blood in urine or stools, or red pinpoint spots on skin.
- Stress the importance of avoiding accidental cuts from sharp objects because excessive bleeding or infection may occur.
- Encourage patient to drink plenty of fluids to increase urine output and help excrete uric acid.
- Suggest that patient with stomatitis eat bland, soft foods served cold or at room temperature to decrease irritation.
- Caution patient to avoid contact sports or other situations that put her at risk for bruising or injury.
- Stress the importance of complying with the dosage regimen and of keeping follow-up medical appointments and appointments for laboratory tests.
- Reassure patient that her hair should grow back after vinblastine therapy has been completed.
- Urge patient to use contraception because of the risk of fetal harm. Instruct her to immediately report becoming pregnant.

vincristine sulfate
Oncovin, Vincasar PFS

Class and Category
Chemical: Vinca alkaloid
Therapeutic: Antineoplastic
Pregnancy category: D

Indications and Dosages

▶ *To treat acute lymphocytic leukemia, Hodgkin's disease or non-Hodgkin's lymphoma, neuroblastoma, or Wilms' tumor*

I.V. INJECTION

Adults. 10 to 30 mcg (0.01 to 0.03 mg)/kg or 400 mcg (0.4 mg) to 1.4 mg/m² over 1 min every wk. Dosage adjusted based on patient's clinical response and presence or severity of toxicity.

Children weighing more than 10 kg. 1.5 to 2 mg/m² over 1 min every wk.

Children weighing 10 kg and less. 50 mcg (0.05 mg)/kg over 1 min every wk.

DOSAGE ADJUSTMENT Dosage decreased by 50% for patients with direct serum bilirubin concentration above 3 mg/dl.

Mechanism of Action

Inhibits the formation of microtubules, which normally contribute to cell structure and movement, thus arresting cells in metaphase. Vincristine is cell-cycle–phase specific for the M phase of cell division.

Incompatibilities

Don't give vincristine with solutions that move pH above or below the range of 3.5 to 5.5. Give only with normal saline solution or D₅W.

Contraindications

Demyelinating form of Charcot-Marie-Tooth syndrome

Interactions

DRUGS

asparaginase, itraconazole, neurotoxic drugs: Possibly additive neurotoxic effects

bleomycin: Increased susceptibility of cancer cells to bleomycin

blood-dyscrasia–causing drugs (such as cephalosporins and sulfasalazine): Increased risk of leukopenia and thrombocytopenia

bone marrow depressants (such as carboplatin and lomustine): Possibly additive bone marrow depression

doxorubicin: Increased risk of myelosuppression when used in combination with vincristine and prednisone

phenytoin: Possibly decreased blood phenytoin level and increased risk of seizures

vaccines, killed virus: Possibly decreased antibody response to vaccine

vaccines, live virus: Possibly decreased antibody response to vaccine, increased adverse effects of vaccine, and severe infection

Adverse Reactions

CNS: Fever, headache, progressive neurotoxicity (including blurred or double vision, decreased reflexes, difficulty walking, neuritic pain, and paresthesia)

CV: Hypertension, hypotension

EENT: Stomatitis

ENDO: Syndrome of inappropriate ADH secretion (SIADH)

GI: Bloating, constipation (severe), diarrhea, nausea, vomiting

GU: Dysuria, polyuria, uric acid nephropathy, urine retention

HEME: Anemia, leukopenia, thrombocytopenia

RESP: Bronchospasm, dyspnea

SKIN: Alopecia, rash

Other: Allergic reaction, hyperuricemia, injection site pain or redness, weight loss

Nursing Considerations

- Follow facility protocols for preparation and handling of antineoplastic drugs and for appropriate disposal of used equipment.
- Be aware that vincristine dosage may vary, depending on dosage schedule and regimen being used.
- Be aware that adverse reactions can vary when vincristine is given in combination therapy. Review information for all drugs administered as part of a specific regimen, including drug interactions and adverse effects.
- Monitor liver function test results; hematocrit, hemoglobin, and platelet count; and leukocyte count (total and differential) before and periodically during treatment, as ordered.
- Monitor the blood uric acid level of patients with a history of gout or renal calculi before and periodically during therapy to detect hyperuricemia. Expect to administer allopurinol, as ordered, to patients with elevated blood uric acid levels to prevent uric acid nephropathy. Be aware that patients already receiving antigout drugs, such as allopurinol, colchicine, probenecid, or sufinpyrazone, may require an adjustment in antigout drug dosage.
- If vincristine solution comes in contact with your skin or mucosa, wash it off thoroughly with warm water. If drug comes in contact with your eye, irrigated the eye thoroughly with water to prevent irritation or corneal ulceration.
- **WARNING** After withdrawing appropriate amount of drug from vial, as ordered, clearly label syringe "Fatal if given in-

TRATHECALLY. FOR I.V. USE ONLY" and place in overwrap. Label overwrap with the same warning and the additional statement "DO NOT REMOVE COVERING UNTIL THE MOMENT OF INJECTION." Don't administer drug intrathecally because potentially fatal paralysis may occur.

- Administer vincristine over a 1-minute period by I.V. bolus, or inject it into a free-flowing I.V. infusion of normal saline solution or D₅W.
- Inspect I.V. site for signs of infiltration and leakage into surrounding tissues. If extravasation occurs, stop the vincristine injection immediately and notify prescriber. Then resume the injection in another vein. Apply warm heat to affected area, and expect to administer a local injection of hyaluronidase, if ordered, to help decrease discomfort and reduce the risk of cellulitis.
- Administer a prophylactic enema or laxative, if ordered, to prevent ileus.
- Monitor patient for hypotension and signs of neurotoxicity, such as paresthesia, decreased reflexes, and weakness. If such signs occur, notify prescriber and expect to decrease dosage or discontinue therapy, as ordered.
- Monitor patients who have, or have recently been exposed to, chicken pox or who have herpes zoster for signs and symptoms of severe generalized disease.
- Be aware that patients who have previously received cytotoxic therapy and those who are receiving concurrent or consecutive radiation therapy are at risk for additive bone marrow depression.
- If patient develops thrombocytopenia, implement protective precautions according to facility policy.
- Assess for signs of infection, such as fever, if patient develops leukopenia. Expect to obtain appropriate specimens for culture and sensitivity testing.
- Store vincristine at 2° to 8° C (36° to 46° F) in a light-resistant container.

PATIENT TEACHING

- Advise patient to immediately report burning at the injection site or other signs or symptoms of extravasation during vincristine therapy.
- Instruct patient who develops bone marrow depression to avoid people with infections. Advise her to report fever, chills, cough, hoarseness, lower back or side pain, or painful or difficult uri-

nation because these signs and symptoms may indicate an infection.

- Instruct patient to avoid touching her eyes or the inside of her nose unless she has washed her hands immediately before doing so.
- Caution patient to avoid receiving immunizations unless approved by prescriber. Urge her to avoid people who have recently received vaccines or to wear a protective mask over her nose and mouth if she must be around them.
- Instruct patient to immediately report unusual bleeding or bruising, black or tarry stools, blood in urine or stool, or red pinpoint spots on skin during vincristine therapy.
- Stress the importance of avoiding accidental cuts from sharp objects, such as razor blades or fingernail clippers, because excessive bleeding or infection may occur.
- Caution patient to avoid contact sports or other situations that put her at risk for bruising or injury.
- Encourage patient to drink fluids to increase urine output and help excrete uric acid; however, caution her not to drink excessive amounts because of the risk of SIADH.
- Suggest that patient with stomatitis eat bland, soft foods served cold or at room temperature to decrease irritation.
- Advise patient to consult prescriber about using a laxative if she develops constipation.
- Reassure patient that her hair should grow back after vincristine therapy has been completed.
- Urge patient to use contraception because of the risk of fetal harm from vincristine therapy. Instruct her to notify prescriber immediately if she becomes pregnant.
- Stress the importance of complying with the dosage regimen and of keeping follow-up medical appointments and appointments for laboratory tests.

voriconazole
Vfend

Class and Category
Chemical: Triazole
Therapeutic: Antifungal
Pregnancy category: D

Indications and Dosages
▶ *To treat invasive aspergillosis; to treat serious fungal infections caused*

by Scedosporium apiospermum *and* Fusarium *species, including* Fusarium solani, *in patients intolerant of or refractory to other therapy*

I.V. INFUSION

Adults and children age 12 and over. *Initial:* 6 mg/kg over 1 to 2 hr at a rate not to exceed 3 mg/kg/hr every 12 hr for 2 doses. *Maintenance:* 4 mg/kg over 1 to 2 hr at a rate not to exceed 3 mg/kg/hr every 12 hr.

▶ *To treat candidemia in nonneutropenic patients and other deep-tissue disseminatinated* Candida *infections involving the abdomen, kidney, bladder wall, skin, or a wound*

I.V. INFUSION

Adults. *Initial:* 6 mg/kg over 1 to 2 hr at no more than 3 mg/kg/hr every 12 hr for two doses. *Maintenance:* 3 to 4 mg/kg over 1 to 2 hr at no more than 3 mg/kg/hr every 12 hr for at least 14 days after symptoms resolve or last positive culture, whichever takes longer.

DOSAGE ADJUSTMENT If patient can't tolerate drug, I.V. maintenance dose may be reduced to 3 mg/kg every 12 hr. For use with phenytoin, maintenance dose may be increased to 5 mg/kg I.V. every 12 hr. For patients with mild to moderate hepatic cirrhosis, standard loading dose should be used but maintenance dose halved for I.V. use.

Mechanism of Action

Prevents fungal ergosterol biosynthesis by inhibiting fungal cytochrome P450–mediated 14 alpha-lanosterol demethylation. The loss of ergosterol in the fungal cell wall renders the fungal cell inactive.

Incompatibilities

Don't infuse into the same line or cannula with other drugs, including parenteral nutrition, to prevent an increase in subvisible particulate matter. Avoid infusion with blood products and any electrolyte supplements. Don't dilute with 4.2% sodium bicarbonate infusion because the mildly alkaline nature of the diluent causes slight degradation of voriconazole after 24 hours of storage at room temperature.

Contraindications

Coadministration with long-acting barbiturates, carbamazepine, CYP3A4 substrates (astemizole, cisapride, pimozide, quinidine, or terfenadine), efavirenz, ergot alkaloids, rifabutin, rifampin, ritonavir, or sirolimus; hypersensitivity to voriconazole or its components; galactose intolerance, glucose-galactose malabsorption, or Lapp lactase deficiency (oral form only contains lactose)

Interactions

DRUGS

benzodiazepines: Possibly prolonged sedative effect of benzodiazepines

calcium channel blockers; HMG-CoA reductase inhibitors, such as lovastatin; omeprazole; sirolimus: Possibly increased plasma concentrations of these drugs, leading to increased risk of adverse reactions and toxicity

carbamazepine, long-acting barbiturates, phenytoin, rifampin: Decreased plasma voriconazole concentration

coumarin, warfarin: Possibly increased PTT

cyclosporine, sirolimus, tacrolimus: Increased serum concentrations of these drugs and increased risk of toxicity, especially nephrotoxicity

CYP3A4 substrates (astemizole, cisapride, pimozide, quinidine, terfenadine): Increased plasma concentrations of CYP3A4 substrates, which may lead to prolonged QT interval and, rarely, torsades de pointes

ergot alkaloids (ergotamine, dihydroergotamine): May increase plasma concentration of ergot alkaloids leading to ergotism

HIV protease inhibitors (amprenavir, nelfinavir, ritonavir, saquinavir), non-nucleoside reverse transcriptase inhibitors (delavirdine, efavirenz): Possibly inhibited metabolism of these drugs and voriconazole

methadone: Increased plasma concentration of methadone, possibly leading to toxicity, including QT-interval prolongation

oral contraceptives: Increased plasma voriconazole level and increased risk of toxicity

rifabutin: Increased rifabutin plasma concentration; decreased voriconazole plasma concentrations

sulfonylureas: Possibly increased plasma concentrations of sulfonylureas and increased risk of hypoglycemia

vinca alkaloids: Possibly increased risk of neurotoxicity

Adverse Reactions

CNS: Chills, dizziness, fever, hallucinations, headache
CV: Chest pain, hypertension, hypotension, peripheral edema, tachycardia, vasodilation
EENT: Abnormal or blurred vision, altered or enhanced visual perception, change in color perception, chromatopsia, dry mouth, eye hemorrhage, photophobia, visual disturbances

GI: Abdominal pain, diarrhea, elevated liver function test results, nausea, vomiting
GU: Abnormal kidney function, acute renal failure, elevated serum creatinine level
HEME: Anemia, leukopenia, pancytopenia, thrombocytopenia
RESP: Respiratory disorders
SKIN: Cholestatic jaundice, erythema multiforme, jaundice, maculopapular rash, photosensitivity, pruritus, rash, Stevens-Johnson syndrome, toxic epidermal necrolysis
Other: Anaphylaxis (I.V. form), elevated alkaline phosphatase, hypokalemia, hypomagnesemia, sepsis

Nursing Considerations

- Use voriconazole cautiously in patients with known hypersensitivity to other azoles and in patients at risk for proarrhythmic events (such as those receiving cardiotoxic chemotherapy or those who have cardiomyopathy or hypokalemia) because some azoles may cause prolong QT interval.
- Obtain specimens for fungal culture and other relevant laboratory studies (including histopathology), as ordered, before giving first dose. Expect to begin drug before test results are known.
- Assess patient's liver function, including bilirubin, as ordered, at start of voriconazole therapy and periodically afterward. Therapy may be discontinued if liver abnormalities occur.
- Check patient's electrolyte levels before start of therapy, as ordered, and correct any imbalances, as prescribed, before administering voriconazole because electrolyte imbalances increase the risk of adverse reactions.
- For I.V. infusion, reconstitute powder with 19 ml of water for injection to obtain 20 ml of concentrate that contains 10 mg/ml of voriconazole. Use a standard 10-ml nonautomated syringe to ensure that exact amount of water is injected into vial.
- Shake the vial until all powder is dissolved.
- Further dilute so that final concentration is not less than 0.5 mg/ml nor more than 5 mg/ml. This requires withdrawing and discarding at least an equal volume of diluent from the infusion bag or bottle before instillation of concentrate.
- Discard partially used vials after mixing. If infusion isn't administered immediately, store at 2° to 8° C (37° to 46° F) for no longer than 24 hours.
- Administer I.V. infusion over 1 to 2 hours at a rate that doesn't exceed 3 mg/kg/hr.

- Monitor renal function, especially serum creatinine level, when administering I.V. form of voriconazole because drug may accumulate in body when creatinine clearance is less than 50 ml/min, increasing the risk of adverse reactions.
- **WARNING** Observe patient receiving I.V. voriconazole closely for anaphylactoid-type reactions—such as flushing, fever, sweating, tachycardia, chest tightness, dyspnea, faintness, nausea, pruritus and rash—which may occur immediately after starting the infusion. Stop the infusion if these reactions occur, and notify prescriber immediately.
- Monitor patient closely throughout therapy for skin rash, which may indicate a serious cutaneous reaction, such as Stevens-Johnson syndrome. If a rash occurs, notify prescriber, and expect that drug may be discontinued.
- Monitor patient closely for elevated levels of cyclosporine, tacrolimus, and warfarin when voriconazole is given with any of these drugs.
- Watch closely for hypoglycemia in diabetic patients who also take sulfonylureas, and check their blood glucose levels regularly.
- Be aware that voriconazole dosage will need to be adjusted when given with phenytoin. Expect to monitor plasma phenytoin levels and observe patient closely for phenytoin-related adverse reactions.
- Assess patient's visual function, including visual acuity, visual field, and color perception, if voriconazole therapy continues longer than 28 days.

PATIENT TEACHING

- Inform female patient of possible risk to fetus, and stress the importance of avoiding pregnancy. Tell her to use an effective form of contraception throughout voriconazole therapy and to notify the prescriber immediately if she is or could be pregnant or of she plans to become pregnant.
- Caution patient not to drive at night and to avoid potentially hazardous activities because drug may cause visual disturbances, including blurring or photophobia.
- Advise patient to avoid exposure to direct sunlight or UV light and to wear sunscreen when outdoors.

W·X·Y·Z

warfarin sodium
Coumadin

Class and Category
Chemical: Coumarin derivative
Therapeutic: Anticoagulant
Pregnancy category: X

Indications and Dosages
▶ *To prevent or treat pulmonary embolism; recurrent MI; thromboembolic complications from atrial fibrillation, heart valve replacement, or MI; and venous thrombosis (and its extension)*
I.V. INJECTION

Adults. *Initial:* 2 to 5 mg daily infused over 1 to 2 min. *Usual:* 2 to 10 mg daily infused over 1 to 2 min. *Maximum:* Determined by target PT and INR results, as prescribed.

DOSAGE ADJUSTMENT For patients with hepatic dysfunction, dosage reduced to 0.1 mg/kg, as prescribed. For elderly patients, dosage possibly reduced based on PT and INR results.

Route	Onset	Peak	Duration
I.V.	Unknown	3 to 4 days	2 to 5 days

Mechanism of Action
Interferes with the liver's ability to synthesize vitamin K-dependent clotting factors, depleting clotting factors II (prothrombin), VII, IX, and X. This action, in turn, interferes with the clotting cascade. By depleting vitamin K-dependent clotting factors and interfering with the clotting cascade, warfarin prevents coagulation.

Incompatibilities
Don't mix warfarin in solution with amikacin sulfate, epinephrine hydrochloride, metaraminol tartrate, oxytocin, promazine hydrochloride, tetracycline hydrochloride, or vancomycin hydrochloride.

Contraindications

Bleeding or bleeding tendencies; blood dyscrasias; cerebral or dissecting aneurysm; cerebrovascular hemorrhage; diverticulitis; eclampsia or preeclampsia; history of warfarin-induced necrosis; hypersensitivity to warfarin or its components; malignant or severe uncontrolled hypertension; malnutrition and emaciation; mental state or condition that leads to lack of patient cooperation; pericardial effusion; pericarditis; polyarthritis; pregnancy; prostatectomy; recent or planned neurosurgery, ophthalmic surgery, or spinal puncture; severe hepatic or renal disease

Interactions

DRUGS

acetaminophen, aminoglycosides, amiodarone, androgens, argatroban, beta blockers, bivalirudin, capecitabine, cephalosporins, chloral hydrate, chloramphenicol, chlorpropamide, cimetidine, clofibrate, corticosteroids, cyclophosphamide, dextrothyroxine, diflunisal, disulfiram, erythromycin, ezetimibe, fluconazole, gemfibrozil, glucagon, hydantoins, ifosfamide, influenza virus vaccine, isoniazid, ketoconazole, lepirudin, loop diuretics, lovastatin, metronidazole, miconazole, mineral oil, moricizine, nalidixic acid, NSAIDs, omeprazole, penicillins, phenylbutazones, propafenone, propoxyphene, proton pump inhibitors, quinidine, quinine, quinolones, salicylates, streptokinase, sulfamethoxazole-trimethoprim, sulfinpyrazone, sulfonamides, tamoxifen, tetracyclines, thyroid hormones, urokinase, valdecoxib, vitamin E: Increased anticoagulant effect of warfarin, increased risk of bleeding

aminoglutethimide, barbiturates, carbamazepine, cholestyramine, dicloxacillin, estrogens, ethchlorvynol, etretinate, glutethimide, griseofulvin, nafcillin, oral contraceptives, rifampin, spironolactone, sucralfate, thiazide diuretics, trazodone, vitamin C, vitamin K: Decreased anticoagulant effect of warfarin

atorvastatin, pravastatin: Increased or decreased anticoagulant effect of warfarin

herbal remedies (including bromelains, danshen, dong quai, garlic, ginkgo biloba, and ginseng): Increased anticoagulant effect of warfarin, increased risk of bleeding

I.V. lipid emulsion, other medical products that contain soybean oil: Possibly decreased vitamin K absorption and increased anticoagulant effect of warfarin

nicotine patch: Altered response to warfarin

FOODS

certain multivitamins, enteral feedings, vitamin-K–rich foods: Decreased effects of warfarin

ACTIVITIES

alcohol use: Increased risk of hypoprothrombinemia

smoking, smoking cessation: Altered response to warfarin

Adverse Reactions

CNS: Coma, intracranial hemorrhage, loss of consciousness, syncope, weakness

CV: Angina, hypotension

EENT: Epistaxis, intraocular hemorrhage

GI: Abdominal cramps and pain, diarrhea, hepatitis, nausea, vomiting

GU: Hematuria, vaginal bleeding (abnormal)

HEME: Anemia, potentially fatal hemorrhage (from any tissue or organ)

SKIN: Alopecia, ecchymosis, jaundice, pallor, petechiae, pruritus, purple-toe syndrome, tissue necrosis

Other: Anaphylaxis

Nursing Considerations

- Reconstitute parenteral warfarin just before administration with 2.7 ml of sterile water for injection to yield 2 mg/ml. Then administer slowly over 1 to 2 minutes through peripheral I.V.
- Avoid I.M. injections during warfarin therapy, if possible, because they can result in bleeding, bruising, and hematoma.
- Monitor international normalized ratio (INR) (daily in acute care setting) and assess for therapeutic effects, as prescribed. Therapeutic INR levels are 2.0 to 3.0 for bioprosthetic heart valve, nonvalvular atrial fibrillation, and venous thromboembolism, and 2.5 to 3.5 after MI and for mechanical heart valve.
- Expect treatment to last up to 12 weeks for bioprosthetic heart valve, 1 to 3 months for nonvalvular atrial fibrillation or venous thromboembolism, and for rest of life after MI and for mechanical heart valve replacement.
- **WARNING** Be aware of the increased risk for intracranial hemorrhage if patient has cerebral ischemia (such as recent transient ischemic attack or minor ischemic CVA) and INR of 3 to 4.5. As prescribed, withhold next warfarin dose and give vitamin K if INR exceeds 4 because of the risk of bleeding.
- Assess for occult bleeding if patient receives I.V. lipid emulsion or other medical product that contains soybean oil. Such products can decrease vitamin K absorption and increase warfarin's anticoagulant effect.

PATIENT TEACHING

- Explain that warfarin therapy aims to prevent thrombosis by decreasing clotting ability while avoiding the risk of spontaneous bleeding.

- Urge patient to keep weekly follow-up appointments for blood tests after discharge until PT and INR levels are stabilized.
- Advise patient to avoid alcohol during warfarin therapy.
- Urge patient to take precautions against bleeding, such as using an electric shaver and a soft-bristled toothbrush. Advise him to continue these precautions for 2 to 5 days after therapy stops, as directed, because anticoagulant effect may persist.
- Caution patient to avoid activities that could cause traumatic injury and bleeding.
- Advise patient to eat consistent amounts of vitamin K–rich foods, such as dark green, leafy vegetables.
- Urge patient to notify prescriber immediately about unusual bleeding and any unexplained symptoms, such as abnormal vaginal bleeding; dizziness; easy bruising; gum bleeding; headache; nosebleeds; prolonged bleeding from cuts; red, black, or tarry stool; red or dark brown urine; swelling; and weakness.
- Advise patient to consult prescriber before taking other drugs—including OTC drugs and herbal remedies—during therapy.
- Instruct female patient of childbearing age to stop taking warfarin and notify prescriber immediately about known or suspected pregnancy.
- Explain that drug may cause reversible purple-toe syndrome and that this syndrome isn't harmful.
- Urge patient to carry medical identification that reveals he's taking warfarin therapy.

zidovudine

Retrovir

Class and Category

Chemical: Synthetic pyrimidine nucleoside analogue
Therapeutic: Antiviral
Pregnancy category: C

Indications and Dosages

▶ *To treat HIV infection*
I.V. INFUSION
Adults and children over age 12 (United States). 1 mg/kg infused over 1 hr five or six times a day. *Maximum pediatric dose:* 160 mg.
Adults and children over age 12 (Canada). 1 to 2 mg/kg in-

fused over 1 hr every 4 hr. *Maximum pediatric dose:* 160 mg.
DOSAGE ADJUSTMENT Adult dosage reduced to 1 mg/kg
every 6 to 8 hr for patients with end-stage renal disease.
▶ *To prevent maternal-fetal HIV transmission*
I.V. INFUSION
Mother. 2 mg/kg infused over 1 hr at the start of labor and de-
livery, followed by 1 mg/kg/hr by continuous infusion until um-
bilical cord is clamped.
Neonate. 1.5 mg/kg infused over 30 min every 6 hr.

Mechanism of Action

Ultimately converted by thymidine kinase and other cellular enzymes to zidovudine triphosphate. Zidovudine triphosphate is incorporated into growing
chains of viral DNA polymerase, an enzyme used in the viral DNA replication
process, thus inhibiting DNA viral replication of HIV.

Incompatibilities

Don't mix zidovudine with biological or colloidal solutions, such
as blood products or protein-containing solutions.

Contraindications

Hypersensitivity to zidovudine or its components

Interactions

DRUGS

atovaquone: Possibly decreased zidovudine clearance and increased
blood zidovudine level
*blood-dyscrasia–causing drugs (such as cephalosporins and sulfasalazine),
bone marrow depressants (such as carboplatin and lomustine):* Increased
risk of additive myelosuppressive effects
clarithromycin: Decreased blood zidovudine level and time to peak
zidovudine concentration
cytotoxic drugs, ganciclovir, interferon alfa: Increased risk of hematologic toxicities
*hepatic glucuronidation–metabolized drugs (such as acetaminophen, as-
pirin, benzodiazepines, cimetidine, indomethacin, morphine, and sulfonamides):* Possibly decreased clearance and toxicity of both drugs
interferons, ribavirin: Increased risk of hepatic decompensation,
neutropenia, and anemia
methadone, rifampin: Possibly altered blood zidovudine level
phenytoin: Possibly decreased blood phenytoin level and decreased
zidovudine clearance

probenecid: Possibly increased blood ziduvodine level and flulike symptoms

ribovirin, stavudine: Possibly antagonized antiviral effect

Adverse Reactions

CNS: Chills, fever, headache, insomnia, tiredness, weakness
EENT: Pharyngitis
GI: Nausea
HEME: Anemia, bone marrow depression, granulocytopenia, leukopenia, neutropenia, platelet count changes
MS: Myalgia
SKIN: Altered skin pigmentation, hyperpigmentation (bluish-brown bands) of nails, pallor
Other: Immune reconstitution syndrome

Nursing Considerations

- Be aware that I.V. infusion of zidovudine is ordered only until oral drug can be administered.
- Dilute ziduvodine with D_5W to a maximum concentration of 4 mg/ml. Use within 8 hours if stored at room temperature or within 24 hours if stored at 2° to 8° C (36° to 46° F) to decrease the risk of microbial contamination. Discard solution if you observe particles or discoloration before administration.
- Administer zidovudine by I.V. infusion at a constant rate over 1 hour; don't administer drug by rapid infusion or by I.M. injection.
- Monitor CBC periodically during zidovudine therapy. Be aware that anemia most commonly occurs after 4 to 6 weeks of therapy and that patient may require dosage adjustment, discontinuation of drug, blood transfusions, or epoetin treatment if hemoglobin level is less than 7.5 g/dl or if granulocyte count is less than 750/mm³.
- Assess patient for dyspnea, tachypnea, or decreased blood bicarbonate level; if she exhibits such findings, expect zidovudine to be discontinued until a diagnosis of lactic acidosis can be ruled out.
- Monitor patient for immune reconstitution syndrome, which may occur during combination antiretroviral therapy that includes zidovudine. During the initial phase of treatment, the syndrome is exhibited by patients developing an inflammatory response to certain infections such as *Mycobactgerium avium* infection, cytomegalovirus, *Pneumocystits jirovecii* (formerly *carinii*) pneumonia or tuberculosis that may require additional therapy.

• Before diluting drug, store it at 15° to 25° C (59° to 77° F) and protect from light.

PATIENT TEACHING

• Advise mothers being treated for HIV infection not to breast-feed infant to prevent transmission of virus.

• Instruct patient to use a condom to decrease the risk of transmitting HIV. Also, urge patient not to share needles with anyone.

• Teach patient proper oral hygiene, and advise her to use a soft-bristled toothbrush to decrease the risk of infection or delayed healing.

• Inform patient who is also receiving cidofovir that zidovudine dosage may need to be adjusted or therapy temporarily discontinued on the day of cidofovir therapy.

• Explain to patient that zidovudine is not a cure for HIV infection. Stress the importance of complying with dosage regimen and of keeping follow-up medical appointments and appointments for laboratory tests.

zinc chloride
(contains 1 mg of elemental zinc per ml for I.V. infusion)

zinc sulfate
1 or 5 mg of elemental zinc per ml for I.V. infusion)
Zinca-Pak

Class and Category
Chemical: Trace element, mineral
Therapeutic: Copper absorption inhibitor, nutritional supplement
Pregnancy category: C

Indications and Dosages
▶ *To prevent zinc deficiency based on U.S. and Canadian recommended daily allowances (RDAs)*
I.V. INFUSION
Adults and children. 2.5 to 4 mg daily added to total parenteral nutrition (TPN) solution. *Maximum:* 12 mg daily.
Children from birth to age 5. 100 mcg/kg daily added to TPN solution.
Premature infants weighing up to 3 kg. 300 mcg/kg daily added to TPN solution.
▶ *To treat zinc deficiency*

I.V. INFUSION

Adults and adolescents. 2.5 to 4 mg daily added to TPN solution. *Maximum:* 12 mg daily.

Children from birth to age 5. 100 mcg/kg daily added to TPN solution.

Premature infants weighing up to 3 kg. 300 mcg/kg daily added to TPN solution.

Mechanism of Action

Needed for proper functioning of more than 200 metalloenzymes (those containing tightly bound zinc atoms as an integral part of their structure), including carbonic anhydrase, carboxypeptidase A, alcohol dehydrogenase, alkaline phosphatase, and RNA polymerase. Zinc also helps maintain nucleic acid, protein, and cell membrane structure and is essential for certain physiologic functions, including cell growth and division, sexual maturation and reproduction, dark adaptation and night vision, wound healing, host immunity, and taste acuity. This mineral also provides cellular antioxidant protection by scavenging free radicals.

In addition, zinc acetate interferes with intestinal absorption of copper and produces a protein that binds with copper, preventing its transfer to the blood. Bound copper is then excreted in stools, thus decreasing copper toxicity in Wilson's disease.

Contraindications

Hypersensitivity to zinc or its components

Interactions

DRUGS

copper supplements: Impaired copper absorption (with large doses of zinc)

oral iron supplements, oral phosphate salts, penicillamine, phosphorus-containing drugs: Decreased zinc absorption

quinolones, tetracyclines: Decreased absorption and possibly decreased effectiveness of these antibiotics

thiazide diuretics: Increased urinary excretion of zinc

zinc-containing preparations: Increased blood zinc level

FOODS

fiber- or phylate-containing foods (such as bran, whole-grain breads, cereal), phosphorus-containing foods (including milk, poultry): Decreased zinc absorption

Adverse Reactions

None with usual dosages

Nursing Considerations

- **WARNING** Don't administer I.V. zinc preparations that contain benzyl alcohol to neonates or premature infants because this preservative may cause a fatal toxic syndrome characterized by metabolic acidosis and CNS, respiratory, circulatory, and renal function impairment.
- Monitor patient receiving long-term zinc therapy for sideroblastic anemia, which may result from zinc-induced copper deficiency and is characterized by anemia, leukopenia, neutropenia, granulocytopenia, and bone marrow problems. Be aware that these effects are reversible after zinc is discontinued.
- Monitor patient with preexisting copper deficiency for exacerbation of this condition; zinc can decrease serum copper level.
- Assess patient for evidence of zinc deficiency, such as growth retardation, hypogonadism, delayed sexual maturation, alopecia, impaired wound healing, skin lesions, immune deficiencies, behavioral disturbances, night blindness, and taste impairment.
- Monitor blood alkaline phosphatase level monthly, as ordered; it may increase.
- Be aware that zinc chloride contains aluminum, which may accumulate to the point of toxicity if the patient's kidney function is impaired. Assess kidney function regularly.

PATIENT TEACHING
- Inform patient that I.V. therapy is only necessary until she is able to take zinc orally.

zoledronic acid

Reclast, Zometa

Class and Category

Chemical: Bisphosphonate
Therapeutic: Antihypercalcemic, bone resorption inhibitor
Pregnancy category: D

Indications and Dosages

▶ *To treat hypercalcemia caused by cancer*
I.V. INFUSION (ZOMETA)
Adults. 4 mg infused over at least 15 min. After 7 days, retreatment with 4 mg if serum calcium level doesn't remain at or re-

turn to normal. *Maximum:* 4 mg/dose.

▶ *As adjunct treatment for patients with multiple myeloma or bony metastasis who are receiving standard antineoplastic therapy and have a creatinine clearance above 60 ml/min/1.73 m²*

I.V. INFUSION (ZOMETA)

Adults. 4 mg infused over at least 15 min every 3 to 4 wk.
DOSAGE ADJUSTMENT If creatinine clearance is 50 to 60 ml/min/1.73 m², dosage decreased to 3.5 mg; if it's 40 to 49 ml/min/1.73 m², dosage decreased to 3.3 mg; and if it's 30 to 39 ml/min/1.73 m², dosage decreased to 3 mg.

▶ *To treat postmenopausal osteoporosis*

I.V. INFUSION (RECLAST)

Adult women. 5 mg infused over at least 15 min yearly.

▶ *To treat Paget's disease of the bone*

I.V. INFUSION (RECLAST)

Adults. 5 mg infused over at least 15 min after 1,500 mg elemental calcium daily in divided doses and 800 international units vitamin D daily has been given for 2 wk.

Mechanism of Action

Inhibits resorption of mineralized bone and cartilage by osteoclasts and induces osteoclast breakdown. In cancer-related hypercalcemia, hyperactive osteoclasts cause bone resorption and release of calcium into the blood, which causes polyuria, GI disruption, progressive dehydration, and decreasing GFR. This, in turn, increases renal calcium resorption and worsens hypercalcemia. Zoledronic acid interrupts this process.

Incompatibilities

Don't mix zoledronic acid with calcium-containing I.V. solutions, such as LR.

Contraindications

Hypersensitivity to zoledronic acid, other bisphosphonates, or their components

Interactions

DRUGS

aminoglycosides: Possibly additive serum calcium–lowering effect
loop diuretics, such as furosemide: Possibly increased risk of hypocalcemia
NSAIDs: Increased risk of nephrotoxicity

Adverse Reactions

CNS: Chills, fever, hyperesthesia, tremor
CV: Atrial fibrillation, bradycardia, hypertension, hypotension
EENT: Blurred vision, conjunctivitis, dry mouth, episcleritis, taste disturbance, uveitis
GI: Nausea, vomiting
GU: Elevated serum creatinine level, hematuria, proteinuria, renal insufficiency or failure
MS: Arthralgia; myalgia; osteonecrosis of the jaw; severe bone, joint, and muscle pain
RESP: Bronchoconstriction
SKIN: Diaphoresis, flushing, urticaria
Other: Anaphylaxis, angioedema, hyperkalemia, hypernatremia, hypocalcemia, hypomagnesemia, hypophosphatemia, infusion site redness and swelling, weight gain

Nursing Considerations

- Be aware that zoledronic acid isn't indicated for hypercalcemia from hyperparathyroidism or other nontumor conditions.
- Make sure patient has had a dental checkup before zoledronic acid starts, especially if patient has cancer; is receiving chemotherapy, head or neck radiation, or a corticosteroid; or has poor oral hygiene because the risk of osteonecrosis is increased in these patients, and invasive dental procedures during zoledronic acid therapy may worsen osteonecrosis.
- Expect to aggressively hydrate hypercalcemic patient with I.V. normal saline solution before and throughout zoledronic acid therapy, as prescribed, to achieve and maintain a urine output of about 2 L daily.
- **WARNING** During hydration, monitor fluid intake and output often and assess patient, especially one with heart failure, for evidence of life-threatening overhydration.
- Reconstitute Zometa by adding 5 ml of sterile water for injection to drug vial to yield a solution that contains 4 mg zoledronic acid. Make sure drug is completely dissolved before withdrawing prescribed dose. Further dilute in 100 ml normal saline solution or 5% dextrose injection, and infuse over at least 15 minutes.
- Be aware that Reclast needs no reconstitution.
- Before giving drug, inspect the reconstituted and diluted solution and discard if particles or discoloration are present.
- Refrigerate reconstituted drug at 2° to 8° C (36° to 46° F) and discard it after 24 hours.

- Give drug as a single I.V. solution in a separate I.V. line.
- **WARNING** Be aware that a single dose of Zometa shouldn't exceed 4 mg and that both Zometa and Reclast should be infused over at least 15 minutes. Infusing more quickly may lead to significant renal function deterioration, which may progress to renal failure.
- **WARNING** Assess patient's renal function, as ordered, before and during zoledronic acid therapy to detect deterioration. For patient with a normal serum creatinine level who develops an increase of 0.5 mg/dl within 2 weeks of receiving drug, expect to withhold next dose until serum creatinine level is within 10% of patient's baseline value. For patient with an abnormal serum creatinine level who develops an increase of 1 mg/dl within 2 weeks of receiving drug, expect to withhold next dose until serum creatinine level is within 10% of baseline value.
- Monitor patient's serum calcium, magnesium, and phosphate levels, as ordered, throughout therapy. If hypocalcemia, hypomagnesemia, or hypophosphatemia occurs, expect to give short-term supplemental therapy, as ordered.
- Assess aspirin-sensitive asthma patients for worsening of respiratory symptoms during zoledronic acid therapy because other bisphosphonates have caused bronchoconstriction in these patients.
- Store drug at 25° C (77° F).

PATIENT TEACHING
- Teach patient the importance of consuming a nutritious diet, including adequate amounts of calcium and vitamin D.
- Advise patient to alert prescriber about muscle or bone pain.
- Instruct patient on proper oral hygiene and on need to notify prescriber before undergoing invasive dental procedures.
- Urge women of childbearing age to report suspected or confirmed pregnancy immediately; zoledronic acid will need to be discontinued.

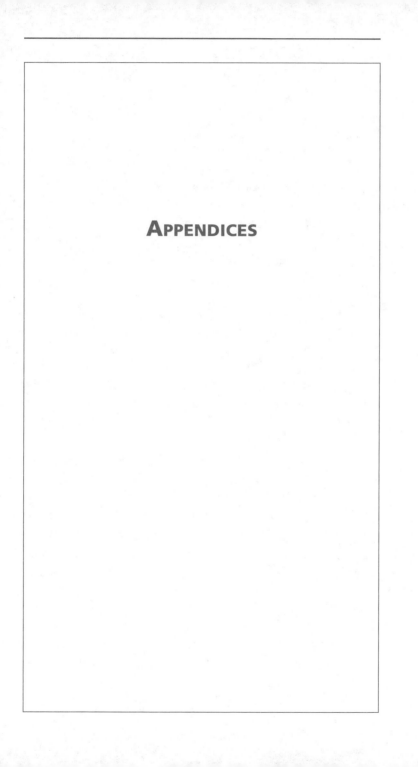

APPENDICES

EQUIANALGESIC DOSES FOR OPIOID AGONISTS

An equianalgesic dose of a synthetic opioid agonist is the dose that produces the same level of analgesia as 10 mg of I.M. or subcutaneous morphine, the principal opioid obtained from opium poppies. If your patient is switched from one opioid to another, expect to use the equianalgesic dose to decrease the risk of adverse reactions while increasing the likelihood of adequate pain relief. The chart below compares equianalgesic doses (oral and parenteral) for adults and children who weigh 50 kg (110 lb) or more.

Opioid agonist	Oral dose	Parenteral dose
codeine	200 mg (not recommended dose)	120 to 130 mg
hydrocodone	30 mg	Not applicable
hydromorphone	7.5 mg	1.5 mg
levorphanol	4 mg	2 mg
meperidine	300 mg	75 to 100 mg
morphine (around-the-clock dosing)	30 mg	10 mg
morphine (single or intermittent dosing)	60 mg	10 mg
oxycodone	30 mg	Not applicable

CALCULATING THE STRENGTH OF A SOLUTION

Most solutions come prepared in the required strength by the pharmacy or medical supply source. But sometimes only the concentrated form is available, and you'll need to dilute the solution or solid to administer the prescribed strength.

When a solid form of a drug is used to prepare a solution, the drug must be completely dissolved. Solid drug forms, such as tablets, crystals, and powders, are considered 100% strength. (An exception to this is boric acid, which is only 5% at full strength.) The final diluted solution is stated in terms of liquid measurement. To prepare a solution, you'll need to add the prescribed solid or liquid form of the drug (the solute) to the prescribed amount of diluent (the solvent). Two of the most common diluents used in the clinical setting are normal saline solution and sterile water.

You can use either of two formulas to calculate the strength of a solution, as shown in the examples below.

Method 1: Calculating percentage and volume
Use the following formula:

$$\frac{\text{Weaker solution}}{\text{Stronger solution}} = \frac{\text{Solute}}{\text{Solvent}}$$

Example: You need to dilute a stock solution of 100% strength to a 5% solution. How much solute will you need to add to obtain 500 ml of the 5% solution?

Calculate as follows:

$$\frac{5\ (\%)\ (\text{Weaker solution})}{100\ (\%)\ (\text{Stronger solution})} = \frac{X\ (g)\ (\text{Solute})}{500\ \text{ml}\ (\text{Solvent})}$$

$$100\ X = (500)(5)\ \text{or}\ 2{,}500$$
$$X = 25\ g$$

Answer: You'll need to add 25 g of solute to each 500 ml of solvent to prepare a 5% solution.

(continued)

CALCULATING THE STRENGTH OF A SOLUTION *(continued)*

Method 2: Calculating percentage and volume

Use the following formula:

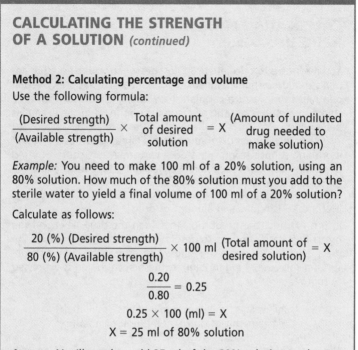

$$\frac{\text{(Desired strength)}}{\text{(Available strength)}} \times \begin{array}{c}\text{Total amount} \\ \text{of desired} \\ \text{solution}\end{array} = X \begin{array}{c}\text{(Amount of undiluted} \\ \text{drug needed to} \\ \text{make solution)}\end{array}$$

Example: You need to make 100 ml of a 20% solution, using an 80% solution. How much of the 80% solution must you add to the sterile water to yield a final volume of 100 ml of a 20% solution?

Calculate as follows:

$$\frac{20\,(\%)\,\text{(Desired strength)}}{80\,(\%)\,\text{(Available strength)}} \times 100\text{ ml}\ \begin{array}{c}\text{(Total amount of} \\ \text{desired solution)}\end{array} = X$$

$$\frac{0.20}{0.80} = 0.25$$

$$0.25 \times 100\,\text{(ml)} = X$$

$$X = 25\text{ ml of 80\% solution}$$

Answer: You'll need to add 25 ml of the 80% solution to the water to yield a final volume of 100 ml of a 20% solution.

CALCULATING PARENTERAL DRUG DOSAGES

You may need to calculate drug dosages when you're asked to administer a drug that is available in one measure, but prescribed in another. To make such calculations, you can use any of the three common methods of ratio and proportion shown in the examples below.

Example: You need to administer a prescribed dose of 1 mg morphine sulfate from a unit-dose cartridge that contains 4 mg per 2 ml. How many milliliters will you need to give to equal the prescribed dose of 1 mg?

Method 1: Using labeled amount of drug

In this method, the proportions between the drug label and the prescribed dose are used to determine ratio and proportion. The drug label, which states the amount of drug in one unit of measure (in this case, 4 mg in 2 ml), is the first ratio and is expressed as follows:

milligrams : milliliter = milligrams : milliliter
4 mg (amount of drug) : 2 ml (unit of measure)

The prescribed dose—in this case, 1 mg—is the second ratio; it must be expressed in the same order and units of measure as the first, as follows:

4 mg : 2 ml = 1 mg : X ml

Calculate as follows:

$$4X = 2$$
$$X = \frac{2}{4}$$
$$X = 0.5 \text{ ml}$$

Answer: You'll need to give 0.5 ml of morphine sulfate to equal the prescribed dose of 1 mg.

CALCULATING PARENTERAL DRUG DOSAGES *(continued)*

Method 2: Using an established formula
Use this formula:

$$\frac{\text{Prescribed dose}}{\text{Dose available}} \times \text{Quantity} \begin{array}{c}\text{(unit of}\\\text{measure)}\end{array} = X \begin{array}{c}\text{(unknown}\\\text{quantity to}\\\text{be given)}\end{array}$$

Calculate as follows:

$$\frac{1 \text{ mg}}{4 \text{ mg}} \times 2 \text{ ml} = X \text{ (number of ml)}$$

$$\frac{4}{2} = 0.5$$

Answer: You'll need to give 0.5 ml of morphine sulfate to equal the prescribed dose of 1 mg.

Method 3: Calculating according to proportion size
To determine the correct amount of morphine sulfate to give using this method, use the following formula:

smaller : greater = smaller : greater
milligrams : milligrams = milliliters : milliliters

Critical thinking leads us to believe that 1 mg is less than 4 mg and that you'll need less than 2 ml to give 1 mg of the drug; therefore, 1 mg goes into the smaller part of the first ratio, and X goes into the smaller part of the second ratio. Set up the proportion as follows:

$$1 \text{ mg} : 4 \text{ mg} = X \text{ (ml)} : 2 \text{ ml}$$

$$4X = 2$$

$$X = \frac{2}{4}$$

$$X = 0.5$$

Answer: You'll need to give 0.5 ml of morphine sulfate to equal the prescribed dose of 1 mg.

CALCULATING I.V. FLOW RATES

When an I.V. solution is delivered by gravity, you must calculate the number of drops needed per minute for proper infusion. To calculate I.V. flow rates, you need to know three things:
- the drip factor—or the number of drops contained in 1 ml for the type of I.V. set you'll be using—which is provided on the individual package label
- the amount and type of fluid that you'll infuse, as prescribed on the physician's order sheet
- the infusion duration time in minutes.

Once you've gathered this information, you can calculate the I.V. flow rate using the following equation:

$$\frac{\text{Total number of ml}}{\text{Total number of min}} \times \text{drip factor (gtt/ml)} = \text{flow rate (gtt/min)}$$

Example 1: If the physician prescribes 1,000 ml of D_5W to infuse over 10 hours, and the drip rate for your administration set is 15 drops (gtt)/ml, calculate as follows:

$$\frac{1,000 \text{ ml}}{10 \text{ hr} \times 60 \text{ min}} \times 15 \text{ gtt/ml} = X \text{ gtt/min}$$

$$\frac{1,000 \text{ ml}}{600 \text{ min}} \times 15 \text{ gtt/ml} = X \text{ gtt/min}$$

$$1.67 \text{ ml/min} \times 15 \text{ gtt/ml} = X \text{ gtt/min}$$

$$25.05 \text{ gtt/min} = X$$

Answer: To infuse, round off 25.05 to 25 gtt/min or according to your institution's policy.

CALCULATING I.V. FLOW RATES *(continued)*

Example 2: If the physician prescribes 500 ml of 0.45NS to infuse over 2 hours, and the drip rate for your administration set is 10 gtt/ml, calculate as follows:

$$\frac{500 \text{ ml}}{2 \text{ hr} \times 60 \text{ min}} \times 10 \text{ gtt/ml} = X \text{ gtt/min}$$

$$\frac{500 \text{ ml}}{120 \text{ min}} \times 10 \text{ gtt/ml} = X \text{ gtt/min}$$

$$4.17 \text{ ml/min} \times 10 \text{ gtt/ml} = X \text{ gtt/min}$$

$$41.7 \text{ gtt/min} = X$$

Answer: To infuse, round off 41.7 to 42 gtt/min or according to your institution's policy.

Note: When a controlled infusion device is being used for I.V. administration, the electronic flow-regulator will either count drops using an electronic eye or use a controlled pumping action to deliver the fluid in milliliters. Your final calculation will be based on the unit of measure used by the device: drops per minute, or milliliters per hour.

I.V. ANTINEOPLASTIC DRUGS

Antineoplastic drugs have become the standard of treatment for most types of cancer today. Most of these drugs work by inhibiting cell proliferation, thereby leading to cell death. They're most effective at killing cells that are actively dividing. Cell-specific antineoplastics exert their actions during one or more phases of the cell cycle. S-phase antineoplastics interfere with DNA synthesis; M-phase drugs interfere with the formation of microtubules and disrupt mitosis. Most antineoplastics impair DNA in one of the following four ways:

• preventing separation of DNA strands
• inhibiting DNA repair
• mimicking DNA bases
• disrupting the triplicate codons or producing oxygen free radicals that damage the DNA.

Antineoplastic drugs are cytotoxic, which means that they affect both neoplastic cells and normal cells. As a result, they may cause serious and sometimes life-threatening adverse reactions. Antineoplastics are most harmful to normal cells that exhibit rapid activity and growth, such as bone marrow tissue, the epithelium of the GI mucosa, and hair follicles. When they suppress bone marrow activity, the patient may develop leukopenia, thrombocytopenia, or anemia. When the drugs affect the GI mucosa, the patient may experience nausea, vomiting, anorexia, bowel dysfunction, and mucosal ulcerations. When they affect the hair follicles, the result is hair loss (alopecia), one of the most common adverse reactions; although not life-threatening, hair loss can be emotionally traumatic for patients, especially women.

Drug Classification

Antineoplastics are classified according to their mechanism of action.

Alkylating drugs, the first drugs developed to fight cancer, are most effective against slow-growing tumors. These agents can damage tissue at the injection site and produce systemic toxicity. They can damage cells during all stages of growth, causing mitotic arrest. Because their actions are not limited to neoplastic cells, they also cause myelosuppression, a predictable adverse reaction. They can also result in secondary tumor development, even years after the initial therapy.

I.V. ANTINEOPLASTIC DRUGS *(continued)*

Antibiotic antineoplastics originated from a genus of fungus-like bacteria called *Streptomyces*. Their classification is based on their origin, not on mechanism of action, toxicity, pharmacokinetics, or varying clinical indications. Many of these drugs bind to specific bases and block DNA synthesis, thus interfering with cell replication.

Antimetabolites are cell-cycle-phase–specific drugs that act by preventing synthesis of nucleotides or inhibiting enzymes by mimicking nucleotides. These drugs tend to be more effective when used in combination.

Antimitotic antineoplastics disrupt the formation of microtubule structures within the cell during mitosis. This breakdown of microtubule production stops the formation of the mitotic spindle, inhibiting cellular reproduction.

Biological response modifiers alter tumor-host metabolic and immunologic relationships.

Antineoplastic enzymes interfere with the breakdown of extracellular asparagine, an endogenous enzyme that leukemic cells depend on for their survival. The rapid depletion of asparagine eventually kills leukemic cells by fragmenting them into membrane-bound particles that are eliminated by phagocytosis.

Hormonal antineoplastics act as agonists to inhibit tumor cell growth or as antagonists to compete with endogenous growth-promoting hormones. Steroid hormones form specific receptor complexes that bind to certain nuclear proteins necessary for DNA transcription.

Miscellaneous antineoplastics act in a variety of ways, such as by destroying microtubules that are essential for tumor cell structure before mitosis and by inhibiting topoisomerase, the enzyme that affects the degree of supercoiling in DNA by cutting one or both strands. This inhibition causes DNA strands to break and synthesizes toxic compounds that inhibit DNA strand repair.

You'll find complete entries for some of the most common I.V. antineoplastics in this book. The following chart lists the generic and common trade names of additional I.V. antineoplastics, which are grouped according to mechanism of action. It also includes FDA-approved indications and the usual adult I.V. dosage for each drug.

(continued)

I.V. ANTINEOPLASTIC DRUGS (continued)

Alkylating drugs

Generic and Trade Names	Indications	Usual Adult Dosages
busulfan Busulfex, Myleran	To prepare for hematopoietic progenitor cell transplantation for chronic myelogenous leukemia	0.8 mg/kg I.V. over 2 hr q 6 hr for 4 days for a total of 16 doses as an adjunct with cyclophosphamide
carmustine (BCNU) BiCNU, Gliadel Wafer	To treat primary brain tumors, Hodgkin's disease, non-Hodgkin's lymphoma, and multiple myeloma	150 to 200 mg/m^2 by slow I.V. infusion as a single dose q 6 to 8 wk; or 75 to 100 mg/m^2 by slow I.V. infusion once daily for 2 days every 6 wk
ifosfamide IFEX	To treat germ cell testicular tumors	1.2 g/m^2 daily by I.V. infusion for 5 days q 3 wk
melphalan (L-phenylalanine mustard)	To treat multiple myeloma	16 mg/m^2 I.V. over 15 min q 2 wk for 4 doses; then at 4 wk
melphalan hydrochloride Alkeran		
mechlorethamine hydrochloride (nitrogen mustard) Mustargen	To treat Hodgkin's disease, non-Hodgkin's lymphoma, and mycosis fungoides	0.4 mg/kg I.V. as a single dose or in divided doses over 2 to 4 days
streptozocin Zanosar	To treat islet cell or pancreatic carcinoma	500 mg/m^2 I.V. for 5 days q 6 wk, or 1,000 mg/m^2 I.V. q wk for 2 wk
thiotepa (TESPA, triethylenethiophosphoramide, TSPA) Thioplex	To treat breast cancer, epithelial ovarian cancer, and Hodgkin's disease	0.3 to 0.4 mg/kg I.V. q 1 to 4 wk, or 0.2 mg/kg for 4 to 5 days q 2 to 3 wk

I.V. ANTINEOPLASTIC DRUGS (continued)

Generic and Trade Names	Indications	Usual Adult Dosages
Antibiotic antineoplastics		
bleomycin sulfate Blenoxane	To treat non-Hodgkin's lymphoma, squamous cell carcinoma, and testicular cancer	0.25 to 0.5 unit/kg or 10 to 20 units/m^2 1 or 2 times/ wk I.V., or 0.25 unit/kg or 15 units/m^2 daily by I.V. infusion over 24 hr
	To treat Hodgkin's disease	0.25 to 0.5 unit/kg I.V. or 10 to 20 units/m^2 1 or 2 times/wk
dactinomycin (actinomycin-D) Cosmegen	To treat Ewing's sarcoma, gestational trophoblastic or Wilms' tumor, rhabdomyo-sarcoma, sarcoma botryoides, and testicular cancer or tumors	15 to 500 mcg/kg daily I.V. for 5 days; may repeat after 3 wk
daunorubicin hydrochloride Cerubidine	To treat acute lymphocytic leukemia	45 mg/m^2 I.V. daily for first 3 days of a 32-day course with vincristine, prednisone, and asparagi-nase
	To treat acute nonlymphocytic leukemia	45 mg/m^2 I.V. daily for first 3 days of first course of combination therapy with cytarabine and first 2 days of second course of combination therapy with cytarabine
daunorubicin, liposomal DaunoXome	To treat AIDS-related Kaposi's sarcoma	40 mg/m^2 I.V. over 60 min q 2 wk

(continued)

I.V. ANTINEOPLASTIC DRUGS *(continued)*

Generic and Trade Names	Indications	Usual Adult Dosages
Antibiotic antineoplastics *(continued)*		
epirubicin hydrochloride Ellence	To treat breast cancer	100 to 120 mg/m^2 by I.V. infusion over 3 to 5 min by a free-flowing I.V. solution as a single dose on day 1 or in divided doses on days 1 and 8; repeated q 3 to 4 wk for 6 cycles in combination with other chemotherapeutic drugs
idarubicin hydrochloride Idamycin	To treat acute nonlymphocytic leukemia	12 mg/m^2/day I.V. over 10 to 15 min for 3 days in combination with cytarabine
mitomycin (mitomycin-C) Mutamycin	To treat gastric or pancreatic cancer	20 mg/m^2 I.V. as a single dose q 6 to 8 wk
pentostatin (2'-deoxycoformycin) Nipent	To treat hairy cell leukemia	4 mg/m^2 by rapid I.V. injection or diluted for infusion over 20 to 30 min as a single dose q other wk
plicamycin (mithramycin) Mithracin	To treat testicular cancer	0.025 to 0.03 mg/kg I.V. daily over 4 to 6 hr for 8 to 10 days
	To treat hypercalcemia and hypercalciuria	0.015 to 0.025 mg/kg I.V. daily over 4 to 6 hr for 3 to 4 days; may repeat dose q wk as needed
Antimetabolites		
cladribine (2-CdA, 2-chloro-deoxyadenosine) Leustatin	To treat hairy cell leukemia	0.1 mg/kg/day by continuous I.V. infusion for 7 days

I.V. ANTINEOPLASTIC DRUGS (continued)

Generic and Trade Names	Indications	Usual Adult Dosages
Antimetabolites (continued)		
cytarabine (ARA-C, cytosine arabinoside) Cytosar, Cytosar-U	To treat acute nonlymphocytic leukemia	Initially, 100 mg/m^2/day by continuous I.V. infusion for 7 days, alone or in combination with other drugs; or 100 mg/m^2 I.V. q 12 hr on days 1 to 7, then consult manufacturer's literature for specific dosage; or high-dose therapy of 2 to 3 g/m^2 I.V over 1 to 3 hr for 2 to 6 days, then consult manufacturer's literature for specific dosage.
	To prevent or treat acute lymphocytic leukemia and chronic myelocytic leukemia	Consult manufacturer's literature for specific dosage.
fludarabine phosphate Fludara	To treat chronic lymphocytic leukemia	25 mg/m^2 I.V. infused over 30 min for 5 days; cycle repeated q 28 days
Antimitotic antineoplastics		
docetaxel Taxotere	To treat breast cancer	60 to 100 mg/m^2 by I.V. infusion over 1 hr q 3 wk
	To treat non–small-cell lung carcinoma	75 mg/m^2 by I.V. infusion over 1 hr q 3 wk
vinorelbine tartrate Navelbine	To treat non–small-cell lung carcinoma	30 mg/m^2 I.V. over 6 to 10 min q wk; or, 25 mg/m^2 I.V. over 6 to 10 min q wk when combined with cisplatin 100 mg/m^2 q 4 wk

(continued)

I.V. ANTINEOPLASTIC DRUGS *(continued)*

Generic and Trade Names	Indications	Usual Adult Dosages
Antineoplastic enzymes		
asparaginase Colaspase, Elspar, Kidrolase (CAN)	To treat acute lymphocytic leukemia	200 international units/kg I.V. daily for 28 days
pegaspargase (PEG-L-asparaginase) Oncaspar	To treat acute lymphoblastic leukemia in adults up to age 21	2,500 international units/m^2 I.V. q 14 days
Biological response modifiers		
aldesleukin (IL-2, interleukin-2) Proleukin	To treat renal cancer and metastatic melanoma	600,000 international units/kg by I.V. infusion over 15 min q 8 hr for 14 doses, followed by 9 days of no drug; then course of 14 doses repeated for total of 28 doses
alemtuzumab Campath	To treat B-cell chronic lymphocytic leukemia	Initially, 3 mg I.V. over 2 hr daily; then 10 mg I.V. over 2 hr daily. For maintenance, 30 mg I.V. over 2 hr three times/wk q other day for up to 12 wk.
denileukin diftitox Ontak	To treat cutaneous or T-cell lymphomas, including mycosis fungoides	9 or 18 mcg/kg/day by I.V. infusion over at least 15 min for 5 days; repeated q 21 days
Miscellaneous antineoplastics		
arsenic trioxide Trisenox	To treat acute promyelocytic leukemia	Induction: 0.15 mg/kg I.V. daily until bone marrow remission. Maximum, 60 doses. Consolidation: Starting 3 to 6 wk after induction is complete, 0.15 mg/kg I.V. daily for 25 doses over up to 5 wk

I.V. ANTINEOPLASTIC DRUGS (continued)

Generic and Trade Names	Indications	Usual Adult Dosages
Miscellaneous antineoplastics (continued)		
dacarbazine DTIC (CAN), DTIC-Dome	To treat Hodgkin's disease	150 mg/m^2 I.V. daily for 5 days with other drugs, possibly repeated q 28 days; or 375 mg/m^2 q 15 days with other drugs
	To treat malignant melanoma	2 to 4.5 mg/kg I.V. daily for 10 days and q 28 days thereafter; or, 250 mg/m^2 I.V. daily for 5 days and q 21 days thereafter
gemcitabine hydrochloride Gemzar	To treat non–small-cell lung carcinoma	1,000 mg/m^2 by I.V. infusion over 30 min on days 1, 8, and 15 every 28 days with cisplatin 100 mg/m^2 on day 28; or 1,250 mg/m^2 I.V. on days 1 and 8 every 21 days with cisplatin 100 mg/m^2 I.V. on day 21
	To treat pancreatic cancer	1,000 mg/m^2 by I.V. infusion over 30 min q wk for 7 wk, followed by 1 wk of no drug; then q wk for 3 wk, followed by 1 wk of no drug; then 4-wk cycle repeated
gemtuzumab ozogamicin Mylotarg	To treat first relapse in patients with CD33-positive acute myeloid leukemia who are age 60 or over and who are not candidates for cytotoxic therapy	9 mg/m^2 by I.V. infusion over 2 hr; repeated in 24 days

(continued)

I.V. ANTINEOPLASTIC DRUGS (continued)

Generic and Trade Names	Indications	Usual Adult Dosages
Miscellaneous antineoplastics (continued)		
mitoxantrone hydrochloride Novantrone	To treat hormone-refractory prostate cancer	12 to 14 mg/m^2 I.V. q 21 days
	To treat acute nonlymphocytic leukemia	12 mg/m^2 by I.V. infusion through free-flowing norml saline solution or D$_5$W over 3 min daily on days 1 and 3 in with cytarabine 100 mg/m^2 daily by continuous I.V. infusion on days 1 to 7; if response is inadequate, second course of same dosage may be given
porfimer sodium Photofrin	To treat esophageal cancer and non–small-cell lung carcinoma	2 mg/kg I.V. over 3 to 5 min, followed by laser light illumination and debridement of tumor; course may be repeated q 30 days three times
topotecan hydrochloride Hycamtin	To treat ovarian cancer and small-cell lung carcinoma	1.5 mg/m^2 I.V. over 30 min daily for 5 days; repeated every 21 days
trastuzumab Herceptin	To treat breast cancer	4 mg/kg I.V. over 90 min, followed by 2 mg/kg I.V. over 30 min q 7 days

ANTINEOPLASTIC DRUGS (continued)

Generic and Trade Names	Indications	Usual Adult Dosages
Miscellaneous antineoplastics (continued)		
velcade Bortezomib	To treat multiple myeloma	1.3 mg/m^2 by I.V. bolus on days 1, 4, 8, and 11 for 2 wk, followed by rest on days 12 through 21. Then repeat 3-wk cycle

BODY MASS INDEX CALCULATION

Body mass index (BMI) is a formula used to determine obesity; it's calculated by dividing a person's weight in kilograms by his height in meters squared (kg/m^2). A BMI of 25 or higher increases your patient's risk of developing hypertension, cardiovascular disease, type 2 diabetes mellitus, and stroke. It also increases the risk that he won't respond effectively to the usual drug dosages. If your patient has an abnormal BMI, be prepared to make dosage adjustments that are individualized based on body weight, as prescribed.

WEIGHT (POUNDS)

HEIGHT (INCHES)																		
58	91	96	100	105	110	115	119	124	129	134	138	143	148	153	158	162	167	172
59	94	99	104	109	114	119	124	128	133	138	143	148	153	158	163	168	173	178
60	97	102	107	112	118	123	128	133	138	143	148	153	158	163	168	174	179	184
61	100	106	111	116	122	127	132	137	143	148	153	158	164	169	174	180	185	190
62	104	109	115	120	126	131	136	142	147	153	158	164	169	175	180	186	191	196
63	107	113	118	124	130	135	141	146	152	158	163	169	175	180	186	191	197	203
64	110	116	122	128	134	140	145	151	157	163	169	174	180	186	192	197	204	209
65	114	120	126	132	138	144	150	156	162	168	174	180	186	192	198	204	210	216
66	118	124	130	136	142	148	155	161	167	173	179	186	192	198	204	210	216	223
67	121	127	134	140	146	153	159	166	172	178	185	191	198	204	211	217	223	230
68	125	131	138	144	151	158	164	171	177	184	190	197	203	210	216	223	230	236
69	128	135	142	149	155	162	169	176	182	189	196	203	209	216	223	230	236	243
70	132	139	146	153	160	167	174	181	188	195	202	209	216	222	229	236	243	250
71	136	143	150	157	165	172	179	186	193	200	208	215	222	229	236	243	250	257
72	140	147	154	162	169	177	184	191	199	206	213	221	228	235	242	250	258	265
73	144	151	159	166	174	182	189	197	204	212	219	227	235	242	250	257	265	272
74	148	155	163	171	179	186	194	202	210	218	225	233	241	249	256	264	272	280
75	152	160	168	176	184	192	200	208	216	224	232	240	248	256	264	272	279	287
76	156	164	172	180	189	197	205	213	221	230	238	246	254	263	271	279	287	295
	19	20	21	22	23	24	25	26	27	28	29	30	31	32	33	34	35	36

BODY MASS INDEX

The table below will help you find your patient's BMI easily. It converts pounds to kilograms and inches to meters, and then it shows the BMI. To use it, simply find the patient's height on either side of the table; then move across the row to the weight that most closely matches your patient's. At the bottom of the column containing the weight, you'll find the BMI for that patient. For example, the BMI for a patient who is 70" tall and weighs 208 lb is 30.

WEIGHT (POUNDS)

																		HEIGHT (INCHES)
177	181	186	191	196	201	205	210	215	220	224	229	234	239	244	248	253	258	**58**
183	188	193	198	203	208	212	217	222	227	232	237	242	247	252	257	262	267	**59**
189	194	199	204	209	215	220	225	230	235	240	245	250	255	261	266	271	276	**60**
195	201	206	211	217	222	227	232	238	243	248	254	259	264	269	275	280	285	**61**
202	207	213	218	224	229	235	240	246	251	256	262	267	273	278	284	289	295	**62**
208	214	220	225	231	237	242	248	254	259	265	270	278	282	287	293	299	304	**63**
215	221	227	232	238	244	250	256	262	267	273	279	285	291	296	302	308	314	**64**
222	228	234	240	246	252	258	264	270	276	282	288	294	300	306	312	318	324	**65**
229	235	241	247	253	260	266	272	278	284	291	297	303	309	315	322	328	334	**66**
236	242	249	255	261	268	274	280	287	293	299	306	312	319	325	331	338	344	**67**
243	249	256	262	269	276	282	289	295	302	308	315	322	328	335	341	348	354	**68**
250	257	263	270	277	284	291	297	304	311	318	324	331	338	345	351	358	365	**69**
257	264	271	278	285	292	299	306	313	320	327	334	341	348	355	362	369	376	**70**
265	272	279	286	293	301	308	315	322	329	338	343	351	358	365	372	379	386	**71**
272	279	287	294	302	309	316	324	331	338	346	353	361	368	375	383	390	397	**72**
280	288	295	302	310	318	325	333	340	348	355	363	371	378	386	393	401	408	**73**
287	295	303	311	319	326	334	342	350	358	365	373	381	389	396	404	412	420	**74**
295	303	311	319	327	335	343	351	359	367	375	383	391	399	407	415	423	431	**75**
304	312	320	328	336	344	353	361	369	377	385	394	402	410	418	426	435	443	**76**
37	**38**	**39**	**40**	**41**	**42**	**43**	**44**	**45**	**46**	**47**	**48**	**49**	**50**	**51**	**52**	**53**	**54**	

BODY MASS INDEX

ABBREVIATIONS

The following abbreviations, which are common to nursing practice, are used throughout the book.

ABG	arterial blood gas
a.c.	before meals
ACE	angiotensin-converting enzyme
ADH	antidiuretic hormone
AIDS	acquired immunodeficiency syndrome
ALT	alanine aminotransferase
ANA	antinuclear antibodies
APTT	activated partial thromboplastin time
AST	aspartate aminotransferase
ATP	adenosine triphosphate
AV	atrioventricular
b.i.d.	twice a day
BUN	blood urea nitrogen
°C	degrees Celsius
cAMP	cyclic adenosine monophosphate
(CAN)	Canadian drug trade name
cap	capsule
CBC	complete blood count
cGMP	cyclic guanosine monophosphate
CK	creatine kinase
Cl	chloride
cm	centimeter
CMV	cytomegalovirus
CNS	central nervous system
COPD	chronic obstructive pulmonary disease
C.R.	controlled-release
CSF	cerebrospinal fluid
CV	cardiovascular
CVA	cerebrovascular accident
D_5W	dextrose 5% in water
$D_{10}W$	dextrose 10% in water
$D_{50}W$	dextrose 50% in water
dl	deciliter
DNA	deoxyribonucleic acid
DS	double-strength
EC	enteric-coated
ECG	electrocardiogram
EEG	electroencephalogram
EENT	eyes, ears, nose, and throat
ENDO	endocrine

ABBREVIATIONS (continued)

E.R.	extended-release
°F	degrees Fahrenheit
FDA	Food and Drug Administration
g	gram
GFR	glomerular filtration rate
GI	gastrointestinal
GU	genitourinary
H_1	histamine$_1$
H_2	histamine$_2$
HDL	high-density lipoprotein
HEME	hematologic
HIV	human immunodeficiency virus
HPV	human papilloma virus
hr	hour
h.s.	at bedtime
HSV	herpes simplex virus
HZV	herpes zoster virus
ICP	intracranial pressure
I.D.	intradermal
IgA	immunoglobulin A
IgE	immunoglobulin E
I.M.	intramuscular
INR	international normalized ratio
I.V.	intravenous
IVPB	intravenous piggyback
kg	kilogram
KIU	kallikrein inactivator unit
L	liter
LA	long-acting
LD	lactate dehydrogenase
LDL	low-density lipoprotein
LOC	level of consciousness
LR	lactated Ringer's solution
M	molar
m^2	square meter
MAO	monoamine oxidase
mcg	microgram
mEq	milliequivalent
mg	milligram
MI	myocardial infarction
min	minute
ml	milliliter
mm	millimeter

(continued)

ABBREVIATIONS *(continued)*

mm^3	cubic millimeter
mmol	millimole
mo	month
MS	musculoskeletal
Na	sodium
NaCl	sodium chloride
NG	nasogastric
NPH	human isophane insulin
NPO	nothing by mouth
NSAID	nonsteroidal anti-inflammatory drug
OTC	over the counter
p.c.	after meals
PCA	patient-controlled analgesia
P.O.	by mouth
P.R.	by rectum
p.r.n.	as needed
PSVT	paroxysmal supraventricular tachycardia
PT	prothrombin time
PTCA	percutaneous transluminal coronary angioplasty
PVC	premature ventricular contraction
q	every
q.i.d.	four times a day
RBC	red blood cell
REM	rapid eye movement
RESP	respiratory
RNA	ribonucleic acid
RSV	respiratory syncytial virus
SA	sinoatrial
sec	second
S.L.	sublingual
S.R.	sustained-release
stat	immediately
SubQ	subcutaneous
supp	suppository
tab	tablet
T_3	triiodothyronine
T_4	thyroxine
t.i.d.	three times a day
USP	United States Pharmacopeia
UTI	urinary tract infection
VLDL	very low-density lipoprotein
WBC	white blood cell
wk	week

INDEX

- **Generic and alternate names:** lowercase initial letter
- **Trade names:** uppercase initial letter
- **Illustrations:** *i* after page number
- **Tables:** *t* after page number

A

abatacept, 1–3
Abbokinase, 739
Abbokinase Open-Cath, 739
Abbreviations, 796–798
abciximab, 3–6
Abelcet, 47
Acetazolam, 6
acetazolamide, 6–9
acetazolamide sodium, 6–9
acetylcysteine, 9–11
Acova, 68
actinomycin-D, 787*t*
Activase, 28
Activase rt-PA, 28
acyclovir sodium, 11–15
Adenocard, 15
Adenoscan, 15
adenosine, 15–17
Adrenalin, 293
adrenaline, 293–296
Adriamycin PFS, 269
Adriamycin RDF, 269
Adrucil, 342
Advate, 62
Adverse reaction, xx
Aerosporin, 641
Aggrastat, 719
Agonists, xix
A-hydroCort, 384
Akineton Lactate, 97
Ak-Zol, 6
alatrofloxacin mesylate, 17–19
aldesleukin, 790*t*
Aldomet, 499
alefacept, 20–22
alemtuzumab, 790*t*

alglucerase, 22–23
Alkeran, 786*t*
Alkylating drugs, 784, 786*t*
Allergic reaction, xx
allopurinol sodium, 23–26
Aloprim, 23
Aloxi, 595
alpha-difluoromethylornithine, 285–286
alpha$_1$–proteinase inhibitor (human), 26–28
Alphanate, 62
alteplase, recombinant, 28–31
Alti-Minocycline, 524
Alti-Valproic, 741
AmBisome, 47
A-methaPred, 502
Amevive, 20
Amicar, 34
amikacin sulfate, 31–34
Amikin, 31
aminocaproic acid, 34–35
aminophylline, 35–38
amiodarone hydrochloride, 38–42
ammonium chloride, 42–43
amobarbital sodium, 43–47
Amphocin, 47
Amphotec, 47
amphotericin B, 47–51
amphotericin B cholesteryl sulfate complex, 47–51
amphotericin B lipid complex, 47–51
amphotericin B liposomal complex, 47–51
ampicillin sodium, 51–55
ampicillin sodium and sulbactam sodium, 55–58

Ampicin, 51
amrinone lactate, 406–408
Amytal, 43
Ana-Guard, 293
Anaphylactic reaction, xx–xxi
Ancef, 124
Anergan 25, 658
Anergan 50, 658
Anexate, 340
Angiomax, 98
anidulafungin, 58–59
Aniflex, 583
anisoylated plasminogen-
    streptokinase activator complex,
    59–62
anistreplase, 59–62
Antagonists, xix–xx
Antibiotic antineoplastics, 785,
    787–788t
antihemophilic factor (human),
    62–66
antihemophilic factor
    (recombinant), plasma/albumin-
    free method (rAHF-PFM), 62–66
antihemophilic factor–von
    Willebrand factor complex
    (human, dried, pasteurized),
    62–66
Antilirium, 633
Antimetabolites, 785, 788–789t
Antimitotic antineoplastics, 785,
    789t
Antinaus 50, 658
Antineoplastic drugs, 784–793
Antineoplastic enzymes, 785,
    790t
antithrombin III, human, 66–68
Anzemet, 259
Apo-Acetazolamide, 6
Apo-Atenol, 71
Apo-Benztropine, 90
Apo-Metoprolol, 509
Apo-Minocycline, 524
Apo-Perphenazine, 615
Apresoline, 382
ARA-C, 789t
Aramine, 487
Aranesp, 215
Aredia, 597

argatroban, 68–70
arsenic trioxide, 790t
asparaginase, 790t
Astramorph PF, 531
AT-III, 66–68
atenolol, 71–73
Ativan, 470
ATnativ, 66
atracurium besylate, 73–75
Atropen, 75
atropine, 75–78
atropine sulfate, 75–78
Avelox, 535
Avelox IV, 535
Azactam, 83
azathioprine, 78–80
azathioprine sodium, 78–80
azithromycin, 80–83
aztreonam, 83–86

B

Bactocill, 585
Bactrim, 199
Banflex, 583
basiliximab, 87–89
BCNU, 786t
Beesix, 671
Benadryl, 253
benzquinamide hydrochloride,
    89–90
benztropine mesylate, 90–93
Betaloc, 509
betamethasone sodium phosphate,
    93–96
Betaxin, 708
Betnesol, 93
Biamine, 708
BiCNU, 786t
Biological response modifiers, 785,
    790t
biperiden lactate, 97–98
bivalirudin, 98–101
Blenoxane, 101, 787t
bleomycin sulfate, 101–104, 787t
Blood products, administering, xxix
Blood types, xxxi
Body mass index calculation,
    794–795t

Boniva, 393
Bortezomib, 793*t*
Bretylate, 105
bretylium tosylate, 105–107, 106*i*
Bretylol, 105
Brevibloc, 313
bumetanide, 107–109
Bumex, 107
Buprenex, 109
buprenorphine hydrochloride,
    109–111
busulfan, 786*t*
Busulfex, 786*t*
butorphanol tartrate, 111–114

C

Caelyx, 274
Calciject, 116
Calcijex, 115
Calcilean, 378
Calciparine, 378
calcitriol, 115–116
calcium chloride, 116–120
calcium gluceptate, 116–120
calcium gluconate, 116–120
Calcium Stanley, 116
Calculating I.V. flow rates, 782–783
Calculating parenteral drug dosages,
    780–781
Calculating the strength of a
    solution, 778–779
Campath, 790*t*
Camptosar, 422
Cancidas, 122
Capastat, 120
capreomycin sulfate, 120–122
Carbacot, 492
carbamide, 737–739
Cardene, 564
Cardene I.V., 564
Cardene SR, 564
Cardizem, 248
carmustine, 786*t*
caspofungin acetate, 122–124, 123*i*
2–CdA, 788*t*
Cefadyl, 157
cefazolin sodium, 124–127

cefepime hydrochloride,
    127–130
Cefizox, 148
cefmetazole sodium, 130–133
Cefobid, 136
cefonicid sodium, 133–136
cefoperazone sodium, 136–139
cefotaxime sodium, 139–142
cefoxitin sodium, 142–144
ceftazidime, 145–148
ceftizoxime sodium, 148–151
ceftriaxone sodium, 151–154
cefuroxime sodium, 154–157
Celestone Phosphate, 93
CellCept Intravenous, 539
cephapirin sodium, 157–160
Ceptaz, 145
Cerebyx, 355
Ceredase, 22
Cerubidine, 787*t*
chloramphenicol sodium succinate,
    160–162
chlordiazepoxide hydrochloride,
    163–165
2–chlorodeoxyadenosine, 788*t*
Chloromag, 473
Chloromycetin, 160
chlorothiazide, 165–167, 166*i*
chlorothiazide sodium, 165–167,
    166*i*
chlorpromazine hydrochloride,
    168–171
cidofovir, 171–174
Cidomycin, 368
cimetidine hydrochloride, 174–176
ciprofloxacin, 176–181
Cipro I.V., 176
cisplatin, 181–185
cladribine, 788*t*
Claforan, 139
Cleocin, 185
clindamycin phosphate, 185–187
coagulation factor VIIa
    (recombinant), 187–189
codeine, 777*t*
codeine phosphate, 189–192
Cogentin, 90
Colaspase, 790*t*
colchicine, 192–194, 193*i*

colistimethate sodium, 195–197
Coly-Mycin M, 195
Compazine, 653
conivaptan hydrochloride, 197–199
Controlled substance schedules, viii
Cordarone, 38
Corlopam, 331
Cortastat, 223
Corvert, 395
Cosmegen, 787*t*
co-trimoxazole, 199–202
Coumadin, 763
Cubicin, 213
Culture, drug dosage and, xxi
cyclophosphamide, 202–206
cyclosporin A, 206–208
cyclosporine, 206–208
cytarabine, 789*t*
Cytosar, 789*t*
Cytosar-U, 789*t*
cytosine arabinoside, 789*t*
Cytovene, 365
Cytovene-IV, 365
Cytoxan, 202

D

dacarbazine, 791*t*
dacliximab, 209–210
daclizumab, 209–210
Dacogen, 219
dactinomycin, 787*t*
Dalacin C Phosphate, 185
Dalalone, 223
Dalgan, 232
Dantrium, 210
Dantrium Intravenous, 210
dantrolene sodium, 210–212
daptomycin, 213–215
darbepoetin alfa, 215–219
daunorubicin, liposomal, 787*t*
daunorubicin hydrochloride, 787*t*
DaunoXome, 787*t*
Dazamide, 6
DDAVP Injection, 221
Decadrol, 223
Decaject, 223
decitabine, 219–221
Demadex, 724

Demerol, 478
denileukin diftitox, 790*t*
2′-deoxycoformycin, 788*t*
Depacon, 741
Depakene, 741
Depakote, 741
Deponit, 567
Deproic, 741
Desired effect, xx
desmopressin acetate, 221–223
Dexacorten, 223
dexamethasone sodium phosphate,
    223–228
Dexasone, 223
DexFerrum, 426
DexIron, 426
Dexone, 223
dexrazoxane, 228–230
dextrose, 230–232
2.5% Dextrose Injection, 230
5% Dextrose Injection, 230
10% Dextrose Injection, 230
20% Dextrose Injection, 230
25% Dextrose Injection, 230
50% Dextrose Injection, 230
60% Dextrose Injection, 230
70% Dextrose Injection, 230
dezocine, 232–235
DFMO, 285–286
D-glucose, 230–232
D.H.E. 45, 246
Diamox, 6
Diamox Sequels, 6
Diazemuls, 235
diazepam, 235–238
diazoxide, 238–240
Didronel, 324
Diflucan, 338
Digibind, 244
digoxin, 241–243
digoxin immune Fab (ovine),
    244–246
dihydroergotamine mesylate,
    246–248
Dihydroergotamine-Sandoz, 246
dihydromorphinone, 387–390
1,25–dihydroxycholecalciferol,
    115–116
Dilantin, 627

Dilaudid, 387
Dilaudid-HP, 387
diltiazem hydrochloride, 248–251, 249*i*
dimenhydrinate, 251–253
Dinate, 251
diphenhydramine hydrochloride, 253–255
Diprivan, 661
dipyridamole, 255–257
disoprofol, 661–663
Diuril, 165
divalproex sodium, 741–744
Dizac, 235
dobutamine hydrochloride, 257–259
Dobutrex, 257
docetaxel, 789*t*
dolasetron mesylate, 259–261
Dom-Proic, 741
dopamine hydrochloride, 261–265
Dopram, 267
Doribax, 265
doripenem, 265–267
doxapram hydrochloride, 267–268
Doxil, 274
Doxine, 671
doxorubicin hydrochloride, 269–274
doxorubicin hydrochloride liposome, 274–278
doxycycline hyclate, 278–281
Dramanate, 251
droperidol, 282–284
Drug absorption, xvi–xvii
Drug administration principles, xxiii–xxxi
Drug classification, xv
Drug distribution, xvii–xviii
Drug excretion, xviii
Drug interaction, xxi
Drug metabolism, xviii
Drug nomenclature, xv
DTIC, 791*t*
DTIC-Dome, 791*t*
Duramorph, 531
Dynacin, 524

E

Edecrin, 321

eflornithine hydrochloride, 285–286
Elderly patients, special considerations and, xxii
Ellence, 788*t*
Elspar, 790*t*
Emend for Injection, 348
Emete-Con, 89
Eminase, 59
enalaprilat, 287–290
enoxaparin sodium, 290–293
Epimorph, 5131
epinephrine, 293–296
epinephrine hydrochloride, 293–296
epirubicin hydrochloride, 788*t*
Epival, 741
EPO, 296–299
epoetin alfa, 296–299
Epogen, 296
epoprostenol sodium, 300–303
Eprex, 296
eptifibatide, 303–305
Equianalgesic doses for opioid agonists, 777
Eraxis, 58
ertapenem sodium, 305–308
Erythrocin, 308
erythromycin gluceptate, 308–313
erythromycin lactobionate, 308–313
erythropoietin alfa, 296–299
erythropoietin, recombinant, 296–299
esmolol hydrochloride, 313–316
esomeprazole magnesium, 316–318
estrogens (conjugated), 318–321
ethacrynate sodium, 321–324
Ethnicity, drug dosage and, xxi
etidronate disodium, 324–325
Etopophos, 325
etoposide, 325–329
etoposide phosphate, 325–329

F

famotidine, 329–331, 330*i*
fenoldopam mesylate, 331–333
fentanyl citrate, 333–336
Ferrlecit, 696
filgrastim, 336–338
Flagyl, 511

Flagyl I.V., 511
Flagyl I.V. RTU, 511
Flexoject, 583
Flolan, 300
Floxin, 577
fluconazole, 338–340
Fludara, 789*t*
fludarabine phosphate, 789*t*
flumazenil, 340–342
fluorouracil, 342–346
Folex, 494
Folex PFS, 494
folic acid, 347–348
Folvite, 347
Fortaz, 145
fosaprepitant dimeglumine, 348–351
foscarnet sodium, 351–355
Foscavir, 351
fosphenytoin sodium, 355–360
5-FU, 342–346
Fungizone Intravenous, 47
furosemide, 360–364

G

Gamimune N 5% S/D, 400
Gamimune N 10% S/D, 400
Gammagard Liquid, 400
Gammagard S/D, 400
Gammagard S/D 0.5 g, 400
Gammar-P IV, 400
Gamunex 10%, 400
ganciclovir sodium, 365–368
Garamycin, 368
gemcitabine hydrochloride, 791*t*
gemtuzumab ozogamicin, 791*t*
Gemzar, 791*t*
Gen-Minocycline, 524
gentamicin sulfate, 368–371
Gliadel Wafer, 786*t*
glucagon, 371–373
Glucagon Diagnostic Kit, 371
Glucagon Emergency Kit, 371
glyceryl trinitrate, 567–570, 568*i*
glycopyrrolate, 373–376
G-Mycin, 368
granisetron hydrochloride, 376–378

granulocyte colony-stimulating factor, 336–338
Gravol, 251

H

Hepalean, 378
heparin calcium, 378–382
heparin co-factor I, 66–68
Heparin Leo, 378
Heparin Lock Flush, 378
heparin sodium, 378–382
Herceptin, 726, 792*t*
Hexadrol Phosphate, 223
Histanil, 658
Hormonal antineoplastics, 785
Humate-P, 62
Humulin R, 415
Hycamtin, 792*t*
hydralazine hydrochloride, 382–384
Hydrate, 251
hydrocodone, 777*t*
hydrocortisone sodium phosphate, 384–387
hydrocortisone sodium succinate, 384–387
Hydrocortone Phosphate, 384
hydromorphone, 777*t*
hydromorphone hydrochloride, 387–390
hyoscyamine sulfate, 390–392
Hyperstat, 238
Hyrexin, 253

I

ibandronate sodium, 393–395
ibutilide fumarate, 395–397
Idamycin, 788*t*
idarubicin hydrochloride, 788*t*
Idiosyncratic response, xx
IFEX, 786*t*
ifosfamide, 786*t*
IGIV, 400–406
Ilotycin, 308
IL-2, 790*t*
imipenem and cilastatin sodium, 397–400

immune globulin intravenous
(human), 400–406
immune serum globulin, 400–406
Imuran, 78
inamrinone lactate, 406–408
Inapsine, 282
Inderal, 664
Indocid PDA, 408
Indocin I.V., 408
indomethacin sodium trihydrate,
408–412
InFeD, 426
infliximab, 412–415
Infusion devices, xxvii–xxviii
Inocor, 406
insulin human injection, buffered
regular, 415–418
insulin human injection, regular,
415–418
insulin injection, regular, 415–418
Integrilin, 303
interferon alfa-2b, recombinant,
418–421
interleukin-2, 790*t*
Intron A, 418
Intropin, 261
Invanz, 305
irinotecan hydrochloride, 422–425
iron dextran, 426–428
iron sucrose, 428–431
ISG, 400–406
isoproterenol hydrochloride,
431–434
Isoptin, 747
Isuprel, 431
I.V. drug administration, principles
of, xxiii–xxxi
Iveegam EN, 400
I.V. flow rates, calculating, 782–783
IVIG, 400–406
I.V. therapy, complications of, xxviii
I.V. therapy, nursing process and,
xxxii–xxxvi
I.V. therapy, teaching patient about,
x–xi

J

Jenamicin, 368

K

Kabikinase, 700
kanamycin sulfate, 435–436
Kantrex, 435
Keppra, 448
ketorolac tromethamine, 437–441
Kidrolase, 790*t*
Kytril, 376

L

labetalol hydrochloride, 441–443
Lanoxin Injection, 241
Lanoxin Injection Pediatric, 241
lansoprazole, 443–445
Largactil, 168
Lasix, 360
Lasix Special, 360
lepirudin, 445–447
Leustatin, 788*t*
Levaquin, 449
levarterenol bitartrate, 573–575
levetiracetam, 448–449
Levo-Dromoran, 454
levofloxacin, 449–453
Levophed, 573
levorphanol, 777*t*
levorphanol tartrate, 454–457
Levothroid, 457
levothyroxine sodium, 457–459
Levsin, 390
Librium, 163
lidocaine hydrochloride, 460–462
lignocaine hydrochloride, 460–462
Lincocin, 462
lincomycin hydrochloride, 462–464
linezolid, 464–467, 465*i*
liothyronine sodium, 467–470
Liquaemin, 378
Lopresor, 509
Lopressor, 509
lorazepam, 470–472
Lovenox, 290
L-phenylalanine mustard, 786*t*
L-thyroxine sodium, 457–459
L-triiodothyronine, 467–470
Luminal, 618

M

magnesium chloride, 473–475
magnesium sulfate, 473–475
mannitol, 476–478
Maxipime, 127
mechlorethamine hydrochloride, 786*t*
Med-Valproic, 741
Mefoxin, 142
Megacillin, 605
melphalan, 786*t*
melphalan hydrochloride, 786*t*
meperidine, 777*t*
meperidine hydrochloride, 478–481
mephentermine sulfate, 481–484
meropenem, 484–486
Merrem I.V., 484
Mestinon, 669
Mestinon-SR, 669
Mestinon Timespans, 669
metaraminol bitartrate, 487–490
methicillin sodium, 490–492
methocarbamol, 492–494
methotrexate (amethopterin), 494–497
methotrexate sodium, 494–497
methoxy polyethylene glycol-epoetin beta, 497–499
methyldopate hydrochloride, 499–502
methylprednisolone sodium succinate, 502–506
metoclopramide hydrochloride, 506–508
metoprolol succinate, 509–511
metoprolol tartrate, 509–511
Metro I.V., 511
metronidazole, 511–513
metronidazole hydrochloride, 511–513
Mexate, 494
Mexate-AQ, 494
Mezlin, 514
mezlocillin sodium, 514–517
micafungin sodium, 517–519
midazolam hydrochloride, 519–522
Migranal, 246
milrinone lactate, 522–524, 523*i*

Minitran, 567
Minocin, 524
minocycline, 524–527
minocycline hydrochloride, 524–527
Miolin, 583
Mio-Rel, 583
Mircera, 497
Mithracin, 788*t*
mithramycin, 788*t*
mitomycin, 788*t*
mitomycin-C, 788*t*
mitoxantrone hydrochloride, 527–531, 792*t*
Monocid, 133
morphine, 777*t*
Morphine Extra-Forte, 531
Morphine Forte, 531
Morphine H.P., 531
morphine sulfate, 531–535
moxifloxacin hydrochloride, 535–539
Mucomyst, 9
Mucosil, 9
Mustargen, 786*t*
Mutamycin, 788*t*
Mycamine, 517
mycophentolate mofetil hydrochloride, 539–542
Myleran, 786*t*
Mylotarg, 791*t*
Myotrol, 583

N

Nafcil, 543
nafcillin sodium, 543–545
nalbuphine hydrochloride, 545–547
Nallpen, 543
nalmefene hydrochloride, 547–549
naloxone hydrochloride, 549–552
Naming drugs, xv–xvi
Narcan, 549
natalizumab, 552–554
Natrecor, 556
Navelbine, 789*t*
Needlestick, preventing, xxix
Nembutal, 611
Neoral, 206

Neosar, 202
neostigmine methylsulfate, 555–556
Neo-Synephrine, 625
nesiritide, 556–559
Nestrex, 671
netilmicin sulfate, 559–561
Netromycin, 559
Neupogen, 336
Nexium I.V., 316
niacin, 561–564
niacinamide, 561–564
nicardipine hydrochloride, 564–567
nicotinic acid, 561–564
Nipent, 788*t*
Nipride, 570
Nitro-Bid, 567
Nitrocot, 567
Nitro-Dur, 567
Nitrogard, 567
nitrogen mustard, 786*t*
nitroglycerin, 567–570, 568*i*
Nitroglyn E-R, 567
Nitroject, 567
Nitrol, 567
Nitrolingual, 567
Nitrong SR, 567
Nitropar, 567
Nitropress, 570
nitroprusside sodium, 570–573
Nitrostat, 567
Nitro-time, 567
norepinephrine bitartrate, 573–575
Norflex, 583
Normodyne, 441
Novantrone, 527, 792*t*
Novo-Atenol, 71
Novo-Cimetine, 174
Novolin ge Toronto, 415
Novolin R, 415
Novometoprol, 509
Novo-Minocycline, 524
NovoSeven, 187
NovoSeven RT, 187
Novo-Valproic, 741
Nubain, 545
Numorphan, 587
Nursing process, I.V. drug therapy
    and, xxxii–xxxvi
Nu-Valproic, 741

O

Octagam 5%, 400
Octostim, 221
octreotide acetate, 575–577
ofloxacin, 577–581, 579*i*
Omnipen-N, 51
Oncaspar, 790*t*
Oncovin, 754
ondansetron hydrochloride,
    581–583
Ontak, 790*t*
Opioid agonists, equianalgesic doses
    for, 777*t*
Orencia, 1
Orfro, 583
Ornidyl, 285
orphenadrine citrate, 583–585
Orphenate, 583
Osmitrol, 476
oxacillin sodium, 585–587
oxycodone, 777*t*
oxymorphone hydrochloride,
    587–590

P

Pacerone, 38
paclitaxel, 591–595
palosetron hydrochloride, 595–597,
    596*i*
2-PAM chloride, 649–651
pamidronate disodium, 597–599
Pantoloc, 600
pantoprazole sodium, 600–602
Parenteral drug dosages, calculating,
    780–781
Parenteral fluids, administering,
    xxix
paricalcitol, 602–605
Patient-controlled analgesia,
    xxviii
Pediatric patients, special
    considerations and, xxii
pegaspargase, 790*t*
PEG-L-asparaginase, 790*t*
penicillin G potassium, 605–607
penicillin G sodium, 605–607
Pentacarinat, 607

Pentam 300, 607
pentamidine isethionate, 607–609
Pentazine, 658
pentazocine lactate, 609–611
Pentids, 605
pentobarbital sodium, 611–614
pentostatin, 788*t*
Pepcid, 329
perphenazine, 615–618
Persantine, 255
pethidine hydrochloride, 478–481
Pfizerpen, 605
PGI$_2$, 300–303
PGX, 300–303
Pharmacodynamics, xviii–xx
Pharmacokinetics, xvi–xviii
Pharmacotherapeutics, xx–xxi
Phenazine 25, 658
Phenazine 50, 658
Phencen-50, 658
Phenergan, 658
Phenerzine, 658
phenobarbital sodium, 618–623
Phenoject-50, 658
phentolamine mesylate, 623–624
L-phenylalanine mustard, 786*t*
phenylephrine hydrochloride, 625–627
phenytoin sodium, 627–633
Photofrin, 792*t*
physostigmine salicylate, 633–635
piperacillin sodium, 635–638
piperacillin sodium and tazobactam sodium, 638–641
Pipracil, 635
Platinol, 181
Platinol-AQ, 181
plicamycin, 788*t*
PMS Benztropine, 90
PMS Perphenazine, 615
PMS-Valproic Acid, 741
Polycillin-N, 51
Polygam S/D, 400
polymyxin B sulfate, 641–644
porfimer sodium, 792*t*
potassium acetate, 644–647
potassium chloride, 644–647
potassium phosphates, 647–649
pralidoxime chloride, 649–651

Pregnancy, special considerations and, xxii
Pregnancy risk categories, vii
Premarin, 318
Prevacid, 443
Prevacid I.V., 443
Prevacid SoluTab, 443
Primacor, 522
Primaxin, 397
Primaxin ADD-Vantage, 397
Primaxin IM, 397
Primaxin IV, 397
Primethasone, 223
Pro-50, 658
procainamide hydrochloride, 651–653
prochlorperazine edisylate, 653–657
Procrit, 296
Procytox, 202
Prolastin, 26
Proleukin, 790*t*
Promacot, 658
Pro-Med 50, 658
Promet, 658
promethazine hydrochloride, 658–661
Pronestyl, 651
propofol, 661–663
propranolol hydrochloride, 664–667
Prorex-25, 658
Prorex-50, 658
prostacyclin, 300–303
Prostaphlin, 585
Prostigmin, 555
protamine sulfate, 667–669
Prothazine, 658
Protonix I.V., 600
Protopam Chloride, 649
Pyri, 671
2–pyridine aldoxime methochloride, 649–651
pyridostigmine bromide, 669–671
pyridoxine hydrochloride, 671–672

Q

quinidine gluconate, 673–675
quinupristin and dalfopristin, 675–678

R

ranitidine hydrochloride,
    678–680
Reclast, 771
recombinant erythropoietin,
    296–299
Refludan, 445
Regitine, 623
Reglan, 506
Regonol, 669
Regular Iletin II, 415
Regular Insulin, 415
Remicade, 412
remifentanil hydrochloride,
    680–683, 682*i*
Remodulin, 729
ReoPro, 3
Resectisol, 476
Retavase, 683
reteplase, 683–685
Retrovir, 766
Revex, 547
Revimine, 261
Rexolate, 698
rG-CSF, 336–338
Rheumatrex, 494
Rh factor, xxxi
Rhophylac, 400
r-HuEPO, 296–299
Rifadin, 685
Rifadin IV, 685
rifampicin, 685–688
rifampin, 685–688
"Rights" of drug administration,
    xxiii–xxv
Rimactane, 685
Rituxan, 688
rituximab, 688–691
Robaxin, 492
Robinul, 373
Rocephin, 151
Rodex, 671
Rofact, 685
Rogitine, 623
Romazicon, 340
Rubex, 269

S

Sandimmune, 206
Sandoglobulin, 400
Sandostatin, 575
SangCya, 206
scopolamine hydrobromide,
    691–693
Selestoject, 93
Septra, 199
Shogan, 658
Simulect, 87
Skelex, 492
sodium bicarbonate, 693–696
sodium ferric gluconate, 696–698
sodium L-triiodothyronine, 467–470
sodium phosphates, 647–649
sodium thiosalicylate, 698–700
Solu-Cortef, 384
Solu-Medrol, 502
Solurex, 223
Solution, calculating strength of,
    778–779
Stadol, 111
Staphcillin, 490
Storzolamide, 6
Streptase, 700
streptokinase, 700–702
streptozocin, 786*t*
Sublimaze, 333
sulfamethoxazole and trimethoprim,
    199–202
Synercid, 675
Synthroid, 457

T

T_3, 467–470
T_4, 457–459
Tagamet, 174
Talwin, 609
Taxol, 591
Taxotere, 789*t*
Tazicef, 145
Tazidime, 145
Tazocin, 638
tenecteplase, 703–705
Tenormin, 71
TESPA, 786*t*

Tham, 735
theophylline ethylenediamine, 35–38
theophylline in dextrose injection, 705–708
thiamine hydrochloride, 708–710
Thioplex, 786*t*
thiotepa, 786*t*
Thorazine, 168
Thrombate III, 66
thyronine sodium, 467–470
thyroxine sodium, 457–459
licar, 710
ticarcillin disodium, 710–713
ticarcillin disodium and clavulanate potassium, 713–716
tigecycline, 716–719
Timentin, 713
tirofiban hydrochloride, 719–721
tissue plasminogen activator, recombinant, 28–31
TNKase, 703
Tobi, 721
tobramycin sulfate, 721–724
Toposar, 325
topotecan hydrochloride, 792*t*
Toprol-XL, 509
Toradol, 437
torsemide, 724–726
Totacillin-N, 51
Total parenteral nutrition, administering, xxx–xxxi
Toxic agents, safe handling of, xxix
Tracrium, 73
Trandate, 441
Transderm-Nitro, 567
trastuzumab, 726–729, 792*t*
treprostinil sodium, 729–731
Tridil, 567
triethylenethiophosphoramide, 786*t*
triflupromazine hydrochloride, 731–735
Trilafon, 615
Trilafon Concentrate, 615
Triostat, 467
Trisenox, 790*t*
tromethamine, 735–736
trovafloxacin mesylate, 17–19
Trovan, 17

Trovan I.V., 17
TSPA, 786*t*
Tusal, 698
Tygacil, 716
Tysabri, 552

U

Ultiva, 680
Unasyn, 55
Unipen, 543
urea, 737–739
Ureaphil, 737
Uritol, 360
urokinase, 739–741

V

Valium, 235
valproate sodium, 741–744
valproic acid, 741–744
Vancocin, 744
vancomycin hydrochloride, 744–747
Vaprisol, 197
Vasotec I.V., 287
Vectrin, 524
Velban, 750
Velbe, 750
Velcade, 793*t*
Velosulin BR, 415
Venofer, 428
Venoglobulin-I, 400
Venoglobulin-S 5%, 400
Venoglobulin-S 10%, 400
Venous access, types of, xxv–xxvii
VePesid, 325
verapamil hydrochloride, 747–750
Versed, 519
Vesprin, 731
Vfend, 758
V-Gan-25, 658
V-Gan-50, 658
Vibramycin, 278
vinblastine sulfate, 750–754
Vincasar PFS, 754
vincristine sulfate, 754–758
vinorelbine tartrate, 789*t*
Vistide, 171